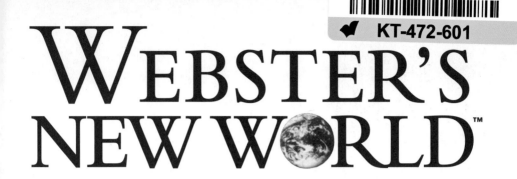

WEBSTER'S NEW WORLD™

Medical Dictionary

Second Edition

From the Doctors and Experts at MedicineNet.com

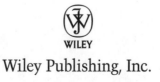

Wiley Publishing, Inc.

Webster's New World™ Medical Dictionary, Second Edition

Published by:
Wiley Publishing, Inc.
909 Third Avenue
New York, NY 10022
www.wiley.com

Published by Wiley Publishing, Inc., New York, NY

Library of Congress Cataloging-in-Publication Data available from publisher.
ISBN: 0-7645-2461-5
Printed in the United States of America
10 9 8 7
2B/SR/QR/QT/IN

Acknowledgments

At MedicineNet.com, we believe that you, the readers, are truly interested in understanding medical topics. Accordingly, we have addressed medical terms with a sensitivity to those who are potentially, acutely, and chronically involved with disease and health issues. Without you, the public, there would be no MedicineNet.com and there would be no *Webster's New World Medical Dictionary, Second Edition*.

On behalf of MedicineNet.com, we wish to thank the staff at John Wiley & Sons, Inc., for bringing this dictionary to those who need it. We also thank the officers of MedicineNet.com who have supported the development of this dictionary.

The excellence of the technical and editorial staffs at MedicineNet.com facilitated the entire project. Dan Griffith and Michael Cupp provided the publishing software development that made it all possible. Cynde Lee has managed the content of MedicineNet.com and maintained communication between editors and writers. Beth Griffith has provided valuable assistance. David Sorenson and Tanya Buchanan from marketing have been most helpful. Donna Whyte's sensitive radar has vigilantly kept us apprised of what information our readers were seeking.

William Shiel cannot thank enough his children, Cara, Daniel, and Tim, who endured the apparent inattentiveness of a distracted father. He acknowledges the endless support and love of his parents, Virginia and William Shiel, as well as his mother-in-law, Helen Stark. With endless love, he thanks his wife, Catherine, whose existence makes him whole.

Frederick Hecht wishes to express his special thanks to his wife, Barbara Hecht, who delayed a needed vacation and took over the selection and production of the daily health news with Cynde Lee for MedicineNet.com so that he could write and revise the entries to this dictionary. He also wishes to thank his children, Rick, Matthew, Maude, Tobias, Kerrie, and Brian, and their spouses and children for their love, support, and input. The major and minor illnesses that we as a family have experienced have contributed a sense of caring to this dictionary.

Thank you all.

— *Frederick Hecht, MD, FAAP, FACMG*

— *William C. Shiel, Jr., MD, FACP*

Editorial Staff

Co-Editors-in-Chief
Frederick Hecht, MD, FAAP
www.MedicineNet.com

William C. Shiel, Jr., MD, FACP
www.MedicineNet.com

Acquisitions Editor
Roxane Cerda

Project Editor
Suzanne Snyder, PhD

Copy Editor
Kitty Jarrett

Assistant Editors
Barbara K. Hecht, PhD
www.MedicineNet.com
Dennis Lee, MD
www.MedicineNet.com

Jay W. Marks, MD
www.MedicineNet.com

Leslie J. Schoenfield, MD, PhD
www.MedicineNet.com

Catherine Shiel, JD
www.MedicineNet.com

Content Manager
Cynde Lee
www.MedicineNet.com

Office & Research Assistants
Beth Griffith
www.MedicineNet.com

Donna Whyte
www. MedicineNet.com

Concept Development
David Sorenson
www.MedicineNet.com

About the Authors

Frederick Hecht, MD, FAAP, Co-Editor-in-Chief

Frederick Hecht, MD, lives in Jacksonville, Florida, and Berkeley, California. He is a pediatrician and medical geneticist and is board certified by the American Board of Pediatrics and the American Board of Medical Genetics. Dr. Hecht was born in Baltimore and raised in nearby Pikesville, Maryland. After graduating from Baltimore Friends School, he attended Dartmouth College in Hanover, New Hampshire, and the Sorbonne at the University of Paris, receiving a bachelor's degree *cum laude* from Dartmouth. He then studied at Middlebury College in Vermont (in French); the Defense Language School (in Russian) in Monterey, California; the University of Maryland (in German); and Boston University (in biomedical sciences) before entering the University of Rochester School of Medicine and Dentistry. He received an MD degree from Rochester with honors. He trained first in pediatrics at Strong Memorial Hospital in Rochester and University Hospital in Seattle, and then in medical genetics at the University of Washington. He has been on the medical school faculty at the Universities of Rochester, Washington, Oregon, Arizona, and Nevada. He has been a traveling fellow of the Royal Society of Medicine in Great Britain. He founded and served as president and director of the Southwest Biomedical Research Institute in Arizona and director of the Genetics Center and Cancer Center, now part of Genzyme, Inc. He has held administrative and research positions, including that of principal investigator for grants and contracts from the National Institutes of Health. Dr. Hecht has taught at a number of medical schools, including the University of Washington, the Oregon Health Sciences University, and Harvard Medical School. Recently, he served as professor of medicine at the University of Nice, France, for 3 years. There he worked in the Laboratory for the Molecular Genetics of Human Cancers, a unit of the CNRS (the French National Center for Scientific Research). He is president of Hecht Associates, consultants in medical genetics. He has served on the editorial boards of medical journal and reviewed articles for distinguished journals, including *Proceedings of the National Academy of Sciences; Nature; Science; New England Journal of Medicine; Pediatrics; Journal of Pediatrics; American Journal of Human Genetics*; and *The Lancet*. He has published extensively and authored and co-authored more than 700 articles and books. Dr. Hecht serves as associate chief editor of Medicine.com and chief editor of MedTerms.com. He was co-editor-in-chief of the first edition of *Webster's New World Medical Dictionary*, published in 2000.

William C. Shiel, Jr., MD, FACP, Co-Editor-in-Chief

William C. Shiel, Jr., MD, FACP, received a bachelor of science degree with honors from the University of Notre Dame. There he was involved in research in radiation biology and received the Huisking Scholarship. After graduating from St. Louis University School of Medicine, he completed his internal medicine residency and rheumatology fellowship at University of California, Irvine. He is board certified in Internal medicine and rheumatology and is a fellow of the American Colleges of Physicians and Rheumatology. Dr. Shiel is in active practice in the field of rheumatology at the Arthritis Center of Southern Orange County, California. He is currently an active associate clinical professor of medicine at University of California, Irvine. He has served as chair of the Department of Internal Medicine at Mission Hospital Regional Medical Center in Mission Viejo, California. Dr. Shiel has authored numerous articles on subjects related to arthritis for prestigious peer-reviewed medical journals, as well as many expert medical-legal reviews. He has lectured in person and on television both for physicians and the community. He is a contributor for questions for the American Board of Internal Medicine and has reviewed board questions on behalf of the American Board of Rheumatology Subspecialty. He served on the Medical and Scientific Committee of the Arthritis Foundation, and he is currently on the Medical Advisory Board of Lupus International. Dr. Shiel is proud to have served as chief editor for MedicineNet.com since its founding in 1996. Dr. Shiel also serves as chief editor of FocusOnArthritis.com. He was co-editor-in-chief of the first edition of *Webster's New World Medical Dictionary*, published in 2000.

Barbara K. Hecht, PhD, Assistant Editor

Dr. Barbara Kaiser-McCaw Hecht is director of Hecht Associates, Inc., consultants in medical genetics based in Jacksonville, Florida. Dr. Hecht lives in Jacksonville and in Berkeley, California. She is board certified in her fields of expertise and is a diplomate of the American Board of Medical Genetics, both in clinical cytogenetics (chromosome genetics) and in medical genetics (genetic counseling). Dr. Hecht earned both her bachelor's and master's degrees in biology from Stanford University. Her master's thesis on cell physiology and radiation was done at Stanford under Prof. Arthur Giese. Following receipt of her master's degree, she was research assistant in the Department of Biology at Stanford. She then worked as an exobiologist for NASA, doing research on the chemistry of extraterrestrial life, with a special interest in Mars. She earned her PhD in biology (genetics) at the University of Oregon, Eugene, under Prof. Edward Novitski. Her doctoral thesis was on the clonal origin of human tumors, using the diseases ataxia-telangiectasia, Burkitt's lymphoma, and ovarian teratomas as models. She did a National Institutes of Health postdoctoral research fellowship in medical genetics under Dr. Robert D. Koler at the Oregon Health Sciences University. Dr. Hecht was research associate both there and at Portland State University. Her subsequent teaching positions included clinical assistant professor of obstetrics and gynecology at the University of Nevada School of Medicine, associate professor of biology at Arizona State University, and professor of medicine at the University of Missouri–Kansas City. She has served on numerous scientific committees and published extensively in a number of fields, including cell biology, biochemistry, human and medical genetics, and oncology. Dr. Hecht was co-founder of the Southwest Biomedical Research Institute (now part of Genzyme, Inc.) in Arizona and served as its senior associate director and director of laboratories. She has held positions in both diagnostic and research genetic laboratories in the United States, Australia, and France. She was recipient of an ARC (French Cancer Society) Fellowship for Cancer Research at the University of Nice, and she was a staff member of the Laboratory for the Molecular Genetics of Human Cancers, a unit of the CNRS (the French National Center for Scientific Research) in France. Dr. Hecht has reviewed articles for distinguished biomedical journals, served on their editorial boards, and published hundreds of scientific and medical articles.

Dennis Lee, MD, Assistant Editor

Dennis Lee, MD, was born in Shanghai, China, and received his college and medical training in the United States. He is fluent in English and three Chinese dialects. He graduated with chemistry departmental honors from Harvey Mudd College. He was appointed president of AOA society at UCLA School of Medicine. He underwent internal medicine residency and gastroenterology fellowship training at Cedars-Sinai Medical Center. Board certified in internal medicine and gastroenterology, Dr. Lee is currently a member of Mission Internal Medical Group, a multispecialty medical group serving southern Orange County, California. Dr. Lee has maintained an interest in technology and medical education. He is a regular guest lecturer at Saddleback College in Orange County, California. Dr. Lee serves as chair of MedicineNet.com.

Jay W. Marks, MD, Assistant Editor

Jay W. Marks, MD, is a board-certified internist and gastroenterologist. He graduated from Yale University School of Medicine and trained in internal medicine and gastroenterology at UCLA/Cedars-Sinai Medical Center in Los Angeles. For 20 years he was associate director of the Division of Gastroenterology at Cedars-Sinai Medical Center and an associate professor of medicine, in residence, at UCLA. At Cedars-Sinai he co-directed the Gastrointestinal Endoscopy Unit, taught physicians during their graduate and postgraduate training, and performed specialized, nonendoscopic gastrointestinal testing. He carried out Public Health Service–sponsored (National Institutes of Health) clinical and basic research into mechanisms of the formation of gallstones and methods for the nonsurgical treatment of gallstones. He is the author of 36 original research manuscripts and 24 book chapters. Dr. Marks presently directs an independent gastrointestinal diagnostic unit where he continues to perform specialized tests for the diagnosis of gastrointestinal diseases. Dr. Marks serves as medical and pharmacy editor of MedicineNet.com. He is also chief editor of FocusOnDigestion.com.

Leslie J. Schoenfield, MD, PhD, Assistant Editor

Leslie J. Schoenfield, MD, PhD, received his undergraduate and medical degrees from Temple University. He completed his residency in internal medicine and gastroenterology at the Mayo Clinic in Rochester, Minnesota, while receiving his PhD in medicine and physiology at the University of Minnesota. He trained further as a National Institutes of Health special fellow at the Karolinska Institute in Sweden and as a research associate at the Fels Research Institute in Philadelphia. He is board certified in internal medicine and gastroenterology. On the faculty of the Mayo Clinic for 7 years, Dr. Schoenfield served as associate professor of medicine and consultant in gastroenterology. He became a professor of medicine in residence at UCLA from 1972 to 1999 (now emeritus). He was the director of gastroenterology at Cedars-Sinai Medical Center for 25 years, where he received the chief Resident's Teaching Award, the President's Award, and the Pioneer of Medicine Award. He is a member of a number of such distinguished scientific societies as the Society for Clinical Investigation and the Western Association of Physicians. He has held numerous offices in regional and national professional societies, culminating in the chairmanship of the Biliary Section of the American Gastroenterological Association. Dr. Schoenfield has lectured frequently at medical centers, societies, and health organizations all over the world. He has an extensive list of published medical research and review articles, has served on several editorial boards, and has reviewed numerous articles for prestigious biomedical journals. Dr. Schoenfield serves as medical editor of MedicineNet.com.

Contributing Authors

Ronald Adamany, M.D., Gastroenterology • Kent Adamson, M.D., Orthopedic Surgery • Leon Baginski, M.D., Obstetrics & Gynecology • Edward Block, M.D., Gastroenterology • James Bredencamp, M.D., Otolaryngology • Yuri Bronstein, M.D., Neurology • Rudolph Brutico, M.D., Pediatrics • Carolyn Janet Crandall, M.D., Internal Medicine & Women's Health • Eric Daar, M.D., Internal Medicine & Infectious Diseases • Steve Ehrlich, M.D., Cardiology • Manuel Fernandez, M.D., Endocrinology • Ronald Gehling, Michael C. Fishbein, M.D., Cardiovascular & Autopsy Pathology • Tse-Ling Fong, M.D., Hepatology • Catherine G. Fuller, M.D., Allergy & Immunology • Ronald Gehling, M.D., Allergy & Immunolgy • Gus Gialamas, M.D., Orthopedic Surgery • Gary W. Gibbon, M.D., Pulmonary Disease & Allergy • Mitchell J. Gitkind, M.D., Gastroenterology • Vay Liang W. Go, M.D., Nutrition • Daniel L. Gomel, M.D., Internal Medicine & Geriatrics • Mark Graber, M.D., Family Practice • Roza Hayduk, M.D., Sleep Medicine • Kendall Ho, M.D., Emergency Medicine • David Kaminstein, M.D., Gastroenterology • Kenneth Kaye, M.D., Pathology • Jillyen E. Kibby, M.A., CCC-A, Audiology • Harley J. Kornblum, M.D., Pediatrics & Neurology • Daniel Lee Kulick, M.D., Internal Medicine & Cardiology • Eric Lee, M.D., Gastroenterology • Margaret Lee, DDS, Dentistry • Stacy E. Lee, M.D., Allergy & Immunology • Michael Lill, M.D., Hematology/Oncology • Arthur H. Loussararian, M.D., Inetrnal Medicine & Cardiology • Ralph Maeda, M.D., Surgery • Dwight Makoff, M.D., Nephrology & Hypertension • Murray Margolis, M.D., Internal Medicine • Randy Martin, M.D., Pulmonary/Infectious Diseases • Ruchi Mathur, M.D., Internal Medicine & Endocrinology • James Meaglia, M.D., Urology • John Mersch, M.D., Pediatrics • Michael Miyamoto, M.D., Cardiology • Zab Mohsenifar, M.D., Internal Medicine & Pulmonary Diseases • John R. Morris, M.D., Orthopedic Surgery • Mim Mulford, M.D., Endocrinology • Mark Scott Noah, M.D., Internal Medicine • Omudhome Ogbru, Pharm.D., Pharmacy • Peter J. Panzarino, Jr. M.D., Psychiatry & Behavioral Medicine • Dennis Philips, M.D., Pediatrics • Donald Pratt, M.D., Internal Medicine • Stefan M. Pulst, M.D., Neurology • Donald Rediker, M.D., Cardiology • Alan Rockoff, M.D., Dermatology • Emmanuel Saltiel, Pharm.D, Pharmacy • Stephen J. Sanders, M.A., CCC-A, Audiology • Michael Santoro, M.D., Gastroenterology • George Schiffman, M.D., Pulmonary • Melvin Shiffman, M.D., Cosmetic Surgery • Lawrence J. Schwartz, M.D., Ophthalmology • David Simon, M.D., Internal Medicine • Robert Simon, M.D., Neurology • Mark Sullivan, M.D., Urology • Alan Szeftel, M.D., Allergy and Immunology/Pulmonary Disease • Bruce Tammelin, M.D., Pulmonary Disease • Michael Truong, M.D., Endocrinology • Theodore Van Dam, M.D., Internal Medicine • John Vierling, M.D., Hepatology • Edward J. White, M.D., General Surgery • Leslie Williams, Ed. D, Psychology • Joseph Y. Wu, M.D., Internal Medicine & Geriatrics • Marilyn A.D. Yee, Pharm. D., Pharmacy • David Zachary, M.D., Family Medicine

Introduction

lexicographer A writer of dictionaries, a harmless drudge.

–Samuel Johnson, 1755

Preparations for this new edition of *Webster's New World Medical Dictionary* began even before the appearance of the first edition in 2000. Like the first edition, this edition has been conceived and developed by the staff of the health information Web site MedicineNet.com. One of the earliest health information sites on the Internet, MedicineNet.com has devoted a number of years to creating an online medical dictionary that now contains a wealth of contemporary medical terms and provides the broad foundation for this book.

To create this new edition of *Webster's New World Medical Dictionary,* we have reviewed every entry in the first edition and have rewritten and strengthened many of those entries. In addition, we have selected new entries from our online medical dictionary for incorporation into this second edition. A unique feature of an online medical dictionary is that it can (and does) evolve rapidly to keep pace with the changes in medicine. We have taken advantage of this to update *Webster's New World Medical Dictionary.*

Like all the medical content from MedicineNet.com, this dictionary was written and edited by physicians, to be used by anyone and everyone concerned about their own health or the health of those who matter to them. All the medical information found on MedicineNet.com has been developed by a network of physicians. The physicians select the topics and review and edit all written content. These physicians also make use of medical specialists and health writers throughout the US. The "About the Authors" pages provide abbreviated biographies of the editors and specialists who contributed content to the MedicineNet.com online dictionary and this book.

Medicine is now advancing with remarkable rapidity on many fronts, and the language of medicine is also continually evolving with remarkable rapidity, commensurate with the changes. Today, there is constant need for communication between and among consumers and providers of health care. There is consequently a need for a high-quality, contemporary medical dictionary.

In the current health care environment, patients and their physicians, nurses, and allied health professionals must be able to discuss the ever-changing aspects of health, disease, and biotechnology. An accurate understanding of medical terminology can assist communication and improve care for patients, and it can help to alleviate the concerns of family members and friends.

The fact that the content of this dictionary is 100 percent physician-produced by MedicineNet.com ensures an unusual degree of professional expertise, reliability, and perspective.

Webster's New World Medical Dictionary, Second Edition is designed in an easy-to-read format with cross-referencing of terms that readers will find helpful. Moreover, from a technical standpoint, the CD-ROM included with this book introduces a dynamic updating capability as well as rapid ease of use for computers in the office or home. The CD-ROM serves to enhance many of the terms found in this dictionary, and it provides an Internet link to MedicineNet.com for readers who want even more detailed information on the latest medical issues.

We hope that you will find *Webster's New World Medical Dictionary, Second Edition* a valuable addition to your family or office library and a source of both information and illumination in any medical situation.

Frederick Hecht, MD, FAAP
William C Shiel, Jr., MD, FACP
Co-Editors-in-Chief

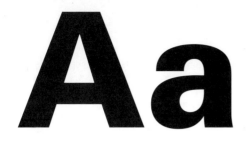

A In genetics, adenine, a member of the adenine-thymine (A-T) base pair in DNA.

a- Prefix indicating the absence or depletion of something: for example, aphagia (not eating) or aphonia (voiceless). The related prefix an- is usually used before a vowel, as in anemia (without blood) and anoxia (without oxygen).

AA **1** Alcoholics Anonymous. **2** Amino acid.

AAAS American Association for the Advancement of Science, a professional organization that publishes the weekly journal *Science.* Pronounced "triple-A-S."

AAFP **1** American Association of Family Physicians, a professional organization for physicians who treat both children and adults. **2** American Academy of Family Physicians, a professional organization for physicians who treat both children and adults.

AAO **1** American Association of Ophthalmology, a professional organization. **2** American Association of Orthodontists, a professional organization. **3** American Academy of Otolaryngology, a professional organization.

AAOS American Academy of Orthopaedic Surgeons, a professional organization. See also *orthopaedics.*

AAP **1** American Academy of Pediatrics, a professional organization for physicians who treat infants, children, adolescents, and young adults. **2** American Academy of Pedodontics, a professional organization. **3** American Academy of Periodontology, a professional organization. **4** American Association of Pathologists, a professional organization.

ab- Prefix indicating from, away from, or off, as in abduction (movement of a limb away from the midline of the body) and abnormal (away from normal).

abdomen The part of the body that contains all the structures between the chest and the pelvis. The abdomen, or belly, is anatomically separated from the chest by the diaphragm, the powerful muscle that spans the body cavity, just below the lungs. See also *abdominal cavity.*

abdomen, acute See *acute abdomen.*

abdominal aorta The final section of the aorta, the largest artery in the body, which begins at the diaphragm as a continuation of the thoracic aorta and ends by splitting in two, to form the common iliac arteries. The abdominal aorta supplies oxygenated blood to all the abdominal and pelvic organs, as well as to the legs. See also *aorta.*

abdominal aortic aneurysm See *aneurysm, abdominal aorta.*

abdominal cavity The cavity within the abdomen. This space between the abdominal wall and the spine contains a number of crucial organs, including the lower part of the esophagus, the stomach, small intestine, colon, rectum, liver, gallbladder, pancreas, spleen, kidneys, ureters, and bladder. See also *abdomen.*

abdominal guarding Tensing of the abdominal wall muscles to guard inflamed organs within the abdomen from the pain of pressure upon them. Abdominal guarding is detected when the abdomen is pressed and is a characteristic finding with inflammation of the inner abdominal (peritoneal) surface due, for example, to appendicitis or diverticulitis. The tensed muscles of the abdominal wall automatically go into spasm to keep the tender underlying tissues from being touched.

abdominal hysterectomy See *hysterectomy, abdominal.*

abdominal muscle One of a large group of muscles in the front of the abdomen that assists in maintaining regular breathing movements, supports the muscles of the spine while lifting, and keeps abdominal organs in place. Abdominal muscles are the target of many exercises, such as sit-ups. The abdominal muscles are informally known as the abs.

abdominal pain Pain in the belly. Abdominal pain can be acute or chronic. It may reflect a major problem with one of the organs in the abdomen, such as appendicitis or a perforated intestine, or it may result from a fairly minor problem, such as excess buildup of intestinal gas.

abducens nerve See *abducent nerve.*

abducent nerve The sixth cranial nerve, which emerges from the skull to operate the lateral rectus muscle. This muscle draws the eye toward the side of the head. Paralysis of the abducent nerve causes inward turning of the eye.

abduction The movement of a limb away from the midline of the body. The opposite of abduction is adduction.

abductor muscle See *muscle, abductor.*

ABG Arterial blood gas, a sampling of the blood levels of oxygen and carbon dioxide within the arteries, as opposed to the levels of oxygen and carbon dioxide in veins. Typically, the acidity (pH) is also simultaneously measured.

abiotrophy Loss of function, or degeneration for reasons unknown.

ablate To remove, from a Latin word meaning "to carry away." See *ablation*.

ablation Removal or excision. Ablation is usually carried out surgically. For example, surgical removal of the thyroid gland (a total thyroidectomy) is ablation of the thyroid.

abnormal Outside the expected norm, or uncharacteristic of a particular patient.

ABO blood group The major human blood group system. The ABO type of a person depends on the presence or absence of two genes, A and B. These genes determine the configuration of the red blood cell surface. A person who has two A genes has red blood cells of type A. A person who has two B genes has red cells of type B. If the person has one A and one B gene, the red cells are type AB. If the person has neither the A nor the B gene, the red cells are type O. It is essential to match the ABO status of both donor and recipient in blood transfusions and organ transplants.

abortifacient A medication or substance that causes pregnancy to end prematurely.

abortion Premature exit of the products of the fetus, fetal membranes, and placenta from the uterus. Abortion can be a natural process, as in a miscarriage; an induced procedure, using medication or other substances that cause the body to expel the fetus; or a surgical procedure that removes the contents of the uterus. See also *dilatation and curettage*.

abortion, habitual The miscarriage of three or more consecutive pregnancies with no intervening pregnancies. Habitual abortion is a form of infertility. Also known as recurrent abortion and multiple abortion.

abortion, multiple See *abortion, habitual*.

abortion, recurrent See *abortion, habitual*.

abortion, spontaneous Miscarriage.

abortive Tending to cut short the course of a disease, as in abortive polio (polio cut short).

abortive polio A minor, abbreviated form of infection with the polio virus. Full recovery occurs in 24 to 72 hours, and the condition does not involve the nervous system or permanent disabilities. See also *polio*.

ABP American Board of Pediatrics, a professional organization for physicians who treat infants, children, adolescents, and young adults.

abrasion 1 A wearing away of the upper layer of skin as a result of applied friction force. See also *scrape*. 2 In dentistry, the wearing away of tooth surfaces.

abruptio placentae Premature separation (abruption) of the placenta from the wall of the uterus, often in association with high blood pressure or preeclampsia. Abruption is a potentially serious problem both for mother and fetus because the area where it occurs bleeds and the uterus begins to contract. Shock may occur. See also *placenta, preeclampsia*.

abs Slang term for the abdominal muscles.

abscess A local accumulation of pus anywhere in the body. See also *boil; pus*.

abscess, perianal An abscess next to the anus that causes tenderness, swelling, and pain on defecation.

abscess, peritonsillar An abscess behind the tonsils that pushes one of the tonsils toward the uvula (the prominent soft tissue dangling from the back of the palate in the back of the mouth). A peritonsillar abscess is generally very painful and associated with difficulty opening the mouth. If a peritonsillar abscess is untreated, the infection can spread deep into the neck, causing airway obstruction and other life-threatening complications.

abscess, skin Medical term for a common boil.

abscission To remove tissue by cutting it away, as in surgery.

absence of the breast See *amastia*.

absence of the nipple See *athelia*.

absinthe An emerald-green liqueur flavored with extracts of the wormwood plant, licorice, and aromatic flavorings in an alcohol base. Absinthe was manufactured, commercialized, and popularized in France in the late 1700s by Henri-Louis Pernod. It was an extremely addictive drink. Prolonged drinking of absinthe causes convulsions, blindness, hallucinations, and mental deterioration. Absinthe has been banned, but something of its taste is still available in such drinks as Greek ouzo and French pastis. Homemade absinthe may still be illicitly consumed in some areas.

absolute CD4 count The number of "helper" T-lymphocytes in a cubic millimeter of blood. The absolute CD4 count is frequently used to monitor the extent of immune suppression in persons with HIV because with HIV, this number declines as the infection progresses. Also known as T4 count.

absorption Uptake. For example, intestinal absorption is the uptake of food (or other substances) from the digestive tract.

abstinence The voluntary self-denial of food, drink, or sex.

abuse, child See *child abuse.*

abuse, elder See *elder abuse.*

a.c. Abbreviation of the Latin phrase *ante cibum,* meaning "before meals." See also Appendix A, "Prescription Abbreviations."

AC joint See *acromioclavicular joint.*

acapnia Lower than normal level of carbon dioxide in the blood. The opposite of acapnia is hypercapnia.

accelerated phase of leukemia Chronic myelogenous leukemia that is progressing. In this phase, the number of immature, abnormal white blood cells in the bone marrow and blood is higher than in the chronic phase but not as high as in the blast phase.

accessory nerve The eleventh cranial nerve, which emerges from the skull and receives an additional (accessory) root from the upper part of the spinal cord. It supplies the sternocleidomastoid and trapezius muscles.

accessory neuropathy A disease of the accessory nerve, paralysis of which prevents rotation of the head away from one or both sides and causes the shoulder to droop. Damage can be confined to the accessory nerve, or it may also involve the ninth and tenth cranial nerves, which exit the skull through the same opening.

accessory placenta See *placenta, accessory.*

acclimatization to altitude The process of adapting to the decrease in oxygen concentration at a specific altitude. A number of changes must take place for the body to operate with decreased oxygen. These changes include increasing the depth of respiration; increasing the pressure in the pulmonary arteries, forcing blood into portions of the lung that are normally not used at sea level; manufacturing additional oxygen-carrying red blood cells; and manufacturing extra 2, 4-DPG, a substance that facilitates the release of oxygen from hemoglobin to the body tissues. Acclimatization generally takes 1 to 3 days and occurs after any significant altitude change above 1,220 meters (approximately 4,000 feet). Acclimatization is the body's natural means of correcting altitude sickness and the rate of acclimatization depends on the altitude, rate of ascent, and individual susceptibility.

accoucheur A male obstetrician. An accoucheuse is a woman obstetrician, or sometimes a midwife.

ACE Angiotensin converting enzyme. ACE converts an angiotensin to its activated form, angiotensin II, enabling it to function.

ACE inhibitor A drug that inhibits ACE. Using an ACE inhibitor relaxes the arteries, not only lowering blood pressure but also improving the pumping efficiency of a failing heart and improving cardiac output in patients with heart failure. ACE inhibitors are therefore used for blood pressure control and congestive heart failure. ACE inhibitors include benazepril (brand name: Lotensin), captopril (brand name: Capoten), lisinopril (brand names: Zestril, Prinivil), quinapril (brand name: Accupril), and ramipril (brand name: Altace). Interestingly, ACE inhibitors were developed from the venom of a Brazilian snake.

acentric chromosome A chromosome that is lacking a centromere (a specialized region of the chromosome to which spindle fibers attach during cell division). As a result, an acentric chromosome is lost when the cell divides. See also *centromere.*

aceruloplasminemia See *ceruloplasmin deficiency.*

acetabulum The cup-shaped socket of the hip joint. The acetabulum is a feature of the pelvis. The head (upper end) of the femur (thighbone) fits into the acetabulum and articulates with it, forming a ball-and-socket joint.

acetaminophen A nonaspirin pain reliever or analgesic. Acetaminophen may be given alone to relieve pain and inflammation or it may be combined with other drugs, as in some migraine medications, which contain acetaminophen, a barbiturate, and caffeine.

acetone A volatile liquid used as an industrial solvent. Acetone is also one of the ketone bodies that is formed when the body uses fat instead of glucose (sugar) for energy. The formation of acetone is usually a sign that cells lack insulin or cannot effectively use the insulin that is available, as occurs in diabetes. Acetone is excreted from the body in the urine.

acetone breath The breath of a person with a lot of acetone in his or her body. Acetone breath smells fruity and is a telltale sign of diabetes. See also *diabetes mellitus.*

acetylcholine A neurotransmitter released by nerves that is essential for communication between the nerves and muscles.

acetylsalicylic acid See *aspirin.*

achalasia A disease of the esophagus that mainly affects young adults. Abnormal function of nerves and muscles of the esophagus causes difficulty swallowing and sometimes chest pain. Regurgitation of undigested food can occur, as can coughing or breathing problems related to entry of food material into the lungs. The underlying problems are weakness of the lower portion of the esophagus and failure of the lower esophageal sphincter to open and allow passage of food. Diagnosis is made by an X-ray, endoscopy, or esophageal manometry. Treatment includes medication, dilation (stretching) to widen the lower part of the esophagus, and surgery to open the lower esophagus. A fairly recent approach involves injecting medicines into the lower esophagus to relax the sphincter.

Achilles tendon One of the longest tendons in the body, a tough sinew that attaches the calf muscle to the back of the calcaneus (heel bone). The name comes from Greek mythology: The hero Achilles was invulnerable to injury except for his heel, which proved his downfall when it was pierced by Paris's arrow. It has also proved, literally, to be the downfall of many athletes who have experienced the sudden pain of its rupture.

Achilles tendonitis Inflammation in the tendon of the calf muscle, where it attaches to the heel bone. Achilles tendonitis causes pain and stiffness at the back of the leg, near the heel. Achilles tendonitis can be caused by overuse of the Achilles tendon, overly tight calf muscles or Achilles tendons, excess uphill running, a sudden increase in the intensity of training or the type of shoes worn to run, or wearing high heels at work and then switching to a lower-heeled workout shoe. Achilles tendonitis causes pain and often swelling over the Achilles tendon. The tendon is tender and may be swollen. There is pain on rising up on the toes and pain with stretching of the tendon. The range of motion of the ankle may be limited. Treatment includes applying ice packs to the Achilles tendon, raising the lower leg, and taking an anti-inflammatory medication. In some severe cases of Achilles tendonitis, a cast may be needed for several weeks. A heel lift insert may also be used in shoes to prevent future overstretching of the Achilles tendon. Exerting rapid stress on the Achilles tendon when it is inflamed can result in rupture of the tendon. Prevention of Achilles tendonitis includes stretching the calf muscles and Achilles tendons carefully before doing vigorous activities. If the Achilles tendons or calf muscles are especially tight, it is a good idea to stretch them twice a day, whether or not sports activities are planned that day.

achlorhydria A lack of hydrochloric acid in the digestive juices in the stomach.

achondroplasia A genetic disorder of bone growth and the most common cause of short stature with disproportionately short arms and legs (known as dwarfism). The individual has a large head with a prominent forehead (frontal bossing); underdevelopment (hypoplasia) of the midface, with cheekbones that lack prominence; and a low nasal bridge with narrow nasal passages. The fingers are short, and the ring and middle fingers diverge to give the hand a trident (three-pronged) appearance. The brain is entirely normal in people with achondroplasia, but complications can damage the brain and spinal cord. Achondroplasia is an autosomal dominant trait, affecting boys and girls equally. Most cases are due to new mutations that appear for the first time in the affected child. Achondroplasia is caused by mutation in the fibroblast growth factor receptor-3 gene (FGFR3), and prenatal diagnosis is possible. See also *dwarfism; dwarfism, hydrochondroplastic.*

acid, pantothenic Vitamin B5. See also Appendix C, "Vitamins."

acid phosphatase An enzyme that acts to liberate phosphate under acidic conditions and is made in the liver, spleen, bone marrow, and prostate gland. Abnormally high serum levels of acid phosphatase may indicate infection, injury, or cancer of the prostate.

acidophilus Bacteria found in yogurt with "live cultures" that can help restore a supportive bacterial environment to an intestinal tract whose normal bacterial population (flora) has been disturbed by disease or antibiotics. Eating yogurt with acidophilus may also be useful in preventing overgrowth of Candida yeast in the intestinal tract, mouth (candidiasis, thrush), and vagina (yeast infection). See also *probiotics.*

acidosis Too much acid in the blood and body. Acidosis is an abnormal condition resulting from the accumulation of acid or the depletion of alkaline reserves. The pH of a body with acidosis is below normal. For a person with diabetes, this can lead to diabetic ketoacidosis. The opposite of acidosis is alkalosis. See also *pH.*

ACL Anterior cruciate ligament.

acne Localized skin inflammation resulting from overactivity of the oil glands at the base of hair follicles or as a response to contact with irritating substances. See also *acne vulgaris.*

acne rosacea   See *rosacea.*

acne vulgaris   The common form of acne, in teens and young adults, that is due to overactivity of the oil (sebaceous) glands in the skin that become plugged and inflamed. Acne typically develops when the oil glands come to life around puberty and are stimulated by male hormones that are produced in the adrenal glands of both boys and girls. Most outbreaks of acne can be treated by keeping the skin clean and avoiding irritating soaps, foods, drinks, and cosmetics. Severe acne and acne in those who are prone to scarring can be treated with topical creams and anti-inflammatory medications. Skin damaged by acne can be improved via treatment by a dermatologist or facial technologist. Techniques include dermabrasion (sanding), removal of scar tissue via laser, and chemical peels. Also known as pimples.

ACOG   American College of Obstetricians and Gynecologists, a professional organization for women's health care providers that also does advocacy work to improve the care of female patients. Pronounced "a cog."

acquired   Not inherited, or present at birth (congenital). For example, AIDS is an acquired, not an inherited, form of immune deficiency.

acquired immunodeficiency disease   See *AIDS.*

acquired mutation   A genetic change that occurs in a single cell after the conception of an individual. That change is then passed along to all cells descended from that cell. Acquired mutations are involved in the development of cancer.

acral-lentiginous melanoma   See melanoma, acral-lentiginous.

acrocentric chromosome   A chromosome in which the centromere is located quite near one end of the chromosome. Humans normally have five pairs of acrocentric chromosomes. Down syndrome is caused by an extra acrocentric chromosome (chromosome 21).

acrocephalosyndactyly   An inherited disorder characterized by abnormalities of the skull, face, hands, and feet. It begins with premature closure of some sutures of the skull (craniosynostosis) and results in a tall peaked head, shallow eye sockets, and underdeveloped cheekbones. With acrocephalosyndactyly, fingers and toes are fused (syndactyly), and the thumbs and big toes have broad ends. Acrocephalosyndactyly is an autosomal dominant trait that affects boys and girls. A parent can transmit the

gene for the disorder, or it can occur due to a new mutation. Surgery is often useful to correct the abnormalities of the skull, face, hands, and feet. See also *Apert syndrome; Crouzon syndrome.*

acrochordon   See *skin tag.*

acrocyanosis   Blueness of the hands and feet, usually due to sluggish circulation.

acrodermatitis enteropathica   A progressive, hereditary disease of children, characterized by the simultaneous occurrence of skin inflammation (dermatitis) and diarrhea. The skin on the cheeks, elbows, and knees is inflamed, as is tissue about the mouth and anus. There is also balding of the scalp, eyebrows, and lashes; delayed wound healing; and recurrent bacterial and fungal infections due to immune deficiency. The key laboratory finding is an abnormally low blood zinc level, reflecting impaired zinc uptake. Treatment with zinc by mouth is curative. Acrodermatitis enteropathica is an autosomal recessive disorder. See also *deficiency, zinc; zinc.*

acromegaly   See *gigantism, pituitary.*

acromioclavicular joint   A gliding joint located between the acromion (a projection of the scapula that forms the point of the shoulder) and the clavicle (the collar bone). It is served and supported by the capsular, superior, and inferior acromioclavicular ligaments; the articular disk; and the coracoclavicular (trapezoid and conoid) ligaments. Abbreviated AC joint.

acrosyndactyly   A condition in which a person has fused or webbed fingers or toes. Acrosyndactyly can be partial or complete, and it can usually be corrected via surgery. It is associated with several birth-defect syndromes. See also *Apert syndrome.*

ACS   American College of Surgeons, a professional organization that administers standards of practice for surgeons. Those who meet the group's standards can call themselves Fellows of the ACS.

actinic   Referring to the ultraviolet (UV) rays from sunlight and UV lamps. Sunburn is an actinic burn. An actinic keratosis is a skin lesion that is the consequence of chronic sun exposure. From the Greek *aktis,* meaning "ray."

actinic keratosis   Rough, scaly patches of skin that are considered precancerous and are due to sun exposure. Prevention is to cut sun exposure and wear sunscreen. Treatments include performing cryosurgery (freezing with liquid nitrogen), cutting the keratoses away, burning them, putting 5-fluorouracil on them, and using photodynamic therapy (injecting into the bloodstream a chemical that collects in actinic keratoses and makes them more sensitive to exposure to a specialized form of light). Also known as solar keratosis and senile keratosis.

active euthanasia The active acceleration of a terminally ill patient's death by use of drugs or other means, with the aid of a physician. Currently, active euthanasia is openly practiced in the Netherlands and in the US state of Oregon. The patient's request to the physician must be voluntary, explicit, and carefully considered, and it must be made repeatedly. Moreover, the patient's suffering must be unbearable and without any prospect of improvement. Suicide for other reasons, whether irrational or rational, is not active euthanasia. The forced killing of an ill or disabled person, as has occurred in eugenics programs, is also not active euthanasia. And although medications administered for pain relief may hasten death, aggressive pain relief is a normal medical decision in terminal care, not in active euthanasia. See also *assisted suicide; eugenics; euthanasia.*

active immunity Immunity produced by the body in response to stimulation by a disease-causing organism or other agent.

activities of daily living Something that a person normally does, including self-care (eating, bathing, dressing, grooming), work, homemaking, and leisure. The ability or inability to perform these activities can be used as a practical measure of ability or disability, and it may be used by insurers and HMOs as a rationale for approving or denying physical therapy or other treatments. Abbreviated ADL.

acuity, auditory The clearness of hearing, a measure of how well a person hears.

acuity test, visual The familiar eye chart test, which measures how well a person can see at various distances.

acuity, visual The clearness of vision, a measure of how well one sees.

acupressure The application of pressure on specific points on the body to control symptoms such as pain or nausea. Similar in concept to acupuncture, but without needles.

acupuncture The practice of inserting needles into specific points on the body with a therapeutic aim, such as to reduce pain or to induce anesthesia without the use of drugs. Traditional Chinese acupuncturists say the practice unblocks the flow of a life force called ch'i; Western researchers believe acupuncture may affect production of endorphins, the body's natural painkillers. In 1997, the National Institutes of Health (NIH) issued a consensus statement stating that "There is sufficient evidence of acupuncture's value to expand its use into conventional medicine."

acupuncturist A person skilled in the practice of acupuncture, who may or may not be credentialed by an accrediting body.

acute Of short duration, rapid, and abbreviated in onset. A condition is termed acute in comparison to a subacute condition, which lasts longer or changes less rapidly; or a chronic condition, which may last almost indefinitely, with virtually no change. Each disease has a unique time scale: An acute myocardial infarction (heart attack) may last a week, whereas an acute sore throat may last only a day or two.

acute abdomen Medical shorthand for the acute onset of abdominal pain. A potential medical emergency, an acute abdomen may reflect a major problem with one of the organs in the abdomen, such as appendicitis (inflamed appendix), cholecystitis (inflamed gallbladder), a perforated ulcer in the intestine, or a ruptured spleen.

acute esophageal stricture See *esophageal stricture, acute.*

acute fatty liver of pregnancy Liver failure in late pregnancy, usually of unknown cause. Abbreviated AFLP. Symptoms include nausea and vomiting, abdominal pain, yellowing of the skin and eyes (jaundice), frequent thirst (polydipsia), increased urination (polyuria), headache, and altered mental state. Laboratory features of AFLP include low blood sugar (hypoglycemia), elevated liver enzymes, and low levels of blood platelets. Untreated AFLP can cause complete liver failure, bleeding due to impaired blood clotting, and death of the mother and fetus. AFLP is treated by delivering the baby as soon as possible, often by inducing early labor. It usually subsides after delivery and does not occur in subsequent pregnancies. In some cases AFLP is associated with an abnormality of fatty-acid metabolism: a deficiency of the enzyme long-chain-3-hydroxyacyl-CoA dehydrogenase (LCHAD). The mother and father have half the normal LCHAD activity, and the fetus has no LCHAD activity. This metabolic disease in the baby's liver causes the fatty liver disease in the mother.

acute HIV infection See *HIV infection, acute.*

acute idiopathic polyneuritis See *Guillain-Barre syndrome.*

acute illness A disease with an abrupt onset and, usually, a short course.

acute leukemia Cancer of the blood cells that characteristically comes on suddenly and, if not treated, progresses quickly. In acute leukemia, the leukemic cells are not able to mature properly.

acute membranous gingivitis A progressive and painful infection of the mouth and throat due to the spread of infection from the gums. Symptoms include ulceration, swelling, and sloughing off of dead tissue from the mouth and throat. Certain germs (including fusiform bacteria and spirochetes) have been thought to be involved, but the actual cause is not yet known. Like most other poorly understood diseases, acute membranous gingivitis goes by many other names, including acute necrotizing ulcerative gingivitis, fusospirillary gingivitis, fusospirillosis, fusospirochetal gingivitis, necrotizing gingivitis, phagedenic gingivitis, trench mouth, ulcerative gingivitis, ulcerative stomatitis, Vincent angina, Vincent gingivitis, Vincent infection, and Vincent stomatitis.

acute mountain sickness The physical effect of being in a high-altitude environment. Abbreviated AMS, it is common at altitudes above 2,440 meters (approximately 8,000 feet). Three-fourths of people have mild symptoms of AMS at altitudes over 3,048 meters (approximately 10,000 feet). Occurrence depends on the altitude, rate of ascent, and individual susceptibility. Symptoms begin 12 to 24 hours after arrival at a new altitude and include headache, dizziness, fatigue, shortness of breath, loss of appetite, nausea, disturbed sleep, and general malaise. These symptoms tend to worsen at night, when the respiratory drive is decreased. Symptoms should subside within 2 to 4 days, and can be treated by using pain medications such as aspirin. Acetazolamide (brand name: Diamox), a drug that allows one to breathe faster and therefore metabolize more oxygen, can also be used to minimize symptoms caused by poor oxygenation. Acetazolamide may be taken prior to travel at high altitudes as a preventive measure. Moderate AMS has the same symptoms as AMS, but the headaches cannot be relieved with medication, and both breathing and coordinated movements become difficult. The only remedies are advanced medications and descent to lower altitudes. Severe AMS is indicated by great shortness of breath at rest, inability to walk, decreased mental status, and fluid buildup in the lungs. Severe AMS requires immediate descent to lower altitudes: 610 to 1,220 meters (approximately 2,000 to 4,000 feet). See also *acclimatization to altitude*.

acute myelogenous leukemia See *leukemia, acute myeloid.*

acute myeloid leukemia See *leukemia, acute myeloid.*

acute myocardial infarction A heart attack that occurs when the heart muscle is suddenly deprived of circulating blood. Abbreviated AMI. See also *heart attack.*

acute nonlymphocytic leukemia See *leukemia, acute myeloid.*

acute otitis media Painful inflammation of the middle ear, typically with fluid in the middle ear, behind a bulging eardrum or a perforated eardrum, often with drainage of pus. The customary treatment is antibiotics for 7 to 10 days. About 90 percent of children respond within the first 48 hours of treatment. After antibiotic treatment, 40 percent are left with some fluid in the middle ear, which can cause temporary hearing loss for up to 6 weeks. In most children, the fluid eventually disappears spontaneously. If a child has a bulging eardrum and is experiencing severe pain, a myringotomy (surgical incision of the eardrum) to release the pus may be done. The eardrum usually heals within a week. Tubes may be placed in the ear to drain fluid. See also *ear infection.*

acute peritonitis See *peritonitis, acute.*

acute-phase protein A protein whose plasma concentrations increase or decrease by 25 percent or more during certain inflammatory disorders. Perhaps the best-known acute-phase protein is C-reactive protein (CRP).

acute respiratory distress syndrome Respiratory failure of sudden onset due to fluid in the lungs (pulmonary edema), following an abrupt increase in the permeability of the normal barrier between the capillaries in the lungs and the air sacs. The muscles of the lungs are forced to work harder, causing labored and inefficient breathing. An abnormally low level of oxygen in the blood (hypoxemia) occurs. Acute respiratory distress syndrome (ARDS) is the most serious response to acute lung injury. The types of acute lung injury that may lead to ARDS include, but are not limited to, aspiration of food or other items into the lungs, inhalation of a toxic substance, widespread infection of the lungs, blood infection (sepsis), and near-drowning. Treatment frequently involves temporary use of a mechanical ventilator to help the patient breathe.

acute thrombocytopenic purpura Sudden onset of low blood platelet levels, with bleeding into the skin and elsewhere. Abbreviated ATP. ATP can have many causes; for example, it can be a potentially serious complication during the acute phase of measles infection.

acyclovir A potent antiviral (brand name: Zovirax) that works against several human herpes viruses, Epstein-Barr virus, herpes zoster, varicella (chickenpox), cytomegalovirus, and other viruses. It is part of the AIDS drug AZT. See also *AZT.*

ad- Prefix indicating toward or in the direction of. For example, adduction is the movement of a limb toward the midline of the body, and adrenal literally means "toward the kidney."

ad lib Abbreviation of the Latin phrase *ad libitum,* meaning "as much as one desires" or "at your discretion." See also Appendix A, "Prescription Abbreviations."

ADA **1** American Dental Association, a professional organization for dentists. Its Council on Dental Education and Commission on Dental Accreditation are responsible for accrediting schools of dentistry and allied professions. **2** American Diabetes Association, a nonprofit health organization that sponsors diabetes research, provides information about diabetes and diabetes prevention to patients and others, and advocates for improved treatment of people with diabetes. **3** Adenosine deaminase.

Adam's apple The familiar feature on the front of the neck that is the forward protrusion of the thyroid cartilage, the largest cartilage of the larynx. It tends to enlarge at adolescence, particularly in males. It is usually said to take its name from the story that a piece of the forbidden fruit stuck in Adam's throat.

ADD **1** Attention deficit disorder. **2** Adenosine deaminase deficiency.

addiction An uncontrollable craving, seeking, and use of a substance such as alcohol or another drug. Dependence is such an issue with addiction that stopping is very difficult and causes severe physical and mental reactions.

Addison's anemia See *anemia, pernicious.*

Addison's disease Long-term underfunction of the outer portion of the adrenal gland. Causes can include physical trauma to the adrenal gland, hemorrhage, tuberculosis, and destruction of the pituitary gland cells that secrete adrenocorticotropic hormone (ACTH), which normally controls the adrenal gland. Addison's disease is characterized by bronzing of the skin, anemia, weakness, and low blood pressure.

adducted thumbs Clasped thumbs, caused by absence of the extensor pollicis longus and/or brevis muscles to the thumb. When associated with mental retardation, it is part of an X-linked syndrome that affects mainly boys. See *MASA syndrome.*

adduction Movement of a limb toward the midline of the body. The opposite of adduction is abduction.

adductor muscle See *muscle, adductor.*

adenine A member of the base pair adenine-thymine (A-T) in DNA.

adenocarcinoma A cancer that develops in the lining or inner surface of an organ and usually has glandular (secretory) properties. More than 95 percent of prostate cancers are adenocarcinomas.

adenoid A mass of lymphoid tissue in the upper part of the throat, behind the nose. When the adenoids are enlarged due to frequent infections, breathing through the nose may become difficult. Surgical removal may be done, often accompanied by removal of the tonsils. Also known as pharyngeal tonsil.

adenoidectomy The surgical removal of the adenoids.

adenoiditis Infection of the adenoids.

adenoma A benign tumor that arises in or resembles glandular tissue. If an adenoma becomes cancerous, it is called an adenocarcinoma.

adenomyoma A nodule that forms around endometrial tissue in cases of adenomyosis. See *adenomyosis.*

adenomyomata Plural form of adenomyoma.

adenomyosis A common, benign condition of the uterus in which the endometrium (the mucous membrane lining the inside of the uterus) grows into the adjacent myometrium (the uterine musculature located just outside the endometrium). The myometrium may respond to this intrusion with muscular overgrowth. If an island of endometrial tissue is contained and circumscribed within the myometrium, it forms an adenomyoma. Also known as endometriosis interna, endometriosis uterina, adenomyosis uteri, and adenomyometritis.

adenosine deaminase An enzyme that plays a key role in salvaging purine molecules. Abbreviated ADA.

adenosine deaminase deficiency A genetic (autosomal recessive) condition that results in severe combined immunodeficiency disease. The first successful gene therapy for this condition in humans was done in 1990, by infusing patients with genetically engineered blood cells.

adenosine triphosphate A nucleotide compound that is of critical importance for the storage of energy within cells and the synthesis of RNA. Abbreviated ATP.

adenovirus One of a group of viruses that can cause infections of the lung, stomach, intestine, and eyes. Symptoms resemble those of the common cold. There are no effective medications for treating adenovirus infection. Adenovirus infection typically does not cause death or permanent problems. More than 40 types of adenoviruses have been recognized, all of which are extremely tiny. Adenoviruses are being used in research as a vehicle for gene therapy and as a vector for vaccines.

ADH   Antidiuretic hormone.

ADH secretion, inappropriate   A disease that results in the inability to produce dilute urine and disturbs normal balance of fluids and electrolytes in the body. Symptoms include nausea, vomiting, muscle cramps, confusion, and convulsions. This syndrome may occur with oat-cell lung cancer, pancreatic cancer, prostate cancer, and Hodgkin's disease, among other disorders.

ADHD   Attention deficit hyperactivity disorder.

adhesion   The union of two opposing tissue surfaces. This term is often used to refer to the sides of a wound, as well as to scar tissue strands that can form at the site of a previous operation, such as within the abdomen after a laparotomy.

adhesive capsulitis   A condition in which a person has constant severe limitation of the range of motion of the shoulder due to scarring around the shoulder joint. Adhesive capsulitis is an unwanted consequence of rotator cuff disease that involves damage to the rotator cuff. The affected joint is characteristically painful and tender to palpation. Physical therapy and cortisone injections are often helpful. Surgery is used in advanced cases. Also known as frozen shoulder.

adipose   Fatty. Adipose refers to tissue made up of mainly fat cells such as the yellow layer of fat beneath the skin. From the Latin *adeps,* meaning "fat."

adiposis dolorosa   See *Dercum disease.*

adjuvant   A substance that helps and enhances the pharmacological effect of a drug or increases the ability of an antigen to stimulate the immune system.

adjuvant chemotherapy   Chemotherapy given after removal of a cancerous tumor. Many chemotherapy drugs are most effective after the main tumor has been removed and any remaining cancer is in small amounts (microscopic metastases).

adjuvant therapy   Any treatment that is given in addition to the primary (initial) treatment.

ADLs   Activities of daily living.

adnexa   Latin word used to refer to appendages. For example, in gynecology the adnexa are the appendages of the uterus, namely the ovaries, the Fallopian tubes, and the ligaments that hold the uterus in place.

adrenal gland   A small gland located on top of the kidney. The adrenal glands produce hormones that help control heart rate, blood pressure, the way the body uses food, the levels of minerals such as sodium and potassium in the blood, and other functions.

adrenal medulla   See *medulla, adrenal.*

adrenaline   A substance produced within the adrenal gland, synonymous with epinephrine. It is a sympathomimetic catecholamine that quickens the heart beat, strengthens the force of the heart's contraction, and opens up the bronchioles in the lungs, among other effects. The secretion of adrenaline is part of the human "fight or flight" response to fear, panic, or perceived threat. Also known as epinephrine.

adult hemoglobin   See *hemoglobin A.*

adult-onset diabetes   Non-insulin-dependent, or type 2, diabetes, the most common form of diabetes mellitus. Unlike insulin-dependent, or type 1, diabetes patients, in whom the pancreas makes no insulin, adult-onset diabetes patients produce some insulin, sometimes even large amounts. However, their bodies do not produce enough insulin or their body cells are resistant to the action of insulin. People with this form of diabetes can sometimes control their disease by losing weight through diet and exercise. Otherwise, they may need to combine insulin or another diabetes medication with diet and exercise. Generally, adult-onset diabetes occurs in people who are over age 40, and most of the people who have this type of diabetes are overweight.

adult-onset Still's disease   Still's disease that begins in adulthood rather than in childhood. See also *Still's disease.*

adult respiratory distress syndrome   See *acute respiratory distress syndrome.*

advance directive   A document drawn up by a patient or, in some cases, the patient's representative to set treatment preferences and to designate a surrogate decision maker should the patient become unable to make medical decisions. Advance directives include the living will, power of attorney, and health care proxy. See also *DNR.*

adverse event   In pharmacology, any unexpected or dangerous reaction to a drug or vaccine.

aer-, aero-   Prefix indicating air or gas, such as aerogastria (excess stomach gas).

aerobic   Requiring oxygen. Aerobic bacteria require oxygen to grow. Aerobic exercise requires increased oxygen intake, as manifest by an increase in the associated rate of breathing.

aerobic exercise   Brisk exercise that promotes the circulation of oxygen through the blood. Examples include running, swimming, and bicycling.

aerophagia   From the Greek words *aer,* meaning "air," and *phagein,* meaning "to eat," a common cause of stomach gas. Everyone swallows small amounts of air when eating or drinking. However, activities such as rapid eating or drinking, gum chewing, smoking, and wearing ill-fitting dentures may cause a significant increase in swallowed air.

aerosinusitis   Sinus troubles, particularly with pain, due to changing atmospheric pressures. Aerosinusitis is the cause of sinus pain when going up or down in a plane. Also known as barosinusitis and sinus barotrauma.

aerosol   A fine spray or mist. Medications in aerosol form can be administered via a nebulizer and inhaled.

aerotitis   Middle ear problems due to changing atmospheric pressures, as when a plane descends to land. Symptoms include ear pain, ringing ears, diminished hearing and, sometimes, dizziness. Also known as aerotitis media, barotitis, barotitis media, and otic barotrauma.

Aesculapius   The ancient Roman god of medicine, whose staff with a snake curled around it is commonly used as a symbol of medicine. Followers of Aesculapius established temples of healing called asclepions, where the sick rested while proper remedies were revealed to temple priests in their dreams. According to mythology, Aesculapius' children included Hygeia, the goddess of health, and Panaceia, the goddess of healing.

affective disorder   A psychiatric disorder that affects the control of mood. See *bipolar disorder; cyclothymia; depression; seasonal affective disorder.*

afferent   Carrying toward. A vein is an afferent vessel because it carries blood from the body toward the heart. The opposite of afferent is efferent.

afferent nerve   A nerve that carries impulses toward the central nervous system.

afferent vessel   A vessel that carries blood toward the heart. A vein or venule.

AFLP   Acute fatty liver of pregnancy.

AFO   Ankle-foot orthosis.

AFP   Alpha-fetoprotein.

African tapeworm   See *Taenia saginata.*

African tick typhus   See *typhus, African tick.*

afterbirth   The placenta and the fetal membranes that are normally expelled from the uterus after the birth of a baby. See also *placenta.*

aftercare   Medical care and instructions for patients after leaving a medical facility.

agammaglobulinemia   Total or near-total absence of infection-fighting proteins belonging to the class called gamma globulins. Agammaglobulinemia can be due to certain genetic diseases or caused by acquired diseases, including AIDS.

agenesis   Lack of development. For example, agenesis of a toe means the toe failed to form.

agenesis of the gallbladder   A condition in which the gallbladder fails to develop. It occurs in 1 in about every 1,000 people, usually without additional birth defects.

agenesis, sacral   See *caudal regression syndrome.*

agent, antihypertensive   See *antihypertensive.*

agent, anti-infective   See *anti-infective.*

age-related macular degeneration   See *macular degeneration.*

ageusia   An inability to taste sweet, sour, bitter, or salty substances. People who can taste sweet, sour, bitter, or salty substances but have a reduced ability to do so are said to have hypogeusia.

aggressive fibromatosis   See *desmoid tumor.*

agnosia   An inability to recognize sensory inputs such as light, sound, and touch). Agnosia is typically a result of brain injury. For example, damaging the back part of the brain can cause visual agnosia (inability to properly recognize objects by sight).

agonist   A substance that acts like another substance and therefore stimulates an action. Agonist is the opposite of antagonist. Antagonists and agonists are key players in the chemistry of the human body and in pharmacology.

agoraphobia   An abnormal and persistent fear of public places or open areas, especially those from which escape could be difficult or in which help might not be immediately accessible. Persons with agoraphobia frequently also have panic disorder. The severity of agoraphobia is highly variable. People with mild agoraphobia often live normal lives by avoiding anxiety-provoking situations. In the most severe cases, the victims may be incapacitated and homebound. Agoraphobia tends to start in the mid to late 20s, and the onset may appear to be triggered by a traumatic event. From the Greek *agora*, meaning "marketplace," and *phobos*, meaning "fear."

agranulocytosis A marked decrease in the number of granulocytes. Agranulocytosis results in frequent chronic bacterial infections of the skin, lungs, throat, and other areas. It can be an inherited genetic condition or acquired as, for example, in leukemia. See also *agranulocytosis, infantile genetic; granulocytopenia; severe congenital neutropenia.*

agranulocytosis, infantile genetic An inherited condition characterized by a lack of neutrophils, a type of white blood cell that is important in fighting infection, and a predisposition to frequent bacterial infections. In the past, three-fourths of infantile genetic agranulocytosis patients died before 3 years of age. Also known as Kostmann disease or syndrome and genetic infantile agranulocytosis. See also *agranulocytosis; granulocytopenia; severe congenital neutropenia.*

agreement, arbitration See *arbitration agreement.*

Aicardis syndrome A rare genetic disorder that occurs only in females and is caused by congenital absence of the corpus callosum, a large bundle of nerves that connects the left and right sides of the brain. Features include epilepsy that emerges in infancy and is difficult to control, vision problems due to maldeveloped retinas, developmental delay, and sometimes physical deformities of the spine, face, and/or heart. Treatment includes medication for epilepsy and surgery for physical problems. See also *epilepsy; seizure disorders.*

AID Artificial insemination by donor.

AIDS Acquired immunodeficiency syndrome, a syndrome that is due to infection with the human immunodeficiency virus (HIV), with ensuing compromise of the body's immune system. Features include deficiency of certain types of leukocytes, especially T cells; infection with any of a number of opportunistic infections that take advantage of the impaired immune response, such as tuberculosis, bacterial pneumonia, human herpes virus, or toxoplasmosis; certain types of cancer, particularly Kaposi sarcoma; inability to maintain body weight (wasting); and in advanced cases, AIDS dementia complex. Diagnosis of AIDS in most countries requires a positive HIV test, accompanied by other symptoms. Treatment for AIDS has advanced rapidly. Antiviral, antibacterial, and immune-boosting medications, among other treatments, are part of current treatment protocols.

AIDS dementia complex A brain disorder that occurs in people with AIDS, causing loss of thinking capacity and affecting the ability to function in a social or occupational setting. The exact mechanism by which HIV triggers AIDS dementia complex has not been determined, but it may result from HIV infection of cells in the brain or from an inflammatory reaction to such an infection. Another possibility is opportunistic infection of the brain by any of many viruses known to cause neuropsychiatric symptoms. AIDS dementia complex is considered an AIDS-defining illness—that is, one of the serious illnesses that occurs in HIV-positive individuals and warrants an AIDS diagnosis, according to the definition of AIDS by the Centers for Disease Control and Prevention (CDC).

AIDS-related complex A term used in the early years of the AIDS epidemic to describe people with HIV infection who had only mild symptoms of illness, such as swollen lymph glands. It is rarely used today. Abbreviated ARC.

airway The path that air follows to get into and out of the lungs. The mouth and nose are the normal entry and exit ports for the airway. Entering air then passes through the back of the throat (pharynx) and continues through the voice box (larynx), down the trachea, to finally pass through the bronchi.

airway obstruction Partial or complete blockage of the breathing tubes to the lungs due to the presence of foreign bodies, allergic reactions, infections, anatomical abnormalities, trauma, or other causes. The onset of respiratory distress may be sudden, with only a cough for a warning. There is often agitation in the early stages. Other signs include labored, ineffective breathing, until the person is no longer breathing (apneic). Loss of consciousness occurs if the obstruction is not relieved. Treatment of airway obstruction due to a foreign body includes the Heimlich maneuver for adults, a series of five abdominal thrusts for children over 1 year of age, and a combination of five back blows with the flat of the hand and five abdominal thrusts with two fingers on the upper abdomen for infants.

AKA Above-the-knee amputation, generally performed when the leg is not medically viable or to prevent disease in the tissues above the knee.

akasthisia An intense internal sensation of physical restlessness and jumpiness. A person with akasthisia looks and feels uncomfortable if he or she tries to be still. Akasthisia can be a side effect of some psychiatric medications.

akinesia The state of being without movement.

akinetic Related to the loss of the normal ability to move the muscles.

akinetic epilepsy See *epilepsy, akinetic.*

akinetic mutism See *mutism, akinetic.*

alanine aminotransferase An enzyme that is normally present in liver and heart cells. Abbreviated ALT. ALT is released into blood when the liver or heart is damaged; some medications can raise ALT levels. Also known as serum glutamic pyruvic transaminase (SGPT).

alb- Prefix from the Latin word *albus,* meaning "white."

albinism A pigmentation disorder characterized by partial or total lack of the pigment melanin in the skin, hair, and iris. Albinism is caused by an autosomal recessive gene and can occur in people of any ethnic background. People with albinism have delicate skin that sunburns and develops skin cancer easily, and they may suffer from eye disorders as well. Albinism may be partial or complete (tyrosinase-negative albinism). See also *Hermansky-Pudlak syndrome; vitiligo.*

albinism with hemorrhagic diathesis and pigmented reticuloendithelial cells See *Hermansky-Pudlak syndrome.*

albino A person with albinism. The term was first applied by the Portuguese to people in West Africa, who may have had partial or complete albinism.

albuginea Tough white fibrous tissue. The tunica albuginea of the testis, for example, is the layer of dense whitish inelastic tissue that surrounds the testis.

albumin The main protein in human blood and the key to regulating the osmotic pressure of blood. Chemically, albumin is soluble in water, precipitated by acid, and coagulated by heat.

albuminuria More than the normal amount of albumin in the urine. Albuminuria can be a sign that protein is leaking through the kidney, most often through the glomeruli, or a sign of significant kidney disease. It may also be the harmless result of vigorous exercise. Also known as proteinuria.

alcohol An organic substance formed when a hydroxyl group is substituted for a hydrogen atom in a hydrocarbon. The type of alcohol used in alcoholic beverages, ethanol, derives from fermenting sugar with yeast. After alcohol is ingested, the body converts it to sugar-based fuel. Alcohol acts as a central nervous system depressant, and it has many medicinal uses. It may be part of solutions used as preservatives, antiseptics, or medications.

alcohol abuse Use of alcoholic beverages to excess, either on individual occasions (binge drinking) or as a regular practice. For some individuals—children or pregnant women, for example—almost any amount of alcohol use may be legally considered "alcohol abuse," depending on local laws. Heavy alcohol abuse can cause physical damage and death.

alcohol poisoning A condition in which a toxic amount of alcohol has been consumed, usually in a short period of time. The individual may become extremely disoriented, unresponsive, or unconscious, with shallow breathing. Because alcohol poisoning can be deadly, emergency treatment is necessary.

alcohol use in pregnancy The consumption of alcohol during pregnancy, which can damage the fetus. See also *fetal alcohol effect; fetal alcohol syndrome.*

Alcoholics Anonymous A free self-help organization founded to assist people addicted to alcohol in breaking old behavior patterns and gaining support for living a sober lifestyle.

alcoholism Physical dependence on alcohol to the extent that stopping alcohol use would bring on withdrawal symptoms. In popular and therapeutic parlance, the term may also be used to refer to ingrained drinking habits that cause health or social problems. Treatment requires first ending the physical dependence and then making lifestyle changes that help the individual avoid relapse. In some cases, medication and hospitalization are necessary. Alcohol dependence can have many serious effects on the brain, liver, and other organs of the body, some of which can lead to death.

aldosterone A hormone produced by the outer portion (cortex) of the adrenal gland. Aldosterone regulates the balance of water and electrolytes in the body, encouraging the kidney to excrete potassium into the urine and retain sodium, thereby retaining water. It is classified as a mineralocorticoid hormone.

aldosteronism See *Conn syndrome.*

alexia Loss of the ability to read or understand the written word, due either to brain damage that disconnects these functions or to temporary dysfunction caused by unusual electrical or chemical activity in the brain.

alienist French term for a psychologist, a psychiatrist, or another practitioner who cares for the mentally ill.

alkaline phosphatase An enzyme that liberates phosphate under alkaline conditions and is made in liver, bone, and other tissues. Alkaline phosphatase can be measured in a routine blood test. Abnormally high serum levels of alkaline phosphatase may indicate bone disease, liver disease, or bile duct obstruction.

alkalosis   Relatively too much base in the blood and body, an abnormal condition resulting from the accumulation of base or the depletion of acid. The pH of an alkalotic body measures above normal. The opposite of alkalosis is acidosis.

allele   An alternative form of a gene.

allergen   A substance that can cause an allergic reaction. Common allergens include ragweed pollen, animal dander, and mold.

allergic conjunctivitis   Inflammation of the whites of the eyes (conjunctivae), with itching, redness, and tearing, due to allergy.

allergic granulomatosis   See *Churg-Strauss syndrome.*

allergic reaction   A hypersensitive immune response to a substance. An allergic reaction can occur when the immune system attacks a normally harmless substance. The immune system calls upon a protective antibody called immunoglobulin E (IgE) to fight these invading substances. Although everyone has some IgE, an allergic person has an unusually large army of IgE defenders. These IgE antibodies engage and attack the invading allergens. In the melee, cells called mast cells are injured or irritated. The mast cells then release a variety of strong chemicals, including histamine, into the tissues and blood. These chemicals are very irritating and cause itching, swelling, and fluid leakage from nearby cells. They may also cause muscle spasms and can lead to lung, airway, and throat tightening, as is found in asthma, as well as to loss of voice. They are also the cause of allergic rhinitis and some cases of pink eye (conjunctivitis). See also *allergic conjunctivitis; allergic rhinitis; anaphylactic shock; asthma.*

allergic rhinitis   Medical term for hay fever, an allergic reaction that mimics a chronic cold. Symptoms include nasal congestion, a clear runny nose, sneezing, nose and eye itching, and tearing of the eyes. Postnasal dripping of clear mucus frequently causes a cough, loss of smell is common, and loss of taste occurs occasionally. Nosebleeds may occur if the condition is severe. Also known as June cold and summer cold.

allergic rhinitis, perennial   Allergic rhinitis that occurs throughout the year.

allergic rhinitis, seasonal   Allergic rhinitis that occurs during a specific season.

allergic salute   The characteristic gesture of a person with allergic rhinitis: rubbing his or her nose with the index finger.

allergic vasculitis   See *Churg-Strauss syndrome.*

allergy   Hypersensitivity of the body's immune system in response to exposure to specific substances (antigens), such as pollen, bee stings, poison ivy, drugs, or foods. See also *allergic reaction; anaphylactic shock.*

allergy desensitization   Stimulation of the immune system with gradually increasing doses of the substances to which a person is allergic, the aim being to modify or stop the allergic response by reducing the strength of the immunoglobulin E (IgE) and its effect on the mast cells. This form of treatment is very effective for allergies to pollen, mites, animal dander, and stinging insects, including bees, hornets, yellow jackets, wasps, velvet ants, and fire ants. Allergy immunotherapy may take 6 months to 1 year to become effective, and injections are usually required for 3 to 5 years.

allergy scratch test   See *allergy skin test.*

allergy skin test   A test in which a small drop of the suspected allergy-provoking substance (allergen) is placed on the skin and the skin is then gently scratched through the drop with a sterile needle. If the skin reddens and, more importantly, if it swells, the test is read as positive, and allergy to that substance is considered probable.

allergy to cockroaches   An allergic reaction to tiny protein particles shed or excreted by cockroaches. Asthma can be due to exposure to cockroach allergens. Removing cockroach allergens from the home is not an easy job, but it can go far in reducing the frequency and severity of asthma and other allergic reactions.

alopecia   Baldness. Temporary alopecia may occur as a result of chemotherapy. Permanent alopecia may result from any of several conditions, including common male-pattern baldness. Radiation therapy administered to the head can also cause permanent alopecia due to irreversible damage to the hair follicles. See also *alopecia areata; alopecia capitis totalis; alopecia universalis; alopecia, traumatic.*

alopecia areata   Patchy baldness that typically begins with hair loss on discrete areas of the scalp and sometimes progresses to complete baldness and even loss of body hair. The hair loss tends to be rapid and asymmetrical. The characteristic diagnostic finding is "exclamation point" hairs; these short, broken hairs are narrower closer to the scalp, and therefore look like exclamation points. Alopecia areata affects both males and females and, most often, children and young adults. It appears to be caused by an autoimmune mechanism, wherein the body's own immune system attacks the hair follicles and disrupts normal hair formation. Alopecia areata is sometimes associated with allergic disorders, thyroid disease, vitiligo, lupus, rheumatoid arthritis, ulcerative colitis, and other conditions, and some forms may be genetically transmitted. In about half of the cases, hair regrows within a year without treatment. The longer the period of time of hair loss, the less chance that the hair will regrow.

alopecia capitis totalis Loss of all scalp hair, with normal hair elsewhere on the body remaining.

alopecia, traumatic Hair loss caused by injury to the scalp. Common causes include the use of caustic hair straighteners, especially those that include lye as an ingredient; stress traction injury from tight rollers and braiding; overheating of the hair shafts; and compulsive pulling out of hair (trichotillomania). Vigorous combing, chemical bleaches, and some styling products can further irritate the scalp, increasing the rate of hair loss. Traumatic alopecia commonly occurs on both sides of the scalp, and the broken-off hairs are frequently visible. In the US, traumatic alopecia is a common form of hair loss in African-American women. Treatment for traumatic alopecia involves discontinuation of all styling practices that may be causing the hair and scalp injury. Partial or complete regrowth of hair may follow, although permanent loss of hair can occur if the roots of the hair have been severely damaged. The risk of scalp injury can be minimized by using "natural" hair styles, choosing styling products carefully, using looser and larger wrappings and braids to reduce scalp and hair tension, applying any chemicals to the hair only, and unbraiding hair at least every 2 weeks.

alopecia universalis Loss of all hair on the entire body.

alpha-1 antitrypsin deficiency An inherited disorder characterized by a lack of the alpha-1 antitrypsin protease inhibitor. Alpha-1 antitrypsin deficiency leads to damage of various organs, especially the lung and liver. Symptoms may become apparent at a very early age or anytime later, manifesting as shortness of breath due to emphysema or as liver symptoms such as jaundice, fatigue, fluid in the abdomen, mental changes, or gastrointestinal bleeding. There are several options for treatment of the lung disease, including replacement of the missing alpha-1 antitrypsin. Avoidance of smoking and of other lung irritants is an important part of management. Treatment of the liver disease is a well-timed liver transplant. Also known as protease inhibitor 1 deficiency.

alpha cell, pancreatic A type of cell found in areas within the pancreas called the islets of Langerhans. Alpha cells make and release glucagon, which raises the level of glucose (sugar) in the blood.

alpha error The statistical error made in testing a hypothesis when it is concluded that a result is positive but it really is not. Also known as false positive.

alpha-fetoprotein A plasma protein normally produced by a fetus, principally in the fetus's liver, the fetal gastrointestinal (GI) tract, and the yolk sac, a structure temporarily present during embryonic development. Abbreviated AFP. The level of AFP is typically high in the fetus's blood. It goes down after birth. By 1 year of age, it is virtually undetectable. During pregnancy, AFP crosses the placenta from the fetal circulation and appears in the mother's blood. The level of AFP in the mother's blood (the maternal serum AFP, or MSAFP) provides an opportunity to screen for a number of disorders, including open neural tube defects (such as anencephaly and spina bifida), Down syndrome, and other chromosome abnormalities. MSAFP tends to be high in the presence of open neural tube defects and low in Down syndrome. After infancy, renewed AFP production can be stimulated by some diseases in the liver, such as viral hepatitis and cirrhosis. AFP is also made by primary liver tumors (hepatomas) and by germ cell tumors (teratocarcinoma and embryonal cell carcinomas). A person's serum AFP level can therefore be used to help detect these conditions and monitor their treatment.

alpha interferon One of the three main classes of interferons, which are specialized proteins (lymphokines) produced by the body in response to an infection that interfere with the multiplication of viruses in cells. The other two main classes are called beta interferon and gamma interferon. See also *interferon; interferon therapy.*

Alpha Omega Alpha An honor society, the medical school equivalent of Phi Beta Kappa.

alpha thalassemia See *thalassemia, alpha.*

Alport syndrome A hereditary condition characterized by kidney disease, deafness, and sometimes eye defects. Alport syndrome involves inflammation of the kidney (nephritis), often progressing to kidney failure, and sensory nerve hearing loss. Alport syndrome affects both sexes in successive generations. The kidney disease becomes evident via recurrent microscopic or gross blood in the urine as early as childhood, and it usually appears earlier in males than in females. Progression to kidney failure is gradual and usually occurs in males before 50 years of age.

ALS Amyotropic lateral sclerosis, Lou Gehrig's disease.

ALT Alanine aminotransferase.

alternative medicine   Healing arts not generally taught in Western medical schools and not typically practiced in Western hospitals. The term *alternative medicine* is used to cover a wide variety of practices, ranging from the use of traditional Chinese medicine to healing prayer. Some alternatives that appear to be effective have been embraced by mainstream physicians, who may mix them with Western practices: This practice is known as "complementary medicine." Some other alternative therapies are useless or even potentially harmful. See *acupressure; acupuncture; aromatherapy; biofeedback; bodywork; chiropractic; craniosacral therapy; dietary supplement; guided imagery; herbal remedy; homeopathy; iridology; massage; naturopathy; orthomolecular medicine; osteopathy; vision therapy.*

altitude, acclimatization to   See *acclimatization to altitude.*

altitude, high   2,400 to 3,600 meters (approximately 8,000 to 12,000 feet) above sea level. Very high altitude is 3,600 to 5,400 meters (approximately 12,000 to 18,000 feet) above sea level, and extremely high altitude is over 5,400 meters (approximately 18,000 feet) above sea level.

altitude illness   See *altitude sickness.*

altitude sickness   Sickness caused by being at a high altitude, usually above 2,400 meters (approximately 8,000 feet). The cause of altitude sickness is a matter of oxygen physiology. At sea level the concentration of oxygen is about 21 percent, and the barometric pressure averages 760 mm Hg. As altitude increases, the concentration remains the same, but the number of oxygen molecules per breath is reduced. At 5,400 meters (approximately 12,000 feet) above sea level, the barometric pressure is only 483 mm Hg, so there are roughly 40 percent fewer oxygen molecules per breath. In order to oxygenate the body effectively, the breathing rate must increase. This extra ventilation increases the oxygen content in the blood—but not to sea level concentrations. Because the amount of oxygen required for activity is the same at high altitude as at sea level, the body must adjust to having less oxygen. In addition, high altitude and lower air pressure cause fluid to leak from the capillaries, which can cause fluid buildup in the lungs and the brain. Prevention measures for altitude sickness include avoiding or retreating from high-altitude areas, gradual acclimatization, and medication. The acclimatization process is inhibited by dehydration, overexertion, and the use of alcohol and other depressant drugs. Preventive medications include acetazolamide (brand name: Diamox) and dexamethasone (a steroid). See also *acclimatization to altitude; acute mountain sickness.*

alveolus   A tiny air sac in the lungs. The plural is alveoli.

Alzheimer's disease   A progressive degenerative disease of the brain that leads to dementia. On a cellular level, Alzheimer's disease is characterized by the finding of unusual helical protein filaments in nerve cells (neurons) of the brain. These odd, twisted filaments are called neurofibrillary tangles. On a functional level, Alzheimer's disease involves degeneration of the cortical regions, especially the frontal and temporal lobes, of the brain. There is currently no cure for Alzheimer's disease, but new medications and therapies appear to slow its progress and improve the patient's ability to function.

AMA   American Medical Association, a professional organization for physicians that sets widely accepted standards of practice and ethics and that publishes the weekly journal *JAMA* (*Journal of the American Medical Association*).

amastia   A rare condition wherein the normal growth of the breast or nipple does not occur. Unilateral amastia (absence of one breast) is often associated with absence of the pectoral muscles. Bilateral amastia (absence of both breasts) is associated in 40 percent of cases with multiple birth defects involving other parts of the body. See also *amazia.*

amaurosis fugax   A symptom that is often described as a shade coming down over the eye. Amaurosis fugax is a partial or complete loss of sight that is temporary. This temporary interference with vision is usually related to arteriosclerosis in the blood vessels that supply the brain. It can also occur with excessive acceleration, as in flight.

amaurotic familial idiocy   An outdated term for Tay-Sachs disease (TSD). See *Tay-Sachs disease.*

amazia   A condition wherein the breast tissue is absent, but the nipple is present. Amazia is typically a result of radiation or surgery.

amblyopia, nocturnal   Night blindness, also known as day sight. See *nyctanopia.*

ambulance   Today, a special vehicle equipped with medications and devices intended to stabilize patients while speeding them to a hospital. In its original sense, this term denoted a mobile field hospital.

ambulatory   Able to walk about, not bedridden or immobile.

ambulatory care   Medical care provided on an outpatient basis, including diagnosis, observation, treatment, and rehabilitation services.

ameba A single-celled, protozoan organism that constantly changes shape. Amebae can infect the bowels, causing diarrhea. They can also infect the liver, causing abscesses to form.

amebiasis The state of being infected with amebae, especially with the ameba Entamoeba histolytica.

amebic colitis Amebic dysentery with ulcers in the colon due to infection with the ameba Entamoeba histolytica. This single-celled parasite is transmitted to humans via contaminated water and food.

amebic dysentery Inflammation of the intestine due to infection with the ameba Entamoeba histolytica. Amebic dysentery can be accompanied by amebic infection of the liver and other organs.

amelanotic melanoma See *melanoma, amelanotic.*

amelioration Improvement in a patient's condition, or the activity of making an effort to correct, or at least make more acceptable, conditions that are difficult to endure.

amenorrhea See *menstruation, cessation of.*

amenorrhea, physiologic The cessation of menstruation for completely normal reasons. The lack of menstruation during pregnancy and lactation are forms of physiologic amenorrhea.

amenorrhea, primary The failure of menstruation to occur at puberty.

amenorrhea, secondary The cessation of menstruation for abnormal reasons. Causes include anorexia nervosa, disease of the female reproductive tract, and overexercise. Secondary amenorrhea can also be caused by certain medications, notably the birth control medication medroxyprogesterone (brand name: Depo-Provera); in this case, amenorrhea is an expected effect.

American Type Culture Collection The world's premier biological culture repository, and a key resource for medical research. Abbreviated ATCC. Although it is little known to the general public, ATCC provides medical and other biological scientists a reliable source of more than 60,000 authenticated, viable cultures of everything from cultured cell lines to recombinant DNA for use in the lab.

AMI Acute myocardial infarction.

amine A chemical compound containing nitrogen. Amines are derived from ammonia.

amino acid One of the 20 building blocks from which proteins are assembled. Isoleucine, leucine, lysine, phenylalanine, threonine, tryptophan, and valine are deemed "essential" amino acids because the human body cannot make them and they must be obtained in the diet. Amino acids are sometimes taken orally in supplement form.

amino acid screen A screening blood or urine test that returns information about the levels of amino acids. An amino acid screen is useful in diagnosing certain conditions, including the inborn errors of amino acid metabolisms such as phenylketonuria (PKU).

aminotransferase An enzyme that catalyzes the transfer of an amino group from a donor molecule to a recipient molecule. The donor molecule is usually an amino acid and the recipient molecule is usually an alpha-2 keto acid. Two of the best-known enzymes in this class are serum glutamic oxaloacetic transaminase (SGOT) and serum glutamic pyruvic transaminase (SGPT), both of which are normally found primarily in cells in the liver and heart. SGOT and SGPT are released into the bloodstream as the result of liver or heart damage, and so are used as liver and heart tests. Also known as transaminase. SGOT is also known as aspartate aminotransferase (AST), and SGPT is also known as alanine aminotransferase (ALT).

amitriptyline A tricyclic antidepressant drug (brand name: Elavil) prescribed to treat depression, chronic pain, migraines, eating disorders, and a wide variety of other conditions. See also *tricyclic antidepressant.*

AML See *leukemia, acute myeloid.*

amnesia An impairment to or lack of memory. Antegrade amnesia refers to a lack of memory of events occurring after a traumatic event, whereas retrograde amnesia refers to lack of memory of events that occurred before the event.

amniocentesis A prenatal diagnostic procedure in which a long needle is used to obtain amniotic fluid from within the uterus. This fluid can be used for genetic and other diagnostic tests. Informally known as amnio.

amnion A thin membrane that surrounds the fetus during pregnancy. The amnion is the inner of the two fetal membranes (the chorion is the outer one), and it contains the amniotic fluid.

amniotic fluid The fluid bathing a fetus within the uterus, which serves as a shock absorber.

amoeba Alternative spelling for ameba, used mainly in the UK. See also *ameba.*

amphetamine A drug that has a stimulant effect on the central nervous system that can be both physically and psychologically addictive when overused. Amphetamine has been much abused recreationally. The street term "speed" refers to stimulant drugs such as amphetamine.

amplification An event that produces multiple copies of a gene or of any sequence of DNA. Gene amplification plays a role in cancer. Amplification can occur in vivo (in the living individual) or in vitro (in the laboratory).

ampulla of Vater A small projection into the duodenum through which bile and pancreatic secretions flow to mix with food for digestion.

amputation Removal of part or all of a body part that is enclosed by skin. For example, removal of part of a finger or an entire finger would be termed an amputation. Removal of an appendix, on the other hand, would not be termed amputation. A person who has undergone an amputation is called an amputee. Amputation usually takes place during surgery in a hospital operating room. Amputation can occur at an accident site, the scene of an animal attack, or a battlefield. Amputation is also performed as a surgical procedure. It is typically performed to prevent the spread of gangrene as a complication of frostbite, injury, diabetes, arteriosclerosis, or any other illness that impairs blood circulation. It is also performed to prevent the spread of bone cancer and to curtail loss of blood and infection in a person who has suffered severe, irreparable damage to a limb. When performing an amputation, surgeons generally cut above the diseased or injured area so that a portion of healthy tissue remains to cushion bone. Sometimes the location of a cut may depend in part on its suitability to be fitted with an artificial limb, or prosthesis. From the Latin word *amputare,* meaning "to excise" or "to cut out."

AMS 1 Atypical measles syndrome. 2 Acute mountain sickness.

amygdala An almond-shaped structure within the basal ganglia of the brain that is believed to affect the sense of smell, mood, emotion, instinctive behavior, and short-term memory.

amyloidosis A group of diseases that result from the abnormal deposition of a particular protein, called amyloid, in various tissues of the body. Amyloid protein can be deposited in a localized area, and it may not be harmful or it may affect only a single tissue of the body. This form of amyloidosis is called localized amyloidosis. Amyloidosis that affects tissues throughout the body is referred to as systemic amyloidosis. Systemic amyloidosis can cause serious changes in virtually any organ of the body. Amyloidosis can occur as its own entity or secondarily, as a result of another illness, including multiple myeloma, chronic infections (such as tuberculosis or osteomyelitis), or chronic inflammatory diseases (such as rheumatoid arthritis and ankylosing spondylitis).

amyotrophic lateral sclerosis A progressive chronic disease of the motor neurons (the nerves that derive from the spinal cord). These nerves are responsible for supplying electrical stimulation to the muscles, which is a necessary process for the movement of body parts. Abbreviated ALS. ALS is progressive and usually fatal in 2 to 7 years, due to intercurrent illnesses that strike as the body becomes weaker. ALS occurs most often in adults over 50. The cause of ALS is unknown. It is sometimes called Lou Gehrig's disease, after a great baseball player who was its best-known victim.

an- See *a-.*

ANA 1 Antinuclear antibody. 2 Antinuclear antibody screen, a blood test that detects antinuclear antibodies. The ANA test reveals different patterns, depending on how the cell nucleus is stained in the laboratory: homogeneous, or diffuse; speckled; nucleolar; and peripheral, or rim. Although these patterns are not specific for any one illness, certain illnesses can more frequently be associated with some patterns. For example, the nucleolar pattern is commonly seen in the disease scleroderma. The speckled pattern is seen in many conditions and in persons who have no autoimmune disorder. ANAs are found in approximately 5 percent of the normal population, usually in low titers (low levels). Titers lower than 1:80 are less likely than higher titers to be significant. Even higher titers are often insignificant in persons over 60. ANA results must be interpreted in the specific context of an individual patient's symptoms and other test results. 3 Antineuronal antibody screen, a test that searches for antibodies to brain tissue in the bloodstream. Their presence is a general indicator for lupus and some other autoimmune inflammatory diseases.

anaerobic Not requiring oxygen. Anaerobic bacteria, for instance, do not require oxygen to grow.

anal fissure A tear in the anal canal, one of the most common causes of red blood in the stool.

anal itching Irritation of the skin at the exit of the rectum, accompanied by the desire to scratch. The intensity of anal itching is increased by moisture, pressure, and abrasion caused by clothing and sitting. At its most intense, anal itching causes intolerable discomfort. It may be caused by irritating chemicals in food (as in spices, hot sauces, and peppers); irritation due to frequent liquid stools, as in diarrhea; diseases, such as diabetes mellitus or HIV infection, that increase the possibility of yeast infections; and psoriasis. Other causes of anal itching include hemorrhoids, anal fissures, abnormal local growth of anal skin (anal papillae), and skin tags. Treatment is directed first toward relieving the burning and soreness, including cleaning and drying the anus thoroughly, avoiding leaving soap in the anal area, showering gently without directly rubbing or irritating the skin, and using moist pads rather than toilet paper to clean the anus after bowel movements. Local application of cortisone cream may help. If anal itching persists, an examination by a physician can rapidly identify most causes of anal itching. Also known as pruritus ani.

analgesia The inability to feel pain.

analgesic A drug that relieves pain.

analysis In psychology, a term for conversation-based therapeutic processes used to gain understanding of complex emotional or behavioral issues.

anaphylactic shock A widespread and extremely serious allergic reaction that can result in death. Symptoms include dizziness, loss of consciousness, labored breathing, swelling of the tongue and breathing tubes, blueness of the skin, low blood pressure, and heart failure. Immediate emergency treatment is required, for example, administration of antivenom in the case of bee or wasp stings. See also *allergic reaction.*

anaphylactoid purpura A form of blood vessel inflammation that affects small capillaries in the skin and the kidneys. It results in skin rash associated with joint inflammation (arthritis) and cramping pain in the abdomen. Anaphylactoid purpura frequently follows a bacterial or viral infection of the throat or breathing passages, and it is an unusual reaction of the body's immune system to this infection. It occurs most commonly in children. Generally a mild illness that resolves spontaneously, anaphylactoid purpura can sometimes cause serious problems in the kidneys and bowels. Treatment is directed toward the most significant area of involvement. Joint pain can be relieved with anti-inflammatory medications, such as aspirin or ibuprofen. Some patients may require steroid medications, such as prednisone. Also known as Henoch-Schonlein purpura (HSP).

anaphylaxis An allergic reaction. In severe cases, anaphylaxis can include potentially deadly anaphylactic shock. See also *allergic reaction; anaphylactic shock.*

anastomosis The connection of normally separate parts. An anastomosis may be naturally occurring or it may be created during embryonic development, surgery, or trauma, or by pathological means. An anastomosis

may, for example, connect two blood vessels, or it may connect the healthy sections of the colon or rectum after a cancerous or otherwise diseased portion has been surgically removed. A gastrojejunal anastomosis connects the stomach directly with the jejunum.

anat. Abbreviation for anatomy.

anatomy The study of human or animal form, by observation or examination of the living being, examination or dissection of dead specimens, or microscopic examination.

anatomy, gross The study of structures that can be seen with the naked eye. Known among medical students simply as "gross."

anatomy, microscopic The study of normal structures under the microscope. Also known as histology. Known among medical students simply as "micro."

anatripsis The use of friction as a treatment modality for a medical condition. Anatripsis may or may not also involve the application of a medicament.

Anderson-Fabry disease See *Fabry disease.*

androgen A group of hormones, including androsterone, that promotes the development and maintenance of male sex characteristics. Androgen production is stimulated by the hormone testosterone. See also *testosterone.*

android pelvis See *male pelvis.*

androsterone A male sex hormone that is found in the blood and urine of men and women. It is seven times weaker than testosterone.

anemia The condition of having a lower-than-normal number of red blood cells or quantity of hemoglobin, which diminishes the capacity of the blood to carry oxygen. Patients with anemia may feel tired, fatigue easily, appear pale, develop palpitations, and become short of breath. Children with chronic anemia are prone to infections and learning problems. The main processes leading to anemia are hemorrhage (as in intestinal bleeding and menstruation), hemolysis (excessive destruction of red blood cells, as in Rh disease of the newborn), underproduction of red blood cells (as in leukemia and other bone marrow diseases and after chemotherapy), and underproduction of normal hemoglobin (as in sickle cell anemia and in iron deficiency anemia). Women are more likely than men to have anemia because of their loss of blood each month through menstruation. Iron deficiency anemia is common and in adults is most often due to chronic blood loss, which can be due to menstruation or small amounts of repeated bleeding. In children, anemia is mainly due to insufficient iron in the diet. Anemia is also often due to gastrointestinal bleeding caused by medications, including such common drugs as aspirin and ibuprofen.

anemia, Addisonian　See *anemia, pernicious.*

anemia, aplastic　Anemia due to failure of the bone marrow to produce red and white blood cells as well as platelets. Aplastic anemia frequently occurs without a known cause. Known causes include exposure to chemicals (for example, benzene, toluene in glues, insecticides, solvents), drugs (for example, chemotherapy drugs, gold, seizure medications, antibiotics), viruses (for instance, HIV, Epstein-Barr), radiation, immune conditions (for example, systemic lupus erythematosus, rheumatoid arthritis), pregnancy, paroxysmal nocturnal hemoglobinuria, and inherited disorders (for example, Fanconi anemia).

anemia, Cooley　See *thalassemia.*

anemia, Fanconi　See *Fanconi anemia.*

anemia, iron deficiency　Anemia due to a lack of iron. Iron is necessary to make hemoglobin, the molecule in red blood cells that is responsible for the transport of oxygen. In iron deficiency anemia, the red cells are small (microcytic) and pale (hypochromic). Characteristic features of iron deficiency anemia in children include failure to thrive and increased infections. Iron deficiency anemia can be treated with iron supplements and iron-containing foods. Food sources of iron include meat, poultry, eggs, vegetables, and cereals, especially those fortified with iron. Iron supplements may also be taken, although they should never be given to children without a physician's recommendation.

anemia, Mediterranean　See *thalassemia.*

anemia, pernicious　A blood disorder caused by a lack of vitamin B12. Abbreviated PA. Patients with PA do not produce intrinsic factor (IF), a substance that allows the body to absorb vitamin B12. In patients with PA, the blood contains large, immature, nucleated cells (megaloblasts) that are forerunners of red blood cells. PA is thus a type of megaloblastic anemia. PA can be treated by injection of vitamin B12: oral administration will not work because people with PA cannot absorb orally administered vitamin B12. PA may be genetic; one form is inherited as an autosomal recessive trait. The IF gene has been localized to chromosome 11. The word *pernicious* means highly injurious, destructive, or deadly, and PA was once quite deadly. Today, fortunately, it is not. Also known as Addison's anemia.

anemia, refractory　Anemia that is unresponsive to treatment.

anemia, sickle cell　A genetic blood disorder caused by the presence of an abnormal, sickle-shaped form of hemoglobin. These hemoglobin molecules tend to aggregate after unloading oxygen, forming long, rod-like structures that force the red cells to assume a sickle shape. Unlike normal red cells, which are usually smooth and malleable, the sickle red cells cannot squeeze through small blood vessels. When the sickle cells block small blood vessels, the organs are deprived of blood and oxygen. This leads to periodic episodes of pain and damages the vital organs. Sickle red cells die after only about 10 to 20 days, instead of the usual 120 days or so. Because they cannot be replaced fast enough, the blood is chronically short of red cells, causing anemia. The gene for sickle cell anemia must be inherited from both parents for the illness to occur in children. A child with only one copy of the gene may have sickle-cell traits but no symptoms of illness. Sickle cell disease affects millions of people. It is particularly common among people whose ancestors came from sub-Saharan Africa, Spanish-speaking regions (South America, Cuba, Central America), Saudi Arabia, India, and Mediterranean countries, such as Turkey, Greece, and Italy. In the US, sickle cell disease occurs at birth in about 1 in every 500 African-Americans and 1 in every 1,000 to 1,400 Hispanic-Americans. It is believed that the sickle-cell error in the hemoglobin gene results from a genetic mutation that occurred many thousands of years ago, when malaria epidemics caused the death of great numbers of people. In areas where malaria was a problem, people with one sickle hemoglobin gene—and who therefore carried the sickle cell trait—had a survival advantage. See also *sickle cell trait.*

anencephaly　Absence of the cranial vault and of most or all of the cerebral hemispheres of the brain. Anencephaly is due to imperfect development of the neural tube, the structure that gives rise to the central nervous system, during very early pregnancy. The upper end of the neural tube fails to close. Anencephaly is a lethal malformation. The risk of all neural tube defects, including anencephaly, is decreased if the mother's diet during pregnancy contains ample folic acid. See also *neural tube defect.*

anesthesia　Loss of feeling or awareness, as when an anesthetic is administered before surgery.

anesthesiologist　A physician or, less often, a dentist who is specialized in the practice of anesthesiology.

anesthesiology　The branch of medicine specializing in the use of drugs or other agents that cause insensibility to pain.

anesthetic A substance that causes lack of feeling or awareness, dulling pain to permit surgery and other painful procedures.

anesthetic, epidural An anesthetic injected into the epidural space surrounding the fluid-filled sac (the dura) around the spine. It partially numbs the abdomen and legs. Most commonly used during childbirth.

anesthetic, general An anesthetic that puts a person to sleep.

anesthetic, local An anesthetic that causes loss of feeling in a part of the body.

anesthetist A nurse or technician trained to administer anesthetics.

aneuploidy A condition in which a person has one or a few chromosomes above or below the normal chromosome number. For example, three copies of chromosome 21, which is characteristic of Down syndrome, is a form of aneuploidy.

aneurysm A localized widening (dilatation) of an artery, a vein, or the heart. At the point of an aneurysm, there is typically a bulge. The wall of the blood vessel or organ is weakened and may rupture.

aneurysm, abdominal aortic A balloon-like swelling in the wall of the aorta within the abdomen. This swelling weakens the aorta's wall and, because of the great volume of blood flowing under high pressure in the aorta, it can rupture. An abdominal aortic aneurysm should be monitored by ultrasound. Surgery is recommended if the aneurysm is more than 5.5 centimeters (2.2 inches) in diameter or if a smaller aneurysm is enlarging with unusual rapidity.

aneurysm, aortic An aneurysm of the largest artery in the body, the aorta, involving that vessel in its course above the diaphragm (thoracic aortic aneurysm) or, more commonly, below the diaphragm (abdominal aortic aneurysm). Because of the volume of blood flowing under relatively high pressure within the aorta, a ruptured aneurysm of the aorta is a catastrophe. See also *aneurysm, abdominal aortic; aneurysm, thoracic.*

aneurysm, arterial An aneurysm involving an artery.

aneurysm, arteriosclerotic An aneurysm that occurs because a vessel wall is weakened by arteriosclerosis. Also known as atherosclerotic aneurysm.

aneurysm, berry A small aneurysm that looks like a berry and classically occurs at the point at which a cerebral artery departs from the circular artery (the circle of Willis) at the base of the brain. Berry aneurysms frequently rupture and bleed.

aneurysm, brain An aneurysm of a blood vessel in the brain, usually due to a defect in the vessel at birth or from high blood pressure. Rupture of the aneurysm causes a sudden severe headache, often with nausea, vomiting, decreased consciousness, and can be life threatening.

aneurysm, cardiac An outpouching of an abnormally thin portion of the heart wall. Cardiac aneurysms tend to involve the left ventricle because the blood there is under the greatest pressure.

aneurysm, dissecting An aneurysm in which the wall of an artery rips (dissects) longitudinally. This occurs because bleeding into the weakened wall splits the wall. Dissecting aneurysms tend to affect the thoracic aorta. They are a particular danger in Marfan syndrome.

aneurysm, fusiform An aneurysm that is shaped like a spindle and widens an artery or a vein.

aneurysm, miliary A tiny, millet-seed–sized aneurysm that tends to affect minute arteries in the brain and, in the eye, the retina.

aneurysm, saccular An aneurysm that resembles a small sack. A berry aneurysm is typically saccular.

aneurysm, thoracic An aneurysm of the largest artery in the body, the aorta, involving that vessel in its course within the thorax (chest). Because of the volume of blood flowing under relatively high pressure within the aorta, a ruptured aneurysm of the aorta is a catastrophe. See also *aneurysm, abdominal aortic; aneurysm, aortic.*

aneurysm, venous An aneurysm involving a vein.

aneurysmal bone cyst See *bone cyst, aneurysmal.*

angiitis Inflammation of the walls of small blood vessels. Also known as vasculitis.

angiitis, allergic granulomatous See *Churg-Strauss syndrome.*

angina Chest pain due to an inadequate supply of oxygen to the heart muscle. The pain is typically severe and crushing, and it is characterized by a feeling of pressure and suffocation just behind the breastbone.

angina pectoris See *angina.*

angina, Prinzmetal Chest pain due to a coronary artery spasm, a sudden constriction of one of the vessels that supply the heart muscle with blood that is rich in oxygen. This spasm deprives the heart muscle of blood and oxygen. Treatments include beta-blocker medications and, classically, nitroglycerin to open up the coronary arteries. Also known as variant angina. See also *coronary artery spasm.*

angina, variant   See *angina, Prinzmetal.*

angina, Vincent   See *acute membranous gingivitis.*

angioedema   A skin condition that resembles hives but affects a deeper skin layer. See also *angioedema, hereditary.*

angioedema, hereditary   A genetic form of angioedema. Persons with it are born lacking C1 esterase inhibitor, a protein that normally inhibits the activation of a cascade of proteins. Without this inhibitor protein, angioedema occurs, resulting in recurrent attacks of swollen tissues, pain in the abdomen, and swelling of the voice box (larynx), which can compromise breathing. The diagnosis of hereditary angioedema is confirmed by finding subnormal blood levels of C1 esterase inhibitor. Treatment and prevention options include antihistamines and male steroids (androgens). Also known as hereditary angioneurotic edema. See also *angioedema.*

angiogenesis   The process of developing new blood vessels. Angiogenesis is important during the normal development of the embryo and fetus. It also appears to be important during tumor formation. Certain proteins secreted by tumors, including angiostatin and endostatin, appear to interfere with the blood supply that tumors need.

angiogram   An X-ray image of blood vessels. The vessels can be seen because a contrast dye within them blocks the X-rays from developing an imaging film.

angioid streaks   Tiny breaks in the elastin-filled tissue in the retina in the back of the eye. Angioid streaks are seen in patients with pseudoxanthoma elasticum, a rare disorder of degeneration of the elastic fibers with tiny areas of calcification in the skin, retinae, and blood vessels, and they are visible during an examination using an ophthalmoscope. Angioid streaks can be associated with blindness.

angiokeratoma corporis diffusum universale   See *Fabry disease.*

angioneurotic edema, hereditary   See *angioedema, hereditary.*

angiopathy   A disease of the arteries, veins, and capillaries. There are two types of angiopathy: microangiopathy and macroangiopathy. In microangiopathy, the walls of small blood vessels become so thick and weak that they

bleed, leak protein, and slow the flow of blood. For example, diabetics may develop microangiopathy with thickening of capillaries in many areas, including the eye. In macroangiopathy, fat and blood clots build up in the large blood vessels, stick to the vessel walls, and block the flow of blood. Macroangiopathy in the heart is coronary artery disease; in the brain, it is cerebrovascular disease. Peripheral vascular disease is macroangiopathy that affects, for example, vessels in the legs.

angioplasty   A procedure in which a balloon-tipped catheter is used to enlarge a narrowing in a coronary artery. Also known as percutaneous transluminal coronary angioplasty (PTCA).

angiosarcoma   A form of tissue cancer (sarcoma) that arises in the lining of blood vessels in the skin, breast, liver, spleen, bone, lung, and heart. Angiosarcomas tend to be aggressive, recur locally, and spread widely. Predisposing factors include lymphedema (as from a radical mastectomy), radiotherapy, foreign materials (such as steel and plastic) in the body, and environmental agents (such as arsenic solutions used to spray grapevines and vinyl chloride in the plastic industry).

angiostatin   A fragment of a protein, plasminogen, that is involved in blood clotting. Angiostatin is normally secreted by tumors, and it appears to halt the process of developing new blood vessels, which is necessary to tumor development. Angiostatin may represent the prototype for a new class of cancer-treatment agents.

angiotensin   A family of peptides that constrict blood vessels. Narrowing the diameter of the blood vessels causes blood pressure to rise.

angiotensin converting enzyme   See *ACE.*

angle-closure glaucoma   Increased pressure in the anterior (front) chamber of the eye due to blockage of the normal circulation of fluid within the eye. The blockage occurs at the angle of the anterior chamber, which is formed by the junction of the cornea and the iris. When the iris retracts and thickens (when the pupil of the eye is wide open), it blocks the drainage pathway for fluid in the eye. This causes the pressure in the eye to soar, which can damage the optic nerve and lead to blindness. The elevated pressure should ideally be detected before the appearance of other symptoms of angle-closure glaucoma, so the pressure is routinely checked during eye exams. Symptoms of acute angle-closure glaucoma include severe eye and facial pain, nausea and vomiting, blurred vision, and a halo effect around lights. Acute angle-closure glaucoma is an emergency because optic nerve damage and vision loss can occur within hours of its onset. Angle-closure glaucoma tends to affect people born with a narrow angle between the cornea and iris. See also *glaucoma.*

anhidrosis   Lack of sweating. Anhidrosis creates a dangerous inability to tolerate heat.

anisocoria   A condition in which the left and right pupils of the eyes are not of equal size. Although pupils may appear to open (dilate) and close (constrict), the iris is really the prime mover: The pupil is merely the absence of iris. The size of the pupil determines how much light is let into the eye. With anisocoria, the larger pupil lets more light enter the eye. There are many causes of anisocoria, including eye injury or infection and swelling within the brain.

ankle   A complex structure made up of two joints: the true ankle joint and the subtalar joint. The ankle's movement is constrained and controlled by ligaments, including the anterior tibiofibular ligament, which connects the tibia to the fibula; the lateral collateral ligaments, which attach the fibula to the calcaneus to give the outside of the ankle stability; and the deltoid ligaments on the inside of the ankle, which connect the tibia to the talus and calcaneus to provide medial stability to the ankle. The ankle is commonly taken to be the ankle joint proper plus the surrounding region, including the lower end of the leg and the tarsus, the start of the flat of the foot. See also *ankle joint.*

ankle-foot orthosis   A brace, usually made of plastic, that is worn on the lower leg and foot to support the ankle, hold the foot and ankle in the correct position, and correct foot drop. Abbreviated AFO. Also known as foot drop brace.

ankle joint   A joint that is composed of three bones: the tibia, the fibula, and the talus. The ankle joint is responsible for the up-and-down motion of the foot. The subtalar joint is under the ankle joint, and it consists of the talus on top and calcaneus on the bottom. The subtalar joint is responsible for the side-to-side motion of the foot.

ankle pain   Pain in the ankle joint. The ankle is a hinged joint, so there are many potential causes for ankle pain. Ankle sprains resulting from accident or misuse range in severity from mild, resolving within 24 hours to those requiring surgical repair. Tendonitis of the ankle is inflammation of one or more tendons in the ankle, and it may be caused by trauma or certain forms of arthritis.

ankyloglossia   A minor birth defect in which the flap of membrane attached to the underside of the tongue (frenum) is too short. This shortened frenum limits the mobility of the tongue. Ankyloglossia is also called tongue tie, from the folk belief that the anomaly causes feeding and speech problems. A child cannot feed or speak

properly because the tongue is "tied." This antiquated belief is untrue.

ankylosing spondylitis   A form of chronic inflammation of the spine and the sacroiliac joints. The sacroiliac joints are located in the low back, where the sacrum (the bone directly above the tailbone) meets the iliac bones (the bones on either side of the upper buttocks). Chronic inflammation in these areas causes pain and stiffness in and around the spine. Over time, chronic spinal inflammation (spondylitis) can lead to a complete cementing together (fusion) of the vertebrae, a process called ankylosis. Ankylosing spondylitis can sometimes be seen in patients with psoriasis and inflammatory bowel disease (colitis).

ankyrin deficiency   A genetic disorder of the red blood cell membrane. Ankyrin deficiency is the cause of hereditary spherocytosis. See also *spherocytosis, hereditary.*

ANLL   Acute nonlymphocytic leukemia.

annexin   One of a family of proteins that bind calcium and phospholipids.

annexin V   A substance that normally forms a shield around certain phospholipid molecules in the blood, blocking their entry into coagulation (clotting) reactions. Annexin V is thought to be a cause of antiphospholipid syndrome.

anomaly   Any deviation from normal, out of the ordinary. In medicine, an anomaly is usually something that is congenitally abnormal.

anomaly, congenital   A birth defect. A minor congenital anomaly is an unusual anatomic feature such as a short second toe that is of no serious medical or cosmetic consequence. By contrast, a major congenital anomaly is a defect such as a cleft palate that is of serious medical or cosmetic consequence.

anorexia   A decreased appetite or an aversion to food, resulting in disturbed eating habits and weight loss. Anorexia may be caused by some medications and medical conditions, particularly in elderly or hospitalized patients. See also *anorexia nervosa.*

anorexia nervosa   An eating disorder characterized by extreme attempts to control the diet and/or an aversion to food. It affects young women most often, but it may also be seen in men, children, and older adults. Symptoms can include extreme weight loss, weakness, and dulling of hair and skin. In some cases, anorexia nervosa may be a form of obsessive-compulsive disorder. Treatment includes medication, therapy, dietary counseling and, in extreme cases, hospitalization. Untreated anorexia can cause organ failure and death. See also *body dysmorphic disorder; bulimia nervosa; obsessive-compulsive disorder.*

anosmia   The failure of the development of or the loss of the sense of smell.

anotia   The absence from birth of the external, visible part of the ear (the auricle).

anoxia   A deficiency of oxygen.

ant, fire   See *fire ant.*

ant sting   See *fire ant.*

ant, velvet   See *velvet ant.*

antagonist   A substance that acts against and blocks an action. Antagonist is the opposite of agonist. Antagonists and agonists are key players in the chemistry of the human body and in pharmacology.

antenatal diagnosis   See *prenatal diagnosis.*

anterior   The front. For example, the breastbone is part of the anterior surface of the chest. Opposite of posterior. See also Appendix B, "Anatomic Orientation Terms."

anterior cruciate ligament   A ligament in the knee that crosses from the underside of the femur to the top of the tibia. Abbreviated ACL. Injuries to the ACL can occur in a number of situations, including sports, and can be quite serious, sometimes requiring surgery. See also *knee.*

anterior pituitary   See *pituitary, anterior.*

anteroposterior   From front to back. Abbreviated AP. When a chest X-ray is taken with the patient's back against the film plate and the X-ray machine in front of the patient, it is referred to as an AP view. The opposite of AP is posteroanterior (PA). See also Appendix B, "Anatomic Orientation Terms."

anthracosis   See *black lung disease.*

anthrax   A highly infectious disease that normally affects animals, especially ruminants (such as cattle, sheep, and horses), but that can be transmitted to humans by contact with infected animals or their products or by biologic warfare. The agent of anthrax is the bacterium Bacillus anthracis. Its spores can resist destruction and remain viable for years. Anthrax is treated with antibiotics such as penicillin, tetracycline, erythromycin, and ciprofloxin (brand name: Cipro). Three forms of disease are caused by anthrax: cutaneous anthrax, inhalation anthrax, and gastrointestinal anthrax. See also *anthrax, cutaneous; anthrax, gastrointestinal; anthrax, inhalation.*

anthrax, cutaneous   Anthrax infection of the skin. The most common form of anthrax, cutaneous anthrax starts as a red-brown raised spot that enlarges and has redness, blistering, and hardening in the area of the spot. The center of the spot then shows an ulcer crater with blood-tinged drainage and the formation of a black crust (an eschar). The glands in the area become swollen (enlarged lymph nodes), and the patient may have muscle aching and pain, headache, fever, nausea, and vomiting.

anthrax, gastrointestinal   Anthrax infection of the gastrointestinal tract, now very rare but deadly. Gastrointestinal anthrax is caused by eating contaminated meat.

anthrax immunization   A series of six injections over a 6-month period, followed by annual booster shots, given to military personnel and others (including veterinarians who work with large animals) who are at high risk of anthrax exposure.

anthrax, inhalation   Anthrax infection of the lungs, also known as pulmonary anthrax, that is due to the inhalation of anthrax spores. The inhaled spores multiply rapidly in the lymph nodes in the chest. A person infected with inhalation anthrax experiences local bleeding and tissue death (necrosis) in these lymph nodes, and the disease spreads to the adjacent lung tissue. The first symptoms are subtle, gradual, and somewhat flu-like, including rising fever. In a few days, severe respiratory distress occurs, followed by shock and coma. Prompt recognition and treatment are paramount. Even with treatment, the patient may die. Once called woolsorters' disease.

anthrax toxin   The toxic substance secreted by the bacterium *Bacillus anthracis,* the cause of the disease anthrax.

anti-angiogenesis drug   A drug, such as angiostatin or endostatin, that halts the development of new blood vessels (angiogenesis).

antibiotic   A substance produced by one microorganism that selectively inhibits the growth of another. Synthetic antibiotics, usually chemically related to naturally occurring antibiotics, are made to accomplish comparable tasks. Antibiotics are used to treat bacterial infections. See also *cephalosporin antibiotics; penicillin.*

antibiotic resistance   The ability of bacteria and other microorganisms to resist the effects of an antibiotic to which they were once sensitive. Antibiotic resistance is a major concern of overuse of antibiotics. Also known as drug resistance.

antibody A specialized immune protein (an immunoglobulin) produced because of the introduction of an antigen into the body. An antibody possesses the remarkable ability to combine with the antigen that triggered its production. The production of antibodies is a major function of the immune system and is carried out by a type of white blood cell called a B cell, or a B lymphocyte. Antibodies can be triggered by, and directed toward, foreign proteins, microorganisms, or toxins. Some antibodies are autoantibodies and are actually directed against a patient's own tissues. See also *immune system*.

antibody, antinuclear See *antinuclear antibody*.

anticholinergic Related to opposing the actions of the neurotransmitter acetylcholine. Anticholinergic drugs inhibit the transmission of parasympathetic nerve impulses, thereby reducing spasms of smooth muscles (for example, muscles in the bladder).

anticholinergic side effect A symptom in the set of side effects from anticholinergic medications that include dry mouth and related dental problems, blurred vision, tendency toward overheating (hyperpyrexia), and in some cases, dementia-like symptoms.

anticipation The progressively earlier appearance and increased severity of a disease from generation to generation. The phenomenon of anticipation was once thought to be an artifact, but a biological basis for it has been discovered in a number of genetic disorders, such as myotonic dystrophy and Huntington disease.

anticoagulant An agent that is used to prevent the formation of blood clots. Anticoagulants have various uses. Some are used for the prevention or treatment of disorders characterized by abnormal blood clots and emboli. Anticoagulant drugs include intravenous heparin, which acts by inactivating thrombin and several other clotting factors that are required for a clot to form, and oral anticoagulants such as warfarin and dicumarol, which act by inhibiting the liver's production of vitamin K–dependent factors that are crucial to clotting. Anticoagulant solutions are also used for the preservation of stored whole blood and blood fractions and to keep laboratory blood specimens from clotting.

antidepressant A medication that prevents or reduces the symptoms of clinical depression. Some antidepressants may also be prescribed for their other medical effects, including increasing blood flow within the brain and treating chronic pain. See also *MAO inhibitor; SSRI; tricyclic antidepressant*.

antidiuretic hormone A peptide hormone made in the hypothalamus and released at the base of the brain by the nearby pituitary gland. Abbreviated ADH. ADH prevents the production of dilute urine and is therefore an antidiuretic. It can also stimulate contraction of arteries and capillaries, and it may have effects on mental function. Also known as vasopressin. See also *ADH secretion, inappropriate; pituitary, posterior*.

antiDNAse B A blood test for antibodies to the streptococcus B bacteria.

antidote A drug that counteracts a poison.

antifungal A medication that limits or prevents the growth of yeasts and other fungal organisms.

antigen A substance that the immune system perceives as being foreign or dangerous. The body combats an antigen with the production of an antibody.

antigen, prostate specific See *prostate specific antigen test*.

antihistamine A drug that opposes the action of histamine released during an allergic reaction by blocking the action of the histamine on the tissue. Antihistamines do not stop the formation of histamine; rather, they protect tissues from some of its effects. Antihistamines frequently cause dry mouth and sleepiness. Some antihistamines are nonsedating. Antihistamine side effects that may occur include urine retention in males and increased heart rate.

antihypertensive A medication or another substance that reduces high blood pressure (hypertension).

anti-infective An agent that is capable of acting against infection, either by inhibiting the spread of an infectious agent or by killing the infectious agent outright.

antinuclear antibody An unusual antibody that is directed against the structures within the nucleus of a cell. Abbreviated ANA. ANAs are found in patients whose immune systems attack their own body tissues (autoimmunity), such as patients with systemic lupus erythematosus, rheumatoid arthritis, juvenile diabetes mellitus, and pulmonary fibrosis. ANAs can also be found in patients with chronic infections and cancer, and many medications—including procainamide (brand name: Procan SR), hydralazine, and phenytoin (brand name: Dilantin)—can stimulate their production. See also *ANA; autoimmune disorder*.

antioxidant A substance that reduces damage due to oxygen (damage), such as that caused by free radicals. Well-known antioxidants include a number of enzymes and other substances, such as vitamin C, vitamin E, and beta carotene, that are capable of counteracting the damaging effects of oxidation. Antioxidants are also commonly added to food products such as vegetable oils and prepared foods to prevent or delay their deterioration from the action of air. Antioxidants may possibly reduce the risks of cancer. Antioxidants clearly slow the progression of age-related macular degeneration.

antiphospholipid syndrome An immune disorder characterized by the presence of abnormal antibodies in the blood. Abbreviated APS. APS is associated with abnormal blood clotting, migraine headaches, recurrent pregnancy loss, and low blood platelet counts (thrombocytopenia). The abnormal antibodies are directed against phospholipids (fats that contain phosphorous). APS can occur by itself (primary APS) or be caused by an underlying condition (secondary APS), such as systemic lupus erythematosus. About one-third of persons with primary APS have heart-valve abnormalities. Antiphospholipid antibodies reduce the levels of annexin V, and this reduction is thought to be a possible mechanism underlying the increased tendency of blood to clot and the propensity to pregnancy loss in APS. Examples of antiphospholipid antibodies are cardiolipin antibody and lupus anticoagulant. See also *annexin V.*

antiplatelet agent A medication that reduces the tendency of platelets in the blood to clump and clot. Aspirin is an antiplatelet agent.

antiseptic Discouraging the growth of microorganisms. Commonly refers to antiseptic preparations used during medical procedures or used to maintain sanitary conditions in nursing homes, barbershops, tattoo parlors, and other facilities where unchecked microorganism growth could result in disease. See also *aseptic.*

antispasmodic A medication that relieves, prevents, or lowers the incidence of muscle spasms, especially those of smooth muscle.

antitoxin **1** An antibody that is naturally produced to counteract a toxin, such as a toxin from a bacterial infection or snake bite. **2** An antibody from the serum of an animal stimulated with specific antibodies that is administered to humans or other animals to provide passive immunity to a disease. Such antitoxins are of short-term value only and are used for treatment rather than prevention.

antiviral agent A medication or another agent that kills viruses or inhibits their capability to reproduce.

antro-duodenal motility study A study designed to detect and record the contractions of the muscles of the stomach and duodenum in order to diagnose motility disorders of the stomach and small intestine. A tube is

passed through the nose, throat, esophagus, and stomach, until the tip lies in the small intestine. The tube senses when the muscles of the stomach and small intestine contract and squeeze it. The contractions are recorded by a computer and analyzed.

antrum A general term for a nearly closed cavity or chamber. For example, the antrum of the stomach (gastric antrum) is a portion before the outlet, which is lined by mucosa and does not produce acid. The paranasal sinuses can be referred to as the frontal antrum, ethmoid antrum, and maxillary antrum.

anus The opening of the rectum to the outside of the body.

anus, imperforate A birth defect in which the rectum is a blind alley and there is no anus. Imperforate anus occurs in about 1 in 5,000 births, and it can be corrected by surgery.

anxiety A feeling of apprehension and fear, characterized by physical symptoms such as palpitations, sweating, and feelings of stress.

anxiety disorder A chronic condition characterized by an excessive and persistent sense of apprehension, with physical symptoms such as sweating, palpitations, and feelings of stress. Treatments include the comfort offered by understanding the condition, avoiding or desensitizing the exacerbating situations, and medications.

aorta The largest artery in the body, the major conduit from the heart to the body. The aorta arises from the left ventricle of the heart, ascends a little, arches, and then descends through the chest and the abdomen, ending by dividing into two arteries, the common iliac arteries, which go to the legs. Anatomically, the aorta is traditionally divided into the ascending aorta, the aortic arch, and the descending aorta. The descending aorta is, in turn, subdivided into the thoracic aorta, which goes from the heart to above the diaphragm, and the abdominal aorta, which is below the diaphragm. The aorta has branches to the head and neck, the arms, the major organs in the chest and abdomen, and the legs. It supplies them all with oxygenated blood. See also *abdominal aorta; ascending aorta; descending aorta; thoracic aorta.*

aorta, coarctation of the A constriction of the aorta. At the point of coarctation, the sides of the aorta appear to be pressed together. Blood pressure is increased above the constriction, and the flow of blood is impeded below the level of the constriction. Symptoms may not be evident at birth but can develop as soon as the first week after birth, with congestive heart failure or high blood pressure that call for early surgery. The outlook after surgery is usually favorable. Some cases of coarctation of the aorta have been treated with balloon angioplasty.

aortic aneurysm See *aneurysm, aortic.*

aortic arch The second section of the aorta. As it continues from the heart, it gives off the brachiocephalic trunk, and the left common carotid and subclavian arteries. The brachiocephalic trunk splits to form the right subclavian and the right common carotid arteries, which supply blood to the right arm and the right side of the neck and head. The left common carotid artery and left subclavian artery, the second and third branches off the aortic arch, perform parallel functions on the left side.

aortic insufficiency Sloshing of blood back down from the aorta into the left ventricle due to incompetence of the aortic valve. Also known as aortic regurgitation.

aortic regurgitation See *aortic insufficiency.*

aortic stenosis Narrowing (stenosis) of the aortic valve, the valve between the left ventricle of the heart and the aorta. This narrowing impedes the delivery of blood to the body through the aorta and makes the heart work harder. A normal aortic valve has three flaps (cusps), but a stenotic valve may have only one cusp (unicuspid) or two cusps (bicuspid), which are thick, stiff, and stenotic. Some children with aortic stenosis have chest pain, unusual fatigue, dizziness, or fainting. Many have few or no symptoms. The need for surgery depends on the degree of stenosis. Although surgery may enlarge the stenotic valve, the valve remains deformed and eventually may need to be replaced with an artificial one. A procedure called balloon valvuloplasty has been used in some cases of aortic stenosis. Persons with aortic stenosis need medical follow-up all their lives because even mild stenosis may worsen over time.

aortic valve One of the four valves in the heart. The aortic valve is positioned at the beginning of the aorta. It permits blood from the left ventricle to flow into the aorta, and it prevents blood in the aorta from returning to the heart. See also *heart valves.*

aortic valve, bicuspid An abnormal aortic valve with only two cusps. See also *aortic stenosis.*

AP **1** Angina pectoris. **2** Arterial pressure. **3** In endocrinology, anterior pituitary gland. **4** In anatomy, anteroposterior.

Apert syndrome The best-known type of acrocephalosyndactyly, a group of disorders characterized by malformations of the skull, face, hands, and feet. Apert syndrome is inherited as an autosomal dominant trait and is due to a mutation in the fibroblast growth factor receptor 2 (FGFR2) gene on chromosome 10. Different mutations in FGFR2 are responsible for two other genetic diseases, Pfeiffer syndrome and Crouzon syndrome. See also *acrocephalosyndactyly; fibroblast growth factor receptor 2.*

apex The Latin word for summit, the apex is the tip of a pyramidal or rounded structure, such as the lung or the heart. The apex of the lung is indeed its tip—its rounded most superior portion. The apex of the heart is likewise its tip, but it is formed by the left ventricle, so it is essentially the most inferior portion of the heart.

Apgar score An objective score of the condition of a baby after birth. This score is determined by scoring the heart rate, respiratory effort, muscle tone, skin color, and response to a catheter in the nostril. Each of these objective signs receives 0, 1, or 2 points. An Apgar score of 10 means an infant is in the best possible condition. The Apgar score is done routinely 60 seconds after the birth of the infant. A child with a score of 0 to 3 needs immediate resuscitation. The Apgar score is often repeated 5 minutes after birth, and in the event of a difficult resuscitation, the Apgar score may be done again at 10, 15, and 20 minutes. An Apgar score of 0 to 3 at 20 minutes of age is predictive of high morbidity (disease) and mortality. The test is named for its inventor, American anesthesiologist Virginia Apgar.

aphagia Inability to eat.

aphasia Literally, no speech. Aphasia may also be used to describe defects in spoken expression or comprehension of speech.

apheresis The process of removing a specific component from blood that is temporarily removed from the body. Also known as hemapheresis and pheresis. The forms of apheresis include plasmapheresis, harvesting plasma or liquid part of the blood; leukapheresis, harvesting leukocytes or white blood cells; ranulocytapheresis, harvesting granulocytes; lymphocytapheresis, harvesting lymphocytes; lymphoplasmapheresis, harvesting lymphocytes and plasma; and plateletpheresis, harvesting platelets.

aphonia Inability to speak.

apical The adjective for apex, the tip of a pyramidal or rounded structure, such as the lung or the heart. For example, an apical lung tumor is a tumor located at the top of the lung.

aplasia　Failure to develop. See also *atrophy*.

aplasia of the breast　See *amastia*.

aplastic anemia　See *anemia, aplastic*.

apnea　The absence of breathing (respiration).

apnea, sleep　See *sleep apnea*.

apophysitis calcaneus　Inflammation of the growth plate of the calcaneus, the bone at the back of the heel, where the Achilles tendon attaches. Apophysitis calcaneus occurs mainly in older children and adolescents, especially active boys. It can be very painful, although it may be dismissed as "growing pains." Treatment includes activity limitation, medication, shoe inserts, heel lifts, and sometimes casting if it becomes especially severe. Fortunately, it usually disappears as the child gets older. Also known as Sever condition. See also *Achilles tendon*.

apoptosis　A form of cell death in which a programmed sequence of events leads to the elimination of cells without releasing harmful substances into the surrounding area. Apoptosis plays a crucial role in developing and maintaining the health of the body by eliminating old cells, unnecessary cells, and unhealthy cells. The human body replaces perhaps one million cells per second. Too little or too much apoptosis can play a role in many diseases. When apoptosis does not work correctly, cells that should be eliminated may persist and become immortal. For example, in cancer and leukemia. When apoptosis works overly well, it kills too many cells and inflicts grave tissue damage. This is the case in strokes and neurodegenerative disorders such as Alzheimer's, Huntington's, and Parkinson's diseases. Also known as programmed cell death and cell suicide. Strictly speaking, the term *apoptosis* refers only to the structural changes affecting cells, and programmed cell death refers to the complete underlying process, but the terms are often used interchangeably.

appendectomy　Surgical removal of the appendix. An appendectomy is performed because of probable appendicitis.

appendicitis　Inflammation of the appendix, usually associated with infection of the appendix. Appendicitis often causes fever, loss of appetite, and pain. Appendicitis may be suspected because of the medical history and physical examination. The pain of appendicitis is at first not confined to one spot, but as the inflammation extends through the appendix to its outer covering and then to the lining of the abdomen, the pain changes and becomes localized to one small area between the front of the right hip bone and the belly button. If the appendix ruptures and infection spreads throughout the abdomen, the pain becomes diffuse again as the entire lining of the abdomen becomes inflamed. Ultrasonography and computerized tomography may be helpful in diagnosis. Due to the varying size and location of the appendix, and the proximity of other organs to the appendix, it may be difficult to differentiate appendicitis from other intra-abdominal diseases.

appendix　A small outpouching from the beginning of the large intestine.

appendix epididymis　A small cystic projection from the surface of the epididymis (a structure within the scrotum that is attached to the backside of the testis), which represents a remnant of the embryologic mesonephros.

appendix epiploica　A finger-like projection of fat attached to the colon.

appendix testis　A small solid projection of tissue on the outer surface of the testis, which is a remnant of the embryologic mullerian duct.

apposition　**1** The act of adding or accretion. Growth by apposition is characteristic of many tissues in the body by which nutritive matter from the blood is transformed on the surface of an organ into a solid unorganized substance. **2** The act of putting things in juxtaposition or side by side. To lose a pair of apposed teeth is to lose teeth that are next to each other. Also known as juxtaposition.

apraxia　The inability to execute a voluntary motor movement despite being able to demonstrate normal muscle function. Apraxia is not related to a lack of understanding or to any kind of physical paralysis; rather, it is caused by a problem in the cortex of the brain.

apraxia of speech　A severe speech disorder characterized by an inability to speak or a severe struggle to speak clearly. Apraxia of speech occurs when the oral-motor muscles do not or cannot obey commands from the brain or when the brain cannot reliably send those commands. Apraxia of speech is believed to be caused by a difference in or damage to the Broca area in the brain, possibly with inheritable, genetic underpinnings. Children with apraxia can be helped significantly with intensive speech therapy. See also *dyspraxia of speech*.

APS　Antiphospholipid syndrome.

apthous ulcer　See *canker sore*.

aqueduct　A channel for the passage of fluid.

aqueduct of Sylvius　A canal between the third and fourth ventricles in the brain within the system of four communicating cavities that are continuous with the central canal of the spinal cord. The ventricles are filled with cerebrospinal fluid, which is carried by the aqueduct of Sylvius.

aqueduct of the midbrain   See *aqueduct of Sylvius.*

arachnodactyly   A condition in which a person has long, spider-like fingers and toes. Arachnodactyly is a frequent finding in those with Marfan syndrome.

arachnophobia   An abnormal and persistent fear of spiders. Sufferers from arachnophobia experience undue anxiety, even though they realize that the risk of encountering a spider and being harmed by it is small or nonexistent. They may avoid going barefoot and may be especially alert when taking showers or getting into and out of bed. From the Greek *arachne,* meaning "spider," and *phobos,* meaning "fear." In Greek mythology, Arachne was a maiden, a skilled weaver, who challenged Athena to a weaving contest and was turned into a spider for her impertinence.

arbitration agreement   An arrangement in which the patient waives the right to sue the physician and, instead, agrees to submit any dispute to arbitration. Arbitration agreements are legal and binding. The arguments in their favor are that, for patients, the case can be settled faster, and more money can go to the patient (rather than to a lawyer). Physicians can often get a discount on their malpractice insurance if the majority of their patients sign such agreements.

arbovirus   A type of virus transmitted to humans by mosquitoes and ticks. The name *arbovirus* comes from the first words *arthropod* and *borne.* Arbovirus can cause inflammation of the brain (encephalitis). The types of arboviral encephalitis that occur in the US include LaCrosse, eastern equine, western equine, and St. Louis encephalitis, all of which are transmitted by mosquitoes. Another arbovirus, Powassan, transmitted by ticks, is a cause of encephalitis in the northern US. Many other types of arboviral encephalitis occur throughout the world. Most are problems only for travelers to countries where the viruses are endemic. One, the West Nile virus, has made a major entry into the US. It causes West Nile encephalitis, also known as West Nile fever. See also *hemorrhagic fever with renal syndrome.*

ARC   AIDS-related complex.

arch, aortic   See *aortic arch.*

archaea   A unique group of microorganisms that are called bacteria (Archaeobacteria) but are genetically and metabolically different from all other known bacteria. They appear to be living fossils, the survivors of an ancient group

of organisms that bridged the gap in evolution between bacteria and multicellular organisms (eukaryotes).

arcus senilis   A cloudy opaque arc or circle around the edge of the eye, often seen in the eyes of the elderly.

ARDS   Acute respiratory distress syndrome.

areola   **1** The small, darkened area around the nipple of the breast.   **2** The colored part of the iris around the pupil of the eye.   **3** Any small space in a tissue.

arginine   An essential amino acid and a key component of protein that causes the release of human growth hormone. Lack of arginine in the diet impairs growth, and in adult males it decreases the sperm count. Arginine is available in turkey, chicken, and other meats, and as L-arginine in supplements. Babies born without the enzyme phosphate synthetase have arginine deficiency syndrome; adding arginine to their diets permits normal growth and development.

argyria   Silver poisoning, resulting in ashen, gray, discolored skin, and damage to other tissues of the body. Caused by long-term use of silver salts or other preparations containing silver.

arm   In popular usage, the appendage that extends from the shoulder to the hand. However, the medical definition refers to the upper extremity extending from the shoulder only to the elbow, excluding the forearm, which extends from the elbow to the wrist. The arm contains one bone: the humerus.

arm, wrist, and hand bones   See *bones of the arm, wrist, and hand.*

armed tapeworm   See *Taenia solium.*

aromatherapy   A form of alternative medicine in which essential oils or other scents are inhaled to achieve therapeutic benefit. The mechanism of action in aromatherapy is unknown, but recent studies have shown that aromatherapy may be beneficial for some health problems.

arrector pili   A microscopic band of muscle tissue that connects a hair follicle to the dermis. When stimulated, the arrector pili contracts and causes the hair to become more perpendicular to the skin surface, thereby erecting the hair (causing the hair to stand on end). The arrector pili muscle plays a key role in forming goose bumps. See also *goose bumps.*

arrhythmia   An abnormal heart rhythm. With an arrhythmia, the heartbeats may be irregular or too slow (bradycardia), too rapid (tachycardia), or too early. When a single heartbeat occurs earlier than normal, it is called a premature contraction. See also *bradycardia; tachycardia.*

arrhythmia, atrial   An abnormal heart rhythm due to electrical disturbances in the upper chambers of the heart (atria) or the atrioventricular (AV) node "relay station," leading to fast heart beats. Examples of atrial arrhythmias include atrial fibrillation, atrial flutter, and paroxysmal atrial tachycardia.

arrhythmia, ventricular   An abnormally rapid heart rhythm that originates in the lower chambers of the heart (ventricles). Ventricular arrhythmias include ventricular tachycardia and ventricular fibrillation. Both are life-threatening arrhythmias, and they are most commonly associated with heart attacks or scarring of the heart muscle from previous heart attacks.

arterial anastomosis   A joining of two arteries. See also *anastomosis.*

arterial aneurysm   See *aneurysm, arterial.*

arterial blood gas   See *ABG.*

arterial pressure   The pressure of the blood within an artery. Also known as arterial tension and intra-arterial pressure.

arterial tension   See *arterial pressure.*

arteriogram   An X-ray in which an injection of dye shows blood vessels.

arteriole   A small branch of an artery that leads to a capillary. The oxygenated hemoglobin (oxyhemoglobin) makes the blood in arterioles (and arteries) look bright red.

arteriosclerosis   Hardening and thickening of the walls of the arteries. Arteriosclerosis leads to heart attacks and strokes, as well as to peripheral vascular disease. Arteriosclerosis can be categorized as atherosclerosis, medial calcification, hypertensive, or arteriolar sclerosis. See also *atherosclerosis; heart attack; stroke; peripheral vascular disease.*

arteriosclerotic aneurysm   See *aneurysm, arteriosclerotic.*

arteriovenous malformation   See *malformation, arteriovenous.*

arteritis, cranial   A serious disease characterized by inflammation of the walls of arteries. Symptoms include headache, pain in the jaw when repetitively chewing, and tenderness of the scalp, usually over the inflamed arteries

of the sides of the head (temporal area). Less specific symptoms include fatigue, low-grade fever, and weight loss. The muscle aching of polymyalgia rheumatica is seen in one-fourth of patients with cranial arteritis. When the arteries affected by cranial arteritis become inflamed, they can narrow to the degree that the blood flow through them is limited. This can cause serious deficiency of oxygen supply to the tissues that are normally supplied by these arteries. Deficient oxygenation of the eyes or brain can lead to impaired or double vision, blindness, or stroke. Less commonly, inflammation of the blood vessels supplying the arms can lead to arm pain when the arms are used. Patients with cranial arteritis are usually over 50 years of age. The disease is detected by a biopsy of an artery. It is treated with high dose cortisone-related medications. Also known as temporal arteritis and giant cell arteritis. See also *polymyalgia rheumatica.*

arteritis, giant cell   See *arteritis, cranial.*

arteritis, temporal   See *arteritis, cranial.*

artery   A blood vessel that carries blood, rich in oxygen, away from the heart to the body. The oxygenated hemoglobin (oxyhemoglobin) in arterial blood makes it look bright red. Arteries are part of the efferent wing of the circulatory system. See also *carotid artery; ophthalmic artery; radial artery; splenic artery; vertebral artery.*

artery, coronary   See *coronary artery.*

artery spasm, coronary   See *coronary artery spasm.*

arthralgia   Pain in a joint.

arthritis   Inflammation of a joint. When joints are inflamed, they can develop stiffness, warmth, swelling, redness, and pain. There are more than 100 types of arthritis. See also *ankylosing spondylitis; arthritis, degenerative; arthritis, gouty; arthritis, Lyme; psoriatic arthritis; arthritis, Reiter; arthritis, rheumatoid; arthritis, spondylitis; gout; lupus; pseudogout.*

arthritis, degenerative   A type of arthritis caused by inflammation, breakdown, and eventual loss of the cartilage of the joints. Degenerative arthritis is the most common form of arthritis, usually affecting the hands, feet, spine, and large weight-bearing joints, such as the hips and knees. Also known as osteoarthritis and degenerative joint disease.

arthritis, gouty   See *gouty arthritis.*

arthritis in children   Arthritis in children, usually in the form of juvenile/pediatric arthritis or rheumatoid arthritis. See also arthritis, systemic-onset juvenile rheumatoid.

arthritis, Lyme Joint inflammation associated with Lyme disease, a bacterial disease spread by ticks. See also *Lyme disease.*

arthritis, psoriatic See *psoriatic arthritis.*

arthritis, Reiter The combination of inflammation of the joints (arthritis), eyes (conjunctivitis), and the genitourinary and/or gastrointestinal systems. See also *Reiter syndrome.*

arthritis, rheumatoid An autoimmune disease characterized by chronic inflammation of the joints that can also involve inflammation of tissues in other areas of the body, such as the lungs, heart, and eyes. Because it can affect multiple organs of the body, rheumatoid arthritis is referred to as a systemic illness. Although rheumatoid arthritis is a chronic illness, patients may experience long periods without symptoms. Also known as rheumatoid disease.

arthritis, septic Joint inflammation caused by infection from sepsis (blood poisoning) or from infection within the affected joint itself, or as a side effect of infection in other body tissues. Treatment includes antibiotic medications and surgical drainage. Also known as pyarthosis and suppurative arthritis.

arthritis, spondylitis A form of arthritis that causes chronic inflammation of the spine.

arthritis, systemic-onset chronic rheumatoid See *arthritis, systemic-onset juvenile rheumatoid.*

arthritis, systemic-onset juvenile rheumatoid A form of joint disease in children whose systemic signs and symptoms include high intermittent fever, a salmon-colored skin rash, swollen lymph glands, enlargement of the liver and spleen, inflammation of the lungs (pleuritis), and inflammation around the heart (pericarditis). The arthritis itself may not be immediately apparent, but in time it surfaces and may persist after the systemic symptoms are long gone. Also known as systemic-onset chronic arthritis or Still's disease.

arthrocentesis A procedure in which a sterile needle and syringe are used to drain fluid from the joint. This is usually done as an office procedure or at the bedside in the hospital. For certain conditions, medication is put into the joint after fluid removal. The needle is then removed, and a bandage or dressing is applied over the entry point. Joint fluid is typically sent for examination to the lab to determine the cause of the joint swelling, such as infection, gout, or rheumatoid disease. Arthrocentesis can be helpful in relieving joint swelling and pain. Also known as joint aspiration.

arthrogryposis Joint contractures that develop before birth and are evident at birth. With arthrogryposis there is a lack of the normal range of motion in one or more joints. In normal embryonic development, joints can be seen moving by 8 weeks of gestation. This motion of joints is essential to the proper development of the joints and structures around them. Limitation of joint motion before birth leads to joint contractures and arthrogryposis. Prenatal limitation of joint mobility can result from neurologic deficits, muscle defects, connective tissue defects, and fetal crowding (in which there is not enough room for the fetus to move around freely in the womb).

arthrogryposis multiplex congenital A disorder that develops before birth that is characterized by reduced mobility of multiple joints. The range of motion of the joints in the arms and legs is usually limited or fixed. Joints affected may include the shoulders, elbows, wrists, fingers, hips, knees, ankles, and feet. The impairment of joint mobility is often accompanied by overgrowth of fibrous tissue in the joints (fibrous ankylosis). Once thought to be a single disease, arthrogryposis multiplex congenital is now known to be many. The mechanisms responsible for the disease are presumed to be the same as for all arthrogryposis, regardless of the number of joints involved.

arthroscopic Related to arthroscopy.

arthroscopy A surgical technique in which a tube-like instrument is inserted into a joint to inspect, diagnose, and repair tissues. It is most commonly performed in patients with diseases of the knees or shoulders.

arthrosis See *joint.*

articulation **1** In medicine, the joint where bones come together. See also *joint.* **2** In dentistry, the occlusal surfaces of the teeth, where the teeth come together. **3** In speech, the production of intelligible words and sentences by joining together the lips, tongue, palate, and other structures.

articulation disorder A speech disorder involving difficulties in articulating specific types of sounds. Articulation disorders often involve substitution of one sound for another, slurring of speech, or indistinct speech. Treatment is speech therapy.

artificial heart A human-made heart. An artificial heart is a mechanical pump that is used to replace a damaged heart temporarily or permanently.

artificial insemination A procedure in which a fine catheter (tube) is inserted through the cervix into the uterus to directly deposit a sperm sample. The purpose of this relatively simple procedure is to achieve fertilization and pregnancy. Also known as intrauterine insemination (IUI).

artificial insemination by donor A procedure in which a fine catheter (tube) is inserted through the cervix into the uterus to directly deposit a sperm sample from a donor other than the woman's mate. The purpose of this procedure is to achieve fertilization and pregnancy. Abbreviated AID. Also known as heterologous insemination.

artificial insemination by husband A procedure in which a fine catheter (tube) is inserted through the cervix into the uterus to deposit a sperm sample from the woman's mate directly into the uterus. The purpose of this procedure is to achieve fertilization and pregnancy. Abbreviated AIH. Also known as homologous insemination.

artificial pacemaker A device that uses electrical impulses to regulate the heart rhythm or reproduce it. An internal pacemaker is one in which the electrodes to the heart, the electronic circuitry, and the power supply are all implanted internally, within the body. Although there are different types of pacemakers, all are designed to treat a heart rate that is too slow (bradycardia). Pacemakers may function continuously and stimulate the heart at a fixed rate, or they may function at an increased rate during exercise. A pacemaker can also be programmed to detect an overly long pause between heartbeats and then stimulate the heart.

artificial pancreas A machine that constantly measures glucose (sugar) in the blood and, in response to an elevated level of glucose, releases an appropriate amount of insulin. In this respect, an artificial pancreas functions like a natural pancreas.

asbestos A natural material made up of tiny fibers that is used as thermal insulation. Inhalation of asbestos fibers can lead to asbestosis.

asbestosis Scarring of the lungs caused by inhalation of asbestos fibers. When asbestos fibers lodge in the lungs, they promote the development of cancer, such as mesothelioma of the pleura (the lining of the lung) and bronchogenic carcinoma (cancer of the lung). See also *mesothelioma*.

ascaris Intestinal roundworms. Infection with ascaris is referred to as ascariasis.

ascending aorta The first section of the aorta, which starts from the left ventricle of the heart and extends to the aortic arch. The right and left coronary arteries that supply blood to the heart muscle arise from the ascending aorta.

ascites An abnormal buildup of fluid within the abdomen. There are many causes of ascites, including cirrhosis of the liver, cancer within the abdomen, congestive heart failure, and tuberculosis.

ascorbic acid Vitamin C, an essential nutrient found mainly in fruits and vegetables. The body requires ascorbic acid in order to form and maintain bones, blood vessels, and skin. Ascorbic acid also promotes the healing of cuts, abrasions and wounds; helps fight infections; inhibits conversion of irritants in smog, tobacco smoke, and certain foods into cancer-causing substances; appears to lessen the risk of developing high blood pressure and heart disease; helps regulate cholesterol levels; prevents the development of scurvy; appears to lower the risk of developing cataracts; and aids in iron absorption. Ascorbic acid can cause adverse reactions when taken with some drugs.

ASD Atrial septal defect.

aseptic Free from infection, sterile. See also *antiseptic*.

aseptic necrosis See *avascular necrosis*.

ASO Antistreptolysin-O, a blood test that looks for antibodies to the streptococcus A bacteria. Also abbreviated ASLO.

aspartate aminotransferase An enzyme that is normally present in liver and heart cells that is released into the blood when the liver or heart is damaged. Abbreviated AST. The blood levels of AST are elevated when liver damage (for example, from viral hepatitis) or heart damage (for example, from a heart attack) occurs. Some medications can also raise AST levels. Also known as serum glutamic oxaloacetic transaminase (SGOT).

Asperger syndrome A disorder related to autism that is characterized by obsessive interests and behavior, but without speech delay or mental retardation. Other features of Asperger syndrome include physical clumsiness, and/or moderate to severe social deficits. Asperger syndrome is the mildest of and at the highest functioning end of the spectrum of pervasive developmental disorders (the autism spectrum). It is a neurologically based disorder of development, most often of unknown cause, in which there are deviations or abnormalities in three broad aspects of development: social relatedness and social skills, the use of language for communicative purposes, and certain behavioral and stylistic characteristics that involve repetitive or perseverative features and a limited but intense range of interests. Also known as Asperger disorder, and sometimes misdiagnosed as borderline personality disorder, obsessive-compulsive personality disorder, or schizotypal personality disorder. See also *autism*.

aspergillosis Infection with the fungus Aspergillus, seen especially in immunocompromised people in whom there may be invasive pulmonary infection and sometimes dissemination to other tissues, including the brain, the skin, and bones. Aspergillosis also causes allergic sinusitis and allergic bronchopulmonary disease.

Aspergillus A family of fungal organisms and molds, some of which can cause disease.

asphyxia Impaired or impeded breathing.

aspirate To suck in. For example, a patient may aspirate by accidentally drawing material from the stomach into the lungs, and a physician can aspirate fluid from a joint. See also *arthrocentesis; aspiration.*

aspiration 1 Removal of a sample of fluid and cells through a needle. 2 The accidental sucking of food, fluid, vomit, or other foreign material into the lungs.

aspiration, joint See *arthrocentesis.*

aspiration pneumonia Inflammation of the lungs due to aspiration.

aspirin Once the Bayer trademark for acetylsalicylic acid, now the common name for this anti-inflammatory pain reliever.

assay 1 An analysis done to determine the presence and amount of a substance. An assay may be done, for example, to determine the level of thyroid hormones in the blood of a person suspected of being hypothyroid. 2 An analysis done to determine the biologic or pharmacologic potency of a drug. For example, an assay may be done of a vaccine to determine its potency. 3 As a verb, to try or attempt. For example, "She assayed this operation for the first time and was understandably nervous." 4 The act of analyzing a mixture for one or more of its components. 5 The act of judging the value or worth of something.

assistant, physician See *physician assistant.*

assisted living A type of long-term care facility for elderly or disabled people who are able to get around on their own but who may need help with some activities of daily living or simply prefer the convenience of having their meals in a central cafeteria and having nursing staff on call.

assisted suicide Deliberate hastening of death performed by a terminally ill patient, with assistance from a physician, a family member, or another individual. See also *active euthanasia.*

assistive device A device that is designed, made, or adapted to help a person perform a particular task. For example, canes, crutches, walkers, wheelchairs, and shower chairs are all assistive devices. See also *assistive technology.*

assistive technology An assistive device or, more commonly, some kind of electronic or computerized device that helps a disabled person to function more easily in the world. Examples of assistive technology include devices that allow people to control a computer with the mouth, keyboards that can "speak" for mute individuals, and closed-captioning systems that help the hearing impaired enjoy television shows and videos. See also *augmentative communication device.*

association 1 In the study of birth defects (dysmorphology), the nonrandom occurrence in two or more individuals of a pattern of multiple anomalies not known to be a malformation syndrome (such as Down syndrome), a malformation sequence of events, or a field defect, in which all the defects are concentrated in one particular area of the body. An example of an association in dysmorphology is the VATER association. 2 In genetics, the occurrence together of two or more characteristics more often than would be expected by chance alone. Association is to be distinguished from linkage. An example of association involves a feature on the surface of white blood cells, the human leukocyte antigen (HLA) type. HLA type B-27 is associated with an increased risk for a number of diseases, including ankylosing spondylitis, which is 87 times more likely in people with HLA B-27 than in the rest of the population.

Association of American Medical Colleges A nonprofit association of accredited medical schools in the US and Canada that is responsible for the Medical College Admission Test (MCAT), an entrance examination for medical schools.

association, VATER See *VATER association.*

AST Aspartate aminotransferase.

asthma A common lung disorder in which inflammation causes the bronchi to swell and narrow the airways, creating breathing difficulties that may range from mild to life-threatening. Symptoms include shortness of breath, cough, wheezing, and chest tightness. Asthma affects only the bronchi—not the lungs themselves. Chest X-rays are therefore usually negative. The diagnosis of asthma is based on evidence of wheezing and is confirmed with breathing tests. Many allergens and irritants can precipitate attacks of asthma. Avoidance of precipitating factors helps to manage asthma. The narrowing of airways can usually be totally or at least partially reversed with treatment. Treatment may include lifestyle changes, activity reduction, allergy shots, and medications to prevent or reverse the bronchospasm that is characteristic of asthma.

asthma, exercise-induced Asthma triggered by vigorous physical activity. It primarily affects children and young adults because of their high levels of physical activity, but it can occur at any age. Exercise-induced asthma is initiated by respiratory heat exchange, which is the fall in airway temperature during rapid breathing followed by rapid reheating with lowered ventilation. The more heat that is transferred, the cooler the airways become, and the more rapidly the airways rewarm, the more the bronchi are narrowed. Acute attacks can be minimized by warming up before strenuous activity. An inhalator may also be used before exertion. The condition is common and usually treatable. Also known as exercise-induced bronchospasm and thermally induced asthma.

asthma, thermally induced See *asthma, exercise-induced.*

astigmatic A person having astigmatism.

astigmatism A common form of visual impairment in which part of an image is blurred due to an irregularity in the curvature of the front surface of the eye, the cornea, which should be shaped somewhat like a US football. With astigmatism, light rays entering the eye are not uniformly focused on the retina. The result is blurred vision at all distances. Almost everyone has some degree of astigmatism, usually so slight that it causes no problems. Significant astigmatism can cause headaches, eye strain, and seriously blurred vision. Astigmatism is often not detected during routine eye screening in schools. It may coexist with other refractive errors such as nearsightedness and farsightedness. Astigmatism is corrected with slightly cylindrical lenses that have greater light-bending power in one direction than the other. Use of these lenses elongates objects in one direction and shortens them in the other, much like looking into a distorting wavy mirror.

astrocytoma A tumor that begins in the brain or spinal cord from the proliferation of small, star-shaped cells called astrocytes. Astrocytes are normally a type of glial, or supportive, cell. The location of the tumor depends on the age of the patient. Astrocytomas most often are in the cerebrum in adults, whereas in children they arise in the brain stem, cerebrum, and cerebellum. A far-advanced (grade IV) astrocytoma is called a glioblastoma multiforme.

asymptomatic Without symptoms. For example, an asymptomatic infection is an infection with no symptoms.

ataxia Poor coordination and unsteadiness due to the brain's failure to regulate the body's posture and regulate the strength and direction of limb movements. Ataxia is usually due to disease in the brain, specifically in the cerebellum, which beneath the back part of the cerebrum.

ataxia-telangiectasia A progressive neurodegenerative disease characterized by cerebellar ataxia (poor coordination and lack of balance), ocular telangiectasia (red eyes due to widening of small blood vessels in the conjunctiva), and recurrent sinus and pulmonary infections. Abbreviated AT. Patients with AT have a striking predisposition to leukemia and lymphoma and are extremely sensitive to radiation. Other features of AT include difficulty swallowing (which causes choking and drooling) and slowed growth. AT is inherited as an autosomal recessive trait. The gene for AT is on chromosome 11 and is called ATM (ataxia-telangiectasia mutated).

ATCC American Type Culture Collection.

atelectasis Failure of full expansion of the lung at birth, or lung collapse thereafter. Also known as collapsed lung.

atelectasis, primary Failure of full expansion of the lung at birth.

atelectasis, secondary Partial or complete collapse of a previously expanded lung. Secondary atelectasis may occur in a variety of situations, including after chest surgery.

athelia Absence of the nipple. Athelia tends to occur on one side (unilaterally) in children with the Poland syndrome and on both sides (bilaterally) with certain types of ectodermal dysplasia. Athelia also occurs in association with progeria (premature aging). See also *amastia; amazia; Poland syndrome; progeria.*

atherectomy A procedure to remove plaque (atheroma) from the inside of a blood vessel. Atherectomy is done most often in major arteries, such as the coronary, carotid, and vertebral arteries, that have experienced the occlusive effects of atherosclerosis. Atherectomy may be accomplished by various means, including angioplasty, laser surgery, conventional surgical incision, or use of a small drill-tipped catheter. In the US, atherectomy is nicknamed the "Rotorooter" procedure, after a company that cleans out drainage pipes.

atherosclerosis The presence of fatty lipid deposits in the lining (intima) of an artery. Atherosclerosis is a form of arteriosclerosis. See also *arteriosclerosis.*

athetosis Involuntary writhing movements, particularly of the arms and hands. Athetosis is associated with several neurological disorders, such as cerebral palsy and Rett syndrome.

athlete's foot A skin infection caused by a fungus called Trichophyton that thrives within the upper layer of the skin when it is moist, warm, and irritated. The fungus can be found on floors and in socks and clothing, and it can be spread from person to person through contact with these objects. However, without proper growing conditions, athlete's foot fungus will not infect the skin. It can be treated with topical antifungal preparations. Also known as tinea pedis, athlete's foot is a form of ringworm.

atlantoaxial joint The joint between the first (atlas) and second (axis) vertebrae of the neck. The axis features a bony prominence called the odontoid process, about which the atlas rotates. The atlantoaxial joint is a pivot type of joint. It allows the head to turn from side to side. The atlantoaxial joint is supported and strengthened by the capsular, anterior, and posterior atlantoaxial and by the transverse ligaments. Also known as atloaxoid joint.

atlas The first vertebra in the neck. It supports the head. Also known as first cervical vertebra.

atopic dermatitis A skin disease characterized by areas of severe itching, redness, scaling, and loss of the surface of the skin. Atopic dermatitis is the most common of the many types of eczema. Atopic dermatitis is frequently associated with other allergic disorders, especially asthma and hay fever. A defect of the immune system within the skin has been detected in patients who have atopic dermatitis, but the reason for the defect is unknown.

ATP 1 Acute thrombocytopenic purpura. 2 Adenosine triphosphate.

atresia Absence of a normal opening, or failure of a structure to be tubular. Atresia can affect many structures in the body. For example, esophageal atresia is a birth defect in which part of the esophagus is not hollow, and with anal atresia, there is no hole at the bottom end of the intestine.

atria The plural of atrium.

atrial arrhythmia See *arrhythmia, atrial.*

atrial fibrillation See *fibrillation, atrial.*

atrial septal defect A hole in the wall (septum) between the upper chambers of the heart (atria). Abbreviated ASD. ASD is a major class of heart malformation. Normally, when clots in veins break off (embolize), they travel first to the right side of the heart and then to the lungs, where they lodge. When there is an ASD, however, a clot can cross from the right to the left side of the

heart, and then pass into the arteries as a paradoxical embolism. Once a clot is in the arterial circulation, it can travel to the brain, block a vessel there, and cause a stroke. Because of the risk of stroke from paradoxical embolism, even small ASDs should generally be closed.

atrial septum The wall between the right and left atria of the heart.

atrioventricular Pertaining to the upper chambers of the heart (atria) and the lower chambers of the heart (ventricles).

atrioventricular node The electrical relay station between the upper and lower chambers of the heart. Abbreviated AV node. Electrical signals from the atria must pass through the AV node to reach the ventricles. The AV node, which controls the heart rate, is one of the major elements in the cardiac conduction system. The AV node serves as an electrical relay station, slowing the electrical current sent by the sinoatrial (SA) node before the signal is permitted to pass down through to the ventricles. This delay ensures that the atria have an opportunity to fully contract before the ventricles are stimulated. After passing the AV node, the electrical current travels to the ventricles, along special fibers embedded in the walls of the lower part of the heart.

atrium An entry chamber. On both sides of the heart, the atrium is the chamber that leads to the ventricle.

atrophic vaginitis Thinning of the lining (endothelium) of the vagina due to decreased production of estrogen. Atrophic vaginitis may occur with menopause.

atrophy A wasting away or diminution. Muscle atrophy is a decrease in muscle mass, often due to extended immobility.

atropine A drug, made from the belladonna plant, that is administered via injection, eye drops, or in oral form to relax muscles by inhibiting nerve responses.

atropine psychosis A syndrome characterized by dry mouth, blurred vision, forgetfulness, and difficulty with urination that can be caused by the anticholinergic effects of some drugs, particularly antipsychotic medications. Treatment requires reducing or stopping the medication.

attack, vasovagal See *vasovagal reaction.*

attention The act of attending to discrete stimuli in the environment. Learning is most efficient when a person is paying attention. Poor attention can be a key sign of behavior disorders in children.

attention deficit disorder See *attention deficit hyperactivity disorder.*

attention deficit hyperactivity disorder A disorder in which a person is unable to control behavior due to difficulty in processing neural stimuli, accompanied by an extremely high level of motor activity. Abbreviated ADHD. ADHD can affect children and adults, but it is easiest to perceive during schooling. A child with ADHD may be extremely distractible, unable to remain still, and very talkative. ADHD is diagnosed by using a combination of parent and/or patient interview, observation of the patient, and sometimes use of standardized screening instruments. Treatments include making adjustments to the environment to accommodate the disorder, behavior modification, and the use of medications. Stimulants are the most common drugs used, although certain medications developed for high blood pressure and some antidepressants are also effective in some patients.

attenuate To weaken, or to make or become thin.

attenuated virus A weakened, less vigorous virus. An attenuated virus may be used to make a vaccine that is capable of stimulating an immune response and creating immunity but not of causing illness.

atypical Unusual, or not fitting a single diagnostic category.

atypical measles syndrome The modified expression of measles, as may occur in persons who were incompletely immunized against measles or who have compromised immune systems. Abbreviated AMS. AMS begins suddenly with high fever, headache, cough, and abdominal pain. A rash may appear 1 to 2 days later, often beginning on the limbs. Swelling (edema) of the hands and feet may occur. Pneumonia is common and may persist for 3 months or more. See also *measles.*

audiogram A test of hearing at a range of sound frequencies.

audiology The study of hearing.

audiometry The measurement of hearing.

auditory acuity The clarity or clearness of hearing, a measure of how well a person hears. Auditory acuity is measured in order to determine a person's need for a hearing aid.

auditory tube See *Eustachian tube.*

augmentative communication device A physical, mechanical, or electronic device that helps a person with a speech impairment to communicate. Augmentative communication devices range from books of pictures or words that the patient can show to express thoughts, to computers that are capable of synthesizing complex speech.

aura A premonitory sensation that is a symptom of brain malfunction. An aura often occurs before a migraine or seizure. It may consist of flashing lights, a gleam of light, blurred vision, an odor, the feeling of a breeze, numbness, weakness, or difficulty in speaking. Auras may themselves be seizures that affect areas of the brain other than the motor cortex.

aural vertigo, recurrent See *Ménière's disease.*

auricle **1** The principal projecting part of the ear, also known as pinna. **2** Something that is ear-shaped, like the atrium of the heart, which is also referred to as the auricle of the heart.

auricular Of or pertaining to the outer ear, or to something else that is ear-shaped, such as the atrium of the heart.

auricular fibrillation See *fibrillation, atrial.*

auscultate To listen, for diagnostic purposes, to the sounds made by the internal organs of the body. For example, nurses and physicians auscultate the lungs and heart of a patient by using a stethoscope placed on the patient's chest or back.

autism A spectrum of neuropsychiatric disorders characterized by deficits in social interaction and communication and by unusual and repetitive behavior. Some, but not all, people with autism are nonverbal. Autism is normally diagnosed before age 6, and it may be diagnosed in infancy in some cases. The cause of autism is currently unknown, although it is believed to involve an inherited or acquired genetic defect involving multiple chromosomes, possibly including chromosomes 6, 15, 17, and/or the X chromosome. Autism is not caused by emotional trauma, as was once theorized. Autistic or autistic-like behavior may be caused by other neurological conditions—particularly the seizure disorder Landau-Kleffner syndrome—certain forms of encephalitis, and several genetic disorders, including Angelman syndrome and Rett syndrome. Also known as Kanner syndrome or infantile autism. See also *Asperger syndrome; elective mutism; fragile X syndrome; Landau-Kleffner syndrome; Prader-Willi syndrome; Rett syndrome.*

autistic disorder Autism, particularly the most serious form of autism.

autoantibody An antibody that is directed against the patient's own body. Autoantibodies play a causative role in a number of diseases, such as rheumatoid arthritis, systemic lupus erythematosus, and Hashimoto disease.

autoclave A chamber for sterilizing with steam under pressure. The original autoclave was essentially a pressure cooker in which steam tightened the lid.

autogenous Self-produced.

autoimmune disorder A condition in which a misdirected immune system is characterized by the abnormal production of autoantibodies that are directed against the tissues of the body. Autoimmune disorders typically feature inflammation of various tissues of the body and are associated with antinuclear antibodies (ANAs) in the blood. Examples of autoimmune disorders include systemic lupus erythematosus, Sjogren's syndrome, rheumatoid arthritis, polymyositis, scleroderma, Hashimoto's thyroiditis, juvenile (type 1) diabetes mellitus, Addison disease, vitiligo, pernicious anemia, glomerulonephritis, and pulmonary fibrosis. Autoimmune disorders are more frequent in women than in men. It is thought that the estrogen of females may influence the immune system to predispose some women to autoimmune disorders. Furthermore, the presence of one autoimmune disorder increases the chance for developing another simultaneous autoimmune disorder.

autoimmune thyroiditis See *Hashimoto disease*.

autologous In blood transfusion and transplantation, a situation in which the donor and recipient are the same person. Patients scheduled for non-emergency surgery may be autologous donors by donating blood for themselves that will be stored until the surgery. An autologous graft is a graft (such as a graft of skin) that is provided for oneself.

automatism A behavior that is performed without conscious knowledge and that does not appear to be under conscious control. This curious type of behavior occurs in a number of neurological and psychiatric disorders. The neurologic disorders associated with automatism include narcolepsy and some forms of epilepsy. The psychiatric conditions associated with automatism include schizophrenia and fugue states. Automatism involves doing something "automatically" and not remembering afterward how one did it or even that one did it. Also known as automatic behavior. See also *epilepsy; seizure disorders*.

autonomic nervous system A part of the nervous system that regulates key functions of the body, including the activity of the heart muscle; the smooth muscles, including the muscles of the intestinal tract; and the glands. The autonomic nervous system has two divisions: the sympathetic nervous system, which accelerates the

heart rate, constricts blood vessels, and raises blood pressure, and the parasympathetic nervous system, which slows the heart rate, increases intestinal and gland activity, and relaxes sphincter muscles.

autopsy A postmortem examination. Also known as necropsy.

autosomal Pertaining to a chromosome that is not a sex chromosome. People normally have 22 pairs of autosomes (44 autosomes) in each cell, together with 2 sex chromosomes, X and Y in a male and X and X in a female.

autosomal dominant trait A genetic trait that appears in patients who have received one copy of a specific autosomal (nonsex) gene for that particular trait. For example, achondroplasia, Marfan syndrome, and Huntington disease are autosomal dominant traits.

autosomal recessive trait A genetic trait that appears only in patients who have received two copies of a specific autosomal (nonsex) gene for that particular trait, one from each parent. For example, sickle cell anemia and cystic fibrosis are autosomal recessive traits.

autosome Any chromosome other than the X and Y sex chromosomes. People normally have 22 pairs of autosomes (44 autosomes) in each cell.

aux- Prefix indicating growth or increase.

AV **1** Atrioventricular. Relating to the atrium(atria) and ventricle(s) of the heart. **2** Arteriovenous. Relating to an artery(ies) and a vein(s).

AV node Atrioventricular node.

avascular necrosis A condition in which poor blood supply to an area of bone leads to bone death. Abbreviated AVN. Also known as aseptic necrosis and osteonecrosis.

AVM Arteriovenous malformation. See *malformation, arteriovenous*.

avulsion Tearing away. A nerve can be avulsed by an injury, as can part of a bone.

axilla Armpit.

axillary Pertaining to the armpit, the cavity beneath the junction of the arm and the body.

axillary dissection Removal of a portion of the lymph nodes under the arm.

axis The second cervical vertebra. The first cervical vertebra (atlas) rotates around the odontoid process of the axis. See also *atlas; atlantoaxial joint*.

axon A long fiber of a nerve cell (neuron) that acts somewhat like a fiber-optic cable to carry outgoing messages. The neuron sends electrical impulses from its cell body through the axon to target cells. Each nerve cell has one axon. An axon can be over a foot in length. See also *dendrite; neuron.*

Ayurveda India's traditional, natural system of medicine that has been practiced for more than 5,000 years. Ayurveda provides an integrated approach to preventing and treating illness through lifestyle interventions and natural therapies. Ayurvedic theory states that all disease begins with an imbalance or stress in the individual's consciousness. Lifestyle intervention is a major ayurvedic preventive and therapeutic approach.

azotemia A higher-than-normal blood level of urea or other nitrogen-containing compounds. The hallmark test for azotemia is the serum blood urea nitrogen (BUN) level. Azotemia is usually caused by the inability of the kidneys to excrete these compounds.

AZT Azidothymidine, now renamed zidovudine, but still best known by the abbreviation AZT. This antiviral drug is prescribed, usually in combination with protease inhibitors and other drugs, to treat AIDS.

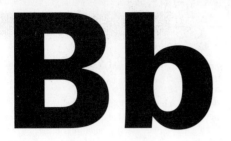

B cell   A type of white blood cell that is important to the immune system. B cells are lymphocytes that mature in the bone marrow (as opposed to T cells, which mature in the thymus). Many B cells go on to become plasma cells and produce antibodies; some B cells mature into memory B cells. B cells are responsible for the production of immunoglobulins and express immunoglobulins on their surfaces. See also *memory B cell; plasma cell.*

B. quintana   See *Bartonella quintana.*

B variant GM2-gangliosidosis   See *Tay-Sachs disease.*

Babinski reflex   An important neurologic test characterized by extension of the big toe while fanning the other toes. The Babinski reflex is obtained by stimulating the external portion (the outside) of the sole of the foot. The examiner begins the stimulation at the heel and goes forward to the base of the toes. Most newborn babies and young infants are not neurologically mature, and they therefore show a Babinski reflex. A Babinski reflex in an older child or an adult is abnormal and is a sign of a problem in the central nervous system (CNS), most likely in the pyramidal tract. A Babinski reflex that is present on one side but not the other is also abnormal, and it can indicate which side of the CNS is involved. Also known as plantar response, big toe sign, and Babinski phenomenon, response, or sign.

baby teeth   See *primary teeth.*

bacillus   A large family of bacteria that are rod-like in shape. They include the bacteria that cause food to spoil, as well as those that are responsible for some diseases. Helpful members of the bacillus family are used to make antibiotics or colonize the human intestinal tract and aid with digestion.

back pain, low   Pain in the lower back area that can relate to problems with the lumbar spine, the discs between the vertebrae, the ligaments around the spine and discs, the spinal cord and nerves, muscles of the low back, internal organs of the pelvis and abdomen, or the skin covering the lumbar area. See also *sciatica.*

backbone   The spine, a flexible row of bones stretching from the base of the skull to the tailbone. See also *vertebral column.*

bacteremia   The presence of live bacteria in the bloodstream. From bacteria and -emia ("in the blood"). Also known as bacillemia. See also *blood culture; septicemia.*

bacteria   Single-celled microorganisms that can exist either as independent (free-living) organisms or as parasites (dependent on another organism for life). Examples of bacteria include Acidophilus, a normal inhabitant of yogurt; Chlamydia, which causes an infection very similar to gonorrhea; Clostridium welchii, the most common cause of gangrene; E. coli, which commonly and benignly lives in colons and, on occasion, can be a dangerous agent of disease; and Streptococcus, the bacterium that causes the common infection of the throat called strep throat. Bacterium is the singular and bacteria the plural (that is, one bacterium, two bacteria). The term was devised in 1847 by the German botanist Ferdinand Cohn, who based it on the Greek bakterion, meaning "a small rod or staff."

bacteria, flesh-eating   See *necrotizing fasciitis.*

bacterial   Of or pertaining to bacteria, as in a bacterial lung infection.

bacterial vaginosis   A vaginal condition characterized by an abnormal vaginal discharge due to an overgrowth of normal bacteria in the vagina. Women with bacterial vaginosis also have fewer than the usual number of vaginal bacteria, called lactobacilli. Symptoms of bacterial vaginosis are vaginal discharge and sometimes a fishy odor. A microscopic sign of bacterial vaginosis is an unusual vaginal cell called a clue cell. Treatment options include oral antibiotics and vaginal gels. Bacterial vaginosis can cause premature labor and delivery, as well as infection of the amniotic fluid and of the uterus after delivery. Therefore, screening and treatment for bacterial vaginosis during pregnancy may be done. The antibiotic treatment is the same in pregnant and nonpregnant women.

bacteriocidal   Capable of killing bacteria. Antibiotics, antiseptics, and disinfectants can all be bactericidal.

bacteriophage   A virus that lives within a bacterium, replicating itself and eventually destroying the bacterial cell. Bacteriophages have been very helpful in the study of bacterial and molecular genetics. They are sometimes simply called phages.

bacteriostatic   Capable of inhibiting the growth or reproduction of bacteria. See also *bacteriocidal.*

bacterium   Singular of bacteria. See also *bacteria.*

bag of waters   The amniotic sac and amniotic fluid.

Baker cyst   A swelling in the space behind the knee (the popliteal space) that is composed of a membrane-lined sac filled with synovial fluid that has escaped from the joint. Also known as synovial cyst of the popliteal space.

balanitis   Inflammation of the rounded head (the glans) of the penis. Inflammation of the foreskin is called posthitis. In the uncircumcised male, balanitis and posthitis generally occur together as balanoposthitis: inflammation of both the glans and foreskin.

balanitis, circinate   A skin inflammation around the penis in males with Reiter syndrome. With circinate balanitis, the skin around the shaft and tip of the penis can become inflamed and scaly. TCortisone creams can be used as treatment. See also *balanitis; keratodermia blennorrhagicum; Reiter syndrome.*

balanoposthitis   Inflammation of both the glans and foreskin. In the uncircumcised male, balanitis and posthitis (inflammation of the foreskin) usually occur together as balanoposthitis. An uncircumcised boy should be taught to clean his penis with care to prevent infection and inflammation of the foreskin and the glans. Cleaning of the penis is done by gently retracting the foreskin, only to the point where resistance is met. Full retraction of the foreskin may not be possible until after age 3. Circumcision and careful cleaning prevent balanoposthitis. See also *balanitis; posthitis.*

baldness   Lack or loss of hair on the scalp. Also known as alopecia. There are many types of baldness, each with a different cause. Baldness may be localized to the front and top of the head, as in the very common type of male-pattern baldness; baldness may be patchy, a condition called alopecia areata; or it may involve the entire head, as in alopecia capitis totalis. See *alopecia; alopecia areata; alopecia capitis totalis; alopecia, traumatic; alopecia universalis.*

ball-and-socket joint   A joint in which the round end of a bone fits into the cavity of another bone. The hip joint is a ball-and-socket joint.

balloon angioplasty   Coronary angioplasty that is accomplished by using a balloon-tipped catheter inserted through an artery in the groin or arm, to enlarge a narrowing in a coronary artery. Angioplasty is successful in opening coronary arteries in 90 percent of patients. Forty percent of patients with successful coronary angioplasty develop recurrent narrowing at the site of balloon inflation. See also *coronary artery disease.*

balloon tamponade   A procedure in which a balloon is inflated within the esophagus or stomach, to apply pressure on bleeding blood vessels, compress the vessels, and stop the bleeding. It is used in the treatment of bleeding veins in the esophagus (esophageal varices) and stomach. The balloon used in the esophagus is shaped like a sausage, whereas the balloon used in the stomach is rounded. Also known as esophagogastric tamponade.

banding of chromosomes   Treatment of chromosomes to reveal characteristic patterns of horizontal bands. Thanks to these banding patterns, which resemble bar codes, each human chromosome is distinctive and can be identified without ambiguity. Banding also permits the detection of chromosome deletions (lost segments), duplications (extra segments), and other structural abnormalities.

barbiturate   A class of drugs that depresses activity in the central nervous system (CNS), including many sleeping pills, sedatives, antispasmodics, and anesthetics. Barbiturates are addictive, carry a high risk of overdose, and should never be used with alcohol or with other CNS depressants.

barium enema   An enema that is given with a white, chalky solution containing barium, in preparation for series of X-ray images of the lower intestine. The barium outlines the intestines on the X-ray film.

barium solution   A liquid that contains barium sulfate, which shows up on X-ray film. Barium solution outlines organs of the body so they can be seen as images on X-ray film.

barium sulfate   An odorless, flavorless barium salt. Barium is a metallic chemical element. See also *barium enema; barium solution; barium swallow.*

barium swallow   A test that involves filling the esophagus, stomach, and small intestines with a barium solution in preparation for an X-ray, to define the anatomy of the upper digestive tract. Also known as upper gastrointestinal series.

barosinusitis   See *aerosinusitis.*

barotitis   See *aerotitis.*

Barr body   A microscopic feature of female cells that is due to the presence of two X chromosomes, one of which is inactive and crumples up.

Barrett esophagus A complication of chronic severe gastrointestinal reflux disease (GERD) that involves a change in the cells that line the bottom of the inner esophagus. The esophagus becomes irritated when the contents of the stomach back up (when reflux occurs). There is a small but definite increased risk of cancer of the esophagus (adenocarcinoma) in people with Barrett esophagus. The diagnosis of Barrett esophagus is made on seeing (through endoscopy) a pink esophageal lining (mucosa) that extends a short distance (usually less than 2.5 inches) up the esophagus from the gastroesophageal junction and finding intestinal type cells (goblet cells) on biopsy of the lining. Treatment is, in general, essentially the same as for GERD both medically (with acid-suppression drugs) and surgically (with fundoplication).

barrier method A birth control method that employs a barrier which prevents sperm from entering the cervix, thereby preventing conception. Condoms and diaphragms are examples of a barrier method. See also *cervical cap; condom; condom, female; diaphragm.*

Bartholin gland One of a pair of glands between the vulva and the vagina that produce lubrication in response to stimulation. Along with a second pair of nearby glands, called the lesser vestibular glands, the Bartholin glands act to aid in sexual intercourse. Also known as greater vestibular gland.

Bartonella henselae See *cat scratch disease.*

Bartonella quintana A parasitic microorganism in the rickettsiae family that can multiply within the gut of a louse and can then be transmitted to humans and cause trench fever. Transmission occurs when infected louse feces are rubbed into abraded skin or into the whites of the eyes. Trench fever was first recognized in the trenches of World War I, and it now occurs among homeless people, injection drug users, street alcoholics, and others who live in cramped, unhygienic quarters. B. quintana is also responsible for a disease called bacillary angiomatosis in people infected with HIV, and for infection of the heart and great vessels (endocarditis) in people with bloodstream infection (bacteremia). The full spectrum of disease caused by B. quintana is still unfolding. Also known as Rochalimaea quintana. See also *trench fever.*

basal cell A small, round cell found in the lower part, or base, of the epidermis.

basal cell carcinoma The most common type of skin cancer, which commonly presents as a sore that seems to get better and then recurs and may start to bleed. Basal cell carcinoma often occurs on the face and neck, where the skin is exposed to sunlight. These tumors are locally invasive and tend to burrow in but not metastasize (spread) to distant locations.

basal ganglia A region of the base of the brain that consists of three clusters of neurons (caudate nucleus, putamen, and globus pallidus) that are responsible for involuntary movements such as tremors, athetosis, and chorea. The basal ganglia are abnormal in a number of important neurologic conditions, including Parkinson's disease and Huntington's disease.

basal metabolic rate The rate of metabolism, as measured by the amount of heat given off when a person is at rest; it is expressed as calories of energy per hour per square meter of skin. The basal metabolic rate can offer clues about underlying health problems. For example, a person with an overly active thyroid has an elevated basal metabolic rate.

basal temperature 1 Usually, a person's temperature on awakening in the morning. Because changes in basal temperature accompany ovulation, basal temperature is often tracked by women who want to ensure or avoid pregnancy. 2 A crude measure of thyroid function that is achieved by taking and comparing basal temperatures. This measure is now superceded by modern thyroid function blood tests. Also known as Broda test.

base A unit of DNA. There are four bases in DNA: adenine (A), guanine (G), thymine (T), and cytosine (C). The sequence of bases (for example, CAG) constitutes the genetic code.

base pair Two DNA bases that are complementary to one another (A and T, or G and C) and join in strands to form the double-helix that is characteristic of DNA.

base sequence The order of nucleotide bases in a DNA molecule.

battered child syndrome A condition in which a person has skeletal fractures, especially multiple injuries of various ages, that result from child abuse. The term battered child syndrome entered medicine in 1962. By 1976, all states in the US had adopted laws mandating the reporting of suspected instances of child abuse. See also *child abuse.*

battle fatigue The World War II name for what is known today as post-traumatic stress disorder (PTSD). See also *post-traumatic stress disorder.*

BCG Bacille Calmette Guérin, a weakened (attenuated) version of a bacterium called Mycobacterium bovis that is closely related to Mycobacterium tuberculosis, the agent responsible for tuberculosis. See *tuberculosis vaccination.*

bedbug A blood-sucking bug in the Cimex family that lives hidden in bedding or furniture and comes out at night to bite its victims.

bedsore A painful, often reddened area of degenerating, ulcerated skin that is caused by pressure and lack of movement and that is worsened by exposure to urine or other irritating substances on the skin. Untreated bedsores can become seriously infected or gangrenous. Bedsores are a major problem for patients who are confined to a bed or wheelchair, and they can be prevented by moving the patient frequently, changing bedding, and keeping the skin clean and dry. Also known as pressure sore, decubitus sore, and decubitus ulcer.

bedwetting Involuntary urination in bed after the usual age of toilet training. Also known as nighttime enuresis and nocturnal enuresis. It may be caused by incomplete development of bladder control, a sleep or arousal disorder, bladder or kidney disease, neurological problems, or psychological causes (such as fear of the dark that prevents the child from leaving the bed). About 20 percent of 5-year-olds wet the bed at least once a month; surprisingly, 1 to 2 percent of teenagers have nighttime enuresis. Treatment depends on the cause and may include education, behavior modification techniques, the use of alarms, bladder-retention training, and medication. See also *enuresis.*

bee sting A sting from a bee or another large stinging insect such as a yellow jacket, hornet, or wasp that can trigger an allergic reaction, up to and including life-threatening anaphylactic shock. Avoidance and prompt treatment are essential for those who are allergic to bee stings. Self-injectible adrenaline can be carried by persons known to be allergic when in risk areas. Hikers should wear long pants and shirts in risk areas. If a person is attacked, he or she should run for shelter, covering the face to prevent airway stings. Treatment depends on the severity of symptoms. Stingers should be removed promptly, and the area should be cleansed with soap and water. Ice packs, pain medications, and anti-itching medications can be helpful in treating local reactions. Victims with more serious symptoms or multiple stings are often hospitalized for observation and treatment. They can require intravenous fluids, oxygen, cortisone medicine, or epinephrine, as well as medications to open the breathing passages. In very severe reactions, the venom is removed from the blood by plasmapheresis or hemodialysis. In selected cases, allergy injection therapy is highly effective for prevention. For those who are not allergic, stings are a minor nuisance unless they occur in multiples. The lethal dose of honeybee venom, for example, is about 19 stings per kilogram of body weight (for example, 1,300 stings for a 150-pound person).

bee sting, Africanized A sting from an Africanized ("killer") bee, a species of large honey bees found in South and Central America, as well as in some parts of the US. This species of bees has an unusual and dangerous natural defense mechanism when disturbed. A loud noise or vibration, such as a barking dog or lawn mower, near a hive may cause the bees to display aggressive behavior. They attack in large numbers and for a longer period of time than is typical of the common European honeybee. As a result, Africanized bees inflict more stings, injecting a higher dosage of bee venom into their victims. See also *bee sting.*

beef tapeworm The most common of the large tapeworms that parasitize people. Beef tapeworm can be contracted from infected beef that is raw or rare. Also known as Taenia saginata.

behavior modification The use of rewards and/or punishments to encourage desirable behavior.

behavioral disorder Technically, a condition characterized by undesirable behavior that is within the patient's control (for example, substance abuse and antisocial behavior). The term is also used as a euphemism for psychiatric disorder.

behaviorism The science of studying and modifying animal or human behavior, often through behavior modification techniques.

Behcet's syndrome A chronic inflammatory disorder that involves the small blood vessels and is classically characterized by a triad of features: ulcers in the mouth, ulcers of the genitalia, and inflammation of the eye (uveitis). The ulcers of the mouth are typically recurring crops of aphthous ulcers. Arthritis is also commonplace with Behcet's syndrome. The cause of Behcet's syndrome is not known. It is more frequent and severe in patients from the Eastern Mediterranean and Asia than in those of European descent.

belching A normal process of releasing through the mouth air that accumulates in the stomach, thereby relieving distention. Upper abdominal discomfort associated with excessive swallowed air may extend into the lower chest, producing symptoms that suggest heart or lung disease.

Bell's palsy Paralysis of the nerve that supplies the facial muscles on one side of the face (the seventh cranial nerve, or facial nerve). Bell's palsy often starts suddenly. The cause may be related to viral infection. Treatment is directed toward protecting the eye on the affected side from dryness during sleep. Massage of affected muscles can reduce soreness. Sometimes cortisone medication, such as prednisone, is given to reduce inflammation during the first weeks of illness. The outlook is generally good; about 80 percent of patients recover within weeks or months.

belly See *abdomen.*

bellybutton The navel or umbilicus; the former site of attachment of the umbilical cord.

benign Not malignant. A benign tumor is one that does not invade surrounding tissue or spread to other parts of the body; it is not a cancer.

benign intracranial hypertension See *pseudotumor cerebri.*

benign partial epilepsy with centro-temporal spikes See *epilepsy, benign rolandic.*

benign prostatic hyperplasia A noncancerous prostate problem in which the normal elements of the prostate gland grow in size and number. Their sheer bulk may compress the urethra, which courses through the center of the prostate, impeding the flow of urine from the bladder through the urethra to the outside. This leads to urine retention and the need for frequent urination. Abbreviated BPH. If BPH is severe enough, complete blockage can occur. BPH generally begins in a man's 30s, evolves slowly, and causes symptoms only after age 50. BPH is very common. Half of men over age 50 develop symptoms of PBH, but only 10 percent need medical or surgical intervention. Watchful waiting with annual medical monitoring is appropriate for most men with BPH. Medical therapy includes drugs such as finasteride and terazosin. Prostate surgery has traditionally been seen as offering the most benefits—and the most risks—for BPH. BPH is not a sign of prostate cancer. Also known as benign prostatic hypertrophy and nodular hyperplasia of the prostate.

benign rolandic epilepsy of childhood See *epilepsy, benign rolandic.*

beriberi Inflammation of multiple nerves (polyneuritis), heart disease (cardiopathy), and edema (swelling) due to a deficiency of thiamine (vitamin B1) in the diet.

Bernard-Soulier syndrome A disorder in which the platelets lack the ability to adequately stick to injured blood vessel walls. Because this is a crucial aspect of the process of forming a blood clot, when it does not happen, abnormal bleeding occurs. Bernard-Soulier syndrome usually appears in the newborn period, infancy, or early childhood, with bruises, nosebleeds (epistaxis), and gum (gingival) bleeding. Problems can occur later, with anything that induces bleeding, such as menstruation, trauma, surgery, or stomach ulcers. Bernard-Soulier syndrome is an inherited disease, transmitted as an autosomal recessive trait. The molecular basis is a deficiency in platelet glycoproteins Ib, V, and IX. There is no specific treatment. Bleeding episodes may require platelet transfusions. The abnormal platelets in the syndrome are usually considerably larger than normal platelets. However, this is not the only syndrome with large platelets. Specific platelet function tests, as well as tests for the glycoproteins common to Bernard-Soulier syndrome, can confirm the diagnosis. Also known as giant platelet syndrome.

berry aneurysm See *aneurysm, berry.*

beta-adrenergic blocking drug See *beta blocker.*

beta blocker A class of drugs that block beta-adrenergic substances such as adrenaline (epinephrine), which is a key agent in the sympathetic portion of the involuntary nervous system. By blocking the action of the sympathetic nervous system on the heart, these agents relieve stress on the heart. They slow the heartbeat, lessen the force with which the heart muscle contracts, and reduce blood vessel contraction in the heart, brain, and body. Beta blockers are used to treat abnormal heart rhythms, specifically to prevent abnormally fast heart rates (tachycardias) or irregular heart rhythms, such as premature ventricular beats. Because beta blockers reduce the demand of the heart muscle for oxygen, they can be useful in treating angina. They have also become important drugs in improving survival after a person has had a heart attack. Due to their effect on blood vessels, beta blockers can lower the blood pressure and are of value in the treatment of hypertension. Other uses include the prevention of migraine headaches and the treatment of familial or hereditary essential tremors. Beta blockers reduce pressure within the eye, probably by reducing the production of the liquid within the eye (aqueous humor), and they are therefore used to lessen the risk of damage to the optic nerve and loss of vision in patients with glaucoma. Beta blockers include acebutolol (brand name: Sectral), atenolol (brand name: Tenormin), bisoprolol (brand name: Zebeta), metoprol (brand names: Lopressor, Lopressor LA, Toprol XL), nadolol (brand name: Corgard), and timolol (brand name: Bloacadren). Beta blockers are also available in combination with diuretics; for example, with bisoprolol and hydrochlorothiazide (brand name: Ziac). Eye-specific beta blockers include timolol ophthalmic solution (brand name: Timoptic) and betaxolol hydrochloride (brand name: Betoptic).

beta carotene   A protective antioxidant vitamin that is a natural component of carrots. See also Appendix C, "Vitamins."

beta cell, pancreatic   A cell that makes insulin and is found in the areas of the pancreas called the islets of Langerhans. Destruction of beta cells causes type 1 (insulin-dependent) diabetes mellitus. See also *diabetes mellitus.*

beta error   The statistical error (said to be "of the second kind," or type II) that is made in testing when it is concluded that something is negative when it really is positive. Also known as false negative.

beta-2 microglobulin   A test that measures the amount of cell destruction present. It is considered to be one of the best ways to measure the progression of HIV-related disease, although it may also indicate cell destruction due to cytomegalovirus or other causes. Results over 5 are considered very significant.

bezoar   A clump or wad of swallowed food or hair. Bezoars can block the digestive system, especially the exit of the stomach. A bezoar composed of hair is called a trichobezoar. A bezoar composed of vegetable materials is called a phytobezoar. A bezoar composed of hair and food is called a trichophytobezoar.

BF   Physician's shorthand for black female.

bi-   Prefix indicating two, as in biceps (a muscle with two heads) or bicuspid (having two flaps or cusps).

bias   In a clinical trial, the effects that may cause an incorrect conclusion. Common examples of bias include advanced knowledge of the treatment being given, strong desire of the researcher for a specific outcome, or improper study design. To avoid bias, a blinded study may be done. See also *blinded study; double-blinded study.*

bicarbonate   In medicine, bicarbonate usually refers to bicarbonate of soda (sodium bicarbonate, baking soda), a white powder that is a common ingredient in antacids. Also, the bicarbonate level is an indirect measure of the acidity of the blood that is determined when electrolytes are tested. The normal serum range for bicarbonate is 22–30 mmol/L.

biceps   A muscle that has two heads, or origins. There is more than one biceps muscle. The biceps brachii is the well-known flexor muscle in the upper arm; it bulges when the arm is bent in a C-shape with the fist toward the forehead. The biceps femoris is in the back of the thigh.

bicornuate   Having two horns or horn-shaped branches. The uterus is normally unicornuate, but it can sometimes be bicornuate.

bicuspid   Having two flaps or cusps.

bicuspid aortic valve   An aortic valve in the heart that has two flaps (cusps) that open and close. A normal aortic valve in the heart has three flaps. There may be no symptoms of bicuspid aortic valve in childhood, but in time the valve may become narrowed (stenotic), making it harder for blood to pass through it, or blood may start to leak backward through the valve (regurgitate). Treatment depends on how the valve is working. For a severely deteriorated valve, replacement surgery may be necessary.

bicuspid valve   See *mitral valve.*

b.i.d.   An abbreviation commonly used on prescriptions that means twice a day. See also Appendix A, "Prescription Abbreviations."

bifid   Split in two.

bifid uvula   See *uvula.*

big toe sign   See *Babinski reflex.*

bilateral   Affecting both sides. For example, bilateral arthritis affects joints on both the left and right sides of the body.

bile   A yellow-green fluid that is made by the liver and stored in the gallbladder. Bile passes through the common bile duct into the duodenum, where it helps digest fat. The principal components of bile are cholesterol, bile salts, and the pigment bilirubin. Cholesterol is normally kept in liquid form by the dissolving action of the bile salts. An increased amount of cholesterol in the bile overwhelms the dissolving capacity of the bile salts and leads to the formation of cholesterol gallstones. Similarly, a deficiency of bile salts promotes cholesterol gallstone formation. Pigment gallstones are frequently associated with chronic infection in the bile, especially in certain Asian countries, where parasitic infection of the bile ducts is common. Patients with blood diseases that cause excessive breakdown of red blood cells can have increased amounts of bilirubin in the bile, thus causing bilirubin gallstones to form. See also *gallstones.*

bile acid resin   A substance that binds in the intestine with bile acids that contain cholesterol and is then eliminated in the stool. The major effect of bile acid resin is to lower LDL-cholesterol by about 10 to 20 percent. Small doses of bile acid resin can produce useful reductions in LDL-cholesterol. Bile acid resin may be prescribed, together with a statin, for patients with heart disease, to reduce cholesterol. When these two drugs are combined, their effects are added together, lowering LDL-cholesterol by over 40 percent. Cholestyramine (brand name:

Questran) and colestipol (Colestid) are the two main bile acid resins currently available. These two drugs are available as powders or tablets. Bile acid resin powders must be mixed with water or fruit juice and taken once or twice (sometimes three times) daily with meals. Tablets must be taken with large amounts of fluids to avoid gastrointestinal symptoms. Side effects may include constipation, bloating, nausea, and gas. Although bile acid resin is not absorbed, it may interfere with the absorption of other medicines if taken at the same time as the other medicines. Therefore, other medications should be taken at least 1 hour before or 4 to 6 hours after a resin.

bile sludge See *biliary sludge*.

bilharzia A schistosome, a trematode worm that parasitizes people. Three main species of these worms—Schistosoma haematobium, S. japonicum, and S. mansoni—cause disease in humans. Larval forms of the parasite live in freshwater snails. When the parasite is liberated from the snail, it burrows into the skin, transforms to the schistosomulum stage, and migrates to the urinary tract (S. haematobium), or liver or intestine (S. japonicum or S. mansoni), where the adult worms develop. Eggs are shed into the urinary tract or the intestine, where they hatch to form another form of the parasite, called miracidia, that can then infect snails again, completing the parasite's life cycle. Adult schistosome worms can seriously damage tissue. Also known as schistosomiasis.

biliary Having to do with the gallbladder, bile ducts, or bile. The biliary system consists of the gallbladder, bile ducts, and bile. See also *bile*.

biliary cirrhosis, primary See *cirrhosis, primary biliary*.

biliary sand A term used by surgeons to describe small particles in bile that are visible to the naked eye and are large enough to be counted easily in a gallbladder that has been removed. Biliary sand may be looked upon as a stage of growth between bilary sludge, which is made up of microscopic particles, and gallstones. The composition of biliary sand varies but is similar to that of gallstones, the most common components being cholesterol crystals and calcium salts. Biliary sand may cause no symptoms, or it may cause intermittent symptoms, including pain in the abdomen, nausea, and vomiting, particularly after a fatty meal. Biliary sand can cause complications, including inflammation of the pancreas (pancreatitis) and inflammation of the gallbladder (cholecystitis). Biliary sand can often be detected by an ultrasound of the abdomen. If patients with biliary sand develop symptoms or complications, gallbladder removal (cholecystectomy) is performed.

biliary sludge Microscopic particulate matter in bile. The composition of biliary sludge varies. The most common particulate components are cholesterol crystals and calcium salts. Biliary sludge has been associated with certain conditions, including rapid weight loss, fasting, pregnancy, the use of certain medications (for example, ceftriaxone, octreotide), and bone marrow or solid organ transplantation. However, it most commonly occurs in individuals with no identifiable conditions. Biliary sludge can be looked upon as microscopic gallstones, although it is not clear at what size the particles in biliary sludge should be considered gallstones. Biliary sludge usually causes no symptoms, and it may appear and disappear over time. It may, however, cause intermittent pain in the abdomen, often with nausea and vomiting. This occurs when the particles obstruct the ducts leading from the gallbladder to the intestine. On occasion, the particles may grow in size to become larger gallstones. Biliary sludge may also cause more serious complications, including inflammation of the pancreas (pancreatitis) and inflammation of the gallbladder (cholecystitis). Biliary sludge can be detected with ultrasound of the abdomen, or by directly examining bile content under a microscope (bile microscopy). If patients with biliary sludge develop symptoms or complications, the gallbladder may be removed.

bilirubin A yellow-orange compound that is produced by the breakdown of hemoglobin from red blood cells.

binge drinking The dangerous practice of consuming large quantities of alcoholic beverages in a single session. Binge drinking carries a serious risk of harm, including alcohol poisoning. See also *alcohol poisoning*.

binge eating disorder An eating disorder characterized by periods of extreme overeating, but not followed by purging behaviors, as in bulimia. Binge eating disorder can occur alone or in conjunction with a lesion of the hypothalamus gland, Prader-Willi disorder, or other medical conditions. It can contribute to high blood pressure, weight gain, diabetes, and heart disease. Treatment may include therapy, dietary education and advice, and medication.

binocular vision The ability to maintain visual focus on an object with both eyes, creating a single visual image. Lack of binocular vision is normal in infants. Adults without binocular vision experience distortions in depth perception and visual measurement of distance.

bio- Prefix indicating living plants or creatures, as in biology (the study of living organisms).

biofeedback A method of treatment that uses a monitor to measure patients' physiologic information of which they are normally unaware. By watching a monitor, patients can learn by trial and error to adjust their thinking and other mental processes in order to control "involuntary" bodily processes such as blood pressure, temperature, gastrointestinal functioning, and brain wave activity. Biofeedback is now used to treat a wide variety of conditions and diseases, including stress, alcohol and other addictions, sleep disorders, epilepsy, respiratory problems, fecal and urinary incontinence, muscle spasms, partial paralysis, muscle dysfunction caused by injury, migraine headaches, hypertension, and a variety of vascular disorders, including Raynaud's phenomenon. The US experimental psychologist Neal E. Miller conducted pioneering work in biofeedback in the 1950s and 1960s. Miller worked to map the physiological bases of the most visceral of human drives, such as fear, hunger, and curiosity. Miller's ideas were revolutionary at the time.

bioflavinoid An antioxidant compound that is found in various plants and is available in supplement form. Once known as vitamin P.

biologic evolution A process mediated by genes that shows a slow rate of change and uses mutations and selection as agents of change. New variants in biologic evolution are often harmful, and when these new variants are transmitted from parents to offspring, this occurs according to classical genetics. Humans require cultural as well as biological evolution. See also *cultural evolution.*

biological response modifier A substance that stimulates the body's response to infection and disease. Abbreviated BRM. The body naturally produces small amounts of BRMs. Some BRMs are made in the laboratory in large amounts for use in treating cancer, rheumatoid arthritis, Crohn's disease, hepatitis, and other diseases. BRMs used in biological therapy include monoclonal antibodies, interferon, interleukin-2 (IL-2), and colony-stimulating factor (CSF, GM-CSF, and G-CSF). Side effects of BRM therapy often include flu-like symptoms, such as chills, fever, muscle aches, weakness, loss of appetite, nausea, vomiting, and diarrhea. Some patients develop a rash, and some bleed or bruise easily. Interleukin therapy can cause swelling. Depending on the severity of these problems, patients may need to stay in the hospital during treatment. The side effects usually go away gradually after treatment stops.

biological therapy Treatment to stimulate or restore the ability of the immune system to fight infection and disease. Biological therapy is thus any form of treatment that uses the body's natural abilities to cause the immune system to fight infection or to protect the body from side effects of treatment. Biological therapy often employs biological response modifiers (BRMs). For example, biological therapy to block the action of a messenger of inflammation, called tumor necrosis factor (TNF), is being used to treat conditions such as Crohn's disease and rheumatoid arthritis. Also known as biotherapy or immunotherapy.

biomarker A biologic feature that can be used to measure the presence or progress of disease or the effects of treatment. For example, prostate specific antigen (PSA) is a biomarker for cancer of the prostate.

biopsy The removal of a sample of tissue for examination under a microscope to check for cancer cells or other abnormalities.

biopsy, endometrial A procedure for sampling the lining of the uterus (the endometrium). Endometrial biopsy is usually done to learn the cause of abnormal uterine bleeding, but it may be used to determine the cause of infertility, test for uterine infections, and even monitor responses to certain medications. The procedure can be done in a physician's office. There are few risks, the most common being cramping and pain. Oral pain medications taken beforehand may help reduce cramping and pain. See also *biopsy.*

biopsy, needle A procedure in which a small amount of tissue is taken for examination by using a hollow needle. See also *biopsy; biopsy, stereotactic needle.*

biopsy, punch See *punch biopsy.*

biopsy, sentinel-lymph-node Examination of the first lymph node that receives lymphatic drainage from a tumor to learn whether that node has tumor cells in it. The sentinel node's identity is determined by injecting around the tumor a tracer substance that travels through the lymphatic system to the first draining node, thereby identifying it. If the sentinel node contains tumor cells, removal of more nodes in the area may be warranted. If the sentinel node is normal, extensive dissection of the regional lymph-node basin is not needed. Sentinel-lymph-node biopsy has become a standard technique for determining the nodal stage of disease in some patients with malignant melanoma. See also *biopsy.*

biopsy, stereotactic needle A procedure in which the spot to be biopsied is located three-dimensionally, the information is entered into a computer, and then the computer calculates the information and positions a needle to remove the biopsy sample. Stereotactic needle biopsy can be done in a properly equipped physician's office, and it carries a minimal amount of pain and risk compared to other types of biopsy. See also *biopsy.*

biotechnology The fusion of biology and technology, the application of biological techniques to product research and development. In particular, biotechnology involves the use by industry of recombinant DNA, cell fusion, and new bioprocessing techniques.

bioterrorism Terrorism using biologic agents. Biological diseases and the agents that might be used for terrorism have been listed by the US Centers for Disease Control and Prevention (CDC). The list includes a number of "select agents" that are potential weapons whose transfer in the scientific and medical communities is regulated, to keep them out of unfriendly hands. These agents include viruses, bacteria, rickettsiae (microorganisms that have traits common to both bacteria and viruses), fungi, and biological toxins and are classified into three categories, according to the degree of danger each agent is felt to pose. Category A biological diseases pose high risk to national security because they can be easily disseminated or transmitted from person to person; cause high mortality, with the potential for major public health impact; might cause public panic and social disruption; and require special action for public health preparedness. Examples of Category A biological diseases include anthrax, botulism, the plague, smallpox, tularemia, and hemorrhagic fever due to the Ebola and Marburg viruses. Category B biological diseases are agents that are moderately easy to disseminate; cause moderate morbidity and low mortality; and require specific enhancements of the CDC's diagnostic capacity and enhanced disease surveillance. Examples of Category B biological diseases include Q fever, Brucellosis, Glanders, Ricin toxin, epsilon toxin of the gas gangrene bacillus, and Staphylococcus enterotoxin B. Category C biological diseases are emerging pathogens that could be engineered for mass dissemination in the future because of their availability; ease of production and dissemination; and potential for high morbidity and mortality and major health impact. Examples of Category C biological diseases include Nipah virus, Hantavirus, tickborne hemorrhagic fever and encephalitis viruses, Yellow fever, and Tuberculosis (multi-drug-resistant TB).

bipolar disorder A disorder, formerly called manic-depressive illness, in which the patient cycles through uncontrollable mood states. Less prevalent than simple clinical depression, bipolar disorders involve cycles of depression, hypomania (elevated mood), mania (extremely elevated mood), and in some cases psychosis. Sometimes the mood switches are dramatic and rapid, but most often they are gradual. Both depression and mania affect thinking, judgment, and social behavior in ways that cause serious problems. For example, unwise business, financial, and personal decisions may be made when an individual is in a manic phase. Bipolar disorder is usually a chronic recurring condition, with serious impairment and suicide common in untreated cases. The

cause is as yet unknown, although bipolar disorders appear to have a strong genetic basis and may be influenced by seasonal patterns, hormones, or viral infection. The diagnostic term bipolar I refers to classic bipolar disorder, which is characterized by episodes of both depression and mania, whereas the term bipolar II refers to a condition with cyclical episodes of clinical depression and perhaps hypomania, but no frank episodes of mania. A strategy that combines medication and psychosocial treatment is optimal for managing bipolar disease. Also known as manic-depressive disease and manic depression. See also *cyclothymia; seasonal affective disorder; depression; mania; mixed mania.*

birth The process of delivering a fetus from the uterus. Normally, the fetus is expelled through the cervix and birth canal with the assistance of rhythmic muscle contractions. Birth may instead be a surgical procedure: a Caesarean section. See also *caesarean section.*

birth control The practice of exercising some level of control over contraception. Birth control methods are many, and they vary in effectiveness. The most effective method is abstinence from sex, followed by oral, injectible, or implanted contraceptives; barrier methods used consistently and with spermicidal gel; and the basal temperature method, if used carefully and consistently. See also *barrier method; cervical cap; coitus interruptus; condom; condom, female; contraceptive; contraceptive, emergency; contraceptive, implanted; Depo-Provera; diaphragm; intrauterine device; natural family planning; oral contraceptive.*

birth control pill See *oral contraceptive.*

birth defect Any defect present in a baby at birth, regardless of whether it is caused by a genetic factor. Birth defects involve many different tissues, including the brain, heart, lungs, liver, bones, and intestinal tract. These defects can occur for many reasons, including genetic conditions and toxic exposures of the fetus (for example, to alcohol). All parents are at risk of having a baby with a birth defect. Birth defects are now the leading cause of infant mortality (death) in the US and many other developed nations. Of all babies, 2 to 3 percent are born with a medically significant birth defect, including heart defects, cleft lip and palate, Down syndrome, and spina bifida. Also known as congenital malformation or congenital anomaly. See also *dysmorphology.*

birthmark A discoloration of the skin that may or may not be raised and is present at birth. Most birthmarks are harmless. Occasionally a specific type of birthmark can be a visible marker for a more serious health problem. See also *café au lait; port-wine stain.*

birthrate   The number of live births divided by the average population, or by the population at midyear. Also known as crude birthrate.

bisexual   An individual who engages in both heterosexual and homosexual sexual relations. Bisexual can also refer to the corresponding lifestyle. In physical biology, bisexual refers to an individual who was born with gonadal tissue of both sexes (that is, both testicular and ovarian tissue). Also known as true hermaphrodite.

bite   In dental terms, how well the teeth fit together (occlude) in the mouth.

bitewing X-ray   A dental X-ray that shows how the teeth fit together on one side of the mouth.

BKA   Below-the-knee amputation. See *amputation.*

Black Death   See *bubonic plague.*

black eye   Bruising of the eyelid and/or the area around the eye as a result of trauma to the eye. Colloquially known as a shiner.

black lung disease   A disease of the lungs that is caused by inhaling coal dust, which in some patients can lead to progressive massive fibrosis of the lungs and severely impaired lung function. Also known as anthracosis and coal miner's pneumoconiosis.

Black Plague   See *bubonic plague.*

blackhead   A familiar term for what is medically called an open comedo. A comedo, the primary sign of acne, consists of a widened hair follicle filled with skin debris, bacteria, and oil called sebum. A blackhead has a wide opening to the skin and is capped with a blackened mass of skin debris. In contrast, a closed comedo, commonly called a whitehead, has an obstructed opening to the skin and may rupture to cause a low-grade skin inflammatory reaction in the area.

bladder   A hollow organ in the lower abdomen that stores urine. The kidneys filter waste from the blood and produce urine, which enters the bladder through two tubes, called ureters. Urine leaves the bladder through another tube, the urethra. In women, the urethra is a short tube that opens just in front of the vagina. In men, it is longer, passing through the prostate gland and then the penis. Also known as urinary bladder and vesical.

bladder cancer   A common form of cancer that begins in the lining of the bladder. The most common warning sign is blood in the urine. Symptoms include pain during urination, frequent urination, and feeling the need to urinate without results. A diagnosis of bladder cancer is supported by findings in the medical history, physical examination, examination of the urine, and intravenous pyelogram (IVP). Confirmation of the diagnosis requires a biopsy, usually using a cystoscope. The bladder is lined with cells called transitional cells and squamous cells. More than 90 percent of bladder cancers begin in the transitional cells, as transitional cell carcinoma. About 8 percent of bladder cancer patients have squamous cell carcinomas. A tumor may grow through the lining into the muscular wall of the bladder and extend into nearby organs such as the uterus or vagina (in women) or the prostate gland (in men). It may also invade the wall of the abdomen. When bladder cancer spreads beyond the bladder, the malignant cells are frequently found in nearby lymph nodes and may have spread to other lymph nodes or other places, including the lungs, liver, or bones. Risk factors for bladder cancer include age (people under 40 rarely get this disease), race (Caucasians are at twice the risk of African-Americans and Hispanic-Americans, with Asian-Americans at least risk), gender (men are two to three times more likely to get bladder cancer), family history of bladder cancer, use of tobacco (which is a major risk factor), occupational exposures (for example, workers in the rubber, chemical, and leather industries, hairdressers, machinists, metal workers, printers, painters, textile workers, and truck drivers), and prior treatment with cyclophosphamide or arsenic. Treatment depends on the growth, size, and location of the tumor. Surgical operations are commonly needed. Chemotherapy, biological therapy, or radiotherapy may also be used.

bladder infection   Infection of the urinary bladder. Some people are at greater risk for bladder infections and other urinary tract infections (UTIs) than others. Women are at greater risk than men; one woman in five develops a UTI during her lifetime. Not everyone with a UTI has symptoms. Common symptoms include a frequent urge to urinate and a painful burning when urinating. Underlying conditions that impair the normal urinary flow can lead to more complicated UTIs. Also known as bacterial cystitis. See also *bladder pain.*

bladder inflammation   Inflammation of the urinary bladder. Also called cystitis. Can be due to infection from bacteria that ascend the urethra to the bladder or for unknown reasons, such as with interstitial cystitis. Symptoms include a frequent need to urinate, often accompanied by a burning sensation. As bladder inflammation progresses, blood may be observed in the urine and the patient may suffer cramps after urination. In young children, attempts to avoid the pain of cystitis can be a cause for daytime wetting (enuresis). Treatment includes avoiding irritants, such as perfumed soaps, near the urethral opening; increased fluid intake; and, for infectious cystitis, antibiotics. Untreated bladder inflammation can lead to scarring and the formation of stones when urine is retained for long periods of time to avoid painful urination.

bladder, overactive A condition in which sudden involuntary contractions of the muscular wall of the bladder cause urinary urgency, immediate and unstoppable needs to urinate. Overactive bladder is a form of urinary incontinence (the unintentional loss of urine) and affects about 1 in 11 adults, particularly older adults. Treatment may include pelvic muscle strengthening, behavioral therapy, and medications. Also called urge incontinence.

bladder pain Pain from the urinary bladder. Among the symptoms of bladder infection are feelings of pain, pressure, and tenderness around the bladder, pelvis, and perineum (the area between the anus and vagina or anus and scrotum), which may increase as the bladder fills and decrease as it empties; decreased bladder capacity; an urgent need to urinate; painful sexual intercourse; and, in men, discomfort or pain in the penis and scrotum.

Blalock-Taussig operation A pioneering operation that is designed to treat children born with the heart malformation tetralogy of Fallot and that is named for the US surgeon Alfred Blalock and the US pediatric cardiologist Helen B. Taussig.

blast An immature blood cell.

blast crisis A phase of advanced leukemia, usually chronic myelogenous leukemia (CML), in which the number of immature, abnormal white blood cells (blasts) in the bone marrow and blood is extremely high. Also known as the blast phase. See also *leukemia.*

blastoma A tumor thought to arise in embryonic tissue. This term is commonly used as part of the name for a tumor, as in glioblastoma and medulloblastoma (types of brain tumors), hepatoblastoma (a liver tumor), nephroblastoma (a Wilms tumor of the kidney), neuroblastoma (a childhood tumor of neural origin), osteoblastoma (a bone tumor), and retinoblastoma (a tumor of the retina in the eye).

bleb See *blister.*

bleeding Loosing blood, usually because of a minor injury to the small blood vessels known as capillaries. In typical cases of bleeding, simply cleaning the site of injury and applying mild pressure or a bandage is sufficient treatment. If bleeding is caused by injury to a major blood vessel, emergency care is necessary. Bleeding through the skin without visible injury (internal bleeding) is a very serious condition and also requires emergency care.

Menstrual bleeding does not involve injury; it is the normal expulsion of uterine contents and does not involve the blood vessels at all. The formal term for bleeding is hemorrhage. See also *hemorrhage; menstruation.*

blepharospasm The involuntary, forcible closure of the eyelids. The first symptoms may be uncontrollable blinking. Only one eye may be affected initially, but eventually both eyes are usually involved. The spasms may leave the eyelids completely closed, causing functional blindness even though the eyes and vision are normal. Blepharospasm is a form of focal dystonia.

blind Unable to see. See also *blindness.*

blinded study A clinical trial of drugs in which the test participants do not know whether they are receiving the product being tested or a placebo (dummy). This blinding is intended to ensure that the study results are not affected by the power of suggestion (the placebo effect). The general principle of blinding can be applied to other types of studies, such as examining slides under a microscope. See also *double-blinded study.*

blindness Loss of useful sight. Blindness can be temporary or permanent, and there are many causes of blindness. Damage to any portion of the eye, the optic nerve, or the area of the brain that is responsible for vision can lead to blindness. Politically correct terms for blindness include visually handicapped, visually impaired, and visually challenged.

blindness, legal A degree of blindness that entitles a person to certain benefits according to the law. The definition of legal blindness varies from country to country. In the US, the definition of legal blindness that is used to determine eligibility for government disability benefits is as follows: **1** visual acuity of 20/200 or worse in the better eye with corrective lenses (20/200 means that a person must be at 20 feet from an eye chart to see what a person with normal vision can see at 200 feet); or **2** visual field restriction to 20 degrees diameter or less (tunnel vision) in the better eye. Note that these criteria do not necessarily indicate a person's ability to function.

blindness, night See *nyctanopia.*

blindness, river See *river blindness.*

blister A collection of fluid underneath the top layer of skin (epidermis). There are many causes of blisters, including burns, friction forces, and diseases of the skin. Also known as bleb and bulla.

Bloch-Sulzberger syndrome See *incontinentia pigmenti.*

blocker, beta   See *beta blocker.*

blood   The red fluid in the body that contains white and red blood cells, platelets, proteins, and other elements. Blood is transported throughout the body by the circulatory system. Blood functions in two directions: away from the heart (arterial blood) and toward the heart (venous blood). Arterial blood is the means by which oxygen and nutrients are transported to tissues, and venous blood is the means by which carbon dioxide is transported to the lungs for removal from the body.

blood–brain barrier   A protective network of blood vessels and cells that filters blood flowing to the brain. The blood–brain barrier normally prevents infectious agents and foreign substances from getting into the brain. Drugs designed to work within the central nervous system have to cross the blood–brain barrier or influence the behavior of a natural substance that can cross the blood–brain barrier, such as a neurotransmitter.

blood cell   One of several different types of cells that make up the blood. The erythrocytes (red blood cells) contain hemoglobin, which carries oxygen in the blood. The leukocytes (white blood cells) are a blood-borne part of the immune system. The platelets help blood to clot. Together, these three types of cells make up about half of the volume of blood. The remainder is made up of plasma. See also *erythrocyte; leukocyte; plasma; platelet.*

blood clot   A mass of coagulated blood. A blood clot can block a major blood vessel, causing stroke or other major trouble.

blood clot, estrogen-associated   A blood clot associated with estrogen therapy. Blood clots are occasional but serious side effects of estrogen therapy. They occur most frequently with high doses of estrogen. Cigarette smokers on estrogen therapy are at a higher risk for blood clots than nonsmokers are. Therefore, patients requiring estrogen therapy are strongly encouraged to quit smoking. See also *estrogen; estrogen replacement therapy.*

blood coagulation   The aggregation of blood platelets and other components to form a semisolid clot. Coagulation takes place due to the influence of the clotting factors fibrinogen, prothrombin, and thrombin, which are normally activated in response to injury. Working together, these substances thicken the blood and produce fibrin, a substance that closes off the wound. When blood coagulates abnormally, dangerous blood clots can enter the bloodstream.

blood conservation   Actions taken during medical treatment and surgery to limit the amount of donor blood needed.

blood count, complete   See *CBC.*

blood culture   A test that is designed to detect microorganisms, such as bacteria and fungi, in blood. A sample of blood obtained using a sterile technique is placed in a culture medium and incubated in a controlled environment. If microorganisms grow, their type can be identified, and they can be tested against different antibiotics for proper treatment of the infection. Because microorganisms may be only intermittently present in blood, a series of blood cultures is often done before the result is considered negative. See also *bacteremia; sepsis; septicemia.*

blood group   An inherited feature on the surface of the red blood cells. A series of related blood types constitutes a blood group system, such as the Rh or ABO system. The frequencies of the ABO and Rh blood types vary from population to population. In the US, the most common type is O+ (meaning O in the ABO system and positive in the Rh system), which is present in 37.4 percent of the population. The frequencies in the US (in descending order) are O+ (37.4 percent), A+ (35.7 percent), B+ (8.5 percent), O- (6.6 percent), A- (6.3 percent), AB+ (3.4 percent), B- (1.5 percent), and AB- (0.6 percent).

blood group, ABO   See *ABO blood group.*

blood in the urine   Blood that appears in the urine. Also known as hematuria. Gross hematuria refers to blood that is so plentiful in the urine that the blood is visible grossly, with just the naked eye. Microhematuria refers to blood in urine that is visible only under a microscope; there is so little blood that it cannot be seen without magnification. Hematuria, whether gross or microscopic, is abnormal and should be further investigated. It may or may not be accompanied by pain. Painful hematuria can be caused by a number of disorders, including infections and stones in the urinary tract. Painless hematuria can also be due to a large number of causes, including cancer.

blood marker   A sign of a disease or condition that can be isolated from a blood sample. For example, the monoclonal antibody D8/17 is a diagnostic sign of pediatric autoimmune disorders associated with strep.

blood poisoning   A bacterial infection of the blood. See also *bacteremia; sepsis; septicemia.*

blood pressure   The pressure of the blood within the arteries. Blood pressure is produced primarily by the contraction of the heart muscle. The measurement of blood pressure is recorded by two numbers. The first number (the systolic pressure) is measured after the heart contracts, and it is the higher number. The second number (the diastolic pressure) is measured before the heart contracts, and it is the lower number. A blood pressure cuff is used to measure pressure. See also *hypertension; hypotension; sphygmomanometer.*

blood pressure, high See *hypertension.*

blood pressure, low See *hypotension.*

blood sugar, high See *hyperglycemia.*

blood sugar, low See *hypoglycemia.*

blood test A test that requires a sample of blood. Some blood tests require only a finger stick, and others require a venipuncture (blood taken from a vein) or blood withdrawn from an artery.

blood thinner An anticoagulant agent; a medication that works against coagulating factors in the blood.

blood titer A blood test that tests for the level, or amount (titer), of something in the blood. For example, a strep titer looks for the level of streptococcus antibodies in the blood.

blood transfusion The transfer of blood or blood components from one person (the donor) into the bloodstream of another person (the recipient). Blood transfusion may be done as a lifesaving maneuver to replace blood cells or blood products lost through bleeding or due to depression of the bone marrow. Transfusion of one's own blood (autologous) is the safest method but requires advanced planning, and not all patients are eligible for it. Directed donor blood allows the patient to receive blood from known donors. Volunteer donor blood is usually most readily available and, when properly tested, has a low incidence of adverse events.

blood urea nitrogen A measure of the urea level in blood. Abbreviated BUN. Diseases that compromise the function of the kidney frequently lead to increased BUN levels.

blood, urinary See *blood in the urine.*

bloody nose See *nosebleed.*

bloody show Literally, the appearance of blood, a classic sign of impending labor. The bloody show consists of blood-tinged mucus created by extrusion and passage of the mucous plug that filled the cervical canal during pregnancy.

blot, Western A technique in molecular biology that is used to separate and identify proteins. It is called a

Western blot merely because it is similar to a Southern blot, which was named after its inventor, the British biologist M.E. Southern. For example, the Western blot assay method is commonly used to diagnose Lyme disease.

Blount disease See *tibia vara.*

blue baby See *cyanosis.*

blush Redness of the skin, typically over the cheeks or neck. Blushing is an involuntary response of the nervous system that leads to widening of the capillaries in the involved skin. A blush is temporary, and it is brought on by excitement, exercise, fever, or embarrassment. Also known as flush.

BM Physician's shorthand for black male.

BMI Body mass index.

BMJ *British Medical Journal,* one of the major general medical journals in the world. BMJ states that it "aims to help doctors everywhere practice better medicine and to influence the debate on health."

BMR Biological response modifier, a substance that modifies the body's response to infection and disease. The body naturally produces small amounts of BMRs. Scientists can produce some of them in the laboratory in large amounts for use in treating cancer, rheumatoid arthritis, and other diseases. BMRs used in biological therapy include monoclonal antibodies, interferon, interleukin-2 (IL-2), and several types of colony-stimulating factor (CSF, GM-CSF, G-CSF). For example, biological therapy to block the action of a messenger of inflammation, called tumor necrosis factor (TNF), is being used to treat conditions such as Crohn's disease and rheumatoid arthritis. Also known as biotherapy and immunotherapy.

board certified In medicine, a description for a physician who has taken and passed a medical specialty examination by one of several recognized boards of specialists. Before obtaining board certification, the physician must become board eligible.

board eligible In medicine, a description for a physician who has completed the requirements for admission to a medical specialty board examination but has not passed that examination. For example, a physician must have 3 years of training in an approved pediatric residency to be eligible for certification by the American Board of Pediatrics.

body dysmorphic disorder A psychiatric disorder characterized by excessive preoccupation with imagined defects in physical appearance. It is classified as an anxiety disorder, and it is believed to be a variant of obsessive-compulsive disorder. Also known as somatoform disorder and dysmorphophobia.

body mass index   A key index for relating weight to height. Abbreviated BMI. BMI is a person's weight in kilograms (kg) divided by his or her height in meters (m) squared. The National Institutes of Health (NIH) now defines normal weight, overweight, and obesity according to BMI rather than the traditional height/weight charts. Overweight is a BMI of 27.3 percent or more for women and 27.8 percent or more for men. Obesity is a BMI of 30 or more for either sex (about 30 pounds overweight). A very muscular person might have a high BMI without health risks.

body type   A somewhat old-fashioned term used to classify the human shape into three primary types: ecto-morphic, mesomorphic, or endomorphic.

bodywork   Any of a number of therapeutic or simply relaxing practices that involve the manipulation, massage, or regimented movement of body parts. Examples include massage, craniosacral therapy, and Pilates. Bodywork may be used as an adjunct to medical treatment, or it may be prescribed as a form of physical therapy for certain conditions.

boil   A skin abscess, a collection of pus that forms inside the body. The main treatments include hot packs and draining (lancing) the boil when it is soft. Antibiotics are usually not very helpful in treating boils. A person who has a fever or long-term illness, such as cancer or diabetes, or is taking medications that suppress the immune system should contact a health care practitioner on developing a boil. Also known as furuncle.

bone   The hard connective tissue that forms the skeleton of the body. It is composed chiefly of collagen fibers that contain calcium phosphate and calcium carbonate. Bones also serve as a storage area for calcium, playing a large role in calcium balance in the blood. The 206 bones in the human body serve a wide variety of purposes. They support and protect internal organs; for example, the ribs protect the lungs. Muscles pull against bones to make the body move. See also *bone marrow*.

bone, breast   See *sternum*.

bone cancer   A malignancy of bone. Primary bone cancer (cancer that begins in bone) is rare, but it is not unusual for cancers to metastasize (spread) to bone from other parts of the body, such as the breast, lung, and prostate. The most common type of primary bone cancer is osteosarcoma, which develops in new tissue in growing bones. Another type of cancer, chondrosarcoma, arises in

cartilage. Ewing's sarcoma begins in immature nerve tissue in bone marrow. Osteosarcoma and Ewing's sarcoma tend to occur in children and adolescents, and chondrosarcoma occurs most often in adults. Pain is the most frequent symptom of primary and metastatic cancer in bone. Tumors that occur in or near joints may cause swelling or tenderness in the affected area. Bone cancer can also interfere with normal movements and can weaken the bones, leading to fractures. Diagnosis of bone cancer is supported by findings of the medical history and examination, blood tests (including measuring the level of the enzyme for the enzyme alkaline phosphatase), and X-ray studies, and it is confirmed by a biopsy. Treatment depends on the type, location, size, and extent of the tumor. Surgery is often the primary treatment. Although amputation of a limb is sometimes necessary for primary bone cancer, chemotherapy has made limb-sparing surgery possible in many cases. Radiation may also be used.

bone, cuboid   The outer bone in the instep of the foot. It is called the cuboid bone because it is shaped like a cube. The cuboid bone is jointed in back with the heel bone (calcaneus) and in front with the bones just behind the fourth and fifth toes (metatarsals).

bone cyst, aneurysmal   A benign lesion in a bone that contains connective tissue and blood inside a thin bony shell. Aneurismal bone cysts act like tumors and expand the bone, and they typically occur in the second decade of life. They can affect any bone in the arms, legs, trunk, or skull. Abbreviated ABC.

bone cyst, simple   A solitary fluid-filled cyst (cavity) in a bone, usually in the shaft of a long bone, especially the humerus, in a child. A simple bone cyst can cause pain in or near the bone. Also known as unicameral bone cyst and solitary bone cyst.

bone density   The amount of bone tissue in a certain volume of bone. Bone density can be measured by using a special X-ray called a quantitative computed tomogram or by dual energy X-ray absorptometry (DEXA) scan.

bone, heel   See *calcaneus*.

bone marrow   The soft blood-forming tissue that fills the cavities of bones and contains fat and immature and mature blood cells, including white blood cells, red blood cells, and platelets. Diseases or drugs that affect the bone marrow can affect the total counts of these cells.

bone marrow aspiration   The removal of a small amount of liquid bone marrow through a needle. The needle is placed through the top layer of bone, and a liquid sample containing bone marrow cells is obtained through the needle by aspirating (sucking) it into a syringe. The suction causes pain for a few moments. Bone marrow aspiration is done to diagnose and follow the progress of various conditions, including anemia and cancer, and to obtain marrow for transplantation.

bone marrow biopsy The removal of a sample of bone marrow and a small amount of bone through a large needle. Two samples are taken. The first is bone marrow by aspiration (suction with a syringe). The second is a core biopsy to obtain bone marrow along with bone fibers. After the needle is removed, this solid sample is pushed out of the needle with a wire. Both samples are examined under a microscope to examine the cells and the architecture of the bone marrow.

bone marrow transplant A procedure in which diseased or damaged bone marrow is replaced with healthy bone marrow. The bone marrow to be replaced may be deliberately destroyed by high doses of chemotherapy and/or radiation therapy. Replacement marrow may come from another person, or the patient's own marrow may be removed and stored before treatment for later use. When marrow from an unrelated donor is used, the procedure is called an allogeneic bone marrow transplantation. If the marrow is from an identical twin, it is termed syngeneic. Autologous bone marrow transplantation uses the patient's own marrow. Abbreviated BMT. See also *transplant*.

bone scan A technique for creating images of bones on a computer screen or on film. A small amount of radioactive material is injected and travels through the bloodstream. It collects in the bones, especially in abnormal areas of the bones, and is detected by an instrument called a scanner. Bone scans are used for the detection and monitoring of disorders that affect the bones, including Paget disease, cancer, infections, and fractures. Bone scanning is also helpful in evaluating and measuring the activity of certain joint diseases.

bone, sesamoid A little bone that is embedded in a joint capsule or tendon; for example, the kneecap (patella).

bone, shin The larger of the two bones in the lower leg. The shin bone is anatomically known as the tibia. Its smaller companion is the fibula.

bones, appendicular See *bones of the arm, wrist, and hand*.

bones, axial See *bones of the head*.

bones, lower extremity See *bones of the leg, ankle, and foot*.

bones of the arm, wrist, and hand There are 64 bones in the upper extremities. They consist of 10 shoulder and arm, 16 wrist, and 38 hand bones. The 10 shoulder and arm bones are the clavicle, scapula, humerus, radius, and ulna on each side. The 16 wrist bones are the scaphoid, lunate, triquetrum, pisiform, trapezium, trapezoid, capitate, and hamate on each side. The 38 hand bones are the 10 metacarpal bones and 28 finger bones (phalanges). Also known as appendicular bones.

bones of the head There are 29 bones in the human head. They include 8 cranial bones, 14 facial bones, the hyoid bone, and 6 ear (auditory) bones. The 8 cranial bones are the frontal, 2 parietal, occipital, 2 temporal, sphenoid, and ethmoid bones. The 14 facial bones are the 2 maxilla, the mandible, 2 zygoma, 2 lacrimal, 2 nasal, 2 turbinate, vomer, and 2 palate bones. The hyoid bone is the horseshoe-shaped bone at the base of the tongue. The 6 small auditory bones (ossicles) are the malleus, incus, and stapes in each ear. Along with the bones of the trunk, also known as axial bones. See also *bones of the trunk*.

bones of the leg, ankle, and foot There are 62 lower extremity bones. They consist of 10 hip and leg, 14 ankle, and 38 foot bones. The 10 hip and leg bones are the innominate, or hip, bone (which is a fusion of the ilium, ischium, and pubis), and the femur, tibia, fibula, and patella (kneecap) on each side. The 14 ankle bones are the talus, calcaneus (heel bone), navicular, cuboid, internal cuneiform, middle cuneiform, and external cuneiform on each side. The 38 foot bones are the 10 metatarsals and 28 toe bones (phalanges).

bones of the skeleton The human body has 206 bones. These consist of 80 axial (head and trunk) bones and 126 appendicular (upper and lower extremity) bones. See also *bones of the arm, wrist, and hand; bones of the head; bones of the leg, ankle, and foot; bones of the trunk*.

bones of the trunk The 51 trunk bones consist of 26 vertebrae, 24 ribs, and the sternum. The 26 vertebrae comprise 7 cervical, 12 thoracic, and 5 lumbar vertebrae, plus the sacrum and the coccyx. The 24 ribs comprise 14 true ribs, 6 false ribs, and 4 floating ribs. The sternum is the breastbone. Along with the bones of the head, also known as axial bones.

bony syndactyly A condition in which the bones of the fingers or toes are joined together. Bony syndactyly is not the same as cutaneous syndactyly, which only involves webbing of the skin between the digits.

bony tarsus A structure that is made up of seven bones situated between the bones of the lower leg and the metatarsus bones of the feet. The seven bones of the bony tarsus are the calcaneus, talus (astragalus), cuboid, and navicular (scaphoid), plus the first, second, and third cuneiform bones. The bony tarsus contributes to the broad, flat framework of the foot.

booster shot An additional dose of a vaccine needed periodically to "boost" the immune system. For example, a booster shot of the tetanus and diphtheria (Td) vaccine is recommended for adults every 10 years.

borborygmus A gurgling, rumbling, or squeaking noise from the abdomen that is caused by the movement of gas through the bowels. Also known as stomach rumbling. The plural is borborygmi.

borderline personality disorder A personality type characterized by difficulty forming and keeping stable relationships, highly emotional or aggressive behavior, impulsivity, and rapid shifts in values, self-image, mood, and behavior.

Bornholm disease A viral infection that is most commonly caused by an enterovirus called Coxsackie B. Symptoms include fever, intense abdominal and chest pain, and headache. The chest pain is caused by inflammation of the tissue lining the lungs, and it is typically worsened by breathing or coughing. The illness usually lasts from 3 to 14 days. Also known as epidemic myalgia and pleurodynia.

botox A highly purified preparation of botulinum toxin A, a toxin produced by the bacterium Clostridium botulinum. Botox is injected, in very small amounts, into specific muscles, as a treatment. It acts by blocking the transmission of nerve impulses to muscles and so paralyzes the muscles. Botox treatment has found a growing number of uses from easing muscle spasms (as, for example, in spastic cerebral palsy) to its increasingly widespread cosmetic use in flattening wrinkles.

bottlefeeding The practice of feeding an infant a substitute for breast milk. Pediatricians generally advise exclusively breastfeeding (that is, breastfeeding with no supplementary formula) for all full-term, healthy infants for the first 6 months of life. However, many infants are bottlefed today, at least in part. For infants to achieve normal growth and maintain normal health, infant formulas must include proper amounts of water, carbohydrate, protein, fat, vitamins, and minerals.

botulism An uncommon but potentially very serious type of food poisoning that produces paralysis of muscles, via a nerve toxin called botulinum toxin (botox) that is manufactured by the bacteria Clostridium botulinum. There are various types of botulism, including food-borne, wound, infant intestinal, and adult intestinal botulism. The symptoms of botulism can range from mild, including transient nausea and vomiting, to severe cases that progress to heart and lung failure and death. Food-borne botulism occurs typically in unrefrigerated or poorly refrigerated foods and foods without preservatives, especially uncooked or half-cooked meats. It can be prevented through careful use of refrigeration and preservative techniques, and the toxin can be destroyed with heat. Clostridium botulin and botulinum toxin might, it is feared, be misused as agents of bioterrorism. See also *bioterrorism; food poisoning.*

boutonneuse See *typhus, African tick.*

bowel The small and large intestine.

bowel disease, inflammatory A group of chronic intestinal diseases characterized by inflammation of the bowel (the small and large intestine). Abbreviated IBD. The most common types of IBD are ulcerative colitis and Crohn's disease. The portion of the intestine that is affected becomes irritated and swollen, and ulcers may form. IBD can be limited to the intestine or associated with disease involving the skin, joints, spine, liver, eyes, and other organs. The cause is not always known, although it can be caused or made worse by infection. Symptoms include abdominal pain and diarrhea. The course of IBD is unpredictable. Symptoms tend to wax and wane, and long remissions and even spontaneous resolution of symptoms are well known. Although people of any age can be affected, IBD is most common in young adults. Treatment involves dietary changes, the use of medicines, and sometimes surgery, depending on the type and course of the disease under care. Effective therapy exists for the majority of cases. Narcotics, codeine, and antidiarrheal medications should be avoided during severe episodes of IBD because they may induce a toxic megacolon. See also *Crohn's disease; colitis, ulcerative.*

bowel disorders and fiber High-fiber diets help delay the progression of and number of bouts with diverticulosis. In many cases, high-fiber diets help reduce the symptoms of irritable bowel syndrome (IBS). It is generally accepted that a diet high in fiber is protective or at least reduces the incidence of colon polyps and colon cancer.

Bowen's disease See *cancer, skin.*

bowlegs A condition in which the legs curve out, leaving a gap between the knees, after infancy. Bowlegs can be corrected with surgery or casting. Also known as genu varum and tibia vara.

BP **1** In genetics, base pair. **2** In general medicine, blood pressure. On a medical chart, you might see "BP90/60 T98.6 Ht60/reg R15," which signifies that the blood pressure (BP) is 90/60 mm Hg, the temperature (T) is 98.6° Fahrenheit, the heart rate (Ht) is 60 beats per minute and regular, and respirations are occurring at 15 per minute.

BPH Benign prostatic hyperplasia, benign prostatic hypertrophy.

brace, foot drop See *ankle-foot orthosis.*

braces, dental Devices used by orthodontists to move teeth or adjust underlying bone. The ideal time for starting orthodontic treatment is between ages 3 and 12 years. Temporomandibular joint (TMJ) problems can also sometimes be corrected with dental braces. Teeth can be moved by removable appliances or by fixed braces. If there is crowding of teeth, some teeth may need to be extracted before braces are applied. Retainers may be necessary long after dental braces are placed, especially in orthodontic treatment of adults.

brachial artery The artery that runs from the shoulder down to the elbow. See also *brachial vein.*

brachial plexus A bundle of nerves that begins in the back of the base of the neck and extends through the axilla. It is formed by the union of portions of the fifth through eighth cervical spinal nerves and the first thoracic spinal nerve. Damage to the brachial plexus can affect nerves supplying the arm and chest.

brachial vein A vein that accompanies the brachial artery between the shoulder and the elbow. The route of the brachial vein is from the elbow up to the shoulder. See also *brachial artery.*

brachy- Prefix indicating short, as in brachycephaly (short head) and brachydactyly (short fingers and toes).

brachycephaly A condition in which the head is unusually short in diameter from front to back. Brachycephaly is frequently a feature in congenital malformation syndromes, including Down syndrome (trisomy 21).

brachydactyly A condition in which the fingers and toes are short and stubby. Brachydactyly is a common finding in malformation sydromes, such as Down syndrome (trisomy 21).

brachytherapy Radiation treatment given by placing radioactive material directly in or near the target, which is often a tumor. Brachytherapy for prostate cancer, for example, is also called interstitial radiation therapy or seed implantation. In brachytherapy for prostate cancer, radioactive seeds are implanted in the prostate. The seeds might be titanium-encased pellets that contain the radioisotope iodine-125.

brady- Prefix indicating slow, as in bradycardia (slow heart rate), bradykinesia (slow ability to start and continue movements), and bradyphrenia (slow thought processes).

bradycardia A slow heart rate, usually defined as less than 60 beats per minute.

bradykinesia A slow ability to start and continue movements, and an impaired ability to adjust the body's position. Bradykinesia can be a symptom of neurological disorders, particularly Parkinson's disease, or a side effect of medications.

bradyphrenia A slow thought processes. Bradyphrenia can be a side effect of certain psychiatric medications.

Braille A system of raised-dot writing for the blind in which each letter is represented as a raised pattern that can be read by touching it with the fingers. In Braille, dot patterns are assigned to letters of the alphabet, punctuation marks, and other symbols. Braille was devised by Louis Braille.

brain The portion of the central nervous system that is located within the skull. It functions as a primary receiver, organizer, and distributor of information for the body. It has a right half and a left half, each of which is called a hemisphere.

brain aneurysm See *aneurysm, brain.*

brain cancer A malignant growth of the brain. See also *brain tumor.*

brain death The permanent, irreversible cessation of all brain functions. Brain death is not the same thing as a coma or vegetative state. The presence of brain death is legally synonymous with death itself in most US states.

brain, fornix of the One of a pair of arching fibrous bands in the brain that connects the two lobes of the cerebrum.

brain malleability See *brain plasticity.*

brain plasticity The phenomenon of change and learning in the adult brain. Also known as brain malleability.

brain stem　The stem-like part of the brain that is connected to the spinal cord. The brain stem controls the flow of messages between the brain and the rest of the body, and it also controls basic body functions such as breathing, swallowing, heart rate, blood pressure, consciousness, and whether one is awake or sleepy. The brain stem consists of the midbrain, pons, and medulla oblongata.

brain stem glioma　A type of brain tumor that involves the glial cells.

brain tumor　A benign or malignant growth in the brain. Primary brain tumors initially form in brain tissue. Secondary brain tumors are cancers that have spread (metastasized) to the brain tissue from tissue elsewhere in the body. Brain tumors can occur in people of any age.

brain ventricle　One of the communicating cavities within the brain. There are four ventricles: two lateral ventricles, the third ventricle, and the fourth ventricle. The lateral ventricles are in the cerebral hemispheres. Each lateral ventricle consists of a triangular central body and four horns. The lateral ventricles communicate with the third ventricle through the interventricular foramen (opening). The third ventricle is a median (midline) cavity in the brain, bounded by the thalamus and hypothalamus on either side. In front, the third ventricle communicates with the lateral ventricles, and in back it communicates with the aqueduct of the midbrain (the aqueduct of Sylvius). The fourth ventricle is the lowest of the four venticles of the brain. It extends from the aqueduct of the midbrain to the central canal of the upper end of the spinal cord, with which it communicates by the two foramina (openings) of Luschka and the foramen of Magendie. The ventricles are filled with cerebrospinal fluid, which is formed by structures, called choroid plexuses, that are located in the walls and roofs of the ventricles.

brain, water on the　See *hydrocephalus*.

branchial cleft cyst　A cavity that is a remnant from embryologic development and is still present at birth in one side of the neck, just in front of the large angulated muscle on either side (the sternocleidomastoid muscle). The cyst may not be recognized until adolescence, when it enlarges its oval shape. Sometimes a branchial cleft cyst develops a sinus or drainage pathway to the surface of the skin, from which mucus can be expressed. Total surgical excision is the treatment of choice. Recurrence is not expected. Also known as branchial cyst.

branchial cyst　See *branchial cleft cyst*.

Braxton Hicks contraction　An irregular contraction of the womb (uterus) that occurs toward the middle of a woman's first pregnancy and earlier, and more intensely, in her subsequent pregnancies. Braxton Hicks contractions tend to occur during physical activity. The uterus tightens for 30 to 60 seconds, beginning at the top of the uterus, and the contraction gradually spreads downward before the uterus relaxes. Although they are said to be painless, Braxton Hicks contractions may be quite uncomfortable and sometimes difficult to distinguish from the contractions of true labor.

BRCA1　A tumor suppressor gene that normally acts to restrain the growth of cells. Mutated forms of BRCA1 and BRCA2 are responsible for about half the cases of inherited breast cancer, especially those that occur in relatively young women. From the words *breast* and *cancer*. See also *breast cancer susceptibility gene*.

BRCA2　A tumor suppressor gene that normally acts to restrain the growth of cells. Mutations of BRCA2, like those of BRCA1, are responsible mainly for hereditary breast cancer. They seldom appear to be involved in sporadic, noninherited breast cancer—the 95 percent of breast cancer that does not run in families. Both BRCA1 and BRCA2 are large, complex genes. From the words *breast* and *cancer*. See also *breast cancer susceptibility gene*.

breakbone fever　See *dengue fever*.

breast　The front of the chest or, more specifically, the mammary gland. The mammary gland is a milk-producing gland that is largely composed of fat. Within the mammary gland are sac-like structures called lobules, which produce the milk, as well as a complex network of branching ducts. These ducts exit from the lobules at the nipple. The lobules and ducts are supported in the breast by surrounding fatty tissue and ligaments. The breast contains blood vessels and lymphatics, but no muscles. The lymphatics are thin channels similar to blood vessels; they do not carry blood, but they collect and carry tissue fluid, which ultimately reenters the bloodstream. Breast fluid drains through the lymphatics into the lymph nodes located in the underarm (axilla) and behind the breastbone (sternum). The appearance of the normal female breast differs greatly among individuals and at different times during a woman's life: before, during, and after adolescence; during pregnancy; during the menstrual cycle; and after menopause. The nipple of the breast becomes erect because of cold, breastfeeding, and sexual activity. The pigmented area around the nipple is called the areola. See also *gland, mammary*.

breast absence　See *amastia*.

breast augmentation Enlargement of the breasts. Breast augmentation may be done by insertion of a silicone bag (prosthesis) under the breast (submammary) or under the breast and chest muscle (subpectoral), after which the bag is filled with saline solution. This prosthesis expands the breast area to give the appearance of a fuller breast (increased cup size).

breast bone See *sternum*.

breast cancer A common form of cancer that begins in the breast. There are many types of breast cancer, and they differ in their capability for spreading to other body tissues (metastasis). Breast cancer can occur in both men and women, although it is more common in women. Some forms of breast cancer are genetic (inherited), and others are linked to exposure to cancer-causing substances, but most cases of breast cancer occur for unknown reasons. Risk factors for breast cancer may include genetic predisposition, as indicated by a history of breast cancer in close relatives; overexposure of the chest to radiation, smoking, childlessness, induced abortion, obesity and diet, and exposure to carcinogenic substances. Breast cancer is diagnosed with self-examination and physician examination of the breasts, mammography, ultrasound testing, and biopsy. Treatment depends on the type and location of the breast cancer, as well as the age and health of the patient. Options may include lumpectomy (removal of the small, cancerous area only), chemotherapy, radiation, and partial or total mastectomy. The American Cancer Society recommends that all women should perform regular breast self-exams and that women should have a baseline mammogram done between the ages of 35 and 40 years. Between 40 and 50 years of age, mammograms are recommended every other year. After age 50, yearly mammograms are recommended. Breast cancer prevention includes diet changes, avoiding carcinogens when possible, and screening. Most breast cancers are treatable when caught early, and survival rates are high. See also *breast cancer susceptibility gene; breast cancer, familial; breast, infiltrating ductal carcinoma of the; breast, infiltrating lobular carcinoma of the; mastectomy*.

breast cancer, familial A form of breast cancer that tends to occur in members of the same family. A number of factors have been identified as increasing the risk of breast cancer. One of the strongest is a history of breast cancer in a relative. About 15 to 20 percent of women with breast cancer have such a family history of the disease, clearly reflecting the participation of inherited (genetic) components in the development of some breast cancers. Dominant breast cancer susceptibility genes, including BRCA1 and BRCA2, appear to be responsible for about 5 percent of all breast cancer. See also *BRCA1; BRCA2; breast cancer susceptibility gene*.

breast cancer, male Breast cancer in men. Male breast cancer is much less common than breast cancer in women. Fewer than 1 percent of persons with breast cancer are male. However, breast cancer is no less dangerous in males than in females. After the diagnosis of breast cancer is made, the mortality rates are virtually the same for men and for women.

breast cancer susceptibility gene An inherited factor that predisposes an individual to breast cancer. Two of these genes, BRCA1 and BRCA2, have been identified. Several other genes (those for Li-Fraumeni syndrome, Cowden disease, Muir-Torre syndrome, and ataxia-telangiectasia) are also known to predispose women to breast cancer. However, because all these known breast cancer susceptibility genes together do not account for more than a minor fraction of breast cancer that clusters in families, it is clear that more breast cancer genes remain to be discovered. See also *BRCA1; BRCA2*.

breast, infiltrating ductal carcinoma of the One of several recognized specific patterns of cancer of the breast, so named because it begins in the cells that form the ducts of the breast. It is the most common form of breast cancer, comprising 65 to 85 percent of all cases. On a mammogram, invasive ductal carcinoma is usually visualized as a mass with fine spikes radiating from the edges (spiculation). It may also appear as a smooth-edged lump in the breast. On physical examination, this lump usually feels much harder or firmer than benign lumps in the breast, which are usually cysts. On microscopic examination, the cancerous cells that are invading and replacing normal breast tissue can be seen.

breast, infiltrating lobular carcinoma of the The second most common type of invasive breast cancer, accounting for 5 to 10 percent of breast cancer. Infiltrating lobular carcinoma starts in the lobules, the glands that secrete milk, and then infiltrates surrounding tissue. On a mammogram, a lobular carcinoma can look similar to a ductal carcinoma. However, on physical examination of the breast, a lobular carcinoma is usually not a hard mass, as a ductal carcinoma is, but rather a vague thickening of the breast tissue. Lobular carcinoma can occur in more than one site in the breast (a multi-centric tumor) or in both breasts at the same time (a bilateral lobular carcinoma).

breast, Paget's disease of The combination of scaly skin on the nipple that resembles eczema and an underlying cancer of the breast. The nipple is inflamed because of the presence of Paget's cells, which are large, irregular cells that are themselves not cancerous but that are almost always associated with cancer in the breast. The cause of the Paget's cells is still a mystery. In Paget's disease, the nipple and areola (the area surrounding the nipple) are typically red, inflamed, and itchy. There may be crusting, bleeding, or ulceration. The nipple may be inverted (turned inward), and there may be a discharge from the nipple. A lump that can be palpated (felt) in the breast is present in almost half of cases. Paget's disease of the breast accounts for a small but significant minority (1 to 4 percent) of all breast tumors. It usually occurs in women in their 50s, but it can occur at a later age. Its occurrence in men is very rare. Also called Paget's disease of the nipple.

breastbone　See *sternum.*

breastfeeding　The highly recommended practice of feeding an infant with the mother's natural milk. Breast milk contains vitamins, minerals, and enzymes that aid the baby's digestion, and immunity factors in breast milk can help infants fight off infections. Breast milk can be expressed, manually or with the assistance of a breast pump, for use while the mother is away, or breastfeeding and formula-feeding can be used together. The activity of breastfeeding has strong benefits for mothers as well as infants: It encourages the release of hormones that improve uterine muscle tone, and it may help to prevent breast cancer. The ability of the breast to produce milk diminishes soon after childbirth without the stimulation of breastfeeding. Also known as nursing. See also *lactation.*

breathing　The process of respiration, during which air is inhaled into the lungs through the mouth or nose due to muscle contraction and then exhaled due to muscle relaxation.

BREC　Benign rolandic epilepsy of childhood. See *epilepsy, benign rolandic.*

breech　The buttocks.

breech birth　Birth of a baby with the buttocks, rather than the head, emerging first. Breech birth is more likely to cause injury to the mother or the infant than head-first birth. In many cases a baby in the breech position can be turned before delivery by using repeated, gentle massage.

bridge　1 A set of one or more false teeth that is supported by a metal framework and used to replace one or more missing teeth. 2 A form of treatment that serves as a transition from a previous form of treatment and is followed with another form, such as in "bridge therapy." 3 Tissue that forms an arc over adjacent tissue(s). For example, heart tissue that has formed over a coronary artery, sometimes physically pinching the artery, is referred to as a myocardial bridge.

Brill-Zinsser disease　Recrudescence (reactivation) of epidemic typhus years after an earlier attack of the disease. Rickettsia prowazekii, the agent that causes epidemic typhus, remains viable for many years. When the host's defenses are down, it can be reactivated. See also *rickettsial disease; typhus, epidemic.*

brittle bone disease　See *osteogenesis imperfecta.*

Broca area　An area of the cerebral motor cortex in the frontal lobe of the brain that is responsible for speech development. Damage to the Broca area can cause speech disorders, including aphasia, apraxia, and dyspraxia. See also *aphasia; apraxia of speech; dyspraxia of speech.*

Broda test　See *basal temperature.*

bronchi　The plural of bronchus.

bronchiole　The tiny branch of air tubes within the lungs that is a continuation of the bronchus. The bronchioles connect to the alveoli (air sacs).

bronchiolitis　A childhood disease characterized by inflammation of the bronchioles, usually due to viral infections.

bronchitis　Inflammation and swelling of the bronchi. Bronchitis can be acute or chronic.

bronchitis, acute　An infection of the bronchi of recent origin, typically characterized by cough, chest discomfort, and production of mucus (sputum). Acute bronchitis is treated with antibiotics.

bronchitis, chronic　A daily cough, accompanied by production of mucus (sputum) for 3 months, that lasts for 2 years in a row. In chronic bronchitis, there is inflammation and swelling of the lining of the airways, leading to narrowing and obstruction of the airways. The inflammation stimulates production of mucus, which can cause further obstruction of the airways. Obstruction of the airways, especially with mucus, increases the likelihood of bacterial lung infections. Chronic bronchitis is common in persons who have smoked for extended periods.

bronchopulmonary dysplasia　A chronic lung disease in infants who received mechanical respiratory support with high oxygenation in the neonatal period.

bronchopulmonary segment　A subdivision of one lobe of a lung, based on the connection to the segmental bronchus. For example, the right upper lobe of the lung has apical, anterior, and posterior segments.

bronchoscope　A thin, flexible instrument that is used to view the air passages to the lung.

bronchoscopy A test that permits the physician to see the breathing passages through a lighted tube.

bronchospasm A temporary narrowing of the airways in the lung. Bronchospasm causes the breathing difficulties seen in asthma. See also *asthma*.

bronchospasm, exercise-induced See *asthma, exercise-induced*.

bronchus A large air tube that begins at the end of the trachea and branches into the lungs. The supporting walls of the bronchus are made up in part of cartilage.

Brown's syndrome An eye abnormality that is present at birth and that is characterized by an inability to elevate the eyeball when trying to move the eyeball to the outside. Brown's syndrome can also be caused by other conditions that affect the normal function of the eye muscles, such as nodules from rheumatoid arthritis or rare tumors in the eye muscle.

Brucellosis An infectious disease characterized by rising and lowering (undulant) fever, sweating, muscle and joint pains, and weakness. Brucellosis is caused by a bacterium called Brucella, which can be transmitted in unpasteurized milk from cattle, sheep, and goats; cheese made from this unpasteurized milk; and contact with diseased animals. Antibiotics are used to treat Brucellosis. Also known as undulant fever.

bruise A traumatic injury of the soft tissues that results in breakage of the local capillaries and leakage of red blood cells. In the skin it can be seen as a reddish-purple discoloration that does not blanch when pressed. When a bruise fades, it becomes green and brown, as the body metabolizes the blood cells in the skin. It is best treated with local application of a cold pack immediately after injury. Also known as contusion.

Brushfield spot A little white spot on the surface of the iris. Brushfield spots are arranged in a ring, concentric with the pupil. These spots occur in normal children but are far more frequent in those with Down syndrome (trisomy 21). Brushfield spots are due to aggregation of a normal iris element (connective tissue). Also called speckled iris.

bruxism Grinding and gnashing of the teeth. Bruxism is due to clenching of the teeth other than in chewing and is associated with forceful lateral or protrusive jaw movements. This results in the grinding or rubbing together of the teeth. Bruxism can injure teeth and cause local pain in the mouth or jaw and may contribute to temporomandibular joint (TMJ) syndrome. From the Greek *brychein*, meaning "to grind or gnash the opposing rows of upper and lower molar teeth."

bubo An enlarged lymph node that is tender and painful. Buboes particularly occur in the groin and armpit (the axillae). These swollen glands are seen in a number of infectious diseases, including gonorrhea, syphilis, tuberculosis, and the eponymous bubonic plague.

bubonic plague An infectious disease that is caused by the bacterium Yersinia pestis and is transmitted to humans from infected rats by the oriental rat flea. It is named for the characteristic feature of buboes (painfully enlarged lymph nodes) in the groin, armpits (axillae), neck, and elsewhere. Other symptoms of bubonic plague include headache, fever, chills, and weakness. Bubonic plague can lead to gangrene (tissue death) of the fingers, toes, and nose. Also called Black Death and Black Plague.

buccal mucosa The inner lining of the cheeks and lips.

bulimia An eating disorder characterized by periods of extreme overeating, often interrupted by periods of anorexia. Bulimia is usually accompanied by self-induced vomiting or other forms of purging, including the use of laxatives, obsessive exercise, or fasting. Bulimia can be life-threatening due to dehydration, and it can cause permanent damage to the bowels, liver, kidney, teeth, and heart. It also raises a person's risk of seizures. It is believed to be closely related to obsessive-compulsive disorder. Treatment may include cognitive behavior therapy, dietary and health education, and antidepressant medication. The full name of the disorder is bulimia nervosa. See also *anorexia nervosa; body dysmorphic disorder; obsessive-compulsive disorder*.

bulla See *blister*.

bullous Characterized by blistering, such as a second-degree burn.

bullous pemphiguoid A disease characterized by tense, blistering eruptions of the skin. It is caused by antibodies abnormally accumulating in a layer of the skin called the basement membrane. Bullous pemphiguoid can be chronic and mild without affecting the general health. It is diagnosed by skin biopsy showing the abnormal antibodies deposited in the skin layer. Treatment is with topical cortisone creams but sometimes requires high doses of cortisone (steroids) taken internally.

bump A raised area resulting from blood leaking from injured blood vessels into the tissues, as well as from the body's response to the injury. A purplish, flat bruise that occurs when blood leaks out into the top layers of skin is referred to as an ecchymosis.

BUN Blood urea nitrogen.

bunion A localized, painful swelling at the base of the big toe. The joint becomes enlarged due to new bone formation, and the toe is often misaligned. Bunions are frequently associated with inflammation of the nearby bursa (bursitis) and degenerative joint disease (osteoarthritis). Bunions most commonly affect women, particularly those who wear tight-fitting shoes and high heels. Treatment includes rest, a change in shoes, foot supports, medications, or surgery.

Burkitt lymphoma A type of non-Hodgkin lymphoma (NHL) that most often occurs in young people between the ages of 12 and 30 and accounts for about half of all childhood NHL. Burkitt lymphoma usually causes a rapidly growing tumor in the abdomen and, less often, tumors in the testis, sinuses, bone, lymph nodes, skin, bone marrow, or central nervous system. Burkitt lymphoma is a tumor of B cell origin. See also *lymphoma, non-Hodgkin's.*

burn Damage to the skin or other body parts caused by extreme heat, flame, contact with heated objects, or chemicals. Burn depth is generally categorized as first, second, or third degree. The treatment of burns depends on the depth, area, and location of the burn, as well as additional factors, such as material that may be burned onto or into the skin. Treatment options range from simply applying a cold pack to emergency treatment to skin grafts.

burn, first degree A superficial burn with similar characteristics to a typical sunburn. The skin is red in color, sensation is intact, and the burn is usually somewhat painful.

burn, second degree A burn severe enough to cause blistering of the skin. The pain of a second-degree burn is usually somewhat more intense than the pain of a first-degree burn.

burn, third degree A burn in which the damage has progressed to the point of skin death. The skin is white and without sensation. In extreme cases damage may extend beyond the skin and into underlying tissue. In these cases the skin may be blackened or burned away. Unless skin grafts are feasible, loss of the affected limb, permanent disfigurement, and even death are likely in such severe cases.

burning mouth syndrome An intense burning sensation on the tongue, often at the tip of the tongue. Burning mouth syndrome tends to develop in "supertasters"—people with an unusually large density of taste buds, each surrounded by pain fibers—and in postmenopausal women, who may lose their ability to sense bitter tastes as a result of burning mouth syndrome. Clonazepam (brand name: Klonopin), an antiseizure drug, is reportedly effective in treating burning mouth syndrome in more than 70 percent of patients.

bursa A closed, fluid-filled sac that functions as a gliding surface to reduce friction between tissues of the body. When a bursa becomes inflamed, the condition is known as bursitis.

bursitis Inflammation of a bursa, causing joint pain and restriction of movement. See also *bursa; bursitis, aseptic; bursitis, calcific; bursitis, elbow; bursitis, hip; bursitis, knee; bursitis, septic; bursitis, shoulder.*

bursitis, aseptic Bursitis that is not due to an infectious condition. Treatment of noninfectious bursitis includes rest, ice, and medications for inflammation and pain.

bursitis, calcific Chronic bursitis with calcification of the bursa. The calcium deposition can occur as long as the inflammation is present.

bursitis, elbow Inflammation of the bursa at the tip of the elbow, called the olecranon bursa. The olecranon bursa is a common site of bursitis.

bursitis, hip Inflammation of a bursa of the hip. There are two major bursae of the hip, which is a common location for bursitis.

bursitis, knee Inflammation of a bursa of the knee. There are three major bursae of the knee, which is a common site for bursitis.

bursitis, septic Inflammation of a bursa due to infection, usually with bacteria. Septic bursitis is treated with antibiotics, aspiration, and surgery. Also known as infectious bursitis.

bursitis, shoulder Inflammation of a bursa of the shoulder. There are two major bursae of the shoulder, which is a common location for bursitis.

butterfly rash A red, flat, butterfly-shaped facial rash over the bridge of the nose. More than half of patients with systemic lupus erythematosus (SLE) develop this characteristic rash. The butterfly rash of lupus is typically painless and does not itch. Along with inflammation in other organs, the rash can be precipitated or worsened by exposure to sunlight. This photosensitivity can be accompanied by a worsening of inflammation throughout the body, causing a flare-up of the disease. A similar rash can also occur in other conditions, such as rosacea. Also known as a malar rash. See also *lupus; lupus, discoid; lupus erythematosis, systemic.*

bypass An operation in which a new pathway is created for the movement of substances in the body.

bypass, cardiopulmonary A bypass of the heart and lungs as, for example, in open heart surgery. In this procedure, blood returning to the heart is diverted through a heart-lung machine (a pump-oxygenator) before being returned to the arterial circulation.

bypass, coronary A form of bypass surgery that can create new routes around narrowed and blocked arteries, permitting increased blood flow to deliver oxygen and nutrients to the heart muscles. Coronary artery bypass graft (CABG) surgery is an option for selected groups of patients with significant narrowings and blockages of the heart arteries. The bypass graft for a CABG can be a vein from the leg or an inner chest-wall artery. CABG surgery is one of the most commonly performed major operations. Coronary artery disease develops because of hardening of the arteries (atherosclerosis) that supply blood to the heart muscle. Diagnostic tests include electrocardiograms (EKGs), stress tests, echocardiographams, and coronary angiographies.

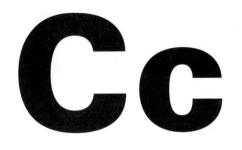

C **1** In genetics, cytosine, a member of the G-C (guanine-cytosine) base pair in DNA. **2** In bioscience, carbon, an essential element in the basic structure of living things.

CA 125 Cancer antigen 125, a protein normally made by certain cells in the body, including those of the Fallopian tubes, the uterus, the cervix, and the lining of the chest and abdominal cavities (the pleura and peritoneum). When CA 125 is found in larger than normal amounts (more than 35 kU/ml), it is considered a marker for cancer.

CA 125 test A test for CA 125 in blood or fluid from the chest or abdomen. The test uses a monoclonal antibody directed against CA 125. When a malignancy is known to be associated with a high CA 125 value, a declining CA 125 level indicates effective therapy, whereas an increasing level indicates tumor recurrence. Because of test variation, small changes are usually not considered significant. A doubling or halving of the previous value would be important. Benign conditions that can raise CA 125 include infections of the lining of the abdomen and chest (peritonitis and pleuritis), menstruation, pregnancy, endometriosis, and liver disease. Benign tumors of the ovaries can also cause abnormal test results.

CABG Coronary artery bypass graft. See *bypass, coronary.*

cachetic Having cachexia. Patients with cancer, AIDS, and other serious chronic diseases may appear cachetic.

cachexia General physical wasting with loss of weight and muscle mass due to a disease. Also known as marasmus.

CAD Coronary artery disease.

caduceus A staff with two snakes entwined about it, topped by a pair of wings. The caduceus was carried by the Greek messenger god Hermes, whose Roman counterpart was Mercury, and is therefore the sign of a herald. By a curious misconception, the caduceus also became the insignia of the US Army Medical Corps and a well-known symbol of physicians and medicine. The Corps should have chosen the symbol of medicine: the rod of Aesculapius, which has only one snake and no wings. No wings were necessary because the essence of medicine was not speed. The single serpent that could shed its skin and emerge in full vigor represented the renewal of youth and health. Interestingly, the ancient caduceus, with its pair of snakes coiled about each other, is reminiscent of the double helix structure of DNA, which was not discovered until modern times.

caesarean section A procedure in which an infant is surgically removed from the uterus rather than being born vaginally. As the name *caesarean* suggests, this is not a new procedure. It was performed in ancient civilizations to salvage a baby upon the death of a nearly full-term pregnant woman. Julius Caesar is said to have been born by this procedure, hence the name. The term *section* in surgery refers to the division of tissue. In the case of a caesarean section, the abdominal wall of the mother and the wall of the uterus are divided in order to extract the baby. Also known as C-section.

caesarean section, lower segment A caesarean section in which the surgical incision is made in the lower segment of the uterus. Abbreviated LSCS.

caesarean section, vaginal birth after A vaginal delivery for a woman who previously had a cesarean section. It was once the rule that after a caesarean section, the next delivery also had to be by caesarean section. Now vaginal delivery after caesarean section is sometimes feasible. Age is one of the factors that need to be considered because women over 30 who try a vaginal delivery after a caesarean section are about three times more likely than younger women to have a uterine rupture. Abbreviated VBAC.

café au lait spot A flat spot on the skin that has a color similar to that of coffee with milk (café au lait) in persons with light skin or that has a darker appearance than the surrounding skin in persons with dark skin. About 10 percent of the general population has café au lait spots, which can be removed with a Yag laser technique. Café au lait spots are normally harmless, but in some cases they are a sign of neurofibromatosis (NF1). The presence of six or more café au lait spots, each of which is 1.5 cm or more in diameter, is diagnostic of NF1. See also *neurofibromatosis; Yag laser surgery.*

caffeine An alkaloid stimulant found naturally in coffee, tea, cocoa (chocolate), and kola nuts (cola) and added to soft drinks, foods, and medicines. A cup of coffee has 100–250 milligrams of caffeine. Black tea brewed for 4 minutes has 40–100 milligrams; green tea has one-third as much caffeine as black tea. In doses of 100–200 milligrams, caffeine can increase alertness, relieve drowsiness, and improve thinking. At doses of 250–700 milligrams per day, caffeine can cause anxiety, insomnia, nervousness, and hypertension. Caffeine is a diuretic and increases urination. It can decrease a person's ability to lose weight because it stimulates insulin secretion, which reduces serum glucose, which increases hunger. Caffeine can help to relieve headaches, so a number of over-the-counter and prescription pain relievers include it as an ingredient, usually with aspirin or another analgesic.

Caffey disease An inflammatory bone disorder seen only in newborn and very young babies, characterized by swelling of soft tissues, irritability, fever, and paleness. Also known as infantile cortical hyperostosis.

calamine An astringent made from zinc carbonate or zinc oxide, customarily used in lotion form to treat skin problems or insect bites that cause itching or discomfort.

calcaneal spur A bony spur, also known as a heel spur, that projects from the back or underside of the heel bone (the calcaneus) and that may make walking painful. Calcaneal spurs are associated with inflammation of the Achilles tendon (Achilles tendinitis), and cause tenderness and pain at the back of the heel, which is made worse by pushing off the ball of the foot. Spurs under the sole (the plantar area) are associated with inflammation of the plantar fascia, which is the bowstring-like tissue that stretches from the heel underneath the sole. These spurs cause localized tenderness and a type of pain that is made worse by stepping down on the heel. Not all calcaneal spurs cause symptoms. Some are discovered on X-rays taken for other purposes. Calcaneal spurs and plantar fasciitis can occur alone, or they can be related to underlying diseases that cause arthritis, such as reactive arthritis and ankylosing spondylitis. Treatment is designed to decrease the inflammation and avoid reinjury. Icing reduces pain and inflammation. Anti-inflammatory agents, such as ibuprofen or injections of cortisone, can help. Heel lifts reduce stress on the Achilles tendon and relieve painful spurs at the back of the heel. Donut-shaped shoe inserts take pressure off plantar spurs. Infrequently, surgery is done on chronically inflamed spurs.

calcaneocuboid joint The joint located in the foot between the calcaneus bone and the cuboid bone. It is a gliding type of joint. The ligaments that serve to support and strengthen this joint are called the capsular, dorsal calcaneocuboid, bifurcated, long plantar, and plantar calcaneocuboid ligaments.

calcaneus The heel bone, a more or less rectangular bone at the back of the foot. Also known as os calcis.

calcific bursitis Chronic inflammation of a bursa (bursitis) that leads to calcium deposition (calcification) of the bursa. The calcification can occur as long as the inflammation is present. See also *bursa; bursitis.*

calcification The process of building bone by suffusing tissues with calcium salts. Also known as ossification.

calcified granuloma A node-like type of tissue inflammation that has a specific appearance under a microscope (granuloma) and contains calcium deposits. Because it usually takes some time for calcium to be deposited in a granuloma, it is generally assumed that a calcified granuloma is an old granuloma, or an old area of inflammation. For example, a calcified granuloma in the lung may be due to tuberculosis contracted years earlier that is now inactive and dormant.

calcinosis An abnormal deposit of calcium salts in body tissues. Examples include the calcifications in the skin from scleroderma and in the muscle from polymyositis.

calcitonin A hormone produced by the thyroid gland that lowers the levels of calcium and phosphate in the blood and promotes the formation of bone. Bone is in a constant state of remodeling. Old bone is removed by cells called osteoclasts, and new bone is added by cells called osteoblasts. Calcitonin inhibits bone removal by the osteoclasts and at the same time promotes bone formation by the osteoblasts. Calcitonin is given in hypercalcemia (high blood calcium) to lower the calcium level; in osteoporosis to increase bone density and decrease the risk of a fracture; and in Paget disease to decrease bone turnover and bone pain. Also known as thyrocalcitonin.

calcium A mineral found mainly in the hard part of bones, where it is stored. Calcium is added to bone by cells called osteoblasts and removed from bone by cells called osteoclasts. Calcium is essential for healthy bones and is also important for muscle contraction, heart action, and normal blood clotting. Food sources of calcium include dairy foods; some leafy green vegetables, such as broccoli and collards; canned salmon; clams; oysters; calcium-fortified foods; and soy foods, such as tofu. According to the National Academy of Sciences, adequate intake of calcium is 1 gram daily for both men and women. The upper limit for calcium intake is 2.5 grams daily.

calcium deficiency A low blood level of calcium (hypocalcemia), which can make the nervous system highly irritable, causing spasms of the hands and feet (tetany), muscle cramps, abdominal cramps, overly active reflexes, and so on. Chronic calcium deficiency contributes to poor mineralization of bones, soft bones (osteomalacia) and osteoporosis, and, in children, rickets and impaired growth.

calcium excess Overly high intake of calcium that can result in elevated blood calcium levels (hypercalcemia), which can cause muscle weakness and constipation, affect the conduction of electrical impulses in the heart (heart block), lead to calcium stones in the urinary tract, impair kidney function through nephrocalcinosis, and interfere with the absorption of iron, predisposing the person to iron deficiency.

calculus A stone, as in the urinary tract, or calcium salt deposits on the teeth. The Latin word *calculus* means "a pebble." Pebbles were once used for counting, from which came the mathematical field of calculus.

calculus, renal See *kidney stone*.

calf The belly or fleshy hind part of the back of the leg below the knee. The calf is made up mainly of the gastrocnemius muscle.

caliper 1 A metal or plastic instrument used to measure the diameter of an object. The skin-fold thickness in several parts of the body can be measured with calipers, as can fat deposits. This measurement is done in medicine, especially in the diagnosis and treatment of obesity, and in physical anthropology. Calipers are also used to measure the diameter of the pelvis in pregnant women to ensure that it is large enough to permit birth. 2 A type of leg splint.

callus 1 A localized, firm thickening of the upper layer of skin as a result of repetitive friction. A callus on the skin of the foot may have become thick and hard from rubbing against an ill-fitting shoe. Calluses of the feet may lead to other problems, such as serious infections. Shoes that fit well can keep calluses from forming on the feet. Also known as keratoma. 2 Hard new bone substance that forms in an area of a bone fracture. It is part of the natural process of bone repair.

calorie A unit of food energy. The word *calorie* is ordinarily used instead of the more precise, scientific term kilocalorie. A kilocalorie represents the amount of energy required to raise the temperature of a liter of water 1° centigrade at sea level. Technically, a kilocalorie represents 1,000 true calories of energy.

Campylobacter jejuni A bacterium that typically infects the bowels. Now the leading cause of bacterial food poisoning, Campylobacter jejuni is most often spread by contact with raw or undercooked poultry. A single drop of juice from a contaminated chicken is enough to make someone sick. Disease caused by Campylobacter jejuni is termed campylobacteriosis. Symptoms tend to start 2 to 5 days after exposure and typically last a week. They resemble the symptoms of viral gastroenteritis—diarrhea, fever, abdominal pain, cramping, nausea, and vomiting—but with campylobacter, fever is typical and the diarrhea is often bloody. Antibiotics can be helpful treatment. Most people who have campylobacteriosis recover completely. However, some suffer long-term consequences, such as arthritis and a condition called Guillain-Barré syndrome. Both are thought to occur when a person's immune system is triggered by the Campylobacter jejuni to attack the person's own body. In arthritis, the attack is mounted against joints, and in Guillain-Barré syndrome, the attack is against nerves and leads to ascending paralysis that typically lasts several weeks and usually requires intensive care.

Canavan disease A progressive, inherited disorder of the central nervous system that is caused by a deficiency of the enzyme aspartoacylase. The signs of Canavan disease usually appear when children are between 3 and 6 months of age. They include developmental delay, significant motor slowness, enlargement of the head (macrocephaly), loss of muscle tone (hypotonia), poor head control, and severe feeding problems. As the disease progresses, seizures, shrinkage of the nerve to the eye (optic atrophy), and often blindness develop, as do heartburn (gastrointestinal reflux) and deterioration of the ability to swallow. Canavan disease is inherited as an autosomal recessive condition, with both parents silently carrying a single Canavan gene and each of their children running a 25 percent risk of receiving both genes and having the disease. Canavan disease is more prevalent among individuals of Eastern European Jewish (Ashkenazi) background than in others. There is currently no cure or effective treatment. Most children with Canavan disease die in the first decade of life. Also known as spongy degeneration of the central nervous system and Canavan-Van Bogaert–Bertrand disease, and by several names of a biochemical nature, including aspartoacylase deficiency, ASPA deficiency, ASP deficiency, aminoacylase 2 deficiency, and ACY2 deficiency.

cancer An abnormal growth of cells that tend to proliferate in an uncontrolled way and, in some cases, to metastasize (spread). Cancer is not one disease; rather, it is a host of more than 100 different and distinctive diseases. A tumor can involve any tissue of the body. Most types of cancer are named for the type of cell or organ in which they start. If a cancer metastasizes, the new tumor bears the same name as the original primary tumor. Skin cancer is the most common type of cancer in both men and women. The second most common types of cancer are prostate cancer in men and breast cancer in women. Lung cancer is the leading cause of death from cancer for both men and women in the US. Cancer is not contagious. *Cancer* is the Latin word for "crab." Also known as malignancy, malignant tumor, and malignant neoplasm. See also *cancer, causes*.

cancer antigen 125 See *CA 125*.

cancer, bladder See *bladder cancer*.

cancer, bone See *bone cancer*.

cancer, brain See *brain cancer.*

cancer, breast See *breast cancer.*

cancer, breast, familial See *breast cancer, familial.*

cancer, breast, susceptibility gene See *breast cancer susceptibility gene.*

cancer, causes Causes of cancer. In most individual cases, the exact cause of cancer is unknown. It's likely that each case represents an interplay of several factors, which may include increased genetic susceptibility; environmental insults, such as chemical exposure or smoking cigarettes; lifestyle factors, including diet; and damage caused by infectious disease. Although they are not causes per se, a number of factors—including gender, race, age, and the health of the patient's immune system—can influence the development of cancer. When common causes for a type of cancer are discovered, this information can be very helpful in prevention and sometimes in treatment. For example, the link between overexposure to the sun and skin cancer is well known, and individuals can easily reduce their risk of skin cancer by avoiding sun tanning and sunburns. Alcohol is associated with an increased risk of cancer of the esophagus, mouth, pharynx, larynx, liver, breast, rectum, and pancreas; one can lower the risk for these malignancies by consuming less alcohol.

cancer, cervical A malignant tumor of the cervix, the lowest part of the uterus, which forms a canal that opens into the vagina. Regular pelvic exams and Pap tests are of great importance and can detect precancerous changes in the cervix. If there is cancer of the cervix, the most common symptom is abnormal bleeding. Cancer of the cervix can be diagnosed by using a Pap test or other procedures that sample the cervix tissue. Precancerous changes in the cervix may be treated with cryosurgery, cauterization, or laser surgery. Cancer of the cervix requires different treatment than cancer that begins in other parts of the uterus. A number of risk factors for cervical cancer have been identified. Women who begin having sexual intercourse before age 18 and have many sexual partners are at increased risk. Furthermore, women whose partners begin having sexual intercourse at a young age and have many sexual partners, especially one who had cervical cancer, are at increased risk. The relevance of sexual history may have to do with the chance of infection with the human papillomaviruses (HPV), a sexually transmitted virus that may trigger cervical cancer. Other risk factors include exposure before birth to the drug diethylstilbestrol (DES), smoking, and immunodeficiency. See also *Pap test.*

cancer, colon A malignant tumor arising from the inner wall of the large intestine (the colon). In the US, colon cancer is the third leading type of cancer in males and the fourth in females. Risk factors for cancer of the colon and rectum (colorectal cancer) include colon polyps, long-standing ulcerative colitis, and genetic family history. Most colorectal cancers develop from polyps. Removal of colon polyps can prevent colorectal cancer. Colon polyps and early colon cancer can have no symptoms. Therefore, regular screening is important, starting at age 50 (or earlier, if added risk factors are present). Diagnosis can be made by barium enema or by colonoscopy, with biopsy confirmation of cancer tissue. Surgery is the most common treatment for colorectal cancer.

cancer, colorectal See *cancer, colon.*

cancer, esophagus See *esophageal cancer.*

cancer, gastric A malignant tumor of the stomach. Gastric cancer can develop in any part of the stomach and can spread from the stomach to other organs. Stomach ulcers do not appear to increase a person's risk of developing stomach cancer. Symptoms of stomach cancer are often vague, such as loss of appetite and weight. Gastric cancer is diagnosed via a biopsy of stomach tissue during an endoscopy. Also called stomach cancer.

cancer, Hodgkin's lymphoma A type of lymphoma (cancer of the lymphatic system). Also known as Hodgkin's disease. The most common symptom is painless swelling of the lymph nodes in the neck, underarm, or groin. Most patients are in their teens or 20s. The diagnosis depends on a biopsy of an enlarged lymph node. Treatment usually includes radiation therapy or chemotherapy. Patients treated for Hodgkin's disease have an increased risk of developing other types of cancer, especially leukemia, later in life. See also *Hodgkin's disease.*

cancer, kidney A malignant tumor of the kidney, which is the main organ responsible for removing from the blood toxins produced during metabolism. Childhood kidney cancer is different from adult kidney cancer. The most common type of childhood kidney cancer is Wilms tumor. The most common type of adult kidney cancer is renal cell cancer (also known as renal adenocarcinoma), which occurs more often in men than in women. A frequent sign of kidney cancer is blood in the urine. The diagnosis of kidney cancer is supported by findings of the medical history and examination, blood, urine, and X-ray tests, and it is confirmed with biopsy. Kidney cancer is treated with surgery, embolization, radiation therapy, hormone therapy, biological therapy, or chemotherapy. See also *cancer, renal cell; Wilms tumor.*

cancer, laryngeal   A malignant tumor of the larynx (the voice box), which is located at the top of the windpipe (trachea). Cancer of the larynx occurs most often in people over the age of 55, especially those who have been heavy smokers. People who stop smoking can greatly reduce their risk. Hoarseness without pain can be a symptom of cancer of the larynx. The larynx can be examined with a viewing tube called a laryngoscope. Cancer of the larynx is usually treated with radiation therapy or surgery. Chemotherapy can also be used for laryngeal cancers that have spread.

cancer, lung   A malignant tumor of the lung, the major organ of respiration. Lung cancer kills more men and women than any other form of cancer. Because the majority of lung cancer is diagnosed at a relatively late stage, only 10 percent of all lung cancer patients are ultimately cured. Eight out of 10 lung cancers are due to damage caused by tobacco smoke. Lung cancers are classified as either small cell or non-small cell cancers. Persistent cough and bloody sputum can be symptoms of lung cancer. Diagnosis of lung cancer can be based on examination of sputum or on tissue examination with biopsy, using bronchoscopy, a needle through the chest wall, or surgical excision.

cancer, male breast   See *breast cancer, male.*

cancer, melanoma   A skin cancer that begins in cells called melanocytes, which normally grow together to form benign (noncancerous) moles. A change in size, shape, or color of a mole can be a sign of melanoma. Melanoma can be cured if it is detected early. If it is not detected early, however, it may spread to other areas of the body, and that can cause death. Diagnosis is confirmed with a biopsy of the abnormal skin. Sun exposure can cause skin damage, which can in turn lead to melanoma. See also *melanoma.*

cancer, multiple myeloma   See *multiple myeloma.*

cancer, myeloma   See *multiple myeloma.*

cancer, non-Hodgkin's lymphoma   See *lymphoma, non-Hodgkin's.*

cancer, oral   A malignant tumor of the mouth area. A sore in the mouth that does not heal can be a warning sign of oral cancer. A biopsy is the only way to determine whether an abnormal area in the oral cavity is cancerous. Oral cancer is almost always caused by tobacco (smoking

and chewing) or alcohol use. Surgery to remove the tumor in the mouth is the usual treatment.

cancer, ovarian   A malignant tumor of the ovary, the egg sac in a female. There are several types of ovarian cancer. Ovarian cancer that begins on the surface of the ovary (epithelial carcinoma) is the most common type. Women who have a family history of ovarian cancer are at an increased risk of developing ovarian cancer. Hereditary ovarian cancer makes up approximately 5 to 10 percent of all cases of ovarian cancer. Three hereditary patterns have been identified: ovarian cancer alone, ovarian and breast cancers, and ovarian and colon cancers. Ovarian cancer is hard to detect early because there usually are no symptoms and the symptoms that do occur tend to be vague. Detection involves physical examination (including pelvic exam), ultrasound, X-ray tests, CA 125 test, and biopsy of the ovary. Most ovarian growths (tumors) in women under age 30 are benign (noncancerous), fluid-filled cysts.

cancer, pancreatic   A malignant tumor of the pancreas. Pancreatic cancer has been called a "silent" disease because early pancreatic cancer usually does not cause symptoms. If the tumor blocks the common bile duct, and bile cannot pass into the digestive system, the skin and whites of the eyes may become yellow (jaundiced), and the urine may become darker as a result of accumulated bile pigment (bilirubin).

cancer, penis   A malignant tumor in which cancer cells are found on the skin of the penis or in the tissues of the penis. It is rare in the US. A physician should be seen if any of the following problems occur: growths or sores on the penis, any unusual liquid coming from the penis (abnormal discharge), or bleeding. The physician examines the penis and feels for any lumps. If warranted, a biopsy is performed. If cancer is found, more tests are done to find out whether the cancer has spread to other parts of the body (staging). Treatment options include surgery, radiation therapy, chemotherapy, and biological therapy. The chance of recovery and choice of treatment depend on the stage of the cancer and the patient's general state of health. Men who are not circumcised at birth may have a higher risk of getting cancer of the penis.

cancer, prostate   A malignant tumor of the prostate, the gland that produces some of the components of semen. Prostate cancer is the second leading cause of death of males in the US. It is often first detected as a hard nodule found during a routine rectal examination. The PSA blood test is a screening test for prostate cancer. Diagnosis of prostate cancer is established when cancer cells are identified in prostate tissue obtained via biopsy. In some patients, prostate cancer is life threatening. In many others, prostate cancer can exist for years without causing any health problems. Treatment options for prostate cancer include observation, radiation therapy, surgery, hormone therapy, and chemotherapy.

cancer, rectal   A malignant tumor arising from the inner wall of the end of the large intestine (rectum). In the US, it is the third leading cause of cancer in males and the fourth in females. Risk factors include heredity, colon polyps, and long-standing ulcerative colitis. Most colorectal cancers develop from polyps in the colon. Removal of these polyps can prevent cancer. Colon polyps and early rectal cancer can have no symptoms, so regular screening is important. Diagnosis can be made by barium enema or by colonoscopy, with biopsy confirmation of cancer tissue. Surgery is the most common treatment.

cancer, renal cell   A malignant tumor that develops in the lining of the renal tubules, which filter the blood and produce urine. Also known as renal cell carcinoma and renal adenocarcinoma. See also *cancer, kidney*.

cancer, skin   A malignant tumor of the outer surface of the body. Skin cancer is the most common cancer in the US. There are many types of skin cancer; the 3 most common types are basal cell carcinoma, squamous cell carcinoma, and the most deadly, melanoma. The main cause of skin cancer is ultraviolet light from sunlight. Tanning lamps are a hazard in this regard. Unexplained changes in the appearance of the skin that last longer than 2 weeks should be evaluated by a physician. The cure rate for skin cancer could be 100 percent if all skin cancers were brought to a physician's attention before they had a chance to spread. See also *basal cell carcinoma; squamous cell carcinoma; melanoma*.

cancer, stomach   See *cancer, gastric*.

cancer symptoms   Symptoms that may be associated with cancer, including changes in bowel or bladder habits, a sore that does not heal, unusual bleeding or discharge, thickening or a lump in the breast or any other part of the body, indigestion or difficulty swallowing, obvious change in a wart or mole, and a nagging cough or hoarseness. These symptoms are not always signs of cancer; they can result from less serious conditions. Some forms of cancer cause little or no discomfort until the disease is far advanced, so it is important to see a physician for regular checkups rather than wait for problems to occur.

cancer, testicular   A malignant tumor of the male sex organ (testicle) that normally produces the hormone testosterone. It is one of the most common cancers in young men. Most testicular cancers are found by men themselves, as lumps in the testicles. The risk of testicular cancer is increased in males whose testicles did not move

down normally into the scrotum during childhood (undescended testicles). When a growth in a testicle is detected, cancer is confirmed after surgical removal of the affected testicle (orchiectomy) and examination of the tissue under a microscope. Testicular cancer is almost always curable if it is found early.

cancer, thyroid   A malignant tumor of the gland in front of the neck that normally produces thyroid hormone, which is important to the normal regulation of the metabolism in the body. There are four major types of cancer of the thyroid gland: papillary, follicular, medullary, and anaplastic. Persons who received radiation to the head or neck in childhood should be examined by a physician for thyroid cancer every 1 to 2 years. The most common symptom of thyroid cancer is a lump, or nodule, that can be felt in the neck. The only certain way to tell whether a thyroid lump is cancer is by examining thyroid tissue obtained via biopsy.

cancer, uterine   A malignant tumor of the uterus (womb), which occurs most often in women between the ages of 55 and 70. Abnormal bleeding after menopause is the most common symptom. Cancer of the uterus is diagnosed based on the results of a pelvic examination, Pap test, biopsy of the uterus, and/or dilation and curettage (D & C).

Candida albicans   A yeast-like fungal organism found in small amounts in the normal human intestinal tract. Normally kept in check by the body's own helpful bacteria, C. albicans can increase in numbers when this balance is disturbed, to cause candidiasis of the intestinal tract or yeast infections of other parts of the body. See also *candidiasis*.

candidiasis   Overgrowth of the yeast called Candida albicans in the gastrointestinal tract or other areas of the body. Vaginal yeast infections; some forms of diaper rash, and other skin rashes that emerge in moist, warm areas of skin; and thrush (white patches inside the mouth and throat) are all forms of yeast infection. Candidiasis tends to develop when the normal balance of intestinal bacteria is upset, as sometimes occurs with the use of antibiotics. Prevention measures include the use of probiotics, and in some cases, dietary changes. Candidiasis can be treated with antifungal medications. Candidiasis is usually a minor and easily addressed problem, but it can be an important problem for those with immune-system disorders, such as AIDS.

canker sore   A small, frequently painful and sensitive crater in the lining of the mouth. Also known as aphthous ulcer. About 20 percent of the population has canker sores at any one time. Sores typically last for 10 to 14 days, and they generally heal without scarring.

cannabis Marijuana (Cannibis sativa), a drug derived from the family of plants that includes hemp. Use of cannabis produces a mild sense of euphoria, as well as impairments in judgment and lengthened response time. Cannabis may be smoked or eaten. Although cannabis use is illegal in most parts of the world, the plant appears to have some potential for medical use, particularly as a palliative for glaucoma and disease-related loss of appetite and wasting, as is often seen in cancer, AIDS, and other illnesses. Some compounds in cannabis have an antiseizure effect. In some areas of the US, individuals whose physicians recommend the medical use of cannabis can obtain special permission.

cannula A hollow tube with a sharp, retractable inner core that can be inserted into a vein, an artery, or another body cavity.

capillary A tiny blood vessel that connects an arteriole (the smallest division of an artery) with a venule (the smallest division of a vein). Although tiny, the capillary is where much action takes place in the circulatory system. The walls of capillaries act as semipermeable membranes that permit the exchange of various substances between the blood stream and the tissues of the body. The substances that are exchanged through the capillary walls include fluids and the gases oxygen and carbon dioxide.

capillary hemangioma See *hemangioma, capillary.*

capitation In US health services, a fixed "per capita" amount that is paid to a hospital, clinic, or physician for each person served. If that person uses few services, the excess amount paid is potential profit for the payee. If the person uses many services, the payee may lose money.

caps Abbreviation for capsules.

carbohydrate One of the three nutrient compounds, along with fat and protein, used as energy sources (calories) by the body. Carbohydrates take the form of simple sugars or of more complex forms, such as starches and fiber. Complex carbohydrates come naturally from plants. Intake of complex carbohydrates, when they are substituted for saturated fat, can lower blood cholesterol. Carbohydrates produce 4 calories of energy per gram. When eaten, all carbohydrates are broken down into the sugar glucose.

carbon monoxide poisoning A potentially deadly condition caused by breathing carbon monoxide gas, which prevents oxygenation of the blood. Common causes of carbon monoxide poisoning include malfunctioning furnaces and the use of kerosene heaters or similar devices in unventilated indoor spaces. Carbon monoxide is also emitted by automobile and other engines, so these should not be run in unventilated spaces, such as closed garages. Inexpensive alarms are available that can detect dangerous buildups of carbon monoxide. The treatment for carbon monoxide poisoning is immediate reoxygenation of the blood in a hospital.

carbuncle A skin abscess (boil) that extends into subcutaneous layers of skin, usually caused by local infection with the bacteria Staphylococcus aureus. Treatment includes antibiotics (typically in the form of topical creams) and, in severe cases, surgical drainage. See also *abscess.*

carcinoembryonic antigen A protein found in many types of cells that is associated with a developing fetus and tumors. Abbreviated CEA.

carcinoembryonic antigen test A blood test for carcinoembryonic antigen (CEA). Conditions that increase CEA include smoking, infection, inflammatory bowel disease, pancreatitis, cirrhosis of the liver, and some benign tumors (in the same organs that have cancers with increased CEA). The normal level is less than 2.5 ng/ml (nanograms per milliliter) in an adult nonsmoker and less than 5.0 ng/ml in a smoker. Benign disease rarely elevates the CEA over 10 ng/ml. The main use of CEA test is as a tumor marker, especially with intestinal cancer. The most common cancers that elevate CEA are in the colon and rectum. Others include cancer of the pancreas, stomach, breast, and lung, as well as certain types of thyroid and ovarian cancer. Levels over 20 ng/ml before therapy are associated with cancer that has already metastasized (spread). CEA tests are useful in monitoring the treatment of CEA-rich tumors. If the CEA is high before treatment, it should fall to normal after successful therapy. A rising CEA level usually indicates progression or recurrence of the cancer, although chemotherapy and radiation therapy can themselves cause a temporary rise in CEA due to death of tumor cells and release of CEA into the blood stream.

carcinogen A substance or an agent that causes cancer. The International Agency for Research on Cancer has classified some 60 substances and processes as probably or definitely being carcinogenic in humans. The agency has divided these substances and processes into three categories: agents (such as arsenic, asbestos, and benzene); mixtures (such as in coal tars, tobacco products, and smoke); and exposure circumstances (such as in aluminum production, shoe manufacturing and repair, and the rubber industry). One of the best-known carcinogens is ionizing radiation.

carcinogenic Having a cancer-causing action.

carcinoma Cancer that begins in the skin or in tissues that line or cover body organs. Examples are carcinoma of the breast, colon, liver, lung, pancreas, prostate, or stomach.

carcinoma in situ Cancer that has stayed in the place where it began and has not spread to neighboring tissues (for example, squamous cell carcinoma in situ).

carcinoma in situ, squamous cell An early stage of skin cancer that develops from squamous cells (the flat, scale-like cells in the outer layer of the skin). The hallmark is a persistent, progressive, slightly raised, red, scaly, or crusted plaque that may occur anywhere on the skin surface or on mucosal surfaces, such as in the mouth. Under a microscope, atypical squamous cells are seen to have proliferated through the whole thickness of the epidermis (the outer layer of the skin) but no further. The classic cause of squamous cell carcinoma in situ is prolonged exposure to arsenic. Today, squamous cell carcinoma occurs most often in the sun-exposed areas of the skin in older white males. Treatment options include freezing of the affected area with liquid nitrogen, cauterization (burning), surgical removal, and chemosurgery. Also known as Bowen disease.

carcinoma, large cell See *large cell carcinoma.*

carcinoma of the breast, infiltrating ductal One of several recognized specific patterns of cancer of the breast, so named because it begins in the cells that form the ducts of the breast. It is the most common form of breast cancer, comprising 65 to 85 percent of all cases. On a mammogram, invasive ductal carcinoma is usually visualized as a mass with fine spikes radiating from the edges (spiculation). It may also appear as a smooth-edged lump in the breast. On physical examination, this lump usually feels much harder or firmer than benign lumps (whether natural structures or cysts) in the breast. On microscopic examination, the cancerous cells are found to have invaded and replaced the normal breast tissue. Treatment may include radiation, chemotherapy, and surgery.

carcinoma of the breast, infiltrating lobular The second most common type of invasive breast cancer, accounting for 5 to 10 percent of breast cancer. Infiltrating lobular carcinoma starts in the glands that secrete milk (lobules) and then invades surrounding tissue. On a mammogram, a lobular carcinoma can look similar to a ductal carcinoma, appearing as a mass with fine spikes radiating from the edges (spiculation). However, on physical examination of the breast, a lobular carcinoma is usually not a hard mass like a ductal carcinoma; rather, it is a vague thickening of the breast tissue. Lobular carcinoma can occur in more than one site in the breast (as a multicentric tumor) or in both breasts at the same time (as bilateral lobular carcinoma). Treatment may include radiation, chemotherapy, and surgery.

carcinoma, squamous cell Cancer that begins in squamous cells, which are thin, flat cells that resemble fish scales. Squamous cells are found in the tissue that forms the surface of the skin, the lining of the hollow organs of the body, and the passages of the respiratory and digestive tracts. See also *carcinoma in situ, squamous cell.*

carcinoma, transitional cell Cancer that develops in the lining of the renal pelvis, ureter, or bladder.

cardiac Having to do with the heart.

cardiac aneurysm See *aneurysm, cardiac.*

cardiac arrest A heart attack in which the heart suddenly stops pumping sufficient blood. A cardiac arrest that results in the death of heart muscle is referred to as a myocardial infarction. See also *myocardial infarction, acute.*

cardiac atrium See *atrium.*

cardiac conduction system The electrical conduction system that controls the heart rate. This system generates electrical impulses and conducts them throughout the muscle of the heart, stimulating the heart to contract and pump blood. Among the major elements in the cardiac conduction system are the sinoatrial node, the atrioventricular (AV) node, and the autonomic nervous system. See also *atrioventricular node; autonomic nervous system; sinoatrial node.*

cardiac defibrillator, implantable A device that is designed to be put in the body to recognize certain types of abnormal heart rhythms (arrhythmias) and correct them by delivering precisely calibrated and timed electrical shocks to restore a normal heartbeat. Defibrillators continuously monitor the heart rhythm in order to detect overly rapid arrhythmias, such as ventricular tachycardia (rapid regular beating of the ventricles, the bottom chambers of the heart) or ventricular fibrillation (rapid irregular beating of the ventricles). These life-threatening ventricular arrhythmias impair the pumping efficiency of the heart, raising the risks of fainting (syncope) and sudden cardiac arrest. Today's implantable defibrillators are about the size of a minicassette and can be implanted with less invasive surgical techniques than were used in the past.

cardiac muscle A type of muscle tissue that is distinguishable from the two other forms of muscle, smooth muscle (that moves internal organs, such as the bowels, and vessels, such as the artery walls) and skeletal muscle (that powers joints) and is found only in the heart. Cardiac muscle is responsible for pumping blood throughout the body.

cardiac output   The amount of blood the heart pumps through the circulatory system in a minute. The amount of blood put out by the left ventricle of the heart in one contraction is called the stroke volume. The stroke volume and the heart rate determine the cardiac output. A normal adult has a cardiac output of 4.7 liters (5 quarts) of blood per minute.

cardiac septum   The dividing wall between the right and left sides of the heart. That portion of the septum that separates the two upper chambers (the right and left atria) of the heart is termed the atrial (or interatrial) septum; the portion that lies between the two lower chambers (the right and left ventricles) of the heart is called the ventricular (or interventricular) septum.

cardiac tamponade   See *tamponade, cardiac.*

cardiac ventricle   See *ventricle, heart.*

cardiologist   A physician who specializes in treating heart disorders.

cardiology   The study and treatment of heart disorders.

cardiomyopathy   Disease of the heart muscle (myocardium).

cardiomyopathy, hypertrophic   A heart defect characterized by increased thickness (hypertrophy) of the wall of the left ventricle, the largest of the four chambers of the heart. Abbreviated HCM. HCM can present at any time in a person's life. It may, in a worst-case scenario, lead to death.

cardiopulmonary   Having to do with both the heart and lungs.

cardiopulmonary bypass   Bypass of the heart and lungs (for example, in open-heart surgery). Blood returning to the heart is diverted through a heart-lung machine (a pump-oxygenator) before it is returned to the arterial circulation. The machine does the work of both the heart and the lungs, by pumping blood and supplying oxygen to red blood cells.

cardiopulmonary resuscitation   A life-saving emergency procedure that involves breathing for the victim and applying external chest compression to make the heart pump. Abbreviated CPR. In the early stages of a heart attack, death can often be avoided if a bystander starts CPR within 5 minutes of the onset of ventricular fibrillation.

When paramedics arrive, medications and/or electrical shock (cardioversion) to the heart can be administered to convert ventricular fibrillation to a normal heart rhythm. Therefore, prompt CPR and rapid paramedic response can improve the chances of survival from a heart attack.

cardiovascular   Relating to the circulatory system, which comprises the heart and blood vessels and carries nutrients and oxygen to the tissues of the body and removes carbon dioxide and other wastes from them. Cardiovascular diseases are conditions that affect the heart and blood vessels and include arteriosclerosis, coronary artery disease, heart valve disease, arrhythmia, heart failure, hypertension, orthostatic hypotension, shock, endocarditis, diseases of the aorta and its branches, disorders of the peripheral vascular system, and congenital heart disease.

cardiovascular system   The heart and blood vessels. Also known as circulatory system.

cardioversion   The conversion of a cardiac rhythm or electrical pattern to another, generally from an abnormal one to a normal one. This conversion can be accomplished by using medications or by electrical cardioversion with a special defibrillator. Also known as countershock.

cardioverter   A defibrillator that is used in cardioversion (the conversion of one cardiac rhythm to another). See also *cardiac defibrillator, implantable.*

carditis   Inflammation of the heart.

care, ambulatory   See *ambulatory care.*

care, managed   See *managed care.*

care, nail   See *nail care.*

care proxy, health   See *health care proxy.*

caries   Dental cavities in the two outer layers of a tooth (the enamel and the dentin). Small caries may not cause pain, and may not be noticed by the patient. Larger caries can collect food, and the inner pulp of the affected tooth can become irritated by bacterial toxins or by foods that are cold, hot, sour, or sweet. The result can be a toothache. Caries are believed to be caused by the Streptococcus bacteria, which produces an enamel-dissolving acid as it devours carbohydrate deposits (plaque) on the teeth. To prevent caries, one should brush and floss the teeth daily, use a bacteriocidal mouthwash, and have regular dental cleanings by a professional. If caries do occur, the eroded area can be cleaned and filled by a dentist to prevent further damage.

carotene, beta See *beta carotene.*

carotenemia An excessive blood level of carotene, which causes a temporary yellowing of the skin (pseudo-jaundice). Carotenemia is most commonly seen in infants fed too much mashed carrots and adults consuming high quantities of carrots, carrot juice, or beta carotene in supplement form.

carotid Pertaining to the carotid artery and the area near that key artery, which is located in the front of the neck.

carotid artery Either of the two key arteries located in the front of the neck, through which blood from the heart goes to the brain. The right and left common carotid arteries are located on each side of the neck. Together, these arteries provide the principal blood supply to the head and neck. The left common carotid artery arises directly from the aorta. The right common carotid artery arises from the brachiocephalic artery, which, in turn, comes off the aorta. Each of the two divides to form external and internal carotid arteries. The external carotids are closer to the surface than the internal carotids, which run deep within the neck. Cholesterol plaque on the inner wall of the carotid artery can lead to a stroke.

carpal tunnel A canal formed by bone and tissues in the palm side of the wrist that provides passage for the median nerve to the hand.

carpal tunnel release A surgical procedure to relieve pressure exerted on the median nerve within the carpal tunnel as a result of carpal tunnel syndrome. Surgical release is performed via a small incision, using conventional surgery techniques or a fiber-optic scope (endoscopic carpal tunnel repair).

carpal tunnel syndrome A type of compression neuropathy caused by compression and irritation of the median nerve in the wrist. The nerve is compressed and irritated within the carpal tunnel, due to pressure from the transverse carpal ligament. Abbreviated CTS. CTS can be due to trauma from repetitive work, such as that of retail checkers and cashiers, assembly line workers, meat packers, typists, writers, and accountants. Other factors predisposing individuals to CTS include obesity, pregnancy, hypothyroidism, arthritis, and diabetes. The symptoms of CTS include numbness, tingling, a "pins and needles" feeling at night in the hand, wrist pain, weakness in the grip, and a feeling of incoordination. In some cases the pain seems to migrate up from the wrist and into the arm, shoulder, and neck. This occurs when the affected person tries to reduce wrist pain by changing posture, in turn stressing new sets of muscles. The diagnosis is suspected based on symptoms, supported by signs on physical examination, and confirmed by nerve conduction testing. Treatment depends on the severity of symptoms and the underlying cause. Early CTS is usually treated by modification of activities, a removable wrist brace, exercises and/or manipulation (massage), and anti-inflammatory medicines. Caught early, CTS is reversible. If numbness and pain continue in the wrist and hand, a cortisone injection into the carpal tunnel can help. Surgery is indicated only when other treatments have failed. In advanced CTS, particularly if there is profound weakness and muscle atrophy (wasting), surgery is done to avoid permanent nerve damage.

carrier test A test designed to detect carriers of a gene for a recessive genetic disorder. For example, carrier testing is done for the sickle cell trait, thalassemia trait, and Tay-Sachs gene.

cartilage Firm, rubbery tissue that cushions bones at joints. A flexible kind of cartilage connects muscles with bones and makes up other parts of the body, such as the larynx and the outside parts of the ears.

casein The main protein found in milk and other dairy products.

cast **1** A protective shell of plaster and bandage that is molded to protect a broken or fractured limb as it heals. **2** An abnormal mass of dead cells that forms in a body cavity. For example, casts of cells that form in the tubules of the kidneys are sometimes detected in urine samples.

casting The application of a molded orthopedic appliance, usually composed of plaster or fiberglass, to immobilize part or all of a limb for the purpose of healing injured tissues.

casting, serial The use of successive casts to reshape deformed or spastic limbs or contracted joints.

castration Removal or destruction of the sex glands. The term is usually used in reference to the testicles, but it also can apply to the ovaries.

CAT scan Computerized axial tomography scan. CAT scanning is a painless process in which a computer generates cross-section views of a patient's anatomy. It can identify normal and abnormal structures, and it can be used to guide procedures. Iodine-containing contrast material is sometimes used in CAT scanning. A patient who is allergic to iodine or contrast materials and is scheduled to have a CAT scan should notify the physician and the radiology staff about the allergy.

cat scratch disease   See *cat scratch fever.*

cat scratch fever   An infection caused by the Bartonella henslae bacteria. Almost half of all domestic cats carry these bacteria and can transmit it to humans through a scratch or bite. Cat scratch fever causes swelling of the lymph nodes, sore throat, fatigue, fever, chills, sweats, vomiting, loss of appetite, and weight loss. There is usually a little bump (a papule), which may be pus-filled (a pustule), at the site of the scratch. In people with immunodeficiency, cat scratch fever can progress to bacillary angiomatosis, a bacterial skin infection that can be treated with the antibiotics rifampin, ciprofloxacin, trimethoprim-sulfamethoxazole, and gentamicin.

catabolism   See *metabolism.*

catalepsy   A body's persistence in unusual postures, with waxy rigidity of the limbs, mutism, and complete inactivity, regardless of outside stimuli, as is sometimes seen in catatonic schizophrenia.

catalyst   A substance that speeds up a chemical reaction but is not consumed or altered in the process. Catalysts are of immense importance in chemistry and biology. All enzymes are catalysts that expedite the biochemical reactions necessary for life. The enzymes in saliva, for example, accelerate the conversion of starch to glucose, doing in minutes what would otherwise take weeks.

cataplexy   A debilitating condition in which a person suddenly feels weak and collapses at times of strong emotion such as during laughter, anger, fear, or surprise. In so collapsing, people with cataplexy may injure themselves. For example, laughter and other emotions may trigger a reflex that can bring many of the muscles of the body to the point of collapse. Cataplexy often affects people who have narcolepsy.

cataract   A clouding or loss of transparency of the lens in the eye. There are many causes of cataracts, including aging, cortisone medication, trauma, diabetes, and other diseases. Cataracts affect most people who live into old age. Symptoms include double or blurred vision and sensitivity to light and glare. A physician can diagnose cataracts by examining the eyes with a viewing instrument. Sunglasses can help to prevent cataracts. See also *cataract surgery.*

cataract surgery   Removal of the clouded (cataractous) lens in its entirety via surgery and replacement of the lens with an intraocular lens (IOL) made of plastic. A typical cataract operation takes about an hour, requires local anesthesia only, and usually does not require hospitalization.

catatonic   In a state of catalepsy. See *catalepsy.*

cath   Medical shorthand for catheter or a procedure using a catheter.

cathartic   A laxative.

catheter   A thin, flexible tube.

catheter, bladder   A flexible plastic tube inserted into the bladder. See also *catheter, Foley; catheter, indwelling bladder.*

catheter, Foley   A flexible plastic tube inserted into the bladder to provide continuous urinary drainage. The Foley catheter has a balloon on the bladder end. After the catheter is inserted in the bladder, the balloon is inflated with air or fluid so that the catheter cannot pull out, but it is retained in the bladder as an indwelling catheter. Removal is accomplished by simply deflating the balloon and slipping the catheter out. See also *catheter, indwelling bladder.*

catheter, indwelling bladder   A catheter inserted into the bladder that remains there to provide continuous urinary drainage. The principal type is the Foley catheter. See also *catheter, Foley.*

catheter, IV   A catheter placed in a vein to provide a pathway for drugs, nutrients, fluids, or blood products. Blood samples can also be withdrawn through an IV catheter.

catheter, oximetry   A catheter used with monitoring equipment that can measure the amount of oxygenated hemoglobin in the bloodstream. See also *catheter, Swan-Ganz.*

catheter, PA   A catheter that is inserted into the pulmonary artery.

catheter, Swan-Ganz   A style of oximetry catheter that is inserted into a major vein under the collarbone or in the neck, threaded through the right side of the heart, and then threaded into the pulmonary artery. Physicians can use monitoring equipment with a Swan-Ganz catheter to measure blood pressure inside the heart and to find out how much blood the heart is pumping.

cauda equina   A bundle of spinal nerve roots that arise from the end of the spinal cord. The cauda equina comprises the roots of all the spinal nerves below the first lumbar (L1) vertebra in the lower back.

cauda equina syndrome   Impairment of the nerves in the cauda equina, characterized by dull pain in the lower back and upper buttocks and lack of feeling (analgesia) in the buttocks, genitalia, and thigh, together with disturbances of bowel and bladder function.

caudad Toward or of the feet (or tail, in embryology). The opposite of cranial. See also Appendix B, "Anatomic Orientation Terms."

caudal regression syndrome A disorder characterized by absence of all or part of the sacrum and dysfunction of the bowels, bladder, and legs. About 20 percent of children with caudal regression are born to mothers with diabetes. Treatment involves surgery to correct these defects, when possible.

caul Folk term for the membranes that surround the fetus in the womb, particularly for the presence of these membranes over the newborn infant's face or head at birth, a relatively common and usually harmless occurrence. In some cultures, the presence of a caul at birth is considered spiritually significant.

cauliflower ear An acquired deformity of the external ear to which wrestlers and boxers are particularly vulnerable, due to trauma. When a blood clot (hematoma) forms under the skin of the ear, the clot disrupts the connection of the skin to the ear cartilage. The cartilage has no other blood supply except from the overlying skin, so if the skin is separated from the cartilage, it is deprived of nutrients and dies. The ear cartilage then shrivels up to form the classic cauliflower ear, so named because the tissue resembles that lumpy vegetable's surface. Treatment involves draining the blood clot through an incision in the ear and then applying a compressive dressing, to sandwich the two sides of the skin against the cartilage. When treated promptly and aggressively, cauliflower ear is unlikely. Delay in diagnosis can lead to cauliflower ear.

causes of cancer See *cancer, causes.*

cauterization The use of heat to destroy abnormal cells. Also known as diathermy and electrodiathermy.

cavernous hemangioma See *hemangioma, cavernous.*

cavernous sinus A large channel of venous blood that creates a cavity (sinus) bordered by the sphenoid bone and the temporal bone of the skull. The cavernous sinus is an important structure because of its location and its contents, which include the third cranial (oculomotor) nerve, the fourth cranial (trochlear) nerve, parts 1 (the ophthalmic nerve) and 2 (the maxillary nerve) of the fifth cranial (trigeminal) nerve, and the sixth cranial (abducens) nerve.

cavernous sinus syndrome A condition characterized by edema (swelling) of the eyelids and the conjunctivae of the eyes, as well as paralysis of the cranial nerves that course through the cavernous sinus. It is caused by a cavernous sinus thrombosis.

cavernous sinus thrombosis A blood clot within the cavernous sinus. A thrombosis in this key crossroads causes cavernous sinus syndrome.

cavity See *caries.*

cavity, abdominal See *abdominal cavity.*

CBC Complete blood count, a set of values of the cellular (formed) elements of blood. CBC measurements are usually determined by specially designed machines that analyze the different components of blood in less than a minute. The values generally included in a CBC are the following:

- The number of white blood cells in a volume of blood. The normal range varies slightly among laboratories but is generally between 4,300 and 10,800 cells per cubic millimeter (cmm).

- The automated white cell differential, which is a machine-generated percentage of the different types of white blood cells, usually split into granulocytes, lymphocytes, monocytes, eosinophils, and basophils.

- Red cell count, which is the number of red blood cells in a volume of blood. The normal range varies slightly among laboratories but is generally between 4.2 and 5.9 million cells/cmm.

- The amount of hemoglobin in a volume of blood. The normal range for hemoglobin is different between the sexes; it is approximately 13–18 g/deciliter for men and 12–16 g/deciliter for women (international units 8.1–11.2 millimoles/liter for men and 7.4–9.9 millimoles/liter for women).

- Hematocrit, the ratio of the volume of red cells to the volume of whole blood. The normal range for hematocrit is different between the sexes and is approximately 45 to 52 percent for men and 37 to 48 percent for women.

- Mean cell volume, which is the average volume of a red cell. This is a calculated value derived from the hematocrit and red cell count, and the normal range is 86–98 femtoliters.

- Mean cell hemoglobin, which is the average amount of hemoglobin in the average red cell. This is a calculated value that is derived from the measurement of hemoglobin and the red cell count. The normal range is 27–32 picograms.

- Mean cell hemoglobin concentration, which is the average concentration of hemoglobin in a given volume of red cells. This is a calculated volume that is derived from the hemoglobin measurement and the hematocrit. The normal range is 32 to 36 percent.

- Red cell distribution width, which is a measurement of the variability of red cell size. Higher numbers indicate greater variation in size. The normal range is 11–15.

- Platelet count, which is the number of platelets in a volume of blood. Platelets are not complete cells; they are actually fragments of cytoplasm from a cell called a megakaryocyte that is found in the bone marrow. Platelets play a vital role in blood clotting. The normal range varies slightly among laboratories but is in the range of 150,000–400,000/cmm (150×109/liter to 400×109/liter).

CBT Cognitive behavior therapy.

CDC The Centers for Disease Control and Prevention, the US agency charged with tracking and investigating public health trends. A part of the US Public Health Services (PHS) under the Department of Health and Human Services (HHS), the CDC is based in Atlanta, Georgia. It publishes key health information, including weekly data on all deaths and diseases reported in the US (in the journal *Morbidity and Mortality Weekly Report*) and travelers' health advisories. The CDC also fields special rapid-response teams to halt epidemic diseases.

CD8 Transmembrane glycoprotein expressed by T-8 cells. See also *T lymphocyte, cytotoxic; T-suppressor cell.*

CD4 Transmembrane glycoprotein, which is expressed by T-4 cells (also known simply as T cells). See also *T cell; T-4 cell.*

CD4 count, absolute See *T-4 count.*

CDH Congenital dislocation of the hip. See *congenital hip dislocation.*

cDNA Complementary DNA.

CEA Carcinoembryonic antigen.

CEA assay CEA test.

cecal Pertaining to the cecum.

cecum The first portion of the large bowel, which is situated in the lower-right quadrant of the abdomen. The cecum receives fecal material from the small bowel (ileum), which opens into it. The appendix is attached to the cecum.

celiac disease, adult See *celiac sprue.*

celiac sprue An immune-system reaction to gluten, a protein found in wheat and related grains. Celiac sprue causes impaired absorption and digestion of nutrients through the small intestine. Symptoms include frequent diarrhea and weight loss. A skin condition called dermatitis herpetiformis can be associated with celiac sprue. The most accurate test for celiac sprue is a biopsy of the small bowel. Treatment involves avoidance of gluten in the diet, and some people must also avoid milk products, which contain a similar protein. Medications are used for refractory (stubborn) sprue. Also known as gluten enteropathy.

cell The basic structural and functional unit of any living thing. Each cell is a small container of chemicals and water wrapped in a membrane. There are 100 trillion cells in a human being, and each contains the entire human genome, all the genetic information necessary to build a human being. This information is encoded within the cell nucleus in 6 billion subunits of DNA called base pairs. These base pairs are packaged in 23 pairs of chromosomes, with 1 chromosome in each pair coming from each parent. Each of the 46 human chromosomes contains the DNA for thousands of individual genes.

cell, alpha See *alpha cell, pancreatic.*

cell, beta See *beta cell, pancreatic.*

cell cloning The process of producing a group of cells that are genetically identical (clones) to a single ancestral cell.

cell cycle The sequence of events within the cell between mitotic (cell) divisions. The cell cycle is conventionally divided into five phases: G0 (the gap); G1, (the first gap); S (the synthesis phase, during which the DNA is synthesized and replicated); G2 (the second gap); and M (mitosis). Cells that are not destined to divide again are considered to be in the G0 phase. The transition from G0 to G1 is thought to commit the cell to completing the cell cycle by dividing.

cell, delta See *delta cell, pancreatic.*

cell, germ The egg or sperm. Each mature germ cell is haploid, meaning that it has a single set of 23 chromosomes that contains half the usual amount of DNA and half the usual number of genes. This makes germ cells notable exceptions to the usual rules governing chromosomes, genes, and DNA.

cell, reproductive   See *cell, germ.*

cellulite   In popular language, deposits of fat that have a cottage cheese–like texture. Medically, cellulite is not considered abnormal.

Centers for Disease Control and Prevention   See *CDC.*

Centigrade   A thermometer scale in which the freezing point of water at sea level is 0°C and the boiling point of water at sea level is 100°C. The Centigrade scale is used in most of the world to indicate the temperature on a thermometer, but the Fahrenheit scale is still in use in the US. This anachronism requires conversion from Centigrade (°C) to Fahrenheit (°F), and vice versa. 1°C = (5/9) (°F–32). 1°F = (9/5) (°C) + 32.

centimorgan   A unit of measure of genetic recombination frequency. Abbreviated cM. One cM is equal to a 1 percent chance that a marker at one genetic locus will be separated from a marker at another locus due to crossing over in a single generation. In humans, 1 cM is equivalent, on average, to 1 million base pairs.

central auditory processing disorder   A neurological disorder in which a person has difficulty properly interpreting sounds received by the ears, particularly the phonemes of speech. Abbreviated CAPD. CAPD can result in difficulties with attention, speech production, and reading.

central core disease of muscle   One of the conditions that produces "floppy baby" syndrome. Central core disease of muscle causes hypotonia (low muscle tone) in a newborn baby, slowly progressive muscle weakness, and muscle cramps after exercise. Muscle biopsy shows a key diagnostic finding of absent mitochondria in the center of many muscle fibers. It is caused by a gene on chromosome 19, involves ryanodine receptor 1, and is inherited as a dominant trait. Abbreviated CCD.

central line   An infusion tube located in or near the heart, which is at the center of the circulatory system. For example, a Swan-Ganz catheter with its tip in the right atrium and ventricle of the heart is a central line.

central nervous system   That part of the nervous system that consists of the brain and spinal cord. Abbreviated CNS. The CNS is one of the two major divisions of the nervous system. The other is the peripheral nervous system (PNS), which is outside the brain and spinal cord. The PNS connects the CNS to sensory organs, such as the eye and ear, and to other organs of the body, muscles, blood vessels, and glands.

central nervous system, spongy degeneration of the   See *Canavan disease.*

central vision   A process in which millions of cells change light into nerve signals that tell the brain what the person is seeing. As a person reads, drives, and performs other activities that require fine, sharp, straight-ahead vision, light is focused onto the macula in the center of his or her retina, the light-sensitive layer of tissue at the back of the eye.

centromere   The "waist" of the chromosome, which is essential for the division and retention of the chromosome in the cell. The centromere is a uniquely specialized region of the chromosome to which spindle fibers attach during cell division.

cephal-   Prefix indicating the head.

cephalgia   Headache.

cephalgia, histamine   See *cluster headache.*

cephalosporin antibiotics   A group of more than 20 antibiotic drugs that are based on compounds originally isolated from the fungus Cephalosporium acremonium. Like all other antibiotics, cephalosporin antibiotics can affect gastrointestinal-tract function and can cause allergic reactions in some people. They may interact with other antibiotics and with anticoagulant medications. See also *antibiotic.*

cephalothoracic lipodystrophy   A disorder characterized by painless symmetrical diffuse deposits of fat beneath the skin of the neck, upper trunk, arms, and legs. The condition is genetic and is inherited as an autosomal dominant trait. Also known as multiple symmetrical lipomatosis, Launois-Bensaude syndrome, Madelung disease, and familial benign cervical lipomatosis.

cerclage   Encirclement with a ring, loop, wire, or ligature. Cerclage can be done around bone fragments to hold them together, but it usually refers to an operation performed on the cervix to prevent a miscarriage.

cerebellum   The portion of the brain that is in the back of the head, between the cerebrum and the brain stem. It is involved in the control of voluntary and involuntary movement.

cerebral   Of or pertaining to the cerebrum or the brain.

cerebral aneurysm   See *aneurysm, brain.*

cerebral fornix   An arching fibrous band in the brain that connects the two lobes of the cerebrum. There are two such bands, each of which is an arched tract of nerves.

cerebral hemisphere One of the two halves of the cerebrum, which is the largest part of the brain.

cerebral palsy An abnormality of motor function (the ability to move and control movements) that is acquired at an early age, usually less than 1 year, and is due to a brain lesion that is nonprogressive. Abbreviated CP. CP is frequently the result of abnormalities that occur while a fetus is developing inside the womb. Such abnormalities may include accidents of brain development, genetic disorders, stroke due to abnormal blood vessels or blood clots, or infection of the brain. In rare instances, obstetrical accidents during particularly difficult deliveries can cause brain damage and result in CP. CP can take three forms: spastic, choreoathetoid, and hypotonic (flaccid). In spastic CP, there is an abnormality of muscle tone in which one or more extremities (arms or legs) are held in a rigid posture. Choreoathetoid CP is associated with abnormal, uncontrollable writhing movements of the arms and/or legs. A child with hypotonic CP appears floppy—like a rag doll. Treatment may include the use of casting and braces to prevent further loss of limb function, speech therapy, physical therapy, occupational therapy, the use of augmentative communication devices, and the use of medications or botulism toxin (botox) injections to treat spasticity.

cerebral ventricle One of a system of four communicating cavities within the brain that are continuous with the central canal of the spinal cord. They include two lateral ventricles in the cerebral hemispheres, each consisting of a triangular central body and four horns. The lateral ventricles communicate with the third ventricle through an opening called the interventricular foramen. The third ventricle, a median (midline) cavity in the brain, is bounded by the thalamus and hypothalamus on either side. In front, the third ventricle communicates with the lateral ventricles, and in back it communicates with the aqueduct of the midbrain (also known as the aqueduct of Sylvius). The fourth ventricle, which is the lowest of the four ventricles of the brain, extends from the aqueduct of the midbrain to the central canal of the upper end of the spinal cord, with which it communicates, through the two foramina of Luschka and the foramen of Magendie. The ventricles are filled with cerebrospinal fluid.

cerebritis Inflammation of the brain.

cerebrospinal fluid A watery fluid that is continuously produced and absorbed and that flows in the ventricles within the brain and around the surface of the brain and spinal cord. Abbreviated CSF. CSF is produced by the choroid plexus, a series of infolded blood vessels that project into the cerebral ventricles, and it is absorbed into the venous system. If production exceeds absorption, CSF pressure rises, and the result is hydrocephalus. This can also occur if the CSF pathways are obstructed, causing the fluid to accumulate. The CSF obtained during a lumbar puncture is analyzed to detect disease.

cerebrovascular accident See *stroke.*

cerebrum The largest part of the brain, which is divided into two hemispheres (halves). The left and right hemispheres are connected by two arching bands of nerves (cerebral fornices). See also *cerebral fornix.*

ceruloplasmin deficiency A genetic disorder that is due to a lack of ceruloplasmin, a protein that is involved in iron transport. The absence of ceruloplasmin leads to the abnormal deposition of iron in the pancreas (causing diabetes), liver (causing cirrhosis), retina (damaging vision), and brain (causing dementia and Parkinson's disease). Aggressive treatment with deferoxamine, a chelating agent that takes up iron, halts the progression of these complications. Also known as aceruloplasminemia.

cervical Having to do with any kind of neck, including the neck on which the head is perched and the neck of the uterus.

cervical cancer See *cancer, cervical.*

cervical cap A specially fitted contraceptive device that bars the entry of sperm into the cervix. The cervical cap is a thimble-shaped dome made of latex rubber and is much smaller than a diaphragm. For best results, a cervical cap is customarily used with spermicidal gel or cream. See also *birth control; contraceptive.*

cervical cerclage The process of encircling a cervix that is abnormally liable to dilate (an incompetent cervix) with a ring or loop to prevent a miscarriage.

cervical intraepithelial neoplasia The growth of abnormal cells on the surface of the cervix. Numbers from one to three (least to most) may be used to describe how much of the cervix contains abnormal cells. Abbreviated CIN.

cervical rib See *rib, cervical.*

cervical vertebrae The upper seven vertebrae in the spinal column, which make up the neck. They are designated C1 through C7, from the top down. See *C1 through C7.*

cervicitis Inflammation of the uterine cervix.

cervix The low, narrow part of the uterus, which forms a canal that opens from the uterus into the vagina. The inner surface of the cervix is covered with mucus. During ovulation, this mucus is specially adapted to speed sperm to the egg. Normally very small, the cervix dilates during birth to permit the newborn's head to emerge.

cervix, incompetent A cervix that is abnormally liable to dilate and so may not be able to keep a fetus from being spontaneously aborted (miscarried).

cesarean section See *caesarean section.*

CFS Chronic fatigue syndrome.

Chagas disease A disease in Central and South America caused by the parasite Trypanosoma cruzi. The parasite can be transmitted through bites from bugs that carry it (known as kissing bugs) or via blood transfusion. It can also be transmitted to the fetus during pregnancy. Soon after infection, there may be symptoms such as swelling of the eye on one side of the face, usually at the bite wound, but many people do not become ill until many years after being infected. Infants and persons with immunodeficiency are at risk of severe infections and complications such as meningitis and heart failure. Also known as American trypanosomiasis. See also *kissing bug.*

chalazion See *cyst, Meibomian.*

CHAMPUS Civilian Health and Medical Program of the Uniformed Services. CHAMPUS is a US federally funded health program that provides beneficiaries with medical care, supplemental to that available in US military and Public Health Service facilities. All CHAMPUS beneficiaries switch to using Medicare at age 65. CHAMPUS is like Medicare in that the government contracts with private parties to administer the program. CHAMPUS was revamped as a managed care system and renamed TRI-CARE, but it is still widely known under its old moniker.

chancre The classic nonpainful ulcer of syphilis that teems with spirochetes. A chancre forms in the first (primary) stage of syphilis, is highly contagious, and can last from 1 to 5 weeks. Syphilis can be transmitted from any contact with a chancre. If a chancre is outside the vagina or on the scrotum of the male, the use of condoms may not help in preventing transmission of syphilis. Likewise, if a chancre is in the mouth, merely kissing an infected individual can spread syphilis. See also *syphilis.*

change of life See *menopause.*

Charcot-Marie-Tooth disease A genetic disease of nerves that is characterized by progressively debilitating weakness, particularly of the limbs. The foremost feature is marked wasting of the distal extremities, particularly the peroneal muscle groups in the calves, resulting in "stork legs." The disease usually weakens the legs before it weakens the arms. Pes cavus (deformity of the foot) is often the first sign of the disease. The disease is one of the most common genetic diseases, and it is the most common genetic disorder of peripheral nerves. Physical therapy can help prevent the wasting of limbs. The disease can be inherited as an autosomal dominant trait, an autosomal recessive trait, or an X-linked trait. There are also sporadic cases in which there is no family history, so the disease is due to a new dominant mutation. Abbreviated CMT. Also known as peroneal muscular atrophy and hereditary motor and sensory neuropathy.

chart, Snellen The familiar eye chart used to measure how well a person sees at various distances. A Snellen chart is imprinted with block letters that decrease in size line by line, corresponding to the distance at which that line of letters is normally visible. The letters on a Snellen chart are called Snellen test type. Each block letter is quite scientific in design, so that at the appropriate distance the letter subtends a visual angle of 5 degrees and each component part subtends an angle of 1 minute.

chase the dragon A practice of heroin use that involves heating heroin and then inhaling it. This practice carries a risk of irreversible brain damage with death in about 20 percent of cases.

cheek The side of the face, which forms the side wall of the mouth. The cheekbone is part of the temporal bone of the skull, and it provides the prominence of the cheek. The term *cheek* also refers to something that has the form of the human cheek, particularly with two laterally paired parts, such as a buttock.

chemical menopause See *menopause, chemical.*

chemical reaction A process in which one substance is transformed into another.

chemokine One of a large group of proteins that act as chemical messengers and were first found attracting white blood cells to areas of inflammation. Chemokines are involved in several forms of acute and chronic inflammation, infectious diseases, and cancer.

chemokine receptor A molecule that receives a chemokine and associated proteins (chemokine docks). Several chemokine receptors are essential co-receptors for the HIV virus.

chemoprevention The use of natural or laboratory-made substances to prevent cancer.

chemotherapy Treatment with drugs to kill cancer cells. Most anticancer drugs are injected into a vein, but some are given by mouth. Chemotherapy is usually systemic treatment, meaning that the drugs flow through the bloodstream to nearly every part of the body. Often, patients who need many doses of IV chemotherapy receive the drugs through a catheter. One end of the catheter is placed in a large vein in the chest, and the other end is outside the body or attached to a small device just under the skin. Chemotherapy is generally given in cycles: A treatment period is followed by a recovery period, another treatment period, and so on. Usually a patient has chemotherapy as an outpatient at a hospital, at a physician's office, or at home. However, depending on what drugs are given and the patient's general health, the patient might need to stay in the hospital for a short time. The side effects of chemotherapy depend mainly on the drugs and doses the patient receives. Generally, anticancer drugs affect cells that divide rapidly, including blood cells, which fight infection, help the blood to clot, and carry oxygen to all parts of the body. When white blood cells are affected by anticancer drugs, patients are likely to develop infections, may bruise or bleed easily, and may have decreased energy. Cells that line the digestive tract also divide rapidly. As a result of chemotherapy, patients can have side effects such as loss of appetite, nausea and vomiting, hair loss or thinning, and mouth sores. For some patients, medicines can be prescribed to help with side effects, especially with nausea and vomiting. Usually these side effects gradually go away during the recovery period or after treatment stops. In some men and women, chemotherapy drugs may result in temporary or permanent loss of the ability to have children. For men, sperm banking before treatment may be considered; women may choose to have eggs extracted and stored. Women's menstrual periods may stop, and women may have hot flashes and vaginal dryness due to induced menopause. Periods may return in young women. In some cases, bone marrow transplantation and peripheral stem-cell support are used to replace bone marrow tissue that has been destroyed by the effects of chemotherapy or radiation therapy. See also *adjuvant chemotherapy; cancer.*

chemotherapy, adjuvant See *adjuvant chemotherapy.*

cherubism A familial (genetic) disorder of childhood that leads to prominence of the lower face and an appearance reminiscent of the cherubs portrayed in Renaissance art. Cherubism is due to a problem in bone formation that is largely limited to the upper and lower jaws (the maxilla and mandible); bone is lost in the jaws and is replaced with excessive amounts of fibrous tissue. These abnormalities often resolve after puberty. Cherubism is inherited as an autosomal dominant condition. Most boys and girls with it have a parent who had cherubism; the few children who have cherubism without a family history are thought to have a new mutation for cherubism. The gene responsible for cherubism is called SH3BP2 (for SH3-domain binding protein 2). Exactly how a mutation in SH3BP2 leads to cherubism is not known.

chest The area of the body located between the neck and the abdomen. The chest contains the lungs, the heart, and part of the aorta. The walls of the chest are supported by the dorsal vertebrae, the ribs, and the sternum. Also known as thorax.

chest film See *chest X-ray.*

chest pain Pain in the chest that can be a result of many things, including angina, heart attack (coronary occlusion), and other important diseases. Chest pain is a warning to seek medical attention, so one should try not to ignore chest pain and "work through it."

chest X-ray A type of X-ray commonly used to detect abnormalities in the lungs. A chest X-ray can also detect some abnormalities in the heart, aorta, and the bones of the thoracic area.

CHF Congestive heart failure.

chickenpox A highly infectious viral disease that is known medically as varicella. It is caused by herpes zoster, a member of the herpes family of viruses. Chickenpox has nothing to do with chicken; the name originated to distinguish this mild pox from smallpox (chicken being used, as in chickenhearted, to mean weak or timid). Chickenpox is not a major matter unless it occurs in an immunodeficient person or the pox become infected with bacteria through scratching. Treatment, other than the use of calamine lotion or other topical solutions to diminish itching, is not normally necessary. However, adults (and sometimes children) can have major problems from chickenpox, including pneumonia and encephalitis (inflammation of the brain) that can lead to difficulty with balance and coordination (cerebellar ataxia). Other serious complications can include ear infections, damaged nerves (palsies), and Reye's syndrome, a potentially fatal complication. In such cases, antiviral medications may be tried. Reinfection with chickenpox is now recognized to be a common event, and reactivation of the chickenpox virus is responsible for shingles. The current aim in the US is to achieve universal immunization of children with the chickenpox vaccine. See also *chickenpox immunization; herpes zoster; neuralgia, postherpetic; shingles.*

chickenpox immunization A vaccination that prevents chickenpox. The vaccination requires only one shot, given at about 1 year of age. If an older person has not had chickenpox, the shot may be given at any time. There have been few significant reactions to the chickenpox vaccine. All children, except those with compromised immune systems or known neurological conditions, should have the vaccination. See also *chickenpox*.

chickenpox rash The itchy rash that characterizes chickenpox, which typically develops in groups of small lesions. Raised red spots arrive first, progressing to blisters that burst to create open sores before crusting over. This process usually starts on the scalp, then the trunk (the area of greatest concentration for the rash), and finally the arms and legs. Any area of skin that is irritated (by diaper rash, eczema, sunburn, and so on) is likely to be hard-hit by the rash. Chickenpox rash is typically very itchy. In rare cases, a person may have chickenpox without the rash. See also *chickenpox*.

chilblain An injury due to cold temperatures that, although painful, causes little or no permanent impairment. It appears as red, swollen skin that is tender and hot to the touch and may itch. This can worsen to an aching, prickly ("pins and needles") sensation, and then numbness. It can develop in only a few hours in skin exposed to cold. The treatment for chilblain is to stop exposure to cold, remove any wet or constrictive clothing, gently wash and dry the injured area, elevate the injured area, cover the injured area with layers of loose warm clothes, and allow the injured area to rewarm. Like other kinds of cold injury, such as trench foot and frostbite, chilblain may occur with and without freezing of body tissues.

child abuse A complex set of behaviors that include child neglect and the physical, emotional, and sexual abuse of children. Although most people think first of physical abuse when they hear the term *child abuse*, physical abuse makes up only 25 percent of reported cases. Physical abuse is defined as physical injury inflicted upon the child with cruel and/or malicious intent, although the law recognizes that in some cases the parent or caretaker may not have intended to hurt the child; rather, the injury may have resulted from excessive discipline or physical punishment. Physical abuse includes punching, beating, kicking, biting, burning, shaking, or otherwise physically harming a child. Fatal injuries can result from many different acts of maltreatment. Such injuries include severe head trauma, shaken baby syndrome, trauma to the abdomen or chest, scalding, burns, drowning, suffocation, and poisoning. Many physically abused children suffer multiple injuries over the years; these injuries may go untreated to cover up for the abuse. Factors that may predispose a caregiver to child abuse include:

- The abuser's childhood. Child abusers often were abused as children.

- Substance abuse. At least half of all child abuse cases involve some degree of alcohol or drug abuse by the caregiver.

- Family stress, particularly if it erupts in spousal abuse. Stress is exacerbated if caregivers do not have outside resources to turn to for help.

- The child. Children at increased risk for child abuse include infants who are felt to be overly fussy, disabled children, and children with chronic diseases.

- Specific trigger events. Events that occur just before many fatal parental assaults on infants and young children include an infant's inconsolable crying, feeding difficulties, a toddler's failed toilet training, and exaggerated parental perceptions of acts of "disobedience" by the child.

- Social forces. Experts debate whether a postulated reduction in religious/moral values coupled with an increase in the depiction of violence by the entertainment and informational media may increase child abuse. Statistically, this seems unlikely because acts now generally thought of as child abuse were both legal and accepted in past times.

Child abuse should always be reported, investigated, and stopped. Along with medical care for any physical injury, treatment possibilities include parenting classes; caregivers' access to support from professionals and the community; home visits from a nurse, social worker, or other professional to reinforce good parenting skills and monitor the child's well-being; and in cases in which these measures fail, temporary or permanent removal of the child from the home. Education is key because many incidents of physical abuse are accidental or occur because parents have not learned effective nonphysical methods of discipline. The best strategy is to prevent child abuse. It's important to note that children were not even granted the same legal status as domesticated animals in regard to protection against cruelty and neglect until the 19th century. In 1962, the term *battered child syndrome* entered medicine. By 1976, all states in the US had adopted laws mandating the reporting of suspected instances of child abuse by health professionals, teachers, and others. See also *child abuse, emotional; child abuse, sexual; child neglect*.

child abuse, emotional The third most frequently reported form of child abuse, accounting for 17 percent of reported cases. It is likely that emotional child abuse is greatly underreported because it can be difficult to detect and document. It includes acts or omissions by the parents or other caregivers that could cause serious behavioral or emotional disorders. In some instances of emotional child abuse, these acts alone, without any harm yet evident in the child's behavior or condition, are sufficient to warrant the intervention of child protective services. For example, the parents/caregivers may use extreme or bizarre forms of punishment, such as confinement of a child in a dark closet. Emotional child abuse is also sometimes termed psychological child abuse, verbal child abuse, and mental injury of a child.

child abuse, psychological See *child abuse, emotional.*

child abuse, sexual The least frequently reported form of child abuse and probably the most underreported type of child maltreatment. Sexual abuse includes fondling a child's genitals, intercourse, incest, rape, sodomy, exhibitionism, and commercial exploitation through prostitution or the production of pornographic materials. Most cases of child sexual abuse involve parents, relatives, or other adults that the child knows well. Sexual abuse committed by strangers, in day-care centers, or in schools is comparatively rare. Diagnosis and treatment of sexual child abuse is complex. Diagnosis involves taking a thorough, nonjudgmental history of the immediate events, as well as reviewing potential similar experiences. This history is often independently done by a physician, a social worker, and the police department to ensure accuracy. A complete physical exam of the child may include taking photographs to document sexual abuse, X-rays, and laboratory tests. Treatment of offenders depends on the situation. In most proven cases, conviction results in imprisonment. Psychiatric treatment, counseling, and reeducation should be provided to all offenders, whether in or out of prison. Pedophiles (people who prefer sex with children) require intense psychological and pharmacological therapy prior to release into the community because of the high rate of repeat offense. Although some offenders can be successfully treated, truly effective treatment has not yet been found for pedophilia. As with all forms of child abuse, prevention is the best policy. Home and school programs that teach recognition of "good touch" and "bad touch" can provide a forum for helping children avoid potentially harmful scenarios. Parents should also be aware of the behavior of other adults in their children's lives and choose licensed day-care centers and schools that have open-door policies regarding parental visitation. See also *pedophilia.*

child abuse, verbal See *child abuse, emotional.*

child health The care and treatment of children. Child health is the purview of pediatrics, which became a medical specialty in the mid-19th century. Before that time the care and treatment of childhood diseases were included within such areas as general medicine, obstetrics, and midwifery.

child neglect The most frequently reported form of child abuse, which involves the failure to provide for the shelter, safety, supervision, and/or nutritional needs of a child. Child neglect can include physical, educational, or emotional neglect. Physical neglect includes refusal of or delay in seeking health care, abandonment, expulsion from the home or refusal to allow a runaway to return home, and inadequate supervision. Educational neglect includes the allowance of chronic truancy, failure to enroll a child of mandatory school age in school, and failure to attend to a special educational need. Emotional neglect includes such actions as marked inattention to the child's needs for affection, refusal of or failure to provide needed psychological care, spouse abuse in the child's presence, and permission of alcohol or other drug use by the child.

childbed fever Fever due to an infection after childbirth, usually of the placental site within the uterus. If the infection involves the bloodstream, it constitutes puerperal sepsis. Childbed fever was once a common cause of death for women of childbearing age, but it is now comparatively rare in the developed world due to improved sanitary practices in midwifery and obstetrics. Also known as childbirth fever and puerperal fever.

childbirth See *labor.*

childbirth fever See *childbed fever.*

childhood 1 The time between birth until adulthood. 2 The time from infancy to the onset of puberty. During childhood, the potential of a unique human person must be nurtured by parents or parent figures.

childhood disintegrative disorder One of the pervasive developmental disorders (PDDs) characterized by apparently normal development for at least the first 2 years after birth, as manifested by the presence of age-appropriate verbal and nonverbal communication, social relationships, play, and adaptive behavior. Children with this disorder display significant loss of previously acquired skills (before age 10 years). This loss may affect expressive or receptive language, social skills or adaptive behavior, bowel or bladder control, play, or motor skills. Childhood disintegrative disorder also involves impairment in social interaction and communication, often with the development of repetitive stereotyped patterns of behavior, interests, and activities, including motor stereotypes and mannerisms. The loss of previously acquired skills distinguishes childhood disintegrative disorder from autism, another PDD. See also *autism; developmental disorder.*

childhood schizophrenia See *schizophrenia, childhood.*

children's immunizations Vaccinations given to children. In the US, it is currently recommended that all children receive vaccination against the following:

- Diphtheria, tetanus, and pertussis (whooping cough), as separate vaccinations or in combination as DPT
- Haemophilus influenzae type B (HIB)
- Hepatitis B
- Measles, mumps, and rubella (German measles), as separate vaccinations or in combination as MMR
- Pneumococcal infections
- Poliovirus
- Tetanus (lockjaw)
- Varicella zoster virus (chickenpox)

Every child in the US should have these vaccinations unless the child has special circumstances, such as a compromised immune system or a neurological disorder.

chimera 1 An imaginary monster made up of incongruous parts. 2 In medicine, a person composed of two genetically distinct types of cells. This may be due to the fusion of two embryos at a very early (blastula) stage. More commonly today, the formation of a chimera is due to transplantation. When bone marrow from one person is used to reconstitute the bone marrow of an irradiated recipient, the recipient becomes a chimera. 3 A viral, bacterial, or other cell that seems to be composed of two genetically distinct strains, as might be seen when genetic engineering techniques are used to enclose therapeutic properties from one cell in another type of cell for delivery.

chiropractic A system of diagnosis and treatment based on the concept that the nervous system coordinates all of the body's functions and that disease results from a lack of normal nerve function. Chiropractic employs manipulation and adjustment of body structures, such as the spinal column, so that pressure on nerves coming from the spinal cord due to displacement (subluxation) of a vertebral body may be relieved. Practitioners believe that misalignment and nerve pressure can cause problems not only in the local area, but also at some distance from it. Chiropractic treatment appears to be effective for muscle spasms of the back and neck, tension headaches,

and some sorts of leg pain. It may or may not be useful for other ailments. Some chiropractors also recommend other forms of treatment, such as massage, diet changes, vitamins and minerals, and herbal supplements. See also *chiropractor.*

chiropractor Someone who practices chiropractic. Becoming a doctor of chiropractic (DC) requires a minimum of 2 years of college and 4 years in a school of chiropractic medicine. Some chiropractors also earn a traditional medical degree (MD) or other additional qualifications. Not all chiropractors are alike in their practice. The International Chiropractors Association believes that patients should be treated by spinal manipulation alone, whereas the American Chiropractic Association advocates a multidisciplinary approach that combines spinal adjustment with other modalities, such as physical therapy, psychological counseling, and dietary measures.

chlamydia The agent of a sexually transmitted disease, a type of bacteria found in the cervix, urethra, throat, or rectum that acts very much like gonorrhea in the way it is spread, the symptoms it produces, and its long-term consequences. Chlamydia is destructive to the Fallopian tubes, causing infertility, tubal pregnancy, and severe pelvic infection. Because it is common for infected women to have no symptoms, chlamydia often goes untreated. Chlamydia is associated with an increased incidence of preterm births. Also, an infant can acquire the disease during passage through the birth canal, leading to eye problems or pneumonia. Chlamydia is one of the reasons newborns are routinely treated with antibiotic eyedrops. Chlamydia can also cause inflammation of the urethra, epididymis, and rectum in men. A chronic form of arthritis, called reactive arthritis, can develop after chlamydia infection.

chloroform A clear, volatile liquid with a strong smell similar to that of ether. Chloroform was once administered by inhalation to produce anesthesia, given to relieve pain, and used as a remedy for cough. It is quite toxic to the kidneys and the liver.

choked disk See *papilledema.*

choking Partial or complete obstruction of the airway, usually due to the presence of food, a toy, or another foreign body in the upper throat or trachea. See also *airway obstruction.*

cholangitis, primary sclerosing See *primary sclerosing cholangitis.*

cholecystitis Inflammation of the gallbladder. Cholecystitis is a complication of gallstones, and it is frequently associated with infection in the gallbladder. Risk factors for cholecystitis include age, obesity, female gender, multiple pregnancies, use of birth control pills, and heredity. The most common symptom is pain in the upper abdomen, although some patients have no symptoms. Diagnosis is usually made with ultrasound of the abdomen. Surgery (standard or laparoscopic) is considered for patients with severe cholecystitis. In some mild cases, medication may be used instead to treat the infection and inflammation and to dissolve the gallstones.

cholera   A devastating disease that is characterized by intense vomiting and profuse watery diarrhea and that rapidly leads to dehydration and often death. Cholera is caused by infection with the bacteria Vibrio cholerae, which may be transmitted via infected fecal matter, food, or water. With modern sanitation, cholera is no longer as common as it once was, but epidemics still occur whenever people must live in crowded and unsanitary conditions, such as in refugee camps. The disease is treated by IV administration of saline solution to rehydrate the patient and with antibiotics to kill the bacteria. Cholera has also been known as Asian cholera, due to its one-time prevalence in that area of the world.

cholescintigraphy   A diagnostic test in which a two-dimensional picture of a radiation source in the biliary system is obtained through the use of radioisotopes. The test is done to examine the biliary system and diagnose obstruction of the bile ducts (for example, by a gallstone or a tumor), disease of the gallbladder, and bile leaks.

cholesterol   The most common type of steroid in the body. Cholesterol has gotten something of a bad name because elevated levels increase the risk for heart and blood vessel disease. However, cholesterol is essential to the formation of bile acids, which aid in the digestion of fats, vitamin D, progesterone, estrogens (estradiol, estrone, estriol), androgens (androsterone, testosterone), mineralocorticoid hormones (aldosterone, corticosterone), and glucocorticoid hormones (cortisol). Cholesterol is also necessary to the normal permeability and function of the membranes that surround cells. Cholesterol is carried in the bloodstream as lipoproteins. A diet high in saturated fats tends to increase blood cholesterol levels, whereas a diet high in unsaturated fats tends to lower blood cholesterol levels. Although some cholesterol is obtained from the diet, most cholesterol is made in the liver and other tissues. The treatment of elevated cholesterol therefore involves not only diet but also weight loss, regular exercise, and medications. After the age of 20, cholesterol testing is recommended every 5 years.

cholesterol gallstone   Stone within the gallbladder that is a result of chronically elevated blood levels of cholesterol (hypercholesterolemia). This can lead to inflammation of the gallbladder (cholecystitis). See also *cholecystitis.*

cholesterol, "bad"   See *LDL cholesterol.*

cholesterol, "good"   See *HDL cholesterol.*

cholesterol, HDL   See *HDL cholesterol.*

cholesterol, high-density lipoprotein   See *HDL cholesterol.*

cholesterol, LDL   See *LDL cholesterol.*

cholesterol, low-density lipoprotein   See *LDL cholesterol.*

cholesterol, lowering with fibrates   Lowering cholesterol levels through the use of cholesterol-lowering drugs that are primarily effective in lowering triglycerides and, to a lesser extent, in increasing HDL levels. Gemfibrozil (brand name: Lopid), the fibrate most widely used in the US, can be very effective for patients with high triglyceride levels. However, it is not particularly effective for lowering LDL. As a result, it is used less often than other drugs in patients with heart disease for whom lowering LDL level is the main goal of treatment. The FDA does not recommend gemfibrozil therapy, by itself, for patients with heart disease. Fibrates are usually given in two daily doses, 30 minutes before the morning and evening meals. If treatment is successful, reductions in triglycerides are in the range of 20 to 50 percent, with increases in HDL of 10 to 15 percent. Fibrates are well tolerated by most patients. Gastrointestinal complaints are the most common side effect, and fibrates appear to increase the likelihood of a patient's developing cholesterol gallstones. Fibrates can increase the effect of medications that thin the blood; this increased effectiveness should be monitored by a physician.

cholesterol, lowering with niacin   Niacin, also known as nicotinic acid, is a water-soluble B vitamin that improves levels of all lipoproteins when given in doses well above the vitamin requirement. Niacin lowers the total cholesterol, LDL cholesterol, and triglyceride levels, while raising the HDL cholesterol level. Niacin can reduce LDL levels by 10 to 20 percent, lower triglyceride levels by 20 to 50 percent, and raise HDL levels by 15 to 35 percent. Most experts recommend starting with the immediate-release form (rather than the timed-release form) of niacin. Niacin is inexpensive and widely accessible without a prescription, but because of potential side effects, it must not be used for cholesterol lowering without being monitored by a physician. Patients are usually started on a low daily dose, which is gradually increased to an average daily dose of 1.5 to 3 grams. A common and troublesome side effect of niacin is flushing, or hot flashes, which is a result of the widening of blood vessels. Most patients develop a tolerance for flushing, and in some patients it can be decreased by taking the drug during or after meals or by the use of aspirin or other similar medications prescribed by a physician. "No-flush" niacin formulations are also available. The effect of high blood pressure medicines may also be increased while one is taking niacin. A patient taking high blood pressure medication should set up a blood pressure monitoring system while getting used to a new niacin regimen. A variety of gastrointestinal symptoms, including nausea, indigestion, gas, vomiting, diarrhea, and the activation of peptic ulcers have been seen in some patients who use niacin. Other major adverse effects include liver problems, gout, and high blood sugar; risk of these complications increases as the dose of niacin increases. The nicotinamide form of niacin does not lower cholesterol levels.

chondromalacia patella See *patellofemoral syndrome.*

chondroplasia The formation of cartilage by specialized cells called chondrocytes.

chondrosarcoma A malignant tumor that arises in cartilage cells (chondroplasts). Chondrosarcoma can be primary or secondary. Primary chondrosarcoma forms in bone and is a disease in children. Secondary chondrosarcoma arises from a preexisting benign defect of cartilage (such as an osteochondroma or enchondroma), usually after age 40. The main treatment is surgery. See also *cartilage; sarcoma.*

chorda tendinea A thread-like band of fibrous tissue that attaches on one end to the edge of the tricuspid and mitral valves of the heart and on the other end to the papillary muscle within the heart. The chorda tendinea serves to anchor the valves.

chorda tympani A branch of the facial nerve (the seventh cranial nerve) that serves the taste buds in the front of the tongue, runs through the middle ear, and carries taste messages to the brain. The chorda tympani is part of one of three cranial nerves involved in taste. The taste system involves a complicated feedback loop, with each nerve acting to inhibit the signals of others. The chorda tympani appears to exert a particularly strong inhibitory influence on other taste nerves, as well as on pain fibers in the tongue. When the chorda tympani is damaged, its inhibitory function is disrupted, leading to less inhibited activity in the other nerves.

chordoma A benign tumor, usually in the lower back, that originates from cells destined to form cartilage. These cells are remnants of the primitive notochord, the flexible rod of cells in the embryo that forms the supporting axis of the body. Chordomas induce bone destruction.

chorea Ceaseless, restless, rapid, complex body movements that look well coordinated and purposeful but are, in fact, involuntary. The term *chorea* is derived from the Greek word *choreia,* which means "dancing" (as is choreography) because chorea was thought to be suggestive of a grotesque dance. See also *Huntington's disease; Sydenham's chorea.*

chorea, Huntington's See *Huntington's disease.*

chorea, Sydenham's See *Sydenham's chorea.*

chorioangioma, placental A benign tumor of a blood vessel in the placenta. Large chorioangiomas can cause complications, including excess amniotic fluid (polyhydramnios), maternal and fetal clotting problems (coagulopathies), premature delivery, toxemia, fetal heart failure, and hydrops (excess fluid) affecting the fetus. Chorioangiomas probably act as shunts between arteries and veins (arteriovenous shunts), leading to progressive heart failure of the fetus. In the presence of placental chorioangioma, labor is usually induced by a physician when the fetus is viable. Alcohol injection into the placental chorioangioma is being tried as a new treatment.

choriocarcinoma A highly malignant tumor that arises from trophoblastic cells within the uterus. Choriocarcinoma may follow any type of pregnancy but is especially likely to occur with a hydatidiform mole. The prognosis for women with metastatic choriocarcinoma has improved with the advent of multidrug chemotherapy. See also *hydatidiform mole.*

chorion The outermost of the two fetal membranes (the amnion is the innermost) that surround the embryo. The chorion develops villi (vascular fingers) and develops into the placenta.

chorionic gonadotropin, human See *human chorionic gonadotropin.*

chorionic villus sampling A procedure for first-trimester prenatal diagnosis. Abbreviated CVS. CVS may be done between the eighth and tenth weeks of pregnancy. The aim is to diagnose severe abnormalities that are present in the fetus. Tissue is withdrawn from the villi of the chorion, a part of the placenta, and then prepared for diagnostic analysis. Abbreviated CVS.

choroiditis An inflammation of the layer of the eye behind the retina, either in its entirety (multifocal choroiditis) or in patches (focal choroiditis). The only symptom is usually blurred vision. Choroiditis is treatment with medications that reduce inflammation. See also *uveitis.*

Christmas disease   See *hemophilia B.*

chromatid   One of the two daughter strands created by the lengthwise division of the f chromosome. The two chromatids are at first joined together by a centromere, and then they separate, with each chromatid becoming a chromosome.

chromatography, gas   An automated technique for separating mixtures of substances in which the mixture to be analyzed is vaporized and carried by an inert gas through a special column and thence to a detection device. Abbreviated GC. The special column can contain an inert porous solid (gas-solid chromatography) or a liquid coated on a solid support (gas-liquid chromatography). The basic aim of GC is to separate each component that was in the mixture so that it produces a different peak in the detection device output, which is graphed on a chart recorder. GC is a valuable tool in biochemistry.

chromatopsia   Colored vision. A condition in which objects appear abnormally colored to the viewer.

chromosome   A carrier of genetic information that is visible under an ordinary light microscope. Each human chromosome has two arms, the p (short) arm and the q (long) arm. These arms are separated from each other only by the centromere, which is the point at which the chromosome is attached to the spindle during cell division. The 3 billion base pairs in the human genome are organized into 24 chromosomes. All genes are arranged linearly along the chromosomes. Generally the nucleus of a human cell contains two sets of chromosomes—one set given by each parent. Each set has 23 single chromosomes: 22 autosomes and an X or a Y sex chromosome. (A normal female has a pair of X chromosomes; a male has an X and Y pair.) A chromosome contains roughly equal parts of protein and DNA. The chromosomal DNA contains an average of 150 million nucleotide building blocks, called bases. DNA molecules are among the largest molecules now known.

chromosome, acentric   A fragment of a chromosome that lacks a centromere, so that the chromosome is lost when the cell divides.

chromosome, acrocentric   A chromosome that has its centromere located near one end of the chromosome. Humans have five pairs of acrocentric chromosomes. Down syndrome is due to an extra acrocentric chromosome (chromosome 21).

chromosome, autosomal   Any chromosome other than a sex chromosome.

chromosome complement   The whole set of chromosomes for a species. In humans, the normal chromosome complement (also known as the karyotype) consists of 46 chromosomes, including the 2 sex chromosomes.

chromosome, dicentric   A chromosome that is abnormal in that it has two centromeres rather than one. Because the centromere is essential for chromosome division, a dicentric chromosome is pulled in opposite directions when the cell divides. This causes the chromosome to form a bridge and then break. Dicentric chromosomes are a cause of chromosome instability.

chromosome disorder   An abnormal condition due to something unusual in an individual's chromosomes. For example, Down syndrome is a chromosome disorder caused by the presence of an extra copy of chromosome 21, and Turner syndrome is most often due to the presence of only a single sex chromosome: one X chromosome.

chromosome inversion   A condition in which a chromosome segment is clipped out, turned upside down, and reinserted back into the chromosome. A chromosome inversion can be inherited from one or both parents, or it may be a mutation that appears in a child whose family has no history of chromosome inversion. An inversion can be "balanced," meaning that it has all the genes that are present in a normal chromosome; or it can be "unbalanced," meaning that genes have been deleted (lost) or duplicated. A balanced inversion causes no problems. An unbalanced inversion is often associated with problems such as developmental delay, mental retardation, and birth defects.

chromosome inversion, paracentric   A type of chromosome rearrangement in which a chromosomal segment that does not include the centromere (and is therefore paracentric) is snipped out of a chromosome, inverted, and inserted back into the chromosome. The feature that makes it paracentric is that both breaks are on the same side of the centromere, so that the centromere is not involved in the rearrangement.

chromosome inversion, pericentric   A basic type of chromosome rearrangement in which a segment that includes the centromere (and is therefore pericentric) is snipped out of a chromosome, inverted, and inserted back into the chromosome. The feature that makes it pericentric is that the breaks are on both sides of the centromere.

chromosome map   The chart of the linear array of genes on a chromosome. The Human Genome Project contributes to the mapping of the human chromosomes. See also *Human Genome Project.*

chromosome, marker An abnormal chromosome that is distinctive in appearance but not fully identified. A marker chromosome is not necessarily a marker for a specific disease or abnormality, but it can be distinguished under the microscope from all the normal human chromosomes. For example, the fragile X (FRAXA) chromosome was once called the marker X.

chromosome, metaphase A chromosome at the stage in the cell cycle at which it is most condensed, easiest to see by itself, and therefore easiest to study. Metaphase chromosomes are often chosen for karyotyping and chromosome analysis.

chromosome, prophase A chromosome at a stage before metaphase in the cell cycle, when the chromosomes are long and often tangled like a ball of twine. Prophase chromosomes may be selected for analysis via resolution chromosome banding when it is important to detect minute details.

chromosome, sex The X or Y chromosome in humans. (Some other species have other sex chromosomes.)

chromosome, X The sex chromosome found twice in normal females and once, along with a Y chromosome, in normal males. The complete chromosome complement (consisting of 46 chromosomes, including the 2 sex chromosomes) is thus conventionally written as 46,XX for chromosomally normal females and 46,XY for chromosomally normal males. The X chromosome not only determines gender but also carries the genetic code for many essential functions in both males and females.

chromosome, Y The sex chromosome found in normal males, together with an X chromosome. Once thought to be a genetic wasteland, the Y chromosome is now known to contain at least 20 genes. Some of these genes are unique to the Y chromosome, including the male-determining gene and male fitness genes that are active only in the testis and that are thought to be responsible for the formation of sperm. Other genes on the Y chromosome have counterparts on the X chromosome, are active in many body tissues, and play crucial "housekeeping" roles within cells.

chromosomes in multiple miscarriages Chromosome abnormalities (such as deletions, additions, or translocations) that are responsible for causing miscarriages. A couple that has had more than one miscarriage has about a 5 percent chance that one member of the couple is carrying an irregular chromosome that is responsible for the miscarriages.

chronic In medicine, lasting a long time. A chronic condition is one that lasts 3 months or more. Chronic diseases are in contrast to those that are acute (abrupt, sharp, and brief) or subacute (within the interval between acute and chronic).

chronic arthritis, systemic-onset juvenile See *Still's disease.*

chronic bronchitis See *bronchitis, chronic.*

chronic fatigue syndrome A debilitating and complex disorder characterized by profound fatigue that lasts 6 months or longer, is not improved by bed rest, and may be worsened by physical or mental activity. Abbreviated CFS. Persons with CFS most often function at a substantially lower level of activity than they were capable of before the onset of the illness. In addition to these key defining characteristics, patients report various nonspecific symptoms, including weakness, muscle pain, impaired memory and/or mental concentration, insomnia, and postexertional fatigue lasting more than 24 hours. In some cases, CFS can persist for years. The cause or causes of CFS have not been identified, and no specific diagnostic tests are available. Moreover, because many illnesses have incapacitating fatigue as a symptom, care must be taken to exclude other known and often treatable conditions before a diagnosis of CFS is made. Also known as chronic fatigue and immune dysfunction syndrome (CFIDS) and myalgic encephalomyelitis (ME).

chronic illness An illness that lasts 3 months or more.

chronic leukemia Cancer of the blood cells that progresses slowly, as opposed to acute leukemia, which progresses quickly. The two major types of chronic leukemia are chronic lymphocytic leukemia (CLL) and chronic myeloid leukemia (CML). See also *leukemia, chronic phase of.*

chronic lymphocytic leukemia See *leukemia, chronic lymphocytic.*

chronic myeloid leukemia See *leukemia, chronic myeloid.*

chronic obstructive lung disease Any disorder that persistently obstructs bronchial airflow. Abbreviated COLD. COLD mainly involves two related diseases: chronic bronchitis and emphysema, both of which cause chronic obstruction of the air that flows through the airways and in and out of the lungs. The obstruction is generally permanent, and it becomes worse over time. In asthma, there is also obstruction of airflow out of the lungs, but the obstruction is usually reversible, and between asthma attacks, the flow of air through the airways is generally good. Also known as chronic obstructive pulmonary disease (COPD).

chronic obstructive pulmonary disease See *chronic obstructive lung disease.*

chronic peritonitis See *peritonitis, chronic.*

chronic phase See *leukemia, chronic phase of.*

chronic tamponade See *tamponade, chronic.*

chronicity The state of being chronic, having a long duration.

Churg-Strauss syndrome A disease characterized by inflammation of the blood vessels in persons with history of asthma or allergy. The symptoms include fatigue, weight loss, inflammation of the nasal passages, numbness, and weakness. The ultimate test for the diagnosis of Churg-Strauss syndrome is a biopsy of involved tissue. Treatment involves stopping inflammation and suppressing the immune system. Also known as allergic granulomatosis and allergic granulomatous angiitis.

chyme A predigested, acidified mass of food that passes from the stomach into the small intestine.

Ci The abbreviation for a Curie, a unit of radioactivity. See also *Curie.*

-cide Suffix indicating killing or killer, as in bactericide (a solution capable of killing bacteria).

ciliary neuralgia See *cluster headache.*

circadian Refers to events occurring within the span of a full 24-hour day, as in a circadian clock.

circadian clock An internal time-keeping system in all organisms. Changes in the external environment, particularly in the light–dark cycle, train this biologic clock. When environmental conditions are constant, rhythms driven by the circadian clock follow a nearly perfect 24-hour pattern. The human circadian clock regulates many daily activities, such as sleep and waking. When a person doesn't follow these natural rhythms, or when the external environment strays from its usual rhythm (as occurs in the long nights and short days of deep winter), the circadian clock must readjust. Rapid environmental changes and problems with circadian clock adjustment are among the causes of jet lag, problems that affect shift workers, some types of sleep disorders, and bipolar disorders, particularly seasonal affective disorder. Genetic researchers have recently identified some of the physical structures

and genes that serve to set and control the circadian clock. See also *bipolar disorder; jet lag; seasonal affective disorder; sleep disorder.*

circinate balanitis See *balanitis, circinate.*

circle of Willis An arterial circle at the base of the brain that is of critical importance. The circle of Willis receives all the blood that is pumped up the two internal carotid arteries that come up the front of the neck and that is pumped from the basilar artery formed by the union of the two vertebral arteries that come up the back of the neck. All the principal arteries that supply cerebral hemispheres of the brain branch off from the circle of Willis.

circulation In medicine, the movement of fluid in a regular or circuitous course. Although circulation does not necessarily refer to the circulation of blood, that is the most common way this word is used in medicine. The circulatory system, composed of the heart and blood vessels, functions to produce circulation. Heart failure is an example of a problem with circulation.

circulation, fetal The blood circulation in the fetus (an unborn baby). Before birth, blood from the fetal heart that is destined for the lungs is shunted away from the lungs through a short vessel called the ductus arteriosus and returned to the aorta. When this shunt is open, it is said to be a patent ductus arteriosus (PDA). The PDA usually closes at or shortly after birth, allowing blood to course freely to the lungs.

circulatory Having to do with circulation, the movement of fluid in a regular or circuitous course.

circulatory system The system that moves blood through the body. The circulatory system is composed of the heart, arteries, capillaries, and veins. This remarkable system transports oxygenated blood from the lungs to the heart and throughout the body via the arteries. The blood goes through the capillaries that are situated between the arteries and veins. Then the blood that has been depleted of oxygen by the body is returned to the lungs and heart via the veins. See also *artery; blood; heart; lung; respiratory system; vein.*

circumcision, female The excision (removal) of part or all of the external female genitalia, including the clitoris, and sometimes extending to the labia. Female circumcision is traditionally practiced in some parts of the Middle East and Africa, particularly Sudan, and it is viewed with disfavor in other parts of the world. Also known as female genital mutilation. See also *clitoridectomy.*

circumcision, male Surgery that removes the protective ring of loose skin (foreskin) that normally covers the glans of the penis. Circumcision dates back to prehistoric times, and it may be performed for religious or cultural reasons, or to promote cleanliness. Newborn circumcision decreases the risk of urinary tract infections and lowers the risk of sexually transmitted diseases, including HIV. It also diminishes the risk for cancer of the penis and lessens the risk for cancer of the cervix in sexual partners.

cirrhosis Liver disease characterized by irreversible scarring of the liver. Alcohol and viral hepatitis, including both hepatitis B and hepatitis C, are among the many causes of cirrhosis. Cirrhosis can cause yellowing of the skin (jaundice), itching, and fatigue. Diagnosis is suggested by physical examination and blood tests, and it can be confirmed by liver biopsy in some patients. Complications of cirrhosis include mental confusion, coma, fluid accumulation (ascites), internal bleeding, and kidney failure. Treatment is designed to limit any further damage to the liver and to prevent complications. Liver transplantation is becoming an important option for patients with advanced cirrhosis.

cirrhosis, primary biliary A liver disease caused by an abnormality of the immune system. Small bile ducts within the liver become inflamed and obliterated. Backup of bile causes intense skin itching and yellowing of the skin (jaundice). Lack of bile decreases absorption of calcium and vitamin D, leading to osteoporosis. Cirrhosis (scarring of the liver) develops over time. See also *cirrhosis.*

Cl The chemical symbol for the element chlorine.

clap Slang term for gonorrhea. See *gonorrhea.*

clasped thumbs and mental retardation See *adducted thumbs.*

claudication Limping. From the Latin *claudicare,* which means "to limp." The Roman emperor Claudius was so named because he limped, probably because of a birth defect.

claudication, intermittent Pain in the calf that comes and goes, typically felt while walking, and usually subsiding with rest. Intermittent claudication can be due to temporary artery narrowing due to vasospasm, permanent artery narrowing due to atherosclerosis, or complete occlusion of an artery to the leg. It is more common in men than in women. It affects 1 to 2 percent of the population under 60 years of age, but it increases to affect more than 5 percent of those over 70. The prognosis is generally favorable because the condition often stabilizes

or improves with time. Conservative therapy is advisable. Walking regularly can sometimes increase the distance that the patient can walk without symptoms. Two drugs that may be prescribed for management of intermittent claudication are pentoxifylline (brand name: Trental) and cilostazol (brand name: Pletal). If conservative therapy is inadequate and claudication is severe and persistent, correction of the narrowing in the affected artery might be suggested, depending on the location and severity of the narrowing in the artery and the underlying medical condition of the patient. Procedures used to correct the narrowing of arteries include surgery, such as bypass grafting; and interventional radiology, such as balloon angioplasty.

claudication, venous Limping and/or pain resulting from inadequate venous drainage.

clavicle See *collarbone.*

clavus See *corn.*

clay-shoveler's fracture See *fracture, clay-shoveler's.*

cleft lip A fissure in the upper lip that is due to failure of the left and right sides of the fetal lip tissue to fuse, an event that should take place by 35 days of uterine age. Cleft lip can be on one side only (unilateral) or on both sides (bilateral). Because failure of lip fusion can impair the subsequent closure of the palatal shelves, cleft lip often occurs in association with cleft palate. It is one of the most common physical birth defects, and it can be corrected with surgery.

cleft palate An opening in the roof of the mouth due to a failure of the palatal shelves to come fully together from either side of the mouth and fuse during the first months of development as an embryo. The opening in the palate permits communication between the nasal passages and the mouth. Surgery is needed to close the palate. Cleft palate can occur alone or in association with cleft lip.

cleft uvula A common minor anomaly that occurs in about 1 percent of Europeans and 10 percent of Native Americans, in which the uvula (the tissue that hangs down at the back of the palate) is cleft. Persons with a cleft uvula should not have their adenoids removed because without the adenoids they cannot achieve proper closure between the soft palate and pharynx while speaking, and they will develop hypernasal speech. Also known as bifid uvula.

cleidocranial dysostosis A genetic disorder of bone development that is characterized by absent or incompletely formed collarbones (a child with this disorder can bring his or her shoulders together, or nearly so) and cranial and facial abnormalities that may include square skull, late closure of the sutures of the skull, late closure of the fontanels, low nasal bridge, delayed eruption of the teeth, and abnormal permanent teeth. The gene for cleidocranial dysostosis has been found on chromosome 6 in band p21 and codes for the transcription factor corebinding factor alpha subunit 1 (CBFA1); mutations of CBFA1 cause this disorder. Also known as cleidocranial dysplasia and craniocleidodysostosis.

click-murmur syndrome   See *mitral valve prolapse.*

clinical   **1** Having to do with the examination and treatment of patients   **2** Applicable to patients. The term comes from the French "clinique" (at the bedside).

clinical cytogenetics   The application of chromosome analysis to clinical medicine. For example, clinical cytogenetic testing is done to look for an extra chromosome 21 in a child who is suspected of having Down syndrome. Clinical cytogenetics emerged around 1960 and today is a specialty that is certified by the American Board of Medical Genetics.

clinical depression   Depressed mood that meets the DSM-IV criteria for a depressive disorder. The term *clinical depression* is commonly used to describe depression that is a type of mental illness—not a normal, temporary mood caused by life events or grieving.

clinical disease   A disease that has recognizable clinical signs and symptoms, as distinct from a subclinical illness, which lacks detectable signs and symptoms. Diabetes, for example, can be a subclinical disease for some years before becoming a clinical disease.

clinical research trial   A study that is intended to evaluate the safety and effectiveness of medications or medical devices by monitoring their effects on large groups of people. Studies may be conducted by government health agencies (such as the National Institutes of Health [NIH]), researchers affiliated with hospital or university medical programs, independent researchers, or individuals from private industry. Usually volunteers are recruited, although in some cases research participants may be paid. Participants are generally divided into two or more groups, including a control group, which does not receive the experimental treatment, receives a placebo (inactive substance) instead of the experimental treatment, or receives a tried-and-true therapy for comparison purposes. Typically, government agencies (such as the Food and Drug Administration [FDA]) approve or disapprove new treatments based on clinical trial results. Although they are important and highly effective in preventing obviously harmful treatments from coming to market, clinical research trials are not always perfect for discovering all side effects, particularly effects associated with long-term

use and interactions between experimental drugs and other medications. For some patients, clinical research trials represent an avenue for receiving promising new therapies that would not otherwise be available. Patients with difficult-to-treat or "incurable" diseases may pursue participation in clinical research trials if standard therapies are not effective.

clinical trial   See *clinical research trial.*

clitoridectomy   The surgical excision (removal) of the clitoris to reduce a woman's ability to be sexually stimulated during intercourse. Also known as female circumcision and female genital mutilation. See also *circumcision, female.*

clitoris   A small mass of erectile tissue in the female that is situated at the anterior apex of the vulva, near the meeting of the labia majora (vulvar lips). Like the penis, the clitoris is highly sensitive to stimulation during sex. The clitoris corresponds to the penis in the male.

CLL   Chronic lymphocytic leukemia. See *leukemia, chronic lymphocytic.*

clone   **1** A replica. For example, a clone can be made of a group of bacteria or a macromolecule such as DNA. **2** A group of cells derived from a single ancestral cell. **3** An individual developed from a single somatic (nongerm) cell from a parent, representing an exact replica of that parent.

clone bank   See *genomic library.*

clone, recombinant   A clone that contains recombinant DNA molecules.

cloning   The process of creating a genetically identical copy.

cloning, cell   The process of producing a group of cells (clones), all genetically identical, from a single ancestral cell.

cloning, DNA   The use of DNA manipulation procedures to produce multiple copies of a single gene or segment of DNA.

cloning, therapeutic   See *therapeutic cloning.*

Clostridium   A genus of bacteria that can survive and thrive in the absence of oxygen. The genus Clostridium contains more than 100 different species, including C. difficile and C. perfringens.

Clostridium difficile   A bacterium that is one of the most common causes of infection of the colon in the US.

Patients taking antibiotics are at risk of becoming infected with C. difficile. Antibiotics disrupt the normal bacteria of the bowel, allowing C. difficile bacteria to become established in the colon. Many persons infected with C. difficile bacteria have no symptoms. These people become carriers of the bacteria and can infect others. In some people, a toxin produced by C. difficile causes diarrhea, abdominal pain, severe inflammation of the colon (colitis), fever, an elevated white blood cell count, vomiting, and dehydration. In severely affected patients, the inner lining of the colon becomes severely inflamed (pseudomembranous colitis). Rarely, the walls of the colon wear away and holes develop (colon perforation), which can lead to a life-threatening infection of the abdomen.

Clostridium perfrigens A bacterium that is the most common cause of gas gangrene, a lethal infection of soft tissue, especially muscle. C. perfringens bacteria are toxin- and gas-producing bacteria. Before the introduction of antibiotics, a significant percentage of battlefield injuries were complicated by gas gangrene. C. perfringens also causes food poisoning and a fulminant form of bowel disease called necrotizing colitis. Formerly known as C. welchii.

Clostridium welchii See *Clostridium perfringens.*

clot-dissolving medication An agent such as plasminogen-activator (t-PA) or streptokinase that is effective in dissolving clots and reopening arteries. For example, clot-dissolving medications may be used in the treatment of heart attacks, to reestablish blood flow to the heart muscle (myocardium). Also known as thrombolytic agents.

clubfoot A common malformation of the foot that is evident at birth. The foot is turned in sharply so that the person seems to be walking on his or her ankle. The medical term for the common ("classic") type of clubfoot is talipes equinovarus. Clubfoot can sometimes be corrected with a combination of surgery, bracing, and physical therapy. When clubfoot cannot be fully corrected, special shoes and braces can help the person achieve a more comfortable gait and avoid stressing and deforming other muscles and bones.

cluster headache A distinctive episodic syndrome of headaches. The most common cluster headache pattern, acute cluster headache, is characterized by one to three short attacks of pain each day around the eyes, clustered over a stretch of one to two months, and followed by a pain-free period that averages 1 year. The other main pattern of cluster headache, chronic or episodic cluster headache, is characterized by the absence of sustained periods of remission, with pain occurring out of the blue or emerging several years after an episodic pattern. The

episodic and acute forms of cluster headache may transform into one another, so it seems they are merely different-appearing patterns of the same disease. Cluster headache looks different and distinct from migraine, although the mechanisms underlying cluster headache and migraine may have a degree of commonality. For example, propranolol is effective in treating migraine but not in treating cluster headache, whereas lithium is beneficial for cluster headache but not migraine. Cluster headache is known by many other names, including ciliary neuralgia, erythroprosopalgia, histamine cephalgia, migrainous neuralgia, Raeder syndrome, spenopalatine neuralgia, and vidian neuralgia.

cluttering A speech disorder characterized by the unwanted repetition of entire words. It resembles stuttering, in which only sounds or parts of words are repeated. See also *speech disorder.*

cM Centimorgan.

CME Continuing medical education, education that physicians are required to obtain in order to earn CME credits to retain their medical licenses. They may do so by taking courses, attending medical conferences where they learn about new developments, or by reading and taking tests.

CML Chronic myeloid leukemia. See *leukemia, chronic myeloid.*

CNA certified nurse aide. See *nurse assistant.*

CNS Central nervous system.

CNS prophylaxis Chemotherapy or radiation therapy to the central nervous system (CNS) as a preventive treatment. CNS prophylaxis is given to kill cancer cells that may be in the brain and spinal cord, even though no cancer has been detected there.

coagulation, blood See *blood coagulation.*

coal miner's pneumoconosis See *black lung disease.*

coarctation A narrowing, stricture, or constriction of an artery. The sides of the vessel at the point of a coarctation appear to be pressed together.

coarctation of the aorta Congenital constriction of the aorta that impedes the flow of blood below the level of the constriction and increases blood pressure above the constriction. Symptoms may not be evident at birth but may develop as soon as the first week after birth, with congestive heart failure or high blood pressure that call for early surgery. If symptoms do not develop, the surgery can be delayed until they do. The outlook after surgery is favorable. Some cases have been treated with balloon angioplasty.

cocaine   A substance derived from the leaves of the coca plant. Cocaine is a bitter, addictive anesthetic substance. Safer anesthetics than cocaine were developed in the 20th century, and cocaine fell into disuse in medicine, although it is still used as an injectable anesthetic by some dentists. Synthetic alternatives, such as procaine, are used far more widely. Tragically, cocaine continues in use as a highly addictive and destructive street drug, an inadvertent contribution by medicine to the contemporary drug culture.

cocci   The plural of coccus.

coccus   A bacterial cell that has the shape of a sphere. Coccus is part of the name of a number of bacteria, such as enterococcus, meningococcus, pneumococcus, staphylococcus, and streptococcus.

coccygeal vertebrae   The three to five (the average number is four) rudimentary vertebrae that make up the coccyx.

coccyx   The small tail-like bone at the bottom of the spine, very near the anus. It is the lowest part of the spinal column. Also known as tailbone.

cochlear implant   A device that is surgically placed (implanted) within the inner ear to help a person with a certain form of deafness to hear. Cochlear implants rarely cure severe or profound deafness, but they can help some hearing-impaired people to distinguish the sounds of language clearly enough to participate in a verbal environment. For children who are congenitally deaf (born deaf), a cochlear implant can markedly increase a preschool child's chances of being able to function effectively in mainstream school classes.

cockroach allergy   A condition that manifests as an allergic reaction when one is exposed to cockroach allergens, tiny protein particles shed or excreted by cockroaches. Asthma can be triggered by exposure to these cockroach allergens. See also *allergy*.

code, genetic   The instructions in a gene that tell the cell how to make a specific protein. A, T, G, and C are the "letters" of the DNA code. They stand for the chemicals adenine, thymine, guanine, and cytosine, respectively, which make up the nucleotide bases of DNA. Each gene's code combines the four chemicals in various ways to spell out three-letter "words" that specify which amino acid is needed at every step in making a protein. The discovery of the genetic code ranks as one of the premiere events of what has been called the golden age of biology (and medicine).

codon   A set of any three adjacent bases in DNA or RNA. There are 64 different codons, of which 61 specify the incorporation of an amino acid into a polypeptide chain; the remaining 3 are stop codons, which signal the ends of polypeptides.

Cogan corneal dystrophy   A disorder in which the cornea shows grayish fingerprint lines, geographic map-like lines, and dots (or microcysts). These lines and dots can be seen on examination with a slit-lamp, which focuses a high-intensity light beam through a slit while the examiner uses a magnifying scope to look at the front of the eye. The disorder is usually without symptoms. However, about 1 patient in 10 has recurrent erosion of the cornea that generally begins after age 30. Under a microscope, a structure called the epithelial basement membrane is abnormal, so the disorder is sometimes called epithelial basement corneal dystrophy. Also known as map-dot-fingerprint type corneal dystrophy and microcystic corneal dystrophy.

Cogan syndrome   Arteritis (also referred to as vasculitis) that involves the ear. Cogan syndrome features not only problems of the hearing and balance portions of the ear but also inflammation of the cornea and often fever, fatigue, and weight loss. Joint and muscle pains can also be present. Less frequently, the arteritis can involve blood vessels elsewhere in the body, as in the skin, kidneys, nerves, and other tissues and organs. Cogan syndrome can lead to deafness or blindness. Treatment is directed toward stopping the inflammation of the blood vessels. Cortisone-related medications, such as prednisone, are often used. Some patients with severe disease can require immunosuppression medications, such as cyclophosphamide (brand name: Cytoxan). Cogan syndrome is extremely rare, and its cause is not known.

cognition   The process of knowing. Cognition includes both awareness and judgment.

cognitive   Having to do with thought, judgment, or knowledge.

cognitive behavior therapy   A therapeutic practice that helps patients recognize and remedy dysfunctional thought patterns. One characteristic technique is exposure and response prevention, in which a patient with a phobia deliberately exposes himself or herself to the feared situation, gradually decreasing the panic response. Cognitive behavior therapy is used to treat obsessive-compulsive disorder, panic disorder, and other biologically based psychiatric illnesses, often in combination with medication. Evidence gathered from brain scans indicates that over time this therapy can sometimes create actual changes in brain and neurotransmitter function. Abbreviated CBT.

cognitive disability   A broad term used to describe such diverse conditions as mental retardation, thought disturbances, and neurological conditions that affect a certain type of perception or mental ability.

cognitive disturbance   Disruption of one's ability to think logically.

cognitive dulling   Loss of mental faculties; difficulty in thinking logically or quickly. Cognitive dulling can occur due to a medical condition or as a side effect of medication.

cognitive science   The study of the mind. Cognitive science is an interdisciplinary science that draws on many fields, including neuroscience, psychology, philosophy, computer science, artificial intelligence, and linguistics. The purpose of cognitive science is to develop models that help explain human perception, thinking, and learning. Its central tenet is that the mind is an information processor. This processor receives, stores, retrieves, transforms, and transmits information. The information and the corresponding information processes can be studied as patterns.

cohort   In a clinical research trial, a group of study participants or patients.

coinsurance   See *copayment*.

coitus   Sexual intercourse.

coitus interruptus   Sexual intercourse in which, as a birth-control measure, the male attempts to withdraw the penis before ejaculation. It is not usually an effective means of birth control because sperm are present in preejaculate fluid produced during intercourse. See also *birth control.*

colchicine   A plant substance that is used in clinical medicine for the treatment of the inflammation of gouty arthritis and in the laboratory to arrest cells during cell division by disrupting the spindles so that their chromosomes can be visualized.

COLD   Chronic obstructive lung disease.

cold, common   A contagious viral upper respiratory tract infection. The common cold can be caused by many different types of viruses, and the body can never build up resistance to all of them. For this reason, colds are a frequent and recurring problem. In fact, kindergarten children average 12 colds per year, and adolescents and adults typically have around 7 colds per year. Going out into cold weather has no effect on the spread of a cold, and antibiotics do not cure or shorten the duration of the common cold.

cold injury   An injury caused by exposure to extreme cold that can lead to loss of body parts and even to death. Examples of cold injury are chilblain, trench foot, and frostbite. Cold injury occurs with and without freezing of body tissues. The young and the elderly are especially prone to cold injury, and alcohol consumption increases the risk of cold injury. It is important not to thaw an extremity if there is a risk of it refreezing. The extremity should be protected from trauma and gradually rewarmed.

cold, June   See *hay fever.*

cold sore   A small sore located on the face or in the mouth that causes pain, burning, or itching before bursting and crusting over. Common locations for cold sores are the lips, chin, cheeks, and nostrils. Cold sores more rarely appear on the gums and the roof of the mouth. Cold sores are caused by herpes simplex type 1 virus, which lies dormant in the body and is reawakened by factors such as stress, sunburn, or fever from a wide range of infectious diseases, including colds. Recurrence is less common after age 35. Sunscreen (SPF 15 or higher) on the lips prevents recurrences of herpes due to sunburn. The virus is highly contagious when fever blisters are present. It is spread by physical contact, such as kissing. Also known as labial herpes, febrile herpes, and fever blister.

cold, summer   See *allergic rhinitis.*

colectomy   An operation to remove all or part of the colon (large intestine). In a partial colectomy, the surgeon removes only part of the colon and a small amount (called a margin) of surrounding healthy tissue. The bowel is then reconnected or an opening of the bowel (ostomy) is created on the abdominal wall to allow the contents of the bowel to exit from the body. Colectomy may be needed for treatment of different types of problems, including diverticulitis, benign polyps of the colon, and cancer of the colon.

colic   An attack of irritability, crying, and apparent abdominal pain in early infancy. Colic is a common condition, occurring in about 1 in 10 babies. An infant with colic often has a rigid abdomen and draws up its legs. Overfeeding, undiluted juices, food allergies, and stress can aggravate colic. Colic usually lasts from early infancy to the third or fourth month of age. Although some experts say colic is not harmful to the baby, it is extremely wearing on parents. Other experts note that very little is known about colic and feel that all efforts should be made to relieve the infant's distress. Treatment can include dietary changes, carefully measured feedings, and extra burping. Parents should not assume that new abdominal pain and loud crying in their baby are colic. It is important for the baby to be seen by a physician to rule out more serious conditions.

colitis Inflammation of the colon (large intestine). There are many forms of colitis, including amebic, Crohn's, infectious, pseudomembranous, spastic, and ulcerative.

colitis, amebic Inflammation of the intestine, with ulcers in the colon, due to infection with an ameba called Entamoeba histolytic. This parasite can be transmitted to humans via contaminated water and food. Symptoms, which include diarrhea, indigestion, nausea, and weight loss, can begin shortly after infection, or the ameba may live in the gastrointestinal tract for months or years before symptoms erupt. Amebic colitis can be treated with medication, including emetine and antibiotics. See also *amebic dysentery; amebiasis.*

colitis, Crohn's Crohn's disease affecting only the colon. Also known as granulomatous colitis. See also *Crohn's disease.*

colitis, granulomatous See *colitis, Crohn's.*

colitis, pseudomembranous Severe inflammation of the inner lining of the colon, usually due to the Clostridium difficile bacterium. Patients taking antibiotics are at particular risk of becoming infected with C. difficile because the natural bacteria of the bowel can usually keep C. difficile at bay but are disrupted by antibiotics. A toxin produced by C. difficile causes colitis symptoms, including diarrhea, abdominal pain, and severe inflammation. Rarely, the walls of the colon wear away and holes develop (colon perforation), which can lead to a life-threatening infection of the abdomen. See also *Clostridium difficile.*

colitis, spastic See *irritable bowel syndrome.*

colitis, ulcerative A common form of inflammatory bowel disease that is characterized by inflammation with ulcer formation in the lining of colon (large intestine). Its cause is unknown. The end of the colon (the rectum) is always involved in ulcerative colitis. When the inflammation is limited to the rectum, the disease is called ulcerative proctitis. The inflammation may extend to varying degrees into the upper parts of the colon. When the entire colon is involved, the terms pancolitis and universal colitis are used. Intermittent rectal bleeding, crampy abdominal pain, and diarrhea can be symptoms of ulcerative colitis. Ulcerative colitis characteristically waxes and wanes. Many patients experience long remissions, even without medication. Ulcerative colitis may mysteriously resolve after a long history of symptoms. Direct visualization (via sigmoidoscopy or colonoscopy) with sampling

of the lining of the bowel is the most accurate diagnostic test. Long-standing ulcerative colitis increases the risk for colon cancer. Ulcerative colitis can also be associated with inflammation in the joints, spine, skin, eyes, liver, and bile ducts. Treatment of ulcerative colitis involves medications and/or surgery; changes in diet can sometimes help.

colitis, universal Ulcerative colitis that involves the entire colon (large intestine).

collagen The principal protein of the skin, tendons, cartilage, bone, and connective tissue. Collagen is an essential part of the framework of the design of our various body tissues.

collagen disease A disease that damages collagen or other components of connective tissue. For example, dermatomyositis and systemic lupus erythematosus are collagen diseases.

collagen injection The practice of injecting collagen into a part of the face or body (often the lips) to make it larger. The effects are long-lasting but not permanent. Collagen injections are usually done by plastic surgeons.

collapsed lung See *atelectasis.*

collarbone A horizontal bone above the first rib that makes up the front part of the shoulder. Also known as the clavicle, the collarbone links the sternum (breastbone) with the scapula, a triangular bone in the back of the shoulder. One end of the collarbone connects to the sternum, forming one side of the sternoclavicular joint. The other end of the collarbone connects to the scapula, there forming one side of the acromioclavicular joint.

collateral 1 In anatomy, a subordinate or accessory part. 2 A side branch, as of a blood vessel or nerve. After a coronary artery occlusion, collateral vessels often develop to shunt blood around the blockage.

collateral knee ligament, lateral A ligament that straps the outside of the knee joint and provides stability and strength to the knee joint.

collateral knee ligament, medial A ligament on the inner side of the knee joint. The medial collateral knee ligament adds stability and strength to the knee joint.

colon The long, coiled, tubelike organ that removes water from digested food. The remaining material, solid waste called stool, moves through the colon to the rectum and leaves the body through the anus. Also known as large bowel and large intestine.

colon cancer See *cancer, colon.*

colon cancer prevention Measures taken to prevent the formation of colon cancer. Colorectal cancer can run in families. The risk of colon cancer is increased for a person whose immediate family member (parent, sibling, or child) had colorectal cancer. It is increased further for a person who has had more than one such relative with colorectal cancer or a family member who has developed colon cancer earlier than 55 years of age. Individuals to whom any of these circumstances apply should undergo colonoscopy every 3 years, starting at an age that is 7 to 10 years younger than when the youngest family member with colon cancer was diagnosed.

colon polyp A benign tumor of the large intestine. Benign polyps do not invade nearby tissue or spread to other parts of the body. Benign polyps can easily be removed during colonoscopy and are not life threatening. If benign polyps are not removed from the large intestine, they can become malignant (cancerous) over time. Most cancers of the large intestine are believed to have developed from polyps.

colonic irrigation See *irrigation of the colon.*

colonoscope A flexible, lighted instrument used to view the inside of the colon.

colonoscopy A procedure whereby a physician inserts a viewing tube (colonoscope) into the rectum for the purpose of inspecting the colon. Polyps can be removed during colonoscopy, and a biopsy can be performed if abnormal areas of the colon are seen.

colony-stimulating factor A laboratory-made agent that is similar to substances in the body that stimulate the production of blood cells. Abbreviated CSF. Treatment with CSF can help blood-forming tissue recover from the effects of chemotherapy and radiation therapy.

colorblindness The inability to perceive colors in a normal fashion. The most common forms of colorblindness are inherited as sex-linked (X-linked) recessive traits. Females are carriers and males are affected. As a result, approximately 1 in 8 males is colorblind, compared to fewer than 1 in 100 females. The most common form of colorblindness is red–green. The second most common form is blue–yellow. A red–green deficit (also known as deuteranomaly, deuteranopia, or Daltonism) is almost always associated with blue–yellow blindness. The most severe form of colorblindness is achromatopsia, the inability to see any color. It is often associated with other eye problems, such as amblyopia (lazy eye), nystagmus, photosensitivity, and extremely poor vision. Testing for colorblindness is commonly performed along with other types of vision screening. Colorblindness is a lifelong condition. It may exclude people from some jobs, such as being a pilot, in which color vision is essential. People with red–green colorblindness may also fail to notice the presence of blood in the urine and stool. See also *monochromatism.*

colorectal Related to the colon and/or rectum.

colorectal cancer See *cancer, colon.*

colostomy An alternative exit from the colon created to divert waste through a hole in the colon and through the wall of the abdomen. A colostomy is commonly performed by severing the colon and then attaching the end leading to the stomach to the skin, through the wall of the abdomen. At the exterior opening (stoma), a bag can be attached for waste removal. The end of the colon that leads to the rectum is closed off and becomes dormant. This is known as a Hartmann colostomy. There are other types of colostomy procedures. Usually a colostomy is performed because of infection, blockage, cancer, or in rare instances, severe trauma of the colon. This is not an operation to be taken lightly; it demands the close attention of both the patient and physician.

colostomy bag A removable, disposable bag that attaches to the exterior opening of a colostomy (stoma) to permit sanitary collection and disposal of bodily wastes.

colostomy, iliac A colostomy in which the exterior opening (stoma) is located on the lower-left side of the abdomen.

colostomy, transverse A colostomy in which the exterior opening (stoma) is located on the upper abdomen.

colostrum A sticky white or yellow fluid secreted by the breasts during the second half of pregnancy and for a few days after birth, before breast milk comes in. It is high in protective antibodies, to give the newborn's immune system a jump-start.

colpo- Prefix referring to the vagina.

colpopexy The use of stitches to bring a displaced vagina back into position against the abdominal wall.

colpoptosis A condition in which the vagina has dropped from its normal position against the abdominal wall.

colporrhaphy Surgical repair of the vagina.

colposcopy A procedure in which a lighted magnifying instrument called a colposcope (or vaginoscope) is used to examine the vagina and cervix.

colpotomy A surgical incision in the vagina.

coma A state of deep, unarousable unconsciousness. A coma may occur as a result of head trauma, disease, poisoning, or numerous other causes. Coma states are sometimes graded based on the absence or presence of reflexive responses to stimuli.

comedo The primary sign of acne, consisting of a widened hair follicle filled with keratin skin debris, bacteria, and sebum (oil). A comedo may be closed or open. A closed comedo (called a whitehead) has an obstructed opening to the skin and may rupture to cause a low-grade inflammatory skin reaction in the area. An open comedo (called a blackhead) has a wide opening to the skin and is capped with a blackened mass of skin debris.

comedones The plural of comedo. See also *comedo.*

comminuted fracture See *fracture, comminuted.*

common bile duct The duct that carries bile from the gallbladder and liver into the duodenum (upper part of the small intestine). The common bile duct is formed by the junction of the cystic duct, from the gallbladder, and the common hepatic duct, from the liver.

common cold See *cold, common.*

communicable disease A disease caused by an infectious organism.

communication disorder A disorder of the speech apparatus and/or of the mental faculties used to speak or communicate by other means. Treatment includes speech therapy and other interventions, as appropriate, for the underlying condition. See also *aphasia; apraxia of speech; articulation disorder; autism; cluttering; speech disorder; stuttering.*

comorbid Occurring together. For example, if a person has both Crohn's disease and stomach ulcers, these are comorbid conditions.

complete blood count See *CBC.*

complete hysterectomy See *hysterectomy, total.*

complete syndactyly See *syndactyly, complete.*

compound fracture See *fracture, compound.*

compound microscope A microscope that consists of two microscopes in series, the first serving as the ocular lens (close to the eye) and the second serving as the objective lens (close to the object to be viewed).

compress Cloth or another material applied under pressure to an area of the skin and held in place for a period of time. A compress can be any temperature, and it can be dry or wet. It may also be impregnated with medication or an herbal remedy. Most compresses are used to relieve inflammation.

compression fracture See *fracture, compression.*

computed tomography scan See *CAT scan.*

computerized axial tomography scan See *CAT scan.*

conception **1** The union of a sperm and an egg to create the first cell of a new organism. The term *conception* has also been used to imply the implantation of the blastocyst, the formation of a viable zygote, and the onset of pregnancy. To conceive a child, a woman must ovulate— release a mature egg from one of her ovaries—and her male reproductive partner must ejaculate tens of millions of mature, motile sperm. Whereas sperm form throughout a man's reproductive life, a woman is born with all the eggs she will ever have. Over the years, her supply is depleted (of about 7 million eggs present at birth, only 400 make it to ovulation) and the remaining eggs age; this aging diminishes the reproductive capacity of the eggs. A sperm must reach and penetrate the egg as it travels from the ovary to the uterus. The fertilized egg must then divide many times, implant in the uterus, and form the placenta that is its lifeline until birth. If the fallopian tubes have been damaged by pelvic infection or there is endometriosis (misplaced growth of the uterine lining), fertilization or implantation may not be possible. A normal menstrual cycle involves the release of an egg once a month. That egg can survive up to 24 hours. The easiest way to know the fertile time is to chart the menstrual cycle on a calendar. A woman is most likely to be fertile 10 to 14 days after the start of menstruation. **2** Related to the formulation or understanding of an idea. See also *pregnancy.*

concussion A traumatic injury to soft tissue, usually the brain, as a result of a violent blow, shaking, or spinning. A brain concussion can cause immediate but temporary impairment of brain functions, such as thinking, vision, equilibrium, and consciousness. After a person has had a concussion, he or she is at increased risk for recurrence. Moreover, after a person has several concussions, less of a blow can cause injury, and the person can require more time to recover.

conditioning **1** Exercise and practice to build up the body for either improved normal performance, as in physical therapy, or in preparation for sports performance. **2** The development of certain predictable behavior as a result of repetitive activity.

conditioning, Pavlovian Use of a system of rewards and punishments to influence behavior. Named after the Russian physiologist Ivan Petrovich Pavlov, who conditioned dogs to respond in what proved to be a predictable manner by giving them rewards.

condom A barrier method of contraception consisting of a sheath made of latex, lambskin, or other material that collects semen and thereby prevents conception. There are both male and female condoms. When not specified, the term *condom* usually refers to a male condom. See also *barrier method; birth control; condom, female; condom, male.*

condom, female A sheath made of plastic or latex that is anchored outside the vagina and lines the interior of the vagina. It collects semen, preventing the semen from reaching the cervix, and thereby preventing conception. It also provides some protection against sexually transmitted diseases, including the HIV virus. A female condom should not be used together with a male condom because they may not both stay in place. See also *barrier method; birth control.*

condom, male A sheath made of latex, lambskin, or other material that is placed over the erect penis before penetration to collect semen, preventing the semen from reaching the cervix, and thereby preventing conception. When used consistently, a condom is a reasonably reliable method of contraception, especially if it is combined with the use of a spermicide or a female barrier method (but not a female condom). Latex condoms also provide some protection against sexually transmitted diseases, including HIV, but lambskin condoms do not protect against HIV. A condom can be used only once. See also *barrier method; birth control.*

conduction system, cardiac See *cardiac conduction system.*

condyloma Wartlike growths around the anus, vulva, or glans penis. There are three major types of condyloma, each of which is sexually transmitted: condyloma acuminatum (warts around the vulva), condyloma latum (a form of secondary syphilis), and condyloma subcutaneum (also known as molluscum contagiosum).

condyloma acuminatum A sexually transmitted disorder characterized by wartlike growths around the vulva. See also *genital wart.*

condyloma latum A form of the secondary stage of syphilis, characterized by wartlike growths around the anus.

condyloma subcutaneum A sexually transmitted disorder characterized by wartlike growths around the anus and genitals that is caused by the virus poxvirus. Also known as molluscum contagiosum.

C1 through C7 The 7 cervical vertebrae of the neck. C1 supports the head and is named atlas, for the Greek god who supported the world. C2 is called the axis because the atlas rotates about the odontoid process, the bony projection of the axis. C7 is sometimes called the prominent vertebra because of its long spine that projects from the back of the vertebral body at the base of the neck.

cone biopsy See *conization.*

cone cell A light-sensitive cell in the retina of the eye. Cone cells absorb light and are essential for distinguishing colors.

congenital A condition that is present at birth, whether or not it is inherited.

congenital aganglionic megacolon See *Hirschsprung disease.*

congenital clasped thumbs with mental retardation See *adducted thumbs.*

congenital defect A birth defect.

congenital dislocation of the hip See *congenital hip dislocation.*

congenital heart disease A malformation of the heart, aorta, or other large blood vessels that is the most frequent form of major birth defect in newborns. Abbreviated CHD. Nearly 1 percent of newborn babies (8 per 1,000) have CHD. There are many types of CHD, including atrial septal defect (ASD), ventricular septal defect (VSD), pulmonary (valvular) stenosis, aortic stenosis, coarctation of the aorta, Tetralogy of Fallot, and transposition of the great arteries. Much of the practice of pediatric cardiology consists of the diagnosis and treatment of CHD. Also known as congenital heart defect, congenital heart malformation, congenital cardiovascular disease, congenital cardiovascular defect, and congenital cardiovascular malformation.

congenital hemolytic jaundice See *spherocytosis, hereditary.*

congenital hip dislocation One of the most common birth defects, characterized by an abnormal formation of the hip joint in which the ball at the top of the thighbone (the head of the femur) is not stable within the socket (acetabulum). The ligaments of the hip joint may also be loose and stretched. The degree of instability at the hip varies. A newborn may have the ball of the hip loosely in the socket (subluxed) or completely dislocated. One of the early signs that a baby has a dislocated hip is a clicking sound when the baby's legs are moved apart. With a full dislocation, the leg "rides up" so that it is shorter than the other leg. The buttocks folds also may not be symmetrical, with more creases on the dislocated side. When the child begins to walk, if the hip problem has not been diagnosed early and treated effectively, he or (more often) she may favor one side or limp. The earlier diagnosis is made, the better. The usual treatment is the use of a device called the Pavlik harness. In up to 97 percent of cases, the Pavlik harness is effective. If it is not, the hip may be positioned into place under anesthesia (closed reduction) and maintained with a body cast (spica). Also known as infantile hip dislocation, congenital dislocation of the hip (CDH), and developmental dysplasia of the hip (DDH).

congenital hypothyroidism   See *cretinism.*

congenital malformation   A physical defect present in a baby at birth that can involve many different parts of the body, including the brain, heart, lungs, liver, bones, and intestinal tract. Congenital malformation can be genetic, it can result from exposure of the fetus to a malforming agent (such as alcohol), or it can be of unknown origin. Congenital malformations are now the leading cause of infant mortality (death) in the US and many other developed nations, and 2 to 3 percent of babies are born with major congenital malformations, such as heart defect, cleft lip and palate, spina bifida, limb defects, and Down syndrome.

congenital neutropenia, severe   See *severe congenital neutropenia.*

congenital ptosis of the eyelids   Drooping of the upper eyelids at birth. The lids may droop only slightly, or they may cover the pupils and restrict or even block vision. Moderate or severe ptosis calls for treatment to permit normal vision development. If congenital ptosis of the eyelids is not corrected, amblyopia (lazy eye) may develop, which can lead to permanently poor vision. Ptosis at birth is often caused by poor development of the eyelid-lifting muscles (levators), which lifts the eyelid. Children with ptosis may tip their heads back into a chin-up position to see underneath the eyelids or raise their eyebrows in an attempt to lift up the lids. Mild or moderate ptosis usually does not require surgery early in life. Treatment usually involves surgery to tighten the levators.

congenital torticollis   See *torticollis, congenital.*

congestive heart failure   Inability of the heart to keep up with the demands on it, with failure of the heart to pump blood with normal efficiency. When this occurs, the heart is unable to provide adequate blood flow to other organs, such as the brain, liver, and kidneys. Abbreviated CHF. CHF may be due to failure of the right or left ventricle, or both. The symptoms can include shortness of breath (dyspnea), asthma due to the heart (cardiac asthma), pooling of blood (stasis) in the general body (systemic) circulation or in the liver's (portal) circulation, swelling (edema), blueness or duskiness (cyanosis), and enlargement (hypertrophy) of the heart. The many causes of CHF include coronary artery disease leading to heart attacks and heart muscle (myocardium) weakness; primary heart muscle weakness from viral infections or toxins, such as prolonged alcohol exposure; heart valve disease causing heart muscle weakness due to too much leaking of blood or causing heart muscle stiffness from a blocked valve; and hypertension (high blood pressure). Rarer causes include hyperthyroidism (high thyroid hormone), vitamin deficiency, and excess use of amphetamines. The aim of therapy is to improve the pumping function of the heart. General treatment includes salt restriction and use of diuretics to get rid of excess fluid, digoxin to strengthen the heart, and other medications. The drug spironolactone (brand name: Aldactone) has been found to be helpful in treating CHF. Its beneficial effects add to the positive effects of ACE inhibitors, another class of drugs commonly relied on in treating heart failure. A pacemaker-like device is also now available to treat heart failure. The implantable device delivers synchronized electrical stimulation to three chambers of the heart, enabling the heart to pump blood more efficiently throughout the body.

conization   Surgery to remove a cone-shaped piece of tissue from the cervix and cervical canal. Conization may be used to diagnose or treat a cervical condition. Also known as cone biopsy.

conjunctiva   A thin, clear, moist membrane that coats the inner surfaces of the eyelids (palpebral conjunctiva) and the outer surface of the eye (ocular, or bulbar, conjunctiva). Inflammation of the conjunctiva is called conjunctivitis (pinkeye).

conjunctivitis   Inflammation of the membrane covering the surface of the eyeball. It can be a result of infection or irritation of the eye, or it can be related to systemic diseases, such as Reiter syndrome. Also known as pinkeye.

conjunctivitis, allergic   Inflammation of the whites of the eyes (the conjunctivae), with itching, redness, and tearing, that is caused by an allergic reaction and frequently accompanied by hay fever.

conjunctivitis arida   See *xerophthalmia.*

Conn syndrome   Overproduction of the hormone aldosterone by a tumor that contains tissue like that in the outer portion (cortex) of the adrenal gland. The excessive aldosterone results in low potassium levels (hypokalemia), underacidity of the body (alkalosis), muscle weakness, excessive thirst (polydipsia), excessive urination (polyuria), and high blood pressure (hypertension). Also known as aldosteronism and hyperaldosteronism.

connectionism A theory of information processing that is based on the neurophysiology of the brain. The basic tenets of connectionism are that signals are processed by elementary units (in this case, neurons), processing units are connected in parallel to other processing units, and connections between processing units are weighted. The weights may be hard-wired, learned, or both, and they represent the strengths of connection (either excitatory or inhibitory) between two units.

connective tissue A material consisting of fibers that form a framework which provides a support structure for body tissues. See also *collagen*.

connective tissue disease A disease (autoimmune or otherwise) that attacks the collagen or other components of connective tissue. Lupus is a connective tissue disease.

connective tissue disease, mixed See *mixed connective tissue disease.*

Conor and Bruch disease See *typhus, African tick.*

consanguinity Close blood relationship, sometimes used to denote human inbreeding. The risks associated with the mating of closely related persons are great. Everyone carries rare recessive genes that, in the company of other genes of the same type, are capable of causing autosomal recessive diseases. First cousins share a set of grandparents, so for any particular gene in one of them, the chance that the other inherited the same allele from the same source is one in eight. For this reason, marriage between first cousins (not to mention closer relatives) is generally discouraged, and in many areas of the world is illegal. Mating between more distant relatives carries lesser risks. In families where a recessive genetic disorder is known or suspected to be present, genetic testing and counseling are advised, even if the level of consanguinity is very low (as, for example, in marriages between third or fourth cousins).

constipation Infrequent and frequently incomplete bowel movements. Constipation is the opposite of diarrhea and is commonly caused by irritable bowel syndrome (IBS), diverticulosis, and medications. Paradoxically, constipation can also be caused by overuse of laxatives. Colon cancer can also narrow the colon and thereby cause constipation. A high-fiber diet can frequently relieve constipation. If the diet is not helpful, medical evaluation is warranted.

continuing medical education See *CME.*

continuous positive airway pressure A treatment for sleep apnea that involves wearing over the face a breathing mask that forces air through the nasal passages at a steady rate, preventing the airway from collapsing during sleep. Abbreviated CPAP. See also *sleep apnea.*

contraceptive Something capable of preventing conception from taking place. See also *barrier method; birth control; cervical cap; condom; condom, female; condom, male; contraceptive, emergency; contraceptive, implanted; Depo-Provera; diaphragm; intrauterine device; Norplant; oral contraceptive.*

contraceptive device, intrauterine See *intrauterine device.*

contraceptive, emergency An oral contraceptive that can be taken after unprotected intercourse. For example, emergency contraceptives may be given to victims of rape as part of aftercare procedures. Also known as the morning-after pill. The current product on the market, Preven, uses four hormone pills, including the hormone levonorgestrel. An emergency contraception treatment was approved in 1999 by the Food and Drug Administration (FDA) for the US market. Its brand name is Plan B.

contraceptive, implanted A time-release contraceptive that is surgically implanted under the skin. At this time, Norplant is the only implantable contraceptive approved for use in the US. See *Norplant.*

contraction The tightening and shortening of a muscle.

contraction, uterine The tightening and shortening of the uterine muscles. During labor, contractions cause the cervix to thin and dilate, and they aid the baby in its entry into the birth canal and then its progress through the birth canal.

contralateral On the other side. The opposite of iposilateral (the same side). For example, a stroke involving the right side of the brain may cause contralateral paralysis of the left leg.

control In research, the group of participants that does not receive the treatment under investigation. The control group may be given a placebo treatment or receive a treatment with known results to permit comparison with the results of the experiment. In lab research that does not use live participants (in vitro research rather than in vivo research), control procedures serve the same purpose as a control group.

contusion   See *bruise.*

copayment   A payment made by an individual who has health insurance, usually at the time a service is received, to offset some of the cost of care. Copayments are a common feature of HMO (health maintenance organization) and PPO (preferred provider organization) health plans in the US. Copayment size may vary depending on the service; generally, low copayments are required for visits to a regular medical provider and higher copayments are required for services received in an emergency room, the latter intended to discourage insured persons from using the emergency room unless it is absolutely necessary. Also known as coinsurance.

COPD   Chronic obstructive pulmonary disease. See *chronic obstructive lung disease.*

coprolalia   The involuntary uttering of obscene, derogatory, or embarrassing words or phrases. Coprolalia is a symptom experienced by about 10 percent of patients with Tourette's syndrome, a tic disorder. Like other tics, coprolalia tends to appear and disappear, and it responds to medication. See also *tic; tic disorder; Tourette's syndrome.*

cords, vocal   See *vocal cords.*

corn   A small callused area of skin caused by local pressure that irritates tissue over a bony prominence. Although the surface area of a corn may be small, the area of hardening actually extends into the deeper layers of skin and flesh. The inside projection of the corn is what causes discomfort. Corns most commonly occur over a toe, where they form what is referred to as hard corns. Between the toes, pressure can form a soft corn of macerated skin, which often yellows. Corns can be softened by soaking them in hot water, with or without softening agents that are available over the counter or by prescription. In some cases, minor outpatient surgery may be used to remove excess corn tissue. Prevention of corns is easier than surgery; it involves simply choosing properly fitted footwear and using commercially available corn pads to prevent further irritation and growth of any corn that may begin to emerge. A corn on the toe may also be called a clavus.

cornea   The clear front window of the eye, which transmits and focuses light into the eye. The cornea is more than a protective film; it is a fairly complex structure that has five layers.

cornea, conical   See *keratoconus.*

corneal dystrophy, Cogan   See *Cogan corneal dystrophy.*

corneal ring, intrastromal   A plastic ring designed to be implanted in the cornea in order to flatten the cornea and thereby correct, or reduce the degree of, nearsightedness (myopia). The ring is placed in the corneal stroma, the middle of the five layers of the cornea.

coronal plane   A vertical two-dimensional imaginary slice through the body from head to foot and parallel to the shoulders.

coronary artery   A vessel that supplies the heart muscle (myocardium) with blood that is rich in oxygen. The coronary arteries encircle the heart in the manner of a crown (in Latin, *corona* means "crown"). Like other arteries, the coronary arteries may be subject to arteriosclerosis (hardening of the arteries). See also *artery.*

coronary artery bypass graft   See *bypass, coronary.*

coronary artery disease   Impedance or blockage of one or more arteries that supply blood to the heart, usually due to atherosclerosis (hardening of the arteries). Abbreviated CAD. A major cause of illness and death, CAD begins when hard cholesterol substances (plaques) are deposited within a coronary artery. The plaques in the coronary arteries can cause the formation of tiny clots that can obstruct the flow of blood to the heart muscle (myocardium), producing symptoms and signs of CAD, including chest pain (angina pectoris), heart attack (myocardial infarction), and sudden death. Treatment for CAD includes bypass surgery, balloon angioplasty, and the use of stents.

coronary artery spasm   A sudden constriction of a coronary artery that deprives the heart muscle (myocardium) of blood and oxygen. This can cause a type of sudden chest pain referred to as variant angina or Prinzmetal angina. Coronary artery spasm can be triggered by emotional stress, medicines, street drugs (particularly cocaine), and exposure to extreme cold. Treatments include the use of beta-blocker medications and, classically, nitroglycerin to permit the coronary arteries to open.

coronary occlusion   Blockage of a coronary artery, which can cause a heart attack. See also *acute myocardial infarction.*

corpora cavernosa   Two chambers that run the length of the penis and are filled with spongy tissue. Blood flows in and fills the open spaces in this spongy tissue to create an erection.

corpus   The body of the uterus.

Corrigan pulse   A pulse that is full and then suddenly collapses. It is usually found in patients with aortic regurgitation, a condition caused by a leaky aortic valve. The left ventricle of the heart ejects blood under high pressure into the aorta. Then the aortic valve normally shuts tight so that blood cannot return to the ventricle. If, however, the aortic valve cannot close completely, the blood in the aorta comes sloshing back into the ventricle, and the pressure and the pulse collapse. Also known as water-hammer pulse.

cortex The outer layer of any organ.

cortex, cerebral The gray outer portion of the cerebrum, the largest part of the brain. Because it has thousands of complex folds, the cerebral cortex has a much larger surface area than one might think. Specific areas of the cerebral cortex govern sensory perception, voluntary response to stimuli, thought, memory, and the unique human capability of consciousness. The white matter of the brain lies within the cerebral cortex, and it carries instructions arising within the cortex to all other parts of the brain and body through an intricate network of nerve fibers.

cortical Having to do with the cortex, the outer layer of an organ.

cortical desmoid tumor See *desmoid, cortical.*

corticosteroid Any of the steroid hormones made by the cortex of the adrenal gland. There are two sets of these hormones: the glucocorticoids, which are produced in reaction to stress and also help in the metabolism of fats, carbohydrates, and proteins; and the mineralocorticoids, which regulate the balance of salt and water within the body.

cortisol A metabolite of the primary stress hormone cortisone. Cortisol is an essential factor in the proper metabolism of starches, and it is the major natural glucocorticoid (GC) in humans.

cortisone A naturally occurring adrenocorticoid hormone that is produced in minute amounts by the adrenal gland. Synthetic cortisone is also available; it is metabolized by the body into cortisol. Uses for synthetic oral, intramuscular, and intravenous cortisone medications include treatment of adrenocortical deficiency and treatment of conditions associated with inflammation. In popular cream form known as hydrocortisone.

coryza A head cold that includes a runny nose.

cosmetic surgeon See *plastic surgeon.*

costal margin The lower edge of the chest (thorax), formed by the bottom edge of the rib cage.

costochondritis Inflammation and swelling of the cartilage of the chest wall, usually involving the cartilage that surrounds the breastbone (sternum) but sometimes including a rib. Costochondritis causes local pain and tenderness of the chest around the sternum. It is sometimes associated with allergies or asthma. Treatment options include anti-inflammatory medications and, in severe cases, corticosteroid injections. Also known as Tietze syndrome.

cough A rapid expulsion of air from the lungs, typically in order to clear the lung airways of fluids, mucus, or other material. Also known as tussis.

cough suppressant A drug used to control coughing, particularly with a dry, nagging, unproductive cough.

coughing syncope See *syncope, coughing.*

Coumadin See *warfarin.*

counseling The therapeutic practice of using discussion to help patients understand and better cope with life's problems or health issues. Areas in which counseling may be used in medicine include nutrition, genetic counseling and family counseling (particularly to help the family cope with a member's illness or death). Counselors may also see individuals or married couples, or they may work with students in a school setting.

counseling, genetic See *genetic counseling.*

counselor A person who practices counseling. Depending on state laws, counselors may or may not be required to hold particular licenses. Credentials used by counselors include MFC (marriage and family counselor) and LMFC (licensed marriage and family counselor). Genetic counselors are certified by the American Board of Medicial Genetics and the American Board of Genetic Counseling.

cousin marriage See *consanguinity.*

cox-1 Cyclooxygenase-1, a protein that acts as an enzyme to speed up the production of certain chemical messengers, called prostaglandins, within the stomach. The prostaglandins work within certain cells that are responsible for inflammation and other functions. For example, they promote the production of the natural mucus lining that protects the inner stomach. Cox-1 is normally present in a variety of areas of the body, including not only the stomach but any other site of inflammation.

cox-1 inhibitor A common anti-inflammatory drug such as aspirin, ibuprofen, and naproxen that blocks the action of both cox-1 and cox-2. Cox-1 inhibitors can reduce inflammation, but they may also decrease the natural protective mucus lining of the stomach. Therefore, these medications can cause stomach upset, intestinal bleeding, and ulcers. In some cases, using a buffered form of a cox-1 inhibitor can eliminate or reduce these adverse effects.

cox-2 Cyclooxygenase-2, a protein that acts as an enzyme to speed up the production of certain chemical messengers, called prostaglandins. Some of these messengers are responsible for promoting inflammation. When cox-2 activity is blocked, inflammation is reduced. Unlike cox-1, cox-2 is active only at the site of inflammation, not in the stomach.

cox-2 inhibitor A type of drug that selectively blocks the cox-2 enzyme. Blocking this enzyme impedes the production of the chemical messengers that cause the pain and swelling of arthritis inflammation. Cox-2 inhibitors do not pose as great a risk of injuring the stomach or intestines as cox-1 inhibitors. Cox-2 inhibitors now on the market include celecoxib (brand name: Celebrex) and rofecoxib (brand name: Vioxx).

CPAP Continuous positive airway pressure.

CPR Cardiopulmonary resuscitation.

crabs Slang for pubic lice, parasitic insects that can infest in the genital area of humans. Pubic lice are usually spread through sexual contact. Rarely, infestation can be spread through contact with an infested person's bed linens, towels, or clothes. The key symptom of pubic lice is itching in the genital area. Lice eggs (nits) or crawling lice can be seen with the naked eye.

cracked-tooth syndrome A toothache caused by a broken tooth (tooth fracture), without associated caries (cavities) or advanced gum disease. Biting on the area of tooth fracture can cause severe, sharp pains. Tooth fractures are usually caused by chewing or biting hard objects, such as hard candies, pencils, nuts, or ice. Sometimes a nearly invisible fracture can be exposed by painting a special dye onto the tooth. Treatment usually involves protecting the tooth with a crown. However, if placing a crown does not relieve pain symptoms, root canal surgery may be necessary.

cradle cap A form of seborrheic dermatitis of the scalp that is usually seen in infants but sometimes found in older children. It is characterized by flaking or scaling of the skin, which may also be reddened.

cramp, writer's A dystonia that affects the muscles of the hand and sometimes the forearm and that only occurs during handwriting. Similar focal dystonias have been called typist's cramp, pianist's cramp, musician's cramp, and golfer's cramp.

cranial Toward (the opposite of caudad) or of the head. See also Appendix B, "Anatomic Orientation Terms."

cranial arteritis See *arteritis, cranial.*

cranial dystonia See *dystonia, cranial.*

cranial nerves The nerves of the brain, which emerge from or enter the skull (the cranium), as opposed to the spinal nerves, which emerge from the vertebral column. There are 12 cranial nerves, each of which is accorded a Roman numeral and a name:

- Cranial nerve I: the olfactory nerve
- Cranial nerve II: the optic nerve
- Cranial nerve III: the oculomotor nerve
- Cranial nerve IV: the trochlear nerve
- Cranial nerve V: the trigeminal nerve
- Cranial nerve VI: the abducent nerve
- Cranial nerve VII: the facial nerve
- Cranial nerve VIII: the vestibulocochlear nerve
- Cranial nerve IX: the glossopharyngeal nerve
- Cranial nerve X: the vagus nerve
- Cranial nerve XI: the accessory nerve
- Cranial nerve XII: the hypoglossal nerve

craniocleidodysostosis See *cleidocranial dysostosis.*

craniofacial disorder A disorder that affects the structure of the skull and face.

craniopharyngioma A type of benign brain tumor that develops from embryonic tissue that forms part of the pituitary gland. Pressure on the pituitary gland by the tumor reduces the availability of the hormone vasopressin, raising the pressure within the cranium. A craniopharyngioma usually includes hard, calcified components within the tumor itself and disrupts normal skull development in its vicinity. Treatment is usually surgery.

craniosacral therapy An alternative therapy in which practitioners attempt to create positive effects by manipulating the bones of the skull and spine, as well as the fascia that underlies muscle tissue. There is little scientific evidence at this time for the value of craniosacral therapy.

craniosynostosis Premature fusion of the sutures between the growth plates in an infant's skull that prevents normal skull expansion. Craniosynostosis involving some but not all of the sutures causes an abnormally shaped skull. Premature closure of all the sutures can cause microcephaly (an abnormally small head), which prevents the normal growth of the brain and results in mental retardation. Early detection of craniosynostosis is therefore of great importance. Treatment is surgery.

craniotomy A surgical operation in which an opening is made in the skull.

cranium The top portion of the skull, which protects the brain. The cranium includes the frontal, parietal, occipital, temporal, sphenoid, and ethmoid bones.

C-reactive protein An acute-phase plasma protein whose blood concentration can rise as high as 1,000-fold with inflammation. Abbreviated CRP. Conditions that commonly lead to marked increases in CRP include infection, trauma, surgery, burns, inflammatory conditions, and advanced cancer. Moderate changes occur after strenuous exercise, heatstroke, and childbirth. Small changes occur after psychological stress and in several psychiatric illnesses. CRP reflects the presence and intensity of inflammation, although an elevation in CRP is not a telltale sign of any particular condition.

cream A water-soluble medicinal preparation applied to the skin. An ointment differs from a cream in that it has an oil base, as opposed to being water-soluble.

crepitus A clinical sign in medicine that is characterized by a peculiar crackling, crinkly, or grating feeling or sound under the skin, around the lungs, or in the joints. Crepitus in soft tissues is often due to gas, most often air, that has penetrated and infiltrated an area where it should not normally be (for example, in the soft tissues beneath the skin). Crepitus in a joint can indicate cartilage wear in the joint space.

CREST syndrome A limited form of scleroderma, a disease of connective tissue that involves the formation of scar tissue (fibrosis) in the skin and sometimes also in other organs of the body. "CREST" is an acronym for Calcinosis (the formation of tiny deposits of calcium in the skin), Raynaud's phenomenon (spasm of the tiny artery vessels that supply blood to the fingers, toes, nose, tongue, or ears), Esophagus (esophageal involvement by the scleroderma), Sclerodactyly (localized thickening and tightness of the skin of the fingers or toes), and Telangiectasias (dilated capillaries that form tiny red areas, frequently on the face and hands and in the mouth, behind the lips).

cretinism Congenital hypothyroidism (underactivity of the thyroid gland at birth), which results in growth retardation, developmental delay, and other abnormal features.

Cretinism can be due to deficiency of iodine in the mother's diet during pregnancy.

Creutzfeldt-Jakob disease A degenerative disease of the brain that causes dementia and, eventually, death. It is believed to be caused by an unconventional transmissible agent called a prion, rather than by bacteria or a virus. Abbreviated CJD. Symptoms of CJD include forgetfulness, nervousness, trembling hand movements, unsteady gait, muscle spasms, chronic dementia, balance disorder, and loss of facial expression. CJD is classified as a spongiform encephalopathy, and it has some relationship to animal diseases in that category, most notably bovine spongiform encephalopathy (mad cow disease). Most cases occur as a result of a random mutation, but inherited forms also exist. In the 1990s, an epidemic of a transmissible CJD variant broke out in Britain, leading to wholesale destruction of English cattle to prevent further cases. In the US, several lots of blood and blood products had to be destroyed when donors later developed CJD. There is neither treatment nor cure for CJD. Also known as Creutzfeldt-Jakob syndrome, Jakob-Creutzfeldt disease, and spastic pseudoparalysis.

crib death See *SIDS*.

crippled A medically outmoded and politically incorrect term that implies a serious loss of normal function through damage or loss of an essential body part or element.

Crohn's colitis Crohn's disease involving only the large intestine (colon). See also *Crohn's disease*.

Crohn's disease A chronic inflammatory disease that primarily involves the small and/or large intestine but that can affect other parts of the digestive system as well. The diagnosis is most commonly made in persons in their teens or 20s. Crohn's disease can be a chronic, recurrent condition, or it can cause minimal symptoms—with or without medical treatment. In mild forms, Crohn's disease causes scattered, shallow, crater-like areas (erosions) called apthous ulcers in the inner surface of the bowel. In more serious cases, deeper and larger ulcers can develop, causing scarring, stiffness, and possibly narrowing of the bowel, sometimes leading to obstruction. Deep ulcers can puncture holes in the bowel wall, leading to infection in the abdominal cavity (peritonitis) and in adjacent organs. Abdominal pain, diarrhea, vomiting, fever, and weight loss can be symptoms. Crohn's disease can also be associated with reddish, tender skin nodules, as well as inflammation of the joints, spine, eyes, and liver. Diagnosis is commonly made by X-ray or colonoscopy. Helpful medications may include anti-inflammatories, immunosuppressors, and antibiotics. Dietary changes can reduce symptoms and increase the patient's comfort level.

Surgery can be necessary in severe cases. Genetic factors contribute to the development of Crohn's disease. Also known as regional enteritis. See also *Crohn's enteritis; Crohn's enterocolitis; Crohn's ileitis; Crohn's ileocolitis.*

Crohn's enteritis   Crohn's disease involving only the small intestine. See also *Crohn's disease.*

Crohn's enterocolitis   Crohn's disease involving both the small and large intestines. See also *Crohn's disease.*

Crohn's ileitis   Inflammation of the ileum (the lowest part of the small intestine) due to Crohn's disease. See also *Crohn's disease.*

Crohn's ileocolitis   Crohn's disease involving the ileum (the lowest portion of the small intestine) and the colon (the large intestine). See also *Crohn's disease.*

cross-section   In anatomy, a transverse cut through a structure or tissue. The opposite is longitudinal section.

cross-sectional study   A study done at one time, not over the course of time. A cross-sectional study might be a study of a disease such as AIDS at one point in time, to learn its prevalence and distribution within the population. Also known as a synchronic study.

cross-training   Doing two or more aerobic activities, such as jogging, bicycling, and swimming, on a regular basis.

crossed embolism   Passage of a clot (thrombus) from a vein to an artery. When clots in veins break off (embolize), they travel first to the right side of the heart and then, normally, to the lungs, where they lodge. The lungs act as a filter to prevent the clots from entering the arterial circulation. However, when there is a hole in the wall between the two upper chambers of the heart (atrial septal defect), a clot can cross from the right side to the left side of the heart and then pass into the arteries. When a clot gets into the arterial circulation, it can travel to the brain, block a vessel there, and cause a stroke (cerebrovascular accident). Because of the risk of stroke from crossed embolism, even small atrial septal defects should generally be closed. Also known as paradoxical embolism.

crossing over   Exchanging genetic material between two paired chromosomes. Crossing over is a way to recombine the genetic material so that each person (except for identical twins) is genetically unique.

crossover study   A type of clinical trial in which the study participants receive each treatment in a random order. With this type of study, every patient serves as his or her own control. Crossover studies are often used when researchers feel it would be difficult to recruit participants willing to risk going without a promising new treatment.

croup   An infection of the larynx, trachea, and bronchial tubes that occurs mainly in children. It is usually caused by viruses but sometimes by bacteria. Symptoms include a cough that sounds like a seal's bark and a harsh crowing sound during inhalation. A low-grade fever (around 100° to 101°F) is common. The child may become very frightened. The major concern with croup is difficulty breathing as the air passages narrow. Treatment may include administration of moist air (as from a humidifier), saltwater nose drops, decongestants and cough suppressants, pain medication, fluids, and, if the infection is bacterial, antibiotics. The breathing of a child with croup should be closely monitored, especially at night, when croup usually gets worse due to prone body position while sleeping. Although most children recover from croup without hospitalization, some may develop life-threatening breathing difficulties. Therefore, close contact with a physician during croup is especially important.

Crouzon syndrome   A hereditary craniofacial disorder characterized by craniosynostosis, small eye sockets that cause the eyes to protrude, a large jaw, and a beaked nose with narrowed breathing passages. Some people with Crouzon syndrome also have sleep apnea, hearing loss, and other difficulties. Treatment involves surgery to correct the craniofacial malformations. Crouzon syndrome is caused by mutations in the gene for fibroblast growth factor receptor-2 (FGFR2). Also known as craniofacial dysostosis. See also *craniosynostosis.*

CRP   C-reactive protein.

cruciate   Cross-shaped.

cruciate ligament   A ligament, such as the ligaments in the knee, that crosses other ligaments. See also *anterior cruciate ligament; posterior cruciate ligament.*

cruciate ligament, anterior   See also *anterior cruciate ligament.*

cruciate ligament, posterior   See *posterior cruciate ligament.*

cryoglobulinemia   The presence in blood of abnormal proteins called cryoglobulins that have the unusual properties of precipitating from the blood serum when it is chilled and redissolving upon rewarming. Cryoglobulins can cause the blood to be abnormally thick, which increases the risk of blood clots forming in the brain (stroke), eyes, and heart. Cryoglobulins can also cause inflammation of blood vessels (vasculitis), which increases the risk of artery blockage. Cryoglobulinemia can also accompany another disease, such as multiple myeloma, dermatomyositis, or lymphoma. Sometimes, small amounts of cryoglobulins are detected in blood samples from people who have no apparent symptoms.

cryopreservation The process of cooling and storing cells, tissues, or organs at very low temperatures to maintain their viability. For example, the technology of cooling and storing cells at a temperature below the freezing point (−196° C) permits high rates of survivability of the cells upon thawing.

cryoprotectant A chemical component of a freezing solution used in cryopreservation to help protect what is being frozen from freeze damage. The chemical glycerol, for example, is commonly used as a cryoprotectant to protect frozen red blood cells.

cryosurgery Treatment performed with an instrument that freezes and destroys abnormal tissue.

crypt In anatomy, variously a blind alley, a tube with no exit, a depression, or a pit in an otherwise fairly flat surface. For example, the tonsillar crypts are little pitlike depressions in the tonsils.

cryptorchidism A condition in which one or both testicles fail to move from the abdomen, where they develop before birth, down into the scrotum. Boys who have had cryptorchidism that was not corrected in early childhood are at increased risk for developing cancer of the testicles. Also known as undescended testicles.

C-section See *caesarean section*.

CSF 1 Cerebrospinal fluid. 2 Colony-stimulating factor.

CT scan See *CAT scan*.

CTL Cytotoxic T lymphocytes. See *T lymphocytes, cytotoxic*.

CTS Carpal tunnel syndrome.

cuboid bone The cube-shaped outer bone in the instep of the foot. The cuboid bone has a joint in back that allows it to articulate posteriorly with the calcaneus (the heel bone). It also has a joint in the front that permits it to articulate anteriorly with the fourth and fifth metatarsals (the bones just behind the fourth and fifth toes).

cul-de-sac In anatomy, a blind pouch or cavity that is closed at one end. Examples include a colonic diverticulum, which is a small bulging sac that pushes outward from the colon wall, as is seen in diverticulosis; and the cecum, the first part of the colon, to which the appendix is attached. The term cul-de-sac is also used specifically

to refer to the rectouterine pouch (the pouch of Douglas), an extension of the peritoneal cavity between the rectum and back wall of the uterus.

culdocentesis The puncture and aspiration (withdrawal) of fluid from the rectouterine pouch (the pouch of Douglas), an extension of the peritoneal cavity between the rectum and back wall of the uterus.

culdoscope The viewing tube (endoscope) introduced through the end of the vagina into the rectouterine pouch (the pouch of Douglas), an extension of the peritoneal cavity between the rectum and back wall of the uterus, in a culdoscopy.

culdoscopy The introduction of a viewing tube (called an endoscope or culdoscope) through the end of the vagina into the rectouterine pouch (the pouch of Douglas), an extension of the peritoneal cavity between the rectum and back wall of the uterus.

cultural evolution Social change mediated by ideas. Cultural evolution shows a rapid rate of change, is usually purposeful and often beneficial, is widely disseminated by diverse means, is frequently transmitted in complex ways, and is enriched by the frequent formation of new ideas and new technologies. Cultural evolution is unique to humans among all forms of life. See also *biologic evolution*.

culture In microbiology, the propagation of microorganisms in a growth medium. Any body tissue or fluid can be evaluated in the laboratory by using culture techniques to detect and identify infectious processes. Culture techniques can be used to determine sensitivity to antibiotics. Cells may also be grown in culture.

curettage Removal of tissue with a curette from the wall of a cavity or another surface. For example, curettage may be done to remove skin cancer. After a local anesthetic numbs the area, the skin cancer is scooped out with a curette. Curettage may also be done in the uterus; dilation and curettage (D&C) refers to the dilation (widening) of the cervical canal to permit curettage of the endometrium, the inner lining of the uterus.

curette spoon-shaped instrument that has a sharp edge. The word curette comes from French and means "scraper." Also spelled curet.

Curie A unit of radioactivity. Specifically, a Curie is the quantity of any radioactive nuclide in which the number of disintegrations per second is 3.7×10 to the 10th power.

Cushingoid Having the constellation of symptoms and signs seen in Cushing's syndrome, caused by an excess of cortisol hormone, particularly facial puffiness and unexplained weight gain. For example, a Cushingoid appearance can result from the extended use of cortisone medications, such as prednisone and prednisolone. See also *Cushing's syndrome.*

Cushing's syndrome   A constellation of symptoms and signs caused by an excess of cortisol hormone. Cushing's syndrome is an extremely complex hormonal condition that involves many areas of the body. Common symptoms are thinning of the skin; weakness; weight gain; bruising; hypertension; diabetes; thin, weak bones (osteoporosis); facial puffiness; and, in women, cessation of menstrual periods. Ironically, one of the most common causes of Cushing's syndrome is the administration of cortisol-like medications for the treatment of diverse diseases. All other cases of Cushing's syndrome are due to the excess production of cortisol by the adrenal gland. This may be caused by an abnormal growth of the pituitary gland, which can stimulate the adrenal gland; a benign or malignant growth within the adrenal gland itself, which produces cortisol; or production within another part of the body (ectopic production) of a hormone that directly or indirectly stimulates the adrenal gland to make cortisol.

cusp   **1** In reference to a heart valve, a triangular segment of the valve, which opens and closes with the flow of blood.   **2** In reference to teeth, a raised area of the biting surface.

cut   An area of severed skin. It is important to wash a cut with soap and water, and keep it clean and dry, but avoid putting alcohol, hydrogen peroxide, or iodine into a cut, which can delay healing. Delay in getting medical care can increase the rate of wound infection. If a cut results from a puncture wound through a shoe, there is a high risk of infection. Redness, swelling, increased pain, and pus draining from the wound also indicate an infection that requires professional care.

cutaneous   Related to the skin.

cutaneous papilloma   See *skin tag.*

cutaneous syndactyly   See *syndactyly, cutaneous.*

cutis anserina   See *goose bumps.*

CVS   Chorionic villus sampling.

cyanosis   A bluish color of the skin and the mucous membranes due to insufficient oxygen in the blood. For example, the lips can develop cynanosis when exposed to extreme cold. Cyanosis can be present at birth, as in a "blue baby," an infant with a malformation of the heart that permits into the arterial system blood that is not fully oxygenated.

cycle, cell   See *cell cycle.*

cycle, menstrual   The monthly progression of changes in the endometrium (the lining of the uterus), which includes the shedding of part of the endometrium and menstruation (monthly vaginal bleeding). This cycle is governed by a complex sequence of hormones that influence fertility and may affect mood and a variety of physical functions. By convention, the menstrual cycle is considered to begin on the first day of menstrual bleeding. See also *menstruation.*

cyclooxygenase-1   See *cox-1.*

cyclooxygenase-1 inhibitor   See *cox-1 inhibitor.*

cyclooxygenase-2   See *cox-2.*

cyclooxygenase-2 inhibitor   See *cox-2 inhibitor.*

cyclophosphamide   A medication (brand name: Cytoxan) that is prescribed primarily to people with autoimmune disorders and certain types of cancer. It can suppress the immune system and kill growing cells.

cyclosporine   An immunosuppressing medication (brand names: Neoral, Sandimmune) that is prescribed chiefly for organ transplant recipients and people with autoimmune disorders.

cyclothymia   A form of bipolar disorder in which the mood swings are less severe than manic depression. See also *bipolar disorder.*

cyst   A closed sac or capsule, usually filled with fluid or semisolid material.

cyst, Baker's   See *Baker's cyst.*

cyst, Meibomian   An inflammation of the oil gland of the eyelid. Also known as chalazion or tarsal cyst.

cyst of the ovary, follicular   A fluid-filled sac in the ovary. A follicular cyst is the most common type of ovarian cyst. It results from the overgrowth of a follicle, the fluid-filled cyst that contains an egg, that does not rupture to release the egg. Normally ovarian cysts resolve with no intervention over the course of days to months. See also *cyst, ovarian.*

cyst, ovarian   A fluid-filled sac in the ovary. The most common type of ovarian cyst is a follicular cyst. Other cysts can contain blood; they are called hemorrhagic or endometrioid cysts. Still other types of ovarian cysts are called dermoid cysts, or ovarian teratomas. These bizarre but usually benign tumors can contain many different body tissues, such as hair, teeth, bone, or cartilage. Most ovarian cysts are never noticed. When a cyst causes symptoms, pain is by far the most common feature. Pain from an ovarian cyst can be caused by rupture of the cyst, rapid growth of the cyst, and spontaneous bleeding into the cyst, or the cyst twisting around its blood supply. Diagnosis is usually made with ultrasound imaging. Blood tests, such as a CA 125 test to help evaluate the potential of cancer, may also be ordered. It should be noted that interpretation of the CA 125 blood test has limitations: Women without cancer may have an elevated CA 125 level, and those with cancer may test negative. Treatment of ovarian cysts depends on the woman's age, the size and type of the cyst, and the cyst's appearance on ultrasound. If a cyst is causing severe pain, is not resolving, or is suspicious in any way, it can be removed through laparoscopy or, if necessary, through an open laparotomy (bikini incision). After a cyst is removed, it should be sent to a pathologist for microscopic examination. For benign cysts, the outcome is usually excellent. See also *cyst of the ovary, follicular; ovarian teratoma.*

cyst, pilonidal An abscess that occurs in the cleft between the buttocks. Pilonidal cysts form frequently in adolescence after long trips that involve sitting, and they may be painful. Treatment frequently involves surgery if not responsive to heat applications and antibiotics.

cyst, sebaceous A rounded, swollen area of the skin formed by an abnormal sac of retained oily excretion (sebum) from the sebaceous glands. See also *glands, sebaceous.*

cyst, synovial, of the popliteal space See *Baker's cyst.*

cyst, tarsal See *cyst, Meibomian.*

cyst, thyroglossal A fluid-filled sac that is present at birth and located in the midline of the neck. A thyroglossal cyst results from incomplete closure of a segment of the thyroglossal duct, a tube-like structure that normally closes as the embryo develops. Also known as thyrolingual cyst.

cyst, thyrolingual See *cyst, thyroglossal.*

cystectomy Surgery to remove the bladder.

cystic acne A localized infection (abscess) that is formed when oil ducts become clogged and infected. Cystic acne is most common in the teenage years. Treatment includes avoiding irritants on the face, including many cleansers and cosmetics, and in some severe cases, use of steroid or antibiotic medication. Cystic acne can cause permanent scarring in severe cases and in those who are prone to forming keloids. See also *acne vulgaris.*

cystic fibrosis A common grave genetic disease that affects the exocrine glands and is characterized by the production of abnormal secretions, leading to mucus buildup that impairs the pancreas and, secondarily, the intestine. Mucus buildup in lungs can impair respiration. Abbreviated CF. Without treatment, CF results in death for 95 percent of affected children before age 5; however, a few long-lived CF patients have survived past age 60. Early diagnosis is of great importance. Early and continuing treatment of CF is valuable. Treatment includes physical therapy to loosen the mucus in the lungs and use of pancreatic enzymes and medications to fight dangerous infections of the lungs. As more people with CF survive childhood, new problems are emerging. For example, in one study, 68 percent of 75 adult women with CF reported leakage of urine within the preceding year. Coughing, sneezing, laughing, and airway clearance provoked the leakage, which worsened when the women's chest disease was most severe. One in 400 couples is at risk for having children with CF. CF is a recessive trait, so the chance of an at-risk couple having a child with CF is 25 percent with each pregnancy. CF is caused by mutations in the CFTR (cystic fibrosis conductance regulator) gene, which is located on chromosome 7.

cysticercosis An infection caused by the pork tapeworm, Taenia solium. Infection occurs when the tapeworm larvae enter the body and form cysts called cysticerci. When cysticerci are found in the brain, the condition is called neurocysticercosis. Cysticercosis is contracted by accidentally swallowing pork tapeworm eggs. Tapeworm eggs are passed in the bowel movement of a person who is infected. These tapeworm eggs are spread through food, water, or surfaces that are contaminated with feces. This can happen by drinking contaminated water or food, or by putting contaminated fingers to the mouth. A person who has a tapeworm infection can reinfect himself or herself. When the tapeworm eggs are inside the stomach, they hatch, penetrate the intestine, travel through the bloodstream, and may develop into cysticerci in the muscles, brain, or eyes. Infection is found most often in rural, developing countries where hygiene is poor and pigs are allowed to roam freely and eat human feces. Cysticercosis is not spread from person to person. However, a person who is infected with the intestinal tapeworm stage of the infection (T. solium) sheds tapeworm eggs in bowel movements. Tapeworm eggs that are accidentally swallowed by another person can cause infection.

cystine An amino acid that is particularly notable because it is the least soluble of all naturally occurring amino acids and because it precipitates out of solution in the heritable disease cystinuria. Cystine tends to precipitate out of urine and form stones (calculi) in the urinary tract, which can obstruct the flow of urine. This obstruction puts pressure back up on the ureter and kidney, causing the ureter to widen (dilate) and the kidney to be compressed. Obstruction also causes the urine to be stagnant, an open invitation to repeated urinary tract infection. Together, pressure on the kidneys and urinary infections result in damage to the kidneys. This damage can progress to renal insufficiency and end-stage kidney disease, requiring renal dialysis or a transplant. See also *cystinuria.*

cystine kidney stones   Kidney stones formed due to an excess of cystine in the urine. Small stones are passed in the urine, but big stones remain in the kidney (nephrolithiasis), impairing the outflow of urine. Medium-size stones can make their way from the kidney into the ureter and lodge there, further blocking the flow of urine. Cystine kidney stones are responsible for all the signs and symptoms of cystinuria. See also *cystinuria.*

cystine transport disease   See *cystinuria.*

cystinuria   A genetic disorder that affects the transport of an amino acid called cystine and results in an excess of cystine in the urine and the formation of cystine kidney stones. Cystinuria is the most common defect in the transport of amino acids. Although cystine is not the only amino acid excreted in excess in cystinuria, it is the least soluble of all naturally occurring amino acids. Signs and symptoms of cystinuria include blood in the urine (hematuria); pain in the side due to kidney pain; intense, cramping pain due to stones in the urinary tract (renal colic); urinary tract disease due to obstruction (obstructive uropathy); and urinary tract infections. There are several genetic types of cystinura. See also *cystine kidney stones.*

cystitis   Inflammation of the bladder. See also *bladder inflammation.*

cystitis, interstitial   Chronic inflammation or irritation of the bladder wall of unknown cause. This inflammation

can lead to scarring and stiffening of the bladder, and even to ulcerations and bleeding. Diagnosis is based on symptoms, findings from cystoscopy and biopsy, and elimination of other treatable causes, such as infection, as suspects. Treatment is aimed at relieving symptoms. Abbreviated IC.

cystoscope   A lighted optical instrument that is inserted through the urethra into the bladder. A cystoscope has two ports: an optical port that permits one to see inside the bladder and a port for insertion of various instruments designed for biopsy, treatment of small bladder tumors, removal of stones from the bladder, and removal of the prostate (prostatectomy).

cystoscopy   A procedure in which a lighted optical instrument called a cytoscope is inserted through the urethra to look at the bladder.

cytogenetics   The study of chromosomes, which are the visible carriers of the hereditary material. Cytogenetics is a fusion science, joining cytology (the study of cells) with genetics (the study of inherited variation).

cytogenetics, clinical   See *clinical cytogenetics.*

cytomegalovirus   A DNA-containing virus from the herpes virus family. Infection with human cytomegalovirus causes mononucleosis and can also cause viral hepatitis and viral pneumonia. Also known as human herpes virus 5 (HHV-5). See also *mononucleosis.*

cytometry, flow   See *flow cytometry.*

cytoplasm   The substance of a cell that lies outside the nucleus.

cytosine   A member of the G-C (guanine-cytosine) pair of bases in DNA.

Cytoxan   See *cyclophosphamide.*

cytotoxic T lymphocytes   See *T lymphocytes, cytotoxic.*

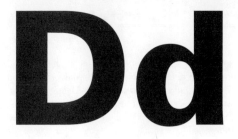

D & C Dilatation and curettage. See also *abortion*.

da Vinci, Leonardo The father of anatomic art, as well as an accomplished architect, scientist, engineer, inventor, poet, sculptor, and painter. Under the secrecy of candlelight necessitated by the church's belief in the sanctity of the human body and a papal decree that forbade human dissection, da Vinci dissected and drew more than 10 human bodies in the cathedral cellar of the mortuary of Santa Spirito. In striking contrast to the pronouncements of Galen and other anatomists, da Vinci recognized that a scientific knowledge of human anatomy could be gained only by dissecting the human body. He injected the blood vessels and cerebral ventricles with wax for preservation, a technique that is still used today. His drawings of the human anatomy have long been considered to be unrivaled.

dactyl-, -dactyl Prefix or suffix denoting the digits (fingers or toes), as in dactylitis (inflammation of a finger or toe).

dactyledema Swelling of a finger or toe.

dactylitis Inflammation of a finger or toe.

dactylomegaly Enlargement of a finger or toe.

dactylospasm A cramp of a finger or toe.

Daily Prayer of a Physician A prayer that is said to have been written by the 12th-century physician–philosopher Moses Maimonides, but possibly penned by German physician Marcus Herz. This prayer is often recited by new medical graduates.

Daltonism See *red-green colorblindness*.

dander Tiny scales shed from human or animal skin or hair. Dander floats in the air, settles on surfaces, and makes up a good portion of household dust. Cat dander is a common cause of allergic reactions.

dandruff A scalp condition that produces white flakes that may be shed and fall from the hair. One cause of dandruff is overworking of the sebaceous glands. Another cause of dandruff is fungus, especially the fungus Pitrosporum ovale. (Most people have this fungus, but people with dandruff have more than the average amount.) To treat dandruff, a person should use a good-quality shampoo (such as Paul Mitchell, Aveda, or Redken). If several weeks of using a good-quality shampoo does not stop the dandruff, the person should use an antifungal shampoo such as Denorex, DHS Targel, ionil-T plus, MG217, Neutrogena T/Gel, Scalpicin, Sebulex, Selsun Blue, Tegrin, or Zircon). The active ingredients approved for dandruff treatment by the US Food and Drug Administration (FDA) include tar, pyrithione zinc, salicylic acid, selenium sulfide, sulfur, and ketoconazole.

dandy fever See *dengue fever.*

Danlos syndrome See *Ehlers-Danlos syndrome.*

Darier disease See *keratosis follicularis.*

daw Abbreviation meaning "dispense as written."

day sight See *nyctanopia.*

DDH Developmental dysplasia of the hip. See *congenital hip dislocation.*

DDX Differential diagnosis.

De Quervain's tenosynovitis Inflammation of the extensor pollicus longus tendon, on the side of the wrist at the base of the thumb. De Quervain's tenosynovitis is typically associated with pain when the thumb is folded across the palm and the fingers are flexed over the thumb as the hand is pulled away from the involved wrist area (the Finklestein sign). Treatment of De Quervain's tenosynovitis includes a combination of rest, splinting, ice, anti-inflammation medication, and/or cortisone injection. Surgery is rarely necessary.

DEA The Drug Enforcement Administration of the US Department of Justice, which regulates interstate commerce in prescription drugs to prevent them from being used as drugs of abuse. Every prescription written in the US bears the DEA number of the prescribing physician.

deafness Partial or complete hearing loss. Levels of hearing impairment vary from a mild to a total loss of hearing. Elderly adults suffer most often from hearing loss. Age-related hearing loss affects 30 to 35 percent of the population between the ages of 65 and 75 years and 40 percent of the population over the age of 75. The most common cause of hearing loss in children is otitis media. A substantial number of hearing impairments are caused by environmental factors such as noise, drugs, and toxins. Deafness can also result from inherited disorders.

deafness, ichthyosis-keratitis See *keratitis-ichthyosis-deafness syndrome.*

deafness with goiter See *Pendred syndrome.*

death, black See *bubonic plague.*

death rate, crude The number of deaths in the population divided by the average population (or the population at midyear). In 1994, for example, the crude death rate per 1,000 population was 8.8 in the US and 7.1 in Australia. A death rate can also be tabulated according to age or cause.

debilitate To impair the strength of or to enfeeble. A chronic progressive disease may debilitate a patient. So may a major surgical procedure, if only temporarily. In either case, the weakness is pervasive. Weakness in an arm or a leg following the removal of a cast is not debilitating, but rather the temporary result of muscle atrophy due to disuse.

deciduous teeth See *primary teeth.*

decongestant A drug that shrinks the swollen membranes in the nose, making it easier for a person to breathe. Decongestants can be taken orally or as nasal spray. Decongestant nasal spray should not be used for more than 5 days without a physician's recommendation, in which case it is usually accompanied by a nasal steroid. Due to a tissue dependence on the medication, many decongestant nasal sprays cause a worsening of symptoms (a rebound effect) when they are taken for too long and then discontinued. Decongestants should not be used by people who have high blood pressure (hypertension) unless they are under a physician's supervision.

decubitus ulcer See *bedsore.*

deep Away from the exterior surface, or farther into the body, as opposed to superficial. For example, the bones are deep to the skin. See also Appendix B, "Anatomic Orientation Terms."

deep vein thrombosis A blood clot in a deep vein in the thigh or leg. The blood clot (thrombus) can break off as an embolus and make its way to the lung, where it can cause respiratory distress and respiratory failure. Even in young, healthy travelers, long stretches of time spent immobilized in the cramped seat of an aircraft with very low humidity sets the stage for formation of blood clots in the leg. Abbreviated DVT. Also known as economy-class syndrome.

defecation syncope See *vasovagal syncope.*

defect, atrial septal See *atrial septal defect.*

defect, enzyme See *enzyme defect.*

defect, ventricular septal See *ventricular septal defect.*

defibrillation The use of a carefully controlled electric shock, administered either through a device on the exterior of the chest wall or directly to the exposed heart muscle, to normalize the rhythm of the heart or restart it.

defibrillator A device that corrects an abnormal heart rhythm by delivering electrical shocks to restore a normal heartbeat.

defibrillator, implantable cardiac See *cardiac defibrillator, implantable.*

deficiency, adenosine deaminase See *adenosine deaminase deficiency.*

deficiency, alpha-1 antitrypsin See *alpha-1 antitrypsin deficiency.*

deficiency, ankyrin See *spherocytosis, hereditary.*

deficiency, calcium See *calcium deficiency.*

deficiency, ceruloplasmin See *ceruloplasmin deficiency.*

deficiency, glucocerebrosidase See *Gaucher disease.*

deficiency, glucose-6-phosphate dehydrogenase See *deficiency, G6PD.*

deficiency, G6PD Deficiency of the enzyme glucose-6-phosphate dehydrogenase (G6PD), the most common enzyme defect of medical importance. In the US, about 10 percent of black males have G6PD deficiency, as do a smaller percentage of black females. G6PD deficiency is also increased in frequency in people of Mediterranean origin (including Italians, Greeks, Arabs, and Jews). The gene that encodes G6PD is on the X chromosome. Males with this enzyme deficiency can develop anemia due to the breakup of their red blood cells when they are first born and any time in life when they are exposed to oxidant drugs, naphthalene moth balls, fava beans, fever, viral and bacterial infections, and diabetic acidosis. Drugs that can cause G6PD deficiency include the antimalarials hydroxychloroquine and primaquine, salicylates, dapsone, sulfonamide antibiotics, nitrofurans, phenacetin, and some vitamin K derivatives.

deficiency, hex-A See *Tay-Sachs disease.*

deficiency, iron A lack of iron, the most common known form of nutritional disorder in the world. Iron is necessary to make hemoglobin, the molecule in red blood cells that is responsible for the transport of oxygen. Iron deficiency results in anemia. In iron deficiency anemia, the red cells are abnormally small (microcytic) and pale (hypochromic). The prevalence of iron deficiency is highest among young children and women of childbearing age (particularly pregnant women). In pregnant women, iron deficiency increases the risk for preterm delivery and delivery of a low-birthweight babies. In children, iron deficiency causes developmental delays, behavioral disturbances, failure to thrive, and increased infections. Iron deficiency is a major problem in developed countries such as the US, Canada, the UK, and Europe. In developing countries, iron deficiency anemia is frequently exacerbated by malaria and worm infections. The treatment of iron deficiency anemia, whether in children or adults, is to add iron supplements and iron-containing foods to the diet. Food sources of iron include meat, poultry, eggs, vegetables, and cereals (especially those fortified with iron). According to the National Academy of Sciences, the recommended dietary allowances of iron are 15 mg per day for women and 10 mg per day for men. However, iron supplements should not be given to children unless a physician recommends them.

deficiency, lactase Lack of the enzyme lactase in the small intestine. Lactase is needed to digest lactose, a sugar found in milk and most other dairy products and also used as an ingredient in other foods. Those with lactase deficiency should check labels carefully. Although most people are born with the ability to make adequate amounts of lactase, the production of lactase normally decreases with age, and there are significant differences in lactase production among ethnic groups. People of African or Asian descent are highly likely to have some degree of difficulty digesting products that contain lactose. The most common symptoms of lactase deficiency are diarrhea, bloating, and gas. Diagnosis may be made through a trial of a lactose-free diet or through special testing. In some cases, other diseases of the intestine may need to be excluded by further medical evaluation. Treatment usually involves avoiding lactose in the diet or taking over-the-counter lactase supplements before eating foods that contain lactose.

deficiency, LCHAD Deficiency of the enzyme long-chain-3-hydroxyacyl-CoA dehydrogenease (LCHAD), an abnormality of fatty acid metabolism. Acute fatty liver of pregnancy (AFLP) has been found to be associated in some cases with LCHAD deficiency. In such cases, both parents have LCHAD activity at half of normal levels, but the fetus has none. The metabolic disease in the baby's liver apparently causes the fatty liver disease in the mother. In cases of AFLP due to LCHAD deficiency, there is a 25 percent or greater risk of AFLP in each pregnancy. See also acute fatty liver of pregnancy.

deficiency, long-chain-3-hydroxyacyl-CoA dehydrogenease See *deficiency, LCHAD.*

deficiency, magnesium Lack of magnesium, which can occur because of inadequate intake or impaired intestinal absorption of magnesium. Low magnesium (hypomagnesemia) levels are often associated with low calcium (hypocalcemia) and potassium (hypokalemia) levels because these nutrients interact with each other. Magnesium deficiency causes increased irritability of the nervous system, as evidenced by spasms of the hands and feet (tetany), muscular twitching and cramps, spasms of the larynx, and other symptoms. Treatment involves ensuring intake and absorption of the recommended dietary allowances of magnesium, currently 420 mg per day for men and 320 mg per day for women. One should not take more than 350 mg per day in supplement form, however.

deficiency, niacin See *pellagra.*

deficiency, protein C See *protein C deficiency.*

deficiency, selenium Lack of the essential mineral selenium, which can cause Keshan disease, a fatal form of cardiomyopathy (disease of the heart muscle) that was first observed in Keshan province in China and has since been found elsewhere. Treatment involves ensuring intake of the recommended dietary allowance of selenium, currently 70 mg per day for men and 55 mg per day for women. Food sources of selenium include seafood; some meats, such as kidney and liver; and some grains and seeds.

deficiency, UDP-glucuronosyltransferase See *Gilbert syndrome.*

deficiency, zinc A deficiency of zinc that is associated with short stature, anemia, increased pigmentation of skin (hyperpigmentation), enlarged liver and spleen (hepatosplenomegaly), impaired gonadal function (hypogonadism), impaired wound healing, and immune deficiency. The key laboratory finding is an abnormally low blood zinc level, reflecting the impaired zinc uptake. One form of zinc deficiency is the hereditary disease acrodermatitis enteropathica. Treatment involves ensuring intake of the recommended dietary allowance of zinc, currently recommended 12 mg per day for women and

10 mg per day for men. Food sources of zinc include meat, eggs, seafood, nuts, and cereals. Longstanding zinc deficiency can lead to chronic diarrhea and inflammation of the skin (dermatitis). See also *acrodermatitis enteropathica.*

deformation A change from the normal size or shape of a structure produced by mechanical forces that distort an otherwise normal structure. Deformations occur most often late in pregnancy and during delivery. For example, a twin pregnancy can cause deformations due to crowding of the twins late in pregnancy. A well-known example of a deformation is molding of the head of a baby born by vaginal delivery. There are usually no significant lasting effects of a deformation. A deformation is different from a malformation in both timing and impact. See also *malformation.*

degeneration, macular See *macular degeneration.*

degenerative arthritis See *arthritis, degenerative.*

degenerative joint disease See *arthritis, degenerative.*

deglutition The act of swallowing, particularly of swallowing food. The muscles of deglutition are the muscles employed in the act of swallowing.

dehydration Excessive loss of body water. Diseases of the gastrointestinal tract that cause vomiting or diarrhea may lead to dehydration. There are a number of other causes of dehydration, including overheating (hyperthermia), prolonged vigorous exercise (as in a marathon), kidney disease, and medications (diuretics). One clue to dehydration is a rapid drop in weight. A loss of more than 10 percent (for example, 15 pounds in a person weighing 150 pounds) in a short period of time is considered severe and may indicate dehydration. Symptoms include increasing thirst, dry mouth, weakness or lightheadedness (particularly when it worsens on standing), and a darkening of or decrease in urination. Severe dehydration can lead to changes in the body's chemistry, kidney failure, and death. The best way to treat dehydration is to prevent it from occurring. Intravenous or oral fluid replacement may be needed in some cases. See also *diarrhea; hyperthermia.*

déjà vu A disquieting feeling of having been somewhere or done something before, even though one has not. Although most people have experienced this feeling at one time or another, in some people sensations of déjà vu are part of a seizure or migraine aura; in others, the sensations are a seizure phenomenon. See also *jamais vu; seizure disorder.*

delay, developmental See *developmental delay.*

deletion Loss of a segment of DNA from a chromosome. A chromosome deletion can cause disease. An example is the cri du chat (cat cry) syndrome, which is due to loss of part of chromosome 5. The opposite of duplication.

delirium tremens A central nervous system symptom of alcohol withdrawal that is seen in chronic alcoholism. Symptoms include uncontrollable trembling, hallucinations, severe anxiety, sweating, and sudden feelings of terror. Abbreviated DTs. DTs can be both frightening and, in severe cases, deadly. Treatment includes observation, comfort care, and in some cases medication.

delivery, breech See *breech birth.*

delivery, footling See *footling birth.*

delivery, vertex See *vertex birth.*

delta cell, pancreatic A type of cell located in tissue that is called the islets of Langerhans in the pancreas. Delta cells make somatostatin, a hormone that inhibits the release of numerous hormones in the body.

delta-storage pool disease See *Hermansky-Pudlak syndrome.*

deltoid The muscle, roughly triangular in shape, that stretches from the clavicle (collarbone) to the humerus, the upper bone of the arm. It is flexed to move the arm up and down from the side.

dementia Significant loss of intellectual abilities, such as memory capacity, that is severe enough to interfere with social or occupational functioning. Criteria for the diagnosis of dementia include impairment of attention, orientation, memory, judgment, language, motor and spatial skills, and function. By definition, dementia is not due to major depression or schizophrenia. Dementia is reported in as many as 1 percent of adults 60 years of age. It has been estimated that the frequency of dementia doubles every 5 years after age 60. Alzheimer's disease is the most common cause of dementia. Other causes include AIDS, alcoholism (in which the dementia is due to thiamine deficiency), brain injury, vascular dementia (damage to the blood vessels leading to the brain), dementia with Lewy bodies (tiny round structures made of proteins that develop within nerve cells in the brain), brain tumors, drug toxicity, encephalitis (infection of brain), Creutzfeldt-Jakob disease, meningitis, Pick disease, syphilis, and thyroid disease (hypothyroidism).

dementia complex, AIDS See *AIDS dementia complex.*

dementia, MELAS See *MELAS syndrome.*

demulcent An agent that forms a soothing, protective film when administered onto a mucous membrane surface. For example, mucilage and oils are demulcents that can relieve irritation of the bowel lining.

demyelination A degenerative process that erodes the myelin sheath that normally protects nerve fibers. Demyelination exposes these fibers and appears to cause problems in nerve impulse conduction that may affect many physical systems. Demyelination is seen in a number of diseases, particularly multiple sclerosis. Diagnosis is by functional observation and by testing for myelin protein in the blood.

dendrite A short, arm-like protuberance from a nerve cell (neuron). Dendrites from juxtaposed neurons are tipped by synapses (tiny transmitters and receivers for chemical messages between the cells). See also *axon; neuron.*

dengue fever An acute mosquito-borne viral illness of sudden onset that usually follows a benign course, with headache, fever, prostration, severe joint and muscle pain, swollen glands (lymphadenopathy), and rash. The presence of fever, rash, and headache (the "dengue triad") is particularly characteristic of dengue. Dengue fever is endemic throughout the tropics and subtropics. Also called breakbone fever, dandy fever, and dengue. Victims of dengue fever often suffer temporary contortions due to the intense joint and muscle pain.

dengue hemorrhagic fever A syndrome caused by the dengue virus that tends to affect children under age 10 and causes abdominal pain, hemorrhage (bleeding), and circulatory collapse (shock). Abbreviated DHF. DHF starts abruptly with high, continuous fever and headache, plus respiratory and intestinal symptoms, including sore throat, cough, nausea, vomiting, and abdominal pain. Shock occurs after 2 to 6 days, with sudden collapse; cool, clammy extremities; weak, thready pulse; and blueness around the mouth (circumoral cyanosis). Other symptoms are bleeding with easy bruising, blood spots in the skin (petechiae), vomiting of blood (hematemesis), blood in the stool (melena), bleeding gums, and nosebleeds (epistaxis). Pneumonia and heart inflammation (myocarditis) may also be present. The mortality rate for those with DHF ranges from 6 to 30 percent. Most deaths occur in children, and infants are at particular risk.

dental braces See *braces, dental.*

dental impaction The pressing together of teeth. For example, molar teeth (the large teeth in the back of the jaw) can be impacted, cause pain, and require pain medication, antibiotics, and surgical removal.

dental pain Pain in or near the mouth that comes from irritation of a nerve to a tooth. The most common cause of toothache is a dental cavity. The second most common is gum disease. Toothache can be caused by a problem that does not originate from a tooth or the jaw.

dentin The hard tissue of the tooth that surrounds the central core of nerves and blood vessels (pulp).

deoxyribonucleic acid See *DNA.*

depilation See *epilation.*

Depo-Provera A contraceptive that is injected and lasts 3 months between doses. Depo-Provera is also used to regulate menstrual cycle in women with uneven or painful menses. It contains the hormonal compound medroxyprogesterone acetate.

depression An illness that involves the body, mood, and thoughts and that affects the way a person eats, sleeps, feels about himself or herself, and thinks about things. Depression is not the same as a passing blue mood. It is not a sign of personal weakness or a condition that can be wished away. People with depression cannot merely "pull themselves together" and get better. Without treatment, symptoms can last for weeks, months, or years. Appropriate treatment, however, can help most people with depression. The signs and symptoms of depression include loss of interest in activities that were once interesting or enjoyable, including sex; loss of appetite, with weight loss, or overeating, with weight gain; loss of emotional expression (flat affect); a persistently sad, anxious, or empty mood; feelings of hopelessness, pessimism, guilt, worthlessness, or helplessness; social withdrawal; unusual fatigue, low energy level, a feeling of being slowed down; sleep disturbance and insomnia, early-morning awakening or oversleeping; trouble concentrating, remembering, or making decisions; unusual restlessness or irritability; persistent physical problems such as headaches, digestive disorders, or chronic pain that do not respond to treatment, and thoughts of death or suicide or suicide attempts. Alcohol or drug abuse may be signs of depression. The principal types of depression are called major depression, dysthymia, and bipolar disease (manic-depressive disease).

depression, bipolar See *bipolar disorder.*

depression, dysthymia See *dysthymia.*

depression, major Depression with a combination of symptoms that interfere with the ability to work, sleep, eat, and enjoy once-pleasurable activities. These disabling episodes of depression can occur once, twice, or several times in a lifetime. See also *depression.*

depression, manic   See *bipolar disorder.*

depression, unipolar   Depressive disease without a manic phase. See *depression.*

depression, winter   See *seasonal affective disorder.*

Dercum disease   A condition characterized by painful fatty tumors (lipomas) beneath the skin. The disease tends to be associated with obesity and is about five times more frequent in females than in males. Onset of symptoms generally occurs in middle age. The fatty tumors are most often located on the trunk and limbs. Also called *adiposis dolorosa.*

dermabrasion   A surgical procedure that involves the controlled scraping away of the upper layers of the skin by using sandpaper or some other mechanical means. The purpose of dermabrasion is to smooth the skin and, in the process, remove small scars (as from acne), moles (nevi), tattoos, or fine wrinkles. Dermabrasion is performed by a dermatologist. Chemical skin peels are an alternative to dermabrasion.

dermatitis   Inflammation of the skin. Dermatitis has many causes, including direct contact with an irritating substance; allergic reaction to an inhaled, ingested, or injected allergen; eczema; or underlying immune disease. Symptoms of dermatitis include redness, itching, and in some cases, blistering. Noneczematous dermatitis is usually caused by direct contact with an irritant. Frequent offenders include detergents, especially those with perfumes; chemicals used in photo development; ammonia from decomposing urine in an infant's diapers (diaper dermatitis); and some types of solvents. Treatment involves identifying and avoiding substances that cause attacks and, during attacks, using topical treatments, such as steroid creams. See also *eczema.*

dermatitis herpetiformis   An intensely itchy skin inflammation caused by an immune reaction to dietary gluten, a protein found in wheat, barley, rye, and related grains. Dermatitis herpetiformis is associated with a disorder of the small intestine called celiac sprue. See also *celiac sprue.*

dermatographism   A common form of hives that appears due to stroking, rubbing, or scratching of the skin, or when tight-fitting clothes rub the skin. Dermatographism occurs in about 5 percent of the population. Dermatographism is not a disease and requires no specific treatment.

dermatologic   Having to do with skin.

dermatologist   A physician who specializes in the diagnosis and treatment of skin problems.

dermatome   **1** A localized area of skin that receives its sensations via a single nerve from a single nerve root of the spinal cord. Shingles (herpes zoster) typically affects one or several isolated dermatomes.   **2** A cutting instrument used for skin grafting or for slicing thin pieces of skin.

dermatomyositis   A chronic inflammatory disease of muscle that is associated with patches of slightly raised reddish or scaly rash. The rash can be on the bridge of the nose, around the eyes, or on sun-exposed areas of the neck and chest. Classically, however, it is over the knuckles. When inflammation of the muscle (myositis) occurs without skin disease, the condition is referred to as polymyositis. Dermatomyositis affects both children and adults, and it is characterized by a rash accompanying or (more often) preceding muscle weakness. The most common symptom is muscle weakness, usually affecting the muscles that are closest to the trunk of the body (proximal). Trouble with swallowing (dysphagia) may occur. Occasionally, the muscles ache and are tender to touch. Some patients develop hardened bumps of calcium deposits under the skin. Treatment commonly involves steroid drugs, such as prednisolone or prednisone. For patients in whom prednisone is not effective, other immunosuppressing drugs, such as azathioprine and methotrexate, may be prescribed. Intravenous immunoglobulin may be effective for severe dermatomyositis. Physical therapy is usually recommended to preserve muscle function and avoid muscle atrophy. Both dermatomyositis and polymyositis can sometimes be associated with cancers, including lymphoma, breast, lung, ovarian, and colon cancer. See also *polymyositis.*

dermatopathy   Any disease of the skin. Also known as dermopathy.

dermatophytic onychomycosis   See *onychomycosis.*

dermis   The lower or inner layer of the two main layers of cells that make up the skin (the other being the epidermis). See also *epidermis; skin.*

dermoid   See *Ovarian teratoma.*

dermoid cyst of the ovary   See *ovarian teratoma.*

dermopathy   See *dermatopathy.*

descending aorta   The part of the aorta that runs down through the chest and the abdomen. The descending aorta starts after the arch of the aorta and ends by splitting into the common iliac arteries that go down toward the thighs. The descending aorta is subdivided into the thoracic aorta and the abdominal aorta. See also *aorta.*

desensitization, allergy See *allergy desensitization.*

designer estrogen An engineered drug that possesses some, but not all, of the actions of estrogen. Also known as selective estrogen-receptor modulator (SERM). For example, raloxifene (brand name: Evista) is classified as a designer estrogen because, like estrogen, it prevents bone loss and lowers serum cholesterol; however, it does not stimulate the endometrial lining of the uterus.

desmoid tumor A benign soft-tissue tumor that does not spread to other parts of the body. Desmoid tumors occur most often in young adults, and they usually involve the limbs or trunk, but they can also arise in the abdomen or thorax. Desmoid tumors are very difficult to remove because they adhere tenaciously to surrounding structures and organs. Surgery has been the traditional main mode of therapy for desmoid tumors, but up to 70 percent of the tumors recur after surgery. Radiation therapy has also been used, as has the combination of surgery and radiation. Although it is somewhat successful, the combination of wide-resection surgery and high-dose radiation represents very aggressive treatment for a benign condition. Limited (low-dose) chemotherapy is a less aggressive treatment for desmoid tumors. A desmoid tumor is also called aggressive fibromatosis because it is locally aggressive and fibrous, like scar tissue.

desmoid tumor, cortical A tumor that arises in embryonic tissue.

desmoplasia The growth of fibrous or connective tissue anywhere in the body.

desmoplastic reaction A reaction that is associated with some tumors and is characterized by the pervasive growth of dense fibrous tissue around the tumor. The formation of scar tissue (adhesion) within the abdomen after abdominal surgery is another type of desmoplastic reaction.

desquamate To shed the outer layers of the skin.

desquamation The shedding of the outer layers of the skin. For example, when the rash of measles fades, desquamation occurs.

deuteranomaly See *colorblindness.*

deuteranopia See *colorblindness.*

development The process of growth and differentiation. The most important stage of human development occurs before birth, as tissues and organs arise from differentiation of cells in the embryo. This process continues until birth, and interruptions in development result in the most serious types of birth defects, such as anencephaly

and spina bifida. The developmental process continues after birth, as an infant or child grows physically, develops basic brain-based abilities such as speech and hand–eye coordination, and learns. Interruptions in any of these processes can result in developmental delay.

development, embryonic See *prenatal development.*

development, fetal See *prenatal development.*

developmental delay A condition in which a child is behind schedule in reaching milestones of early childhood development. This term is often used as a euphemism for mental retardation, which can be less a delay than a permanent limitation of a child's ability to progress.

developmental disorder One of several disorders that interrupt normal development in childhood. A developmental disorder may affect a single area of development (specific developmental disorder) or several areas (pervasive developmental disorder). With early intervention, most specific developmental disorders can be accommodated and overcome. Early intervention is absolutely essential for pervasive developmental disorders, many of which respond to an aggressive approach that may combine speech therapy, occupational therapy, physical therapy, behavior modification techniques, play therapy, and in some cases medication. See also *autism; cerebral palsy; developmental disorder, pervasive; developmental disorder, specific; developmental dyspraxia; dysarthria; dyscalculia; dyslexia.*

developmental disorder, pervasive A class of disorders in which the patient shows impairment in social interaction, imaginative activity, and verbal and nonverbal communication skills, and has a limited number of interests and activities that tend to be repetitive (stereotyped). Abbreviated PDD. All types of PDDs are disorders of the nervous system that are usually evident by age 3. In general, children who have PDDs have difficulty talking, playing with other children, and relating to others, including their family members. The five types of PDD are autistic disorder, Rett syndrome, childhood disintegrative disorder, Asperger syndrome, and "pervasive developmental disorder not otherwise specified." See also *Asperger syndrome; autism; childhood disintegrative disorder; Rett syndrome.*

developmental disorder, specific A disorder that affects only one area of development. For example, dysgraphia is a specific developmental disorder; it is a specific impairment of the ability to write legibly. See also *developmental disorder; developmental disorder, pervasive; dysarthria; dyscalculia; dyslexia.*

developmental dysplasia of the hip See *congenital hip dislocation.*

developmental dyspraxia A pattern of delayed, uneven, or aberrant development of physical abilities during childhood development. The physical abilities affected by developmental dyspraxia can involve gross or fine motor skills. Developmental dyspraxia may be seen alone or in combination with other developmental problems, particularly apraxia or dyspraxia of speech. Treatment is via early intervention, using physical therapy to improve gross motor skills and occupational therapy to assist in fine motor development and sensory integration. See also *apraxia of speech; dyspraxia of speech.*

deviated septum See *nasal septum, deviated.*

device, assistive Any device that is designed, made, and/or adapted to assist a person to perform a particular task that might otherwise be difficult. For example, canes, crutches, walkers, wheelchairs, and shower chairs are all assistive devices. See also *assistive technology; augmentative communication device; device, medical.*

device, intrauterine See *intrauterine device.*

device, medical Broadly defined, any physical item used in medical treatment, from a heart pacemaker to a wheelchair. In insurance parlance, medical device is usually synonymous with assistive device, although it may include items more frequently thought of as medical supplies, such as dressings needed for wound care at home or syringes for self-administration of insulin. Medical devices are not covered by most insurance policies, although they may be available through supplemental insurance or, in some cases, on an inexpensive rental basis through hospitals, clinics, or pharmacies. See also *assistive device.*

dextro- Prefix from the Latin word dexter, meaning "on the right side." For example, a molecule that shows dextrorotation is turning or twisting to the right. The opposite of levo-.

dextrocardia Reversal of the anatomic location of the heart, placing it in the right side of the chest rather than in its normal location on the left. This is a true anatomic reversal, in which the apex (tip) of the heart points to the right instead of the left. Dextrocardia occurs in Kartagener syndrome, an abnormal condition that is present at birth. See also *dextroposition of the heart; Kartagener syndrome.*

dextroposition Moving to the right.

dextroposition of the heart A condition in which the heart is displaced to the right side of the chest, but without any anatomic alteration in the heart itself. Dextroposition occurs when the contents of the left side of the chest shove the heart to the right, or when the contents of the right side of the chest are reduced (for example, by collapse of the right lung) and the heart moves toward the sparsely occupied space on the right. See also *dextrocardia.*

dextrose Glucose, a simple sugar.

DHF Dengue hemorrhagic fever.

Di Ferrante syndrome A rare form of mucopolysaccharidosis. Di Ferrante syndrome is an autosomal recessive genetic disorder. Also known as mucopolysaccharidosis Type IX. See also *mucopolysaccharidosis.*

dia- Prefix meaning through, throughout, or completely, as in diachronic (over a period of time), diagnosis (to completely define the nature of a disease), and dialysis (cleansing the blood by passing it through a special machine).

diabetes See *diabetes mellitus.*

diabetes, adult-onset Type 2 diabetes. See also *diabetes, type 2.*

Diabetes Association, American See *ADA.*

diabetes, brittle See *diabetes, labile.*

diabetes, bronze Diabetes mellitus that occurs as a result of damage to the pancreas from iron deposition of hemochromatosis. See also *diabetes mellitus; hemochromatosis.*

diabetes, childhood Type 1 diabetes. See also *diabetes, type 1.*

diabetes diet Dietary control that is the primary method for treating all forms of diabetes. The goal of diabetes diet changes is to minimize the chance of overloading the body with glucose. Patients with diabetes benefit from eating carefully controlled amounts and types of food at regular intervals throughout the day, rather than at two or three large meals. Soluble fibers, such as oat bran, apples, citrus, pears, peas and beans, and psyllium, slow down the digestion of carbohydrates (sugars), which results in better glucose metabolism. Diabetes patients should avoid consumption of sugary foods and moderate their intake of starches that convert quickly to glucose. Some patients with type 2 diabetes may be successfully treated with diet alone, and patients on insulin can often reduce their insulin requirements by adhering to the appropriate diet. Learning proper eating habits is especially important for children with diabetes (type 1 diabetics), who run the highest long-term risk of severe symptoms.

diabetes, gestational A diabetic condition that appears during pregnancy and usually goes away after the birth of the baby. Gestational diabetes is best controlled via diet. Because a woman's dietary needs increase and change during pregnancy, the services of a professional dietitian and careful monitoring by a midwife, obstetrician, and/or physician with expertise in gestational diabetes are necessary. Gestational diabetes can cause birth complications. One complication is macrosomia, in which the baby is considerably larger than normal due to large deposits of fat; such a baby can grow too large to be delivered through the vagina. Gestational diabetes also increases the risk of hypoglycemia (low blood sugar) and other chemical imbalances such as low serum calcium and low serum magnesium in the baby immediately after delivery. The key to prevention of gestational diabetes is careful control of blood sugar levels in the mother. If the mother maintains normal blood sugar levels, it is less likely that the fetus will develop macrosomia, hypoglycemia, or other chemical abnormalities.

diabetes insipidus A metabolic disorder that mimics symptoms of diabetes mellitus, including increased output of urine and increased thirst. It is caused by a malfunction in the pituitary gland, and can be treated by administering vasopressin, a pituitary hormone. There are two types of diabetes insipidus, central and nephrogenic. Central diabetes insipidus is a lack of ADH production and is due to damage to the pituitary gland or hypothalamus where ADH is produced. Nephrogenic diabetes insipidus is a lack of response of the kidney to the fluid-conserving action of ADH. It can be due to diseases of the kidney (such as polycystic kidney disease), certain drugs (such as lithium), and can also occur as an inherited disorder. In both central and nephrogenic diabetes insipidus, patients excrete extraordinarily large volumes of very dilute urine. Patients feel thirsty and drink large amounts of water to compensate for the water they lose in the urine. The main danger with diabetes insipidus is when fluid intake does not keep pace with urine output, resulting in dehydration and high blood sodium. The treatment of central diabetes insipidus is with vasopressin used as a nasal spray or as tablets. nephrogenic diabetes insipidus does not respond to vasopression treatment. In cases of nephrogenic diabetes insipidus caused by a drug (such as lithium), stopping the drug usually leads to recovery. In cases of hereditary nephrogenic diabetes insipidus, treatment is with fluid intake to match urine output and drugs that lower urine output. Effective treatment is important because the dehydration and high blood sodium can cause brain damage and death. See also *antidiuretic hormone; pituitary, posterior.*

diabetes, insulin-dependent Type 1 diabetes. See also *diabetes, type 1.*

diabetes, insulin-resistant Type 2 diabetes. See also *diabetes, type 2.*

diabetes, labile Type 1 diabetes that is untreated, poorly controlled, or resistant to treatment so that the blood glucose level tends to swing quickly and widely up and down. Also known as brittle diabetes and unstable diabetes. See also *diabetes, type 1.*

diabetes mellitus A chronic condition associated with abnormally high levels of sugar (glucose) in the blood. Absence of, insufficient production of, or autoimmune resistance to the pancreatic hormone insulin causes diabetes. Insulin provides the body with a natural method for oxidizing glucose to provide energy; without enough insulin, glucose builds up in the bloodstream to dangerous levels. The tendency to develop diabetes runs in families, but not all patients have such a family history. Symptoms of diabetes include increased urine output, increased appetite and thirst, unexplained weight loss or fluctuation, and fatigue. Diabetes mellitus is diagnosed through blood sugar testing. Major complications include dangerously elevated blood sugar levels, abnormally low blood sugar levels due to incorrect dosing of diabetes medications, and disease of the blood vessels, which can damage the eyes, kidneys, nerves, and heart. Circulation problems due to blood vessel damage may also endanger the patient's feet and legs, leading in some cases to amputation. When the body cannot use glucose for energy because of inadequate insulin in diabetes, it turns to burning fat as energy. This process creates compounds called ketones. If the blood level of ketones gets too high, the result is a dangerous condition called ketosis that, if unchecked, can cause lethargy, convulsions, coma, and death. Treatment depends on the type of diabetes. Diet is always the primary treatment. Many patients take medications that help to regulate their production and use of insulin. Others may need insulin injections. Insulin can be self-administered via syringe or, more recently, via an almost-painless "gun" device, an external insulin pump, or an internally implanted insulin pump. There are two forms of diabetes mellitus, type 1 (insulin requiring) and type 2 (non-insulin requiring). Approximately 10 percent of the patients with diabetes mellitus have type 1 diabetes; the remaining 90 percent have type 2 diabetes mellitus. Diabetes mellitus is commonly referred to as diabetes, though technically there are two forms of diabetes, diabetes mellitus and diabetes insipidus, which are distinctly different conditions, both of which are characterized by the excessive production of dilute urine. See also *diabetes, type 1; diabetes, type 2.*

diabetes, non-insulin-dependent Type 2 diabetes. See also *diabetes, type 2.*

diabetes, type 1 A chronic condition in which the pancreas makes too little insulin (or no insulin) because the beta cells in the pancreas have been destroyed by the immune system. The body is then not able to effectively use blood glucose (sugar) for energy. The destruction of the beta cells in the pancreas is due to an abnormal immune reaction. The disease tends to occur in childhood, adolescence, or early adulthood (before age 30), but it may appear at any age. The symptoms and signs of type 1 diabetes are great thirst, hunger, a need to urinate often, and loss of weight. Fluctuations in blood glucose levels can lead to blurred vision. Extremely elevated glucose levels can lead to lethargy and coma (diabetic coma). To treat the disease, the person must inject insulin, follow an appropriate diet, exercise daily, and test blood glucose several times daily. This type of diabetes used to be known as juvenile diabetes, juvenile-onset diabetes, and insulin-dependent diabetes. See also *diabetes, type 2; diabetic neuropathy; diabetic retinopathy; diabetic coma; diabetic shock.*

diabetes, type 2   A form of diabetes mellitus in which patients can still produce insulin, but do so relatively inadequately. Type 2 diabetes mellitus occurs mostly in individuals over 30 years old and the incidence increases with age. While there is a strong genetic component to developing this form of diabetes, there are other risk factors: the most significant of which is obesity. There is a direct relationship between the degree of obesity and the risk of developing type 2 diabetes. Symptoms include increased urine output, increased appetite and thirst, unexplained weight loss or fluctuation, and fatigue. Type 2 diabetes mellitus is first treated with weight reduction, a diabetic diet, and exercise. When these measures fail to control the elevated blood sugars, oral medications are used. If oral medications are still insufficient, insulin medications are considered. Also know as non-insulin-dependent diabetes, adult-onset diabetes, or insulin-resistant diabetes. See also *diabetes, type 1; diabetic neuropathy; diabetic retinopathy.*

diabetes, unstable   See *diabetes, labile.*

diabetic coma   Deep unconsciousness that results from uncontrolled diabetes due to the buildup of ketones in the bloodstream. The best treatment is prevention. Careful diet, medication, and insulin dosing, as needed, should prevent ketone buildup. Patients with diabetes and their family members should be aware of the early signs of ketone buildup, including weight loss, nausea, confusion, gasping for breath, a characteristically sweet, chemical odor, similar to that of acetone or alcohol (acetone breath), to the patient's breath, and sometimes sweat. Lethargy, confusion, and convulsions may precede diabetic coma. To prevent death, immediate emergency medical treatment is needed in a hospital setting for patients who show the early signs of incipient diabetic coma.

diabetic nephropathy   Kidney disease associated with long-standing diabetes. It affects the network of tiny blood vessels (the microvasculature) in the glomerulus, a key structure in the kidney that is composed of capillary blood vessels. This structure is critical for blood filtration. Features of diabetic nephropathy include nephrotic syndrome, which is characterized by excessive filtration of protein into the urine (proteinuria), high blood pressure (hypertension), and progressively impaired kidney function. With severe diabetic nephropathy, kidney failure, end-stage renal disease, and the need for chronic kidney dialysis or a kidney transplant may result. Also known as intercapillary glomerulonephritis, Kimmelstiel-Wilson disease, and Kimmelstiel-Wilson syndrome.

diabetic neuropathy   Nerve damage caused by diabetes that leads to numbness and sometimes pain and weakness in the hands, arms, feet, and legs. Diabetic neuropathy can affect the digestive tract, heart, and genitalia. The longer a person has diabetes, the greater the risk of neuropathy. There are four types of diabetic neuropathy: peripheral, autonomic, proximal, and focal. Peripheral neuropathy, the most common, causes pain or loss of feeling in the hands, arms, feet, and legs. Autonomic neuropathy can cause changes in digestion, bowel and bladder control problems, and erectile dysfunction, and it can affect the nerves that serve the heart and control blood pressure. Proximal neuropathy produces pain in the thighs and hips and weakness in the legs. Focal neuropathy can strike any nerve in the body, causing pain or weakness. Treatment of diabetic neuropathy principally involves bringing the blood glucose and glycohemoglobin levels into the normal range. Good foot care is mandatory. Analgesics, low doses of antidepressants, and some anticonvulsant medications may be prescribed for relief of pain, burning, or tingling. Some patients may find that walking regularly, taking warm baths, and using elastic stockings help relieve leg pain due to diabetic neuropathy.

diabetic retinopathy   Disease of the retina caused by diabetes that involves damage to the tiny blood vessels in the back of the eye. Early disease may not cause symptoms. As the disease progresses, it enters its advanced, or proliferative, stage. Fragile, new blood vessels grow along the retina and in the clear, gel-like vitreous that fills the inside of the eye. Without timely treatment, these new blood vessels can bleed, cloud vision, and destroy the retina. Everyone with type 1 or type 2 diabetes is at risk for diabetic retinopathy. Swelling in the portion of the retina that is most sensitive to light (macular edema) makes it hard for a patient to do things like read and drive. As new blood vessels form at the back of the eye, they can bleed and further blur vision. Large hemorrhages tend to happen more than once, often during sleep. There are no early warning signs. Diagnosis of diabetic retinopathy is made during an eye examination that includes a visual acuity test, pupil dilation, ophthalmoscopy (to look in the back of the eye), and tonometry (to check the pressures). The two treatments for diabetic retinopathy are laser surgery, to stop the edema and hemorrhage, and vitrectomy, to remove blood from the back of the eye. It is strongly recommended that all diabetics have eye examinations at least once (ideally twice) a year.

diabetic shock Hypoglycemia (low blood sugar) due to excessive use of insulin or other glucose-lowering medications to lower the blood sugar level in diabetic patients. Symptoms include a sweet, chemical odor on the patient's breath that is similar to that of acetone or alcohol (acetone breath); fatigue, lightheadedness, or fainting; and reddening of the skin in Caucasian patients or darkening of the skin in patients with darker skin. Immediate treatment involves administration of glucose in a prescription sublingual form or in the form of hard candy if nothing else is available. Patients with diabetes and their families should learn the early warning signs of diabetic shock and carry glucose tablets for emergency use. The treatment includes glucagon given by intramuscular injection. Glucagon causes the release of glucose from the liver, and should be part of the emergency kit of a diabetic, especially if the patient uses insulin. Families and friends of those with diabetes need to be taught how to administer glucagon, because obviously the patients will not be able to do it themselves in an emergency situation. Changes in diet, medication, or insulin administration can then be made to prevent future episodes. Also known as an insulin reaction or insulin shock. See also *insulin reaction.*

diachronic Over a period of time. The opposite of synchronic.

diachronic study See *longitudinal study.*

diagnosis Knowledge of the nature of a disease. A patient who speaks of "getting a diagnosis" means learning the medical name for the ailment and gaining an understanding of the condition. Abbreviated dx and Dx. See also *differential diagnosis.*

diagnosis, differential See *differential diagnosis.*

dialysis The process of cleansing the blood by passing it through a special machine. Dialysis is necessary when the kidneys are not able to filter the blood. It gives patients with kidney failure a chance to live productive lives. There are two types of dialysis: hemodialysis and peritoneal dialysis. Each type of dialysis has advantages and disadvantages. Patients can often choose the type of long-term dialysis that best matches their needs. See also *dialysis, peritoneal.*

dialysis machine A machine used in dialysis that filters a patient's blood to remove excess water and waste products when the kidneys are damaged, dysfunctional,

or missing. Blood is drawn through a specially created vein in the forearm, called an arteriovenous (AV) fistula. From the AV fistula, blood is taken to the dialysis machine through plastic tubing. The dialysis machine itself can be thought of as an artificial kidney. Inside, it consists of more plastic tubing that carries the removed blood to the dialyser, a bundle of hollow fibers that forms a semipermeable membrane for filtering out impurities. In the dialyser, blood is diffused with a saline solution called dialysate, and the dialysate is in turn diffused with blood. When the filtration process is complete, the cleansed blood is returned to the patient. Most patients who undergo dialysis because of kidney impairment or failure use a dialysis machine at a dialysis clinic. A session generally takes about 4 hours, and typical patients visit a dialysis clinic one to three times per week. Also, a machine called a peritoneal dialysis machine can be used chronically at home for dialysis, instead of hemodialysis, which eliminates the need for regular dialysis clinic treatments. Using this machine during the day and frequently during sleep, the patient can control his/her own dialysis.

dialysis, peritoneal A dialysis technique that uses the patient's own body tissues inside the belly (abdominal cavity) as a filter. The intestines lie in the abdominal cavity, the space between the abdominal wall and the spine. A plastic tube called a dialysis catheter is placed through the abdominal wall and into the abdominal cavity. A saline fluid called dialysate is then flushed into the abdominal cavity so that it washes around the intestines. The intestinal walls act as a filter between this fluid and the bloodstream. By using different types of solutions, waste products and excess water can be removed from the body through this process.

diaper rash An inflammatory reaction localized to the area of skin usually covered by the diaper. It can have many causes, including infections (yeast, bacterial, or viral), friction irritation, chemical allergies (perfumes, soaps), sweat, decomposed urine, and plugged sweat glands. Most diaper rash problems can be solved by cleansing the skin with nonperfumed, gentle products; changing diapers frequently; and exposing the affected skin area to air. Commercially available diaper rash ointments may be helpful for prevention but may actually cause further irritation if used on the inflamed areas. Also called diaper dermatitis.

diaphragm **1** The muscle that separates the chest (thoracic) cavity from the abdomen. Contraction of the diaphragm helps to expand the lungs when one breathes in air. **2** A specially fitted contraceptive device that covers the cervix to prevent the entry of sperm. For greatest effectiveness, a diaphragm is used with spermicidal gel or cream. See also *birth control; contraceptive.*

diaphragmatic hernia   Passage of a loop of bowel through the diaphragm muscle. This type of hernia occurs as the bowel from the abdomen protrudes (herniates) upward through the diaphragm into the chest (thoracic) cavity.

diarrhea   A common condition that involves unusually frequent or unusually liquid bowel movements and excessive watery evacuations of fecal material. The opposite of constipation. There are myriad infectious and noninfectious causes of diarrhea. Persistent diarrhea is both uncomfortable and dangerous to the health because it can indicate an underlying infection and may mean that the body is not able to absorb some nutrients due to a problem in the bowels. Treatment includes drinking plenty of fluids to prevent dehydration and taking over-the-counter remedies. People with diarrhea that persists for more than a couple days, particularly small children or elderly people, should seek medical attention.

diarrhea and dermatitis, zinc deficiency   See *deficiency, zinc.*

diarrhea, antibiotic-induced   Diarrhea caused by the bacterium Clostridium difficile (C. difficile), one of the most common causes of infection of the large bowel (colon). Patients taking antibiotics are at particular risk of becoming infected with C. difficile. Antibiotics disrupt the normal bacteria of the bowel, allowing C. difficile and other bacteria to become established and overgrow inside the colon. Many infected persons have no symptoms but can become carriers of the bacteria and infect others. In some people, a toxin produced by C. difficile causes diarrhea, abdominal pain, severe inflammation of the colon (colitis), fever, an elevated white blood cell count, vomiting, and dehydration. In severely affected patients, the inner lining of the colon becomes severely inflamed (pseudomembranous colitis). Rarely, the walls of the colon wear away and holes develop (colon perforation), which can lead to a life-threatening infection of the abdomen.

diarrhea, rotavirus   A leading cause of severe diarrhea in infants and young children, often accompanied by fever and dehydration. Treatment includes frequent administration of fluids to prevent dehydration, rest, good nutrition, and in some cases medication. A preventative vaccine has been developed but is not in use at this time. See also *rotavirus.*

diarrhea, travelers'   Illness, including diarrhea, that is associated with travel to a foreign country. Among the causes of travelers' diarrhea are viruses and enterotoxigenic Escherichia coli, which may be transmitted via food or water. Prevention is the best treatment, and it includes drinking bottled water; filtering tap water or, if camping,

water from natural sources; washing fruits and vegetables purchased in local markets with a solution of water and a few drops of bleach; and when possible, choosing restaurants with high standards of sanitation. Treatment includes replacement of fluids and electrolytes (sodium and other ions) lost via diarrhea. In serious cases of persistent travelers' diarrhea, medical care should be sought.

diastolic   Referring to the time when the heart is in a period of relaxation and dilation (expansion), which is called diastole. Diastolic pressure is the minimum arterial pressure during relaxation and dilation of the ventricles of the heart when the ventricles fill with blood. In a blood pressure reading, the diastolic pressure is typically the second number recorded. For example, in a blood pressure reading of 120/80 ("120 over 80"), the diastolic pressure is 80 (that is, 80 mm Hg [millimeters of mercury]). A diastolic murmur is a heart murmur heard during diastole. See also *systolic.*

diathermy   See *cauterization.*

diathesis   An elegant term for a predisposition or tendency. For example, hemorrhagic diathesis means a tendency to bleed.

dicentric chromosome   See *chromosome, dicentric.*

diet   Food and drink. A specific diet can be prescribed for medical reasons according to a certain type, volume, and timing. For examples, specific diets are commonly prescribed for persons affected by hypoglycemia, gout, celiac disease, dermatitis herpetiformis, lactose intolerance, diabetes, hypercholesterolemia, heart disease, kidney disease, and difficulty in swallowing.

dietary supplement   A substance that can be added to the diet, usually in pill, liquid, or powder form, ostensibly to promote health. Dietary supplements range from natural (nonsteroidal) weight-gain concoctions used by bodybuilders, to joint pain relievers, vitamins, herbs, minerals, and salts that claim health benefits. Many dietary supplements are harmless when taken as directed, and the health benefits of some have been substantiated. It is important to tell a physician what supplements are being taken because they can interact with prescription medications, and some are not suitable for people with certain medical conditions.

diethylstilbestrol   The earliest synthetic form of the female hormone estrogen. Abbreviated DES. DES was widely prescribed between 1940 and 1971 to prevent miscarriages. The use of DES during pregnancy declined and was halted when it was found that, when given during the first 5 months of pregnancy, DES can interfere with the development of the fetal reproductive system. Women whose mothers were given DES during pregnancy are at increased risk for an uncommon form of cancer called clear cell adenocarcinoma of the vagina and cervix. Daughters of women who took DES also have an increased risk of having the most common forms of cancer of the cervix. They are also at increased risk of having anatomic abnormalities of the vagina, cervix, and uterus and of having tubal (ectopic) pregnancies, infertility, miscarriages, or premature births. Sons of women who took DES are predisposed to abnormalities of the testicles, such as abnormally small testes and failure of the testes to descend into the scrotum; these abnormalities increase the risk of testicular cancer. People who believe they may have been exposed to DES before birth should inform their physicians of their exposure so that they can be appropriately examined and monitored. DES is still available for prescription in the US for the palliative treatment of breast and prostate cancer.

dietitian   A person trained in the design and management of the diet in health and disease as, for example, in diabetes.

differential diagnosis   Knowledge gained through weighing the probability of one disease against the probability of other diseases that might account for a patient's illness. For example, the differential diagnosis of a runny nose includes allergic rhinitis (hay fever), the abuse of nasal decongestants, and the common cold. Abbreviated DDX. See also *diagnosis.*

differentiation   **1** The process by which cells become progressively more specialized; a normal process by which cells mature. Cells early in development have the potential to develop into many different types of tissues of the body. Differentiation occurs so the specific body tissues can form. Stem cells can, for example, differentiate into secretion in the intestine. Once developed into a specific cell type, the cell has lost its ability to differentiate into a cell for a different tissue.   **2** In cancer, the difference in the maturity (development) of the cancer cells in a tumor. Differentiated tumor cells resemble normal cells and tend to grow and spread at a slower rate than undifferentiated or poorly differentiated tumor cells, which lack the structure and function of normal cells and grow uncontrollably.

diffuse idiopathic skeletal hyperostosis   A form of degenerative arthritis characteristically associated with flowing calcification along the sides of the vertebrae of the spine. Abbreviated DISH. DISH commonly includes inflammation (tendonitis) and calcification of the tendons at their points of attachment to bone. Anti-inflammatory medications (NSAIDs), such as ibuprofen, can be helpful in relieving both pain and inflammation. Also called Forestier disease.

DiGeorge syndrome   A congenital disorder characterized by low blood calcium (hypocalcemia) because of hypoplasia (underdevelopment) of the parathyroid glands needed to control calcium; immunodeficiency due to hypoplasia of the thymus (an organ behind the breastbone in which lymphocytes mature and multiply); and defects involving the outflow tracts from the heart. DiGeorge syndrome is, next to Down syndrome, the most common genetic cause of heart defects present at birth (congenital heart disease). DiGeorge syndrome is caused by a very small deletion (microdeletion) in chromosome band 22q11.2. The key gene that is lost is Tbx-1. Tbx-1 is a master control gene that regulates other genes required for the connection of the heart with the blood circulation. Tbx-1 also controls genes involved in the development of the parathyroid and thymus glands and the shape of the face. Also known as hypoplasia of the thymus and parathyroids and as third and fourth pharyngeal pouch syndrome.

digestive system   The system of organs responsible for getting food into and out of the body and for making use of food to keep the body healthy. The digestive system includes the salivary glands, mouth, esophagus, stomach, liver, gallbladder, pancreas, small intestine, colon, and rectum. The digestive system's organs are joined in a long, twisting tube from the mouth to the anus. Inside this tube is a lining called the mucosa. In the mouth, stomach, and small intestine, the mucosa contains tiny glands that produce juices to help digest food. Two solid organs, the liver and the pancreas (both of which are embryologically derived from the digestive tract), produce digestive juices that reach the intestine through small tubes known as ducts. In addition, parts of other organ systems (for instance, nerves and blood) play a major role in the digestive system.

digit   A finger or toe.

digit, supernumerary   An extra finger or toe.

digital rectal exam   A routine exam in which a physician inserts a lubricated, gloved finger into the rectum and feels for abnormal areas to detect rectal cancer and, in a man, inflammation, enlargement, or cancer of the prostate. A physician can use a rectal exam to detect diseases of the nervous system, which may be indicated by reduction of the normal tone of the muscles of the rectal sphincter.

digitalis   A chemical from the dried leaf of the common foxglove (Digitalis purpurea) plant that is to used to strengthen the force of the heartbeat. The Scottish physician William Withering discovered this use for digitalis in the late 1700s. Digitalis, its components, and their derivatives have long been used to treat congestive heart failure and slow the speeding heart so it is more efficient.

dilatate   In medicine, to enlarge or expand. Also known as dilate.

dilatation   The process of enlargement or expansion. Also known as dilation.

dilate   To stretch or enlarge. Also known as dilatate.

dilating   The widening and opening of an opening, such as the cervix or esophagus. For example, the amount of widening can be described in terms of the number of fingers that could fit in the cervical opening, or it is described in centimeters.

dilation   See dilatation.

dilation and curettage   A minor operation in which the cervix is expanded (dilatated) enough to permit the cervical canal and uterine lining to be scraped with a spoon-shaped instrument called a curette (curettage). Abbreviated D & C. D & C is normally used to remove abnormal material from the uterus, such as unexpelled placental material after birth.

dilation, pupil   A type of eye examination that enables an eye-care professional to see more of the retina, the light-sensitive layer of tissue at the back of the eye. Dilating the pupil permits the retina to be examined for signs of disease. To dilate the pupil, drops are placed into the eye. After the examination, the patient's vision may remain blurred for a while, and the brightness of the sun may be bothersome for several hours.

dilator   A device used to stretch or enlarge an opening. Patients with scarring of the esophagus can require a dilator procedure to open the esophagus for adequate passage of food and fluids.

diphtheria   An acute infectious disease that typically strikes the upper respiratory tract, including the throat. It is caused by infection with the bacteria Corynebacterium diphtheriae. Symptoms include sore throat and mild fever at first. As the disease progresses, a membranous substance forms in the throat that makes it difficult to breathe and swallow. Diphtheria can be deadly. It is one of the diseases that the DT (diphtheria-tetanus), DTP (diphtheria-tetanus-pertussis), and DTaP (diphtheria-tetanus-acellular-pertussis) vaccines are designed to prevent.

diploid   The number of chromosomes in most cells of the body. The diploid in humans is 46, which is twice the haploid number of 23 chromosomes contained in human eggs (ova) and sperm.

diplopia   A condition in which a single object appears as two objects. Also known as double vision.

directive, advance medical   See *advance directive.*

disaster supplies   Items stored in case of emergency, such as a prolonged power outage, earthquake, or flood. Recommended disaster supplies include the following:

- Water. Store at least 3 gallons of water per person (2 quarts for drinking, 2 quarts for food preparation/sanitation × three days). Store it in plastic containers, such as softdrink bottles.

- Food. Store at least a 3-day supply of foods that require no refrigeration, preparation, or cooking (and little or no water). If you must heat food, go to a camping goods store for options that do not require electricity or natural gas. Good choices include ready-to-eat canned meats, fruits, and vegetables; canned juices, milk, and soup (if powdered, store extra water); staples, particularly sugar, salt, and pepper; high-energy foods such as peanut butter, granola bars, and trail mix; vitamin pills; special foods for infants, elderly persons, or persons on special diets; and "comfort foods" such as cookies, hard candy, sweetened cereals, lollipops, instant coffee, and tea.

- First aid kit. Assemble a first aid kit for your home and one for each car. A first aid kit should include sterile adhesive bandages in assorted sizes, four to six 2-inch sterile gauze pads, four to six 4-inch sterile gauze pads, hypoallergenic adhesive tape, three triangular bandages, three rolls of 2-inch sterile roller bandages, three rolls of 3-inch sterile roller bandages, scissors, tweezers, a needle, moist towelettes, antiseptic (cream and/or liquid), thermometer, two tongue depressors, a tube of petroleum jelly or other lubricant, assorted sizes of safety pins, cleansing agent and/or soap, a medicine dropper, two pairs of latex gloves, and sunscreen. Contact your local American Red Cross chapter to obtain a basic first aid manual.

- Nonprescription drugs. Over-the-counter drugs that you might need in an emergency include aspirin or nonaspirin pain relievers, antidiarrhea medication, antacid for stomach upset, syrup of ipecac and activated charcoal (to use if advised by the Poison Control Center), and laxatives.

- Tools and supplies. Keep the items you would most likely need during an evacuation in an easy-to-carry container, such as a large, covered trash container, camping backpack, or duffle bag. These emergency items include mess kits (or paper cups, plates, and plastic utensils), an emergency-preparedness manual, a battery-operated radio with extra batteries, a flashlight with extra batteries, cash or traveler's checks, change, a nonelectric can opener, a utility knife, a small canister fire extinguisher of the ABC type, a tube tent, pliers, tape, a compass, matches in a waterproof container, aluminum foil, plastic storage containers, a signal flare, paper and pencil, needles and thread, a shut-off wrench for turning off household gas and water, a whistle, plastic sheeting, and a map of the area for locating shelters. A map showing the precise location of local shelters may be available in advance from your local emergency-preparedness office.

- Sanitation. Have on hand an adequate supply of toilet paper and/or towelettes, soap, liquid detergent, feminine supplies, personal hygiene items, plastic garbage bags with ties for personal sanitation uses, a plastic bucket with a tight lid, disinfectant, and chlorine bleach.

- Clothing and bedding. Have available at least one complete change of clothing and footwear per person, preferably items that are easy to clean. Depending on your location, you may also need to include sturdy shoes or work boots, hats and gloves, coats and/or rain gear, thermal underwear, blankets or sleeping bags, and sunglasses.

- Special items. Remember family members with special needs, such as infants and elderly or disabled persons. For babies, store an adequate supply of formula, diapers, bottles, powdered milk, and medications. For older children and adults, remember essentials such as heart and high blood pressure medication, insulin and syringes, prescription drugs, denture needs, contact lenses and supplies, extra eyeglasses, and games and books for entertainment. Ask a physician or pharmacist about how to store prescription medications.

- Important documents. Keep these records in a waterproof, portable container: wills, insurance policies, contracts, deeds, stocks and bonds, passports, Social Security cards, immunization records, bank account numbers, credit card account numbers and companies, an inventory of valuable household goods, important telephone numbers, and family records (such as birth, marriage, and death certificates).

This kit should be stored in a convenient place known to all family members, and a smaller version should be stowed in each car trunk. All items should be stored in air-tight plastic bags, and the stored water supply should be changed every 6 months so it stays fresh. Stored food should be rotated every 6 months, and the kit and family needs should be rethought at least once a year. Batteries should be replaced as needed, clothes should be updated as family members' sizes change, and so on.

discharge The flow of fluid from part of the body, such as the nose or vagina.

discoid lupus See *lupus, discoid.*

disease Illness or sickness, often characterized by abnormal sensations (symptoms) and physical findings (signs). For a specific disease, see the specific disease (such as Addison disease) under its alphabetical listing.

disease, metabolic See *metabolic disease.*

disease, obesity-related One of the diseases to which obesity predisposes, including type 2 diabetes; high blood pressure; stroke; heart attack; congestive heart failure; certain forms of cancer, such as prostate and colon cancer; gallstones and gall bladder disease; gout and gouty arthritis; osteoarthritis of the knees, hips, and lower back; sleep apnea; and Pickwickian syndrome.

disease, polygenic A genetic disorder caused by the combined action of more than one gene. Examples of polygenic conditions include some forms of coronary disease, hypertension, asthma, and diabetes. Because such disorders depend on the simultaneous presence of several genes, they are not inherited as simply as single-gene diseases. See also *disease, single gene.*

disease, rickettsial See *rickettsial disease.*

disease, single gene A hereditary disorder caused by a change (mutation) in a single gene. There are thousands of single-gene diseases, including achondroplasia, Huntington's disease, cystic fibrosis, sickle cell anemia, Duchenne muscular dystrophy, and hemophilia. Single-gene diseases typically describe classic simple Mendelian patterns of inheritance (as autosomal dominant, autosomal recessive, and X-linked traits), compared to polygenic diseases, which follow more complex patterns of inheritance. See also *disease, polygenic.*

DISH Diffuse idiopathic skeletal hyperostosis.

disk, choked See *papilledema.*

diskitis Inflammation of the disks between the vertebrae in the spinal column.

diskitis, tuberculous See *tuberculous diskitis.*

disorder, attention deficit See *attention deficit disorder.*

disorder, lymphoproliferative A malignant disease of the lymphoid cells and of cells from the reticuloendothelial system (lymph nodes and drainage tissues that clear inert particles within the body). A patient with lymphoproliferative disorder has proliferation and accumulation of lymphoid cells in the blood and marrow.

disorder, myeloproliferative A malignant disease of certain bone marrow cells, including those that give rise to the red blood cells, the granulocyte (types of white blood cells), and the platelets (which are crucial to blood clotting). The four major myeloproliferative disorders are polycythemia vera, myelofibrosis, thrombocythemia, and chronic myeloidleukemia (CML).

disorder, seasonal affective See *seasonal affective disorder.*

dissect To cut apart or separate tissue, as for anatomical study or in surgery. Also, an artery is said to dissect when its wall is torn, as in a dissecting aneurysm.

dissecting aneurysm See *aneurysm, dissecting.*

dissociation The act of temporarily disconnecting from reality. A person who is dissociating may believe himself or herself to be someone else or may simply experience unusual sensory experiences unrelated to the actual environment. See also *dissociative disorder.*

dissociative disorder A psychiatric disorder characterized by the ability to temporarily disconnect from reality. Multiple personality disorder is a type of dissociative disorder in which, while dissociating, the person believes himself or herself to be another person.

distal The more (or most) distant of two (or more) things. For example, the distal end of the thigh bone is the end of that bone that is by the knee, most distant from the end that is near the hip. The opposite of distal is proximal. See also Appendix B, "Anatomic Orientation Terms."

distal hereditary myopathy See *muscular dystrophy, distal.*

diuresis Excretion of urine, typically in large volumes. See also *diuretic.*

diuretic Something that promotes the formation of urine by the kidney. All diuretics cause a person to "lose water," but they do so by diverse means, including inhibiting the kidney's ability to reabsorb sodium, thus enhancing the loss of sodium and consequently water in the urine (a high-ceiling or loop diuretic); enhancing the excretion of both sodium and chloride in the urine so that water is excreted with them (a thiazide diuretic); or blocking the exchange of sodium for potassium, resulting in excretion of sodium and potassium but relatively little loss of potassium (a potassium-sparing diuretic). Some diuretics work by yet other mechanisms, and some have other effects and uses, such as in treating hypertension. Also known as water pill. Substances in food and drinks, such as coffee, tea, and alcoholic beverages, may act as diuretics.

diuretic, loop A diuretic that works by encouraging the loss of sodium (salt) and water by affecting sodium transport at the loop area of the kidneys. As the sodium is removed, it takes water with it. Loop diuretics are very strong, and they should be used only under constant medical supervision. They can deplete the electrolyte balance, cause dehydration, reduce blood volume, and worsen certain medical conditions. See also *diuretic.*

diuretic, potassium-sparing A diuretic that blocks the exchange of sodium (salt) and potassium, encouraging the excretion of sodium and therefore of water, but generally allowing potassium to be retained. See also *diuretic.*

diuretic, thiazide A diuretic that works by encouraging excretion of both sodium (salt) and chloride. See also *diuretic.*

diurnal Occurring in the daytime. A patient may have a diurnal fever rather than a nocturnal one. Diurnal also refers to something that recurs every day.

diverticula The plural of diverticulum.

diverticulitis Inflammation of diverticula along the wall of the the large intestine (colon). For diverticulitis to occur, there must be diverticulosis. Diverticulosis can occur anywhere in the colon, but is most typical in the sigmoid colon, the S-shaped segment of the colon located in the lower-left part of the abdomen. Diverticulitis can be diagnosed with barium X-rays of the colon or with sigmoidoscopy or colonoscopy. Antibiotics are usually needed to treat acute diverticulitis. Oral antibiotics are sufficient when symptoms are mild. Liquid or low-fiber foods are advised during acute diverticulitis attacks. In severe diverticulitis, with high fever and pain, patients are hospitalized and given intravenous antibiotics. Surgery is necessary for persistent bowel obstruction and for abscesses that do not respond to antibiotics. A high-fiber diet may help delay the progression of diverticulosis and may prevent or reduce bouts of diverticulitis. See also *diverticulosis.*

diverticulitis, bleeding due to Bleeding that is caused by diverticulitis and that typically occurs intermittently over several days. Colonoscopy is usually performed to confirm the diagnosis of diverticulitis and exclude bleeding due to other causes. Thermal probes cannot be used to stop active diverticular bleeding. Therefore, surgical removal of the bleeding diverticula is necessary for those with persistent diverticular bleeding.

diverticulosis The condition of having diverticula, small outpouchings from the large intestine (colon). Diverticulosis can occur anywhere in the colon but is most typical in the sigmoid colon, the S-shaped segment of the colon located in the lower-left part of the abdomen. The incidence of diverticulosis increases with age. As a person ages, the walls of the colon weaken, and this weakening permits the formation of diverticula. By age 80, most people have diverticulosis. A key factor promoting the formation of diverticulosis is elevated pressure within the colon. Pressure within the colon is raised when a person is constipated and has to push down to pass small, hard bits of stool. Most patients with diverticulosis have few or no symptoms, although some have mild symptoms, such as abdominal cramping and bloating. Diverticulosis sets the stage for inflammation and infection of the diverticula (diverticulitis). The best way to avoid developing diverticulosis in the first place is to eat a healthy diet that includes plenty of fiber. A diet that is high in fiber keeps the bowels moving, keeps the pressure in the colon within normal limits, and slows or stops the formation of diverticula. See also *diverticulitis.*

diverticulum A small bulging sac that pushes outward from the colon wall. The plural is diverticula. As a person ages, pressure within the large intestine (colon) causes diverticula. Diverticula can occur throughout the colon but are most common near the end of the S-shaped segment of the colon located in the lower-left part of the abdomen (the sigmoid colon).

diverticulum, Meckel An outpouching of the small bowel. About 1 in every 50 people has a Meckel diverticulum. Meckel diverticula are usually located about 2 feet before the junction of the small bowel and the colon (the large intestine) in the lower-right abdomen. Meckel diverticula can become inflamed, ulcerate, and perforate (break open or rupture), which can cause obstruction of the small bowel. Generally Meckel diverticula that are inflamed or perforated are removed via surgery.

dizziness Painless head discomfort with many possible causes, including disturbances of vision, the brain, the

balance (vestibular) system of the inner ear, or the gastrointestinal system. Dizziness is a medically indistinct term. Laypersons use it to describe a variety of conditions, ranging from lightheadedness or unsteadiness to vertigo. See also *lightheadedness; unsteadiness; vertigo.*

dizziness, anxiety as a cause of One cause of dizziness is overbreathing (hyperventilation) due to anxiety. Relief can be had by breathing in and out of a paper bag to increase the level of carbon dioxide in the blood. In persistent cases, as in repeated panic attacks, antianxiety medication can be helpful.

dizziness, presyncopal Dizziness before fainting. Some symptoms of dizziness, such as "wooziness," feeling as though one is about to black out, and tunnel vision may be presyncopal and are due to insufficient blood flow to the brain. These symptoms are typically worse when standing, improve with lying down, and may be experienced by healthy individuals who rise quickly from a seated or prone position and have a few seconds of disorientation. See also *syncope.*

DMD Duchenne muscular dystrophy. See *muscular dystrophy, Duchenne.*

DNA **1** Deoxyribonucleic acid, one of the two molecules (along with RNA) that encode genetic information. DNA is double-stranded. The two strands are held together by weak hydrogen bonds between base pairs of nucleotides to form a double helix. The double helix looks something like an immensely long ladder twisted into a helix, or coil. The sides of the ladder are formed by a backbone of sugar and phosphate molecules, and the rungs consist of nucleotide bases joined in the middle by the hydrogen bonds. The four nucleotides in DNA contain the bases adenine (A), guanine (G), cytosine (C), and thymine (T). **2** In the UK, an abbreviation for "did not attend," comparable to the US term "no-show" for a patient who missed an appointment.

DNA cloning The use of DNA-manipulation procedures to produce multiple copies of a single gene or segment of DNA. See also *DNA, recombinant.*

DNA, mitochondrial The DNA of the mitochondrion, a structure situated in the cytoplasm of the cell rather than in the nucleus, where all the other chromosomes are located. Abbreviated mtDNA. mtDNA is inherited from the mother. There are 2 to 10 copies of the mtDNA genome in each mitochondrion. mtDNA is a double-stranded, circular molecule. It is very small compared to the chromosomes in the nucleus, and it contains only a limited number of genes. It is specialized in the information it carries, and it encodes a number of the subunits in the mitochondrial respiratory-chain complex that the cell needs in order to respire. Mutations (changes) in mtDNA can cause disease, and they often impair the function of oxidative-phosphorylation enzymes in the respiratory chain, especially in tissues with high energy expenditure, such as brain and muscle tissues. All mtDNA at fertilization comes from the oocyte, so inherited mtDNA mutations are transmitted from the mother to all offspring, both male and female. The higher the level of mutant mtDNA in the mother's blood, the higher the frequency of clinically affected offspring and the more severely those children tend to be affected. Each cell in the body contains different mtDNA populations, and due to the presence of multiple mitochondria in cells, each cell contains several mtDNA copies. This produces tissue variation, so that a mutation in mtDNA versus normal mtDNA can vary widely among tissues in an individual. The percentage of mutant mtDNAs must be above a certain threshold to produce clinical disease, and this threshold varies from tissue to tissue because the percentage of mutant mDNAs needed to cause cell dysfunction varies according to the oxidative requirements of the tissue. See also *mitochondrial diseases.*

DNA polymerase   An enzyme that catalyzes (speeds) the polymerization of DNA. DNA polymerase uses preexisting nucleic acid templates and assembles the DNA from deoxyribonucleotides.

DNA, recombinant   DNA made up of DNA molecules of different origins, joined together by using recombinant DNA technology. A recombinant DNA molecule is constructed (recombined) from segments from two or more different DNA molecules. Under certain conditions, a recombinant DNA molecule can enter a cell and replicate there.

DNA repair   The process by which a cell uses a series of special enzymes to repair mutations (changes) in DNA and restore the DNA to its original state. The DNA is constantly mutating and being repaired. This repair process is controlled by special genes. A mutation in a DNA repair gene can cripple the repair process and cause a cascade of unrepaired mutations in the genome.

DNA repair gene   A gene that is engaged in DNA repair. When a DNA repair gene is altered, mutations pile up throughout the DNA.

DNA repair pathway   The sequence of steps in the repair of DNA. Each step is governed by an enzyme.

DNA replication   A complex process whereby the "parent" strands of DNA in the double helix are separated, and each one is copied to produce a new (daughter) strand. This process is said to be "semiconservative" because one strand from each parent is conserved and remains intact after replication has taken place.

DNA sequence   The precise ordering of the bases (A, T, G, C) from which DNA is composed. Base pairs form naturally only between A and T and between G and C, so the base sequence of each single strand of DNA can be simply deduced from that of its partner strand. The DNA nucleotide code is in triplets, such as ATG; the base sequence of ATG's partner strand would be TAC.

DNR   Do not resuscitate.

D.O.   Doctor of Osteopathy, an osteopathic physician. See also *osteopath; osteopathy.*

do not resuscitate   A directive to not attempt mechanical or manual resuscitation if the patient stops breathing. Abbreviated DNR. See also *advance directive.*

DOB   Date of birth, an abbreviation that is frequently used in medical charting.

doctor   In a medical context, any medical professional with an MD, a PhD, or any other doctoral degree. The term *doctor* is quite unspecific. A doctor may, for example, be a physician, psychologist, biomedical scientist, dentist, or veterinarian. In a nonmedical context, a professor of history might be addressed as doctor, an eminent theologian might be named a doctor of a church, and a person awarded an honorary doctorate by a college or university might also be called a doctor.

doctors' symbol   See *Aesculapius.*

DOE   Department of Energy, one of the US agencies that contributes to the Human Genome Project.

domain   In biomedicine, a discrete portion of a protein that has its own function. The combination of domains in a single protein determines the overall function of the protein.

dominant   A genetic trait that is evident when only one copy of that gene for that trait is present. (As opposed to a recessive trait, which is usually expressed only when two copies of the gene for that trait are present.) Most dominant traits are due to genes located on the autosomes (the nonsex chromosomes). Diseases inherited in an autosomal dominant manner typically affect both males and females and each of their children run a 50 percent chance to receive their disease gene. Autosomal dominant diseases include achondroplasia (dwarfism with short arms and legs), Huntington disease (a form of progressive dementia), and neurofigromatosis (a neurologic disorder with an increased risk of malignant tumors). X-linked dominance is due to genes on the X chromosome. A single copy of the mutant gene on the X chromosome causes the disease in a female. An example is a type of hereditary rickets called hypophosphatemic rickets. See also *autosomal dominant; X-linked dominant.*

dominant, autosomal   See *autosomal dominant.*

dominant, X-linked   See *x-linked dominant.*

donor   The giver of a tissue or an organ, such as a blood donor or kidney donor.

donor insemination   See *artificial insemination by donor.*

dopa-responsive dystonia   A disease characterized by progressive difficulty in walking and in some cases by spasticity. Abbreviated DRD. DRD begins in childhood or adolescence. It can be successfully treated with drugs. Segawa dystonia is an important variant of DRD. Some scientists feel that DRD is not only rare but also rarely diagnosed because it mimics many of the symptoms of cerebral palsy. Medications that affect the chemical nerve transmitter dopa can improve symptoms.

dorsal   Pertaining to the back, or posterior, side of a structure, as opposed to the ventral, or front, side. Some of the dorsal surfaces of the body are the back, buttocks, and calves, and the knuckle side of the hand. See also Appendix B, "Anatomic Orientation Terms."

dorsum   The back or posterior side of a structure. Something that pertains to the dorsum is dorsal.

DOT   Directly observed therapy.

double-blinded study   A medical study in which at least two separate groups receive the experimental medication or procedure at different times, with neither group being made aware of when the experimental medication or procedure has been given. Double-blinded studies are often used when a treatment shows particular promise and the illness involved is serious.

double helix   The structure of DNA, in which two strands of DNA spiral about each other.

double pneumonia   See *pneumonia, double.*

douche   Usually, a stream of water applied to the vagina for cleansing purposes. A douche can use a solution, such as vinegar and water, rather than simple water, and it can be directed at any body cavity or part.

douching   Using water or a medicated solution to clean the vagina and cervix or any other body cavity or part.

Douglas, pouch of   See *pouch of Douglas.*

Dowager's hump   An abnormal outward curvature of the vertebrae of the upper back. Compression of the front portion of the involved vertebrae leads to forward bending of the spine (kyphosis) and creates a hump at the upper back. Dowager's hump is due to osteoporosis changes in the thoracic spine. It may affect men or women. Like most osteoporotic changes, it is often preventable.

Down syndrome   A common birth defect that is usually due to an extra chromosome 21 (trisomy 21). Down syndrome causes mental retardation, a characteristic facial appearance, and multiple malformations. It occurs most frequently in children born to mothers over age 35. It is associated with a major risk for heart problems, a lesser risk of duodenal atresia (partially undeveloped intestines), and a minor but significant risk of acute leukemia. Confirmation of Down syndrome requires chromosome analysis, which is also valuable to rule in or out a translocation (a chromosome rearrangement) that can be heritable and give rise to more cases of Down syndrome in the family. Treatment for Down syndrome includes early intervention to develop the mental and physical capacities to their utmost, speech therapy, and surgery, as needed, to repair malformations. About one-half of children with Down syndrome have heart defects, most often holes between the two sides of the heart (septal defects). Hirschprung's disease (congenital aganglionic megacolon), which can cause intestinal obstruction, occurs more frequently in children with Down syndrome than in other children. With appropriate intervention, most children with Down syndrome live active, productive lives into at least middle age. Most are mildly to moderately retarded, although some have IQs in the low–normal range. Unfortunately, most adults with Down syndrome eventually develop Alzheimer's disease as they grow older. Down syndrome was also once called mongolism, a term now considered out of date, as the disorder has no relationship to Mongolian or Asian heritage. It can occur in any racial or ethnic group.

DPT   Diphtheria-pertussis-tetanus vaccine. Today the more frequent abbreviation is DTP, for diphtheria-tetanus-pertussis vaccine. See also *DTP immunization.*

DRD   See *dopa-responsive dystonia.*

dream   A series of thoughts, visions, and other sensations that occupy the mind in sleep. Dreams occur during that part of sleep when there are rapid eye movements (REM sleep). People have three to five periods of REM sleep per night, which usually come at intervals of 1 to 2 hours and are quite variable in length. An episode of REM sleep might be brief and last just 5 minutes, or it might be much longer. Experiments have shown that a person can communicate with a person who is dreaming. Dreaming is not uniquely human; cats and dogs dream, judging from the physiologic features, and so, apparently, do many other animals. The content of dreams is sometimes the topic of psychoanalysis. Although this method of therapy is less common today than it once was, some physicians still look at dreams as a diagnostic clue to medical disorders. For example, children with bipolar disorder have been found to frequently have a particular type of nightmares, and especially lucid dreams are a side effect of certain medications. These clues indicate that chemicals in the brain, as well as life events and individuals' preoccupations, influence dreams. See also *REM sleep.*

drip   Short for intravenous drip, a device for administering a fluid drop-by-drop into a vein via an intravenous (IV) route.

drug, ACE-inhibitor   See *ACE inhibitor.*

drug activity   A measure of the physiological response that a drug produces. A less active drug produces less response, and a more active drug produces more response.

drug, anti-angiogenesis   See *anti-angiogenesis drug.*

drug, antihypertensive   See *antihypertensive.*

drug, anti-infective   See *agent, anti-infective.*

drug, antiviral   See *antiviral agent.*

Drug Enforcement Administration   See *DEA.*

drug, over-the-counter   A drug for which a prescription is not needed.

drug, prescription   See *prescription drug.*

drug resistance   The ability of bacteria and other microorganisms to withstand a drug that once stalled them or killed them.

drug, teratogenic   See *teratogen.*

drugs during pregnancy, dangerous   See *teratogen.*

dry eyes   See *xerophthalmia.*

dry mouth   See *xerostomia.*

dry skin   See *xeroderma.*

DSM-IV   *Diagnostic and Statistical Manual of Mental Disorders,* 4th edition, the official source on definitions related to mental illness.

DT immunization   A vaccination against diphtheria and tetanus. DT immunization does not protect from pertussis as the DPT and DTaP immunizations do. It is usually reserved for individuals who have had a significant adverse reaction to a DPT shot or who have a personal or family history of seizure disorder or brain disease. See also *diphtheria; tetanus.*

DTaP immunization   Diphtheria-tetanus-acellular-pertussis immunization, a vaccine that, like DPT, protects against diphtheria, pertussis (whooping cough), and tetanus. DTaP is the same as DTP, except that it contains only acellular pertussis vaccine, which is thought to cause fewer of the minor reactions associated with immunization. Acellular pertussis vaccine is also probably less likely than regular pertussis vaccine to cause the more severe reactions occasionally seen following pertussis vaccination. It is currently recommended that DTaP be given at 18 months and at 4 to 6 years of age. See also *diphtheria; pertussis; tetanus.*

DTP immunization   Diphtheria, tetanus, and pertussis (whooping cough) immunization, a vaccine that is given in a series of five shots at 2, 4, 6, and 18 months of age and again at 4 to 6 years of age. Thanks to vaccination programs, diphtheria, tetanus, and pertussis have become less common than they were in the past. However, there are still unvaccinated individuals who are capable of carrying and passing diphtheria and pertussis to others who are not vaccinated. Tetanus bacteria are prevalent in natural surroundings, such as contaminated soil. Children with compromised immune systems or known neurological disorders generally should not receive the DPT immunization, particularly during infancy. See also *DTaP immunization.*

dual diagnosis   A diagnosis of both a mental illness and a substance abuse disorder.

Duchenne muscular dystrophy   See *DMD.*

duct   A walled passageway, such as a lymph duct, that carries fluid from one place to another. Also known as a ductus.

duct, thoracic   See *thoracic duct.*

ductal carcinoma of the breast, infiltrating   See *carcinoma of the breast, infiltrating ductal.*

ductus   See *duct.*

ductus arteriosus   A short vessel through which blood headed from the heart via the pulmonary artery to the lungs is shunted before birth. This blood is shunted away from the lungs and returned to the aorta. When the shunt is open, it is said to be patent. A patent ductus arteriosus (PDA) usually closes at or shortly after birth, and blood is permitted from that moment on to course freely to the lungs. If the ductus stays open, flow reverses, and blood from the aorta is shunted into the pulmonary artery and recirculated through the lungs. The PDA may close later on its own, or it may need to be ligated (tied off) surgically.

due date   The estimated calendar date when a baby is due to be born. Also called the estimated date of confinement (EDC).

dumping syndrome   A group of symptoms, including cramps, nausea, diarrhea, and dizziness, that occur when food or liquid enters the small intestine too rapidly.

duodenal ulcer   A hole (ulcer) in the lining of the beginning of the small intestine (duodenum). Ulcer formation is caused by infection with Helicobacter pylori. Other factors predisposing a person to ulcers include anti-inflammatory medications and cigarette smoking. Ulcer pain may not correlate with the presence or severity of ulceration. Diagnosis is made with barium X-ray or endoscopy. Complications of ulcers include bleeding, perforation, and blockage. Treatment involves using antibiotics to eradicate H. pylori, eliminating risk factors, and preventing complications.

duodenitis   Inflammation of the duodenum, the first part of the small intestine.

duodenum   The first part of the small intestine. The duodenum is a common site for peptic ulcer formation.

duplication, chromosome   The addition of part of another chromosome to a chromosome. This is a common cause of genetic disease. The opposite of deletion.

Dupuytren's contracture   A localized formation of scar tissue in the palm of the hand. The scarring accumulates in a tissue (fascia) beneath the skin of the palm that normally covers the tendons that pull the fingers into a grip. As Dupuytren's contracture progresses, more of the fascia becomes thickened and shortened. Dimpling and puckering of the skin over the area eventually occur. The precise cause of Dupuytren's contracture is not known. However, it is known that it occurs most frequently in patients with diabetes mellitus, seizure disorders (epilepsy), and alcoholism. It also can be inherited. Most patients with Dupuytren's contracture require only stretching exercises with heat application. When the palm is persistently sore with grasping, ultrasound treatments can be helpful. Sometimes local inflammation can be relieved with cortisone injection. For patients with significant fixed flexed posture (contracture) of the fingers from Dupuytren's contracture, surgical procedures can remove the scarred tissue to free the fingers.

durable power of attorney   A type of advance medical directive in which legal documents provide the power of attorney to another person in the case of an incapacitating medical condition. A durable power of attorney allows another person to make bank transactions, sign Social Security checks, apply for disability, or write checks to pay utility bills while an individual is medically incapacitated. Such documents are recommended for any patient who may be unable to make his or her wishes known during a long medical confinement.

DVT   Deep vein thrombosis.

dwarfism   Abnormally short stature, which may be due to a variety of causes. Some forms of dwarfism are hereditary. The Little People of America (LPA) defines dwarfism as a medical or genetic condition that usually results in an adult height of 148 cm (4 feet 10 inches) or shorter, among both men and women. Also known as nanism. Dwarfism is now more correctly called short stature. See also *achondroplasia; dwarfism, pituitary; hypochondroplasia; Seckel syndrome.*

dwarfism, achondroplastic   See *achondroplasia.*

dwarfism, hypochondroplastic   See *hypochondroplasia.*

dwarfism, pituitary   Dwarfism caused by a lack of growth hormone, usually due to malfunction of the anterior pituitary gland. Children with growth hormone deficiency may grow normally for the first 2 to 3 years of life, but they then fall behind their peers in height. Unlike those with other forms of dwarfism, those with pituitary dwarfism are normally proportioned. Pituitary dwarfism can be treated with injections of human growth hormone during childhood. Also known as hypopituitary dwarfism. See also *pituitary, anterior.*

dwarfism, rhizomelic   Dwarfism with shortening especially of the ends of the limbs. See also *achondroplasia; dwarfism.*

dwarfism, Seckel-type   See *Seckel syndrome.*

dwarfism, thanatophoric   A form of short-limbed (micromelic) dwarfism that usually causes death within the first few hours after birth. The bones of the arms and legs are very short. The ribs are also extremely short, and the rib cage is small, leading to respiratory insufficiency and death. See also *achondroplasia; dwarfism; hypochondroplasia.*

dx, DX   Diagnosis.

dys-   Prefix denoting bad or difficult, as in dyspepsia (difficult digestion).

dysarthria   Speech that is characteristically slurred, slow, and difficult to understand. A person with dysarthria may also have problems controlling the pitch, loudness, rhythm, and voice qualities of his or her speech.

Dysarthria is caused by paralysis, weakness, or inability to coordinate the muscles of the mouth. Dysarthria can occur as a developmental disability. It may be a sign of a neuromuscular disorder such as cerebral palsy or Parkinson's disease. It may also be caused by a stroke, brain injury, or brain tumor. Treatment of dysarthria includes intensive speech therapy with a focus on oral-motor skill development.

dyscalculia A specific developmental disability that affects a person's ability to conceptualize and perform mathematics. Mild cases can often be compensated for with use of a calculator, but those with severe dyscalculia need special education services.

dysentery Inflammation of the intestine, with pain, diarrhea, bloody stools, and often a fever above 38.3 degrees C (101°F). The causes of dysentery include bacteria (such as Shigella), protozoa (such as amebae), parasitic worms (such as schistosomes), and viruses. Dysentery can be fatal because it can cause severe dehydration. Treatment includes rapid rehydration, sometimes via IV, and medication.

dysentery, amebic See *amebic dysentery.*

dysfunction, erectile See *erectile dysfunction.*

dysgraphia A specific developmental disability that affects a person's handwriting ability. Problems may include fine-motor-muscle control of the hands and/or processing difficulties. Sometimes occupational therapy is helpful for those with dysgraphia. Most successful students with dysgraphia that does not respond to occupational therapy or extra writing help use a typewriter, computer, or verbal communication.

dyskinesia The presence of involuntary movements, such as the choreaform movements seen in some cases of rheumatic fever or the characteristic movements of tardive dyskinesia. Some forms of dyskinesia are side effects of certain medications, particularly L-dopa and, in the case of tardive dyskinesia, antipsychotic drugs.

dyslexia A specific developmental disability that alters the way the brain processes written material. Because dyslexia is due to a defect in the brain's processing of graphic symbols, it is thought of primarily as a learning disability. The effects of dyslexia vary from person to person. The only common trait among people with dyslexia is that they read at levels significantly lower than are typical for people of their age and intelligence. Dyslexia is different from reading retardation which may, for example, reflect mental retardation or cultural deprivation. Treatment of dyslexia should be directed to the specific learning problems of the affected individual. The usual

course is to modify teaching methods and the educational environment to meet the specific needs of the individual with dyslexia. The outlook for people with dyslexia is mixed. The disability affects such a wide range of people, producing different symptoms and varying degrees of severity, that predictions are hard to make. The prognosis is generally good, however, for individuals whose dyslexia is identified early, who have supportive families and friends and a strong self-image, and who are involved in appropriate remediation programs.

dysmenorrhea See *menstrual cramps.*

dysmorphic feature A body characteristic that is abnormally formed. A malformed ear, for example, is a dysmorphic feature.

dysmorphology The study of human congenital malformations (birth defects), particularly those affecting the anatomy (morphology) of the individual.

dysostosis, cleidocranial See *cleidocranial dysostosis.*

dyspareunia Pain during sexual intercourse. There are many causes of dyspareunia, including vaginal infection or dryness. Treatment is directed toward the underlying cause and vaginal lubricant jelly can be of help.

dyspepsia Indigestion. A condition characterized by upper abdominal symptoms that may include pain or discomfort, bloating, feeling of fullness with very little intake of food (early satiety), feeling of unusual fullness following meals (postprandial fullness), nausea, loss of appetite, heartburn, regurgitation of food or acid, and belching. The term dyspepsia is often used for these symptoms when they are not typical of a well-described disease (for example, gastrointestinal reflux) and the cause is not clear. After a cause for the symptoms has been determined, the term dyspepsia is usually dropped in favor of a more specific diagnosis.

dysphagia Difficulty swallowing. Dysphagia is due to abnormal nerve or muscle control. It is common, for example, after a stroke. Dysphagia can compromise nutrition and hydration and may lead to aspiration pneumonia and dehydration.

dysphonia, spasmodic A disorder that involves the muscles of the throat that control speech. Spasmodic dysphonia causes strained and difficult speaking or breathy and effortful speech. Also known as spastic dysphonia and laryngeal dystonia.

dysphoria Anxiety.

dysplasia Abnormality in form or development. For example, retinal dysplasia is abnormal formation of the retina during embryonic development.

dysplasia, bronchopulmonary Chronic lung disease in infants who have received mechanical respiratory support with high oxygenation in the neonatal period.

dysplasia, cleidocranial See *cleidocranial dysostosis.*

dysplastic nevus A mole whose appearance is different from that of common moles. Dysplastic nevi are generally larger than ordinary moles, and they have irregular borders. Their color is often not uniform. They are usually flat, but parts may be raised above the skin surface. Dysplastic nevi can be precancerous. See *cancer, skin.*

dyspnea Difficult or labored breathing; shortness of breath. Dyspnea is a sign of serious disease of the airway, lungs, or heart. The onset of dyspnea should not be ignored; it is reason to seek medical attention.

dyspnoea See *dyspnea.*

dyspraxia Impaired or painful function of an organ of the body. See also *developmental dyspraxia.*

dyspraxia, developmental See *developmental dyspraxia.*

dyspraxia of speech A developmental disability characterized by difficulty with muscle control, specifically with the muscles involved in producing speech. Dyspraxia of speech is caused by a neurological abnormality that has not yet been pinpointed. Treatment involves intensive speech therapy that concentrates on oral-motor skills. See also *apraxia of speech.*

dysthymia A type of depressive disorder that involves long-term, chronic symptoms that are not disabling but that nonetheless keep a person from full function or from feeling good. Dysthymia is a less severe type of depression than major depression. However, people with dysthymia may also sometimes experience major depressive episodes, suggesting that there is a continuum between dysthymia and major depression. See also *depression; depression, major.*

dystocia Difficult or abnormal labor or delivery.

dystocia, cervical Dystocia caused by mechanical obstruction at the cervix.

dystocia, fetal Dystocia caused by the fetus, due to its size (too big), shape, or position in the uterus.

dystocia, placental Dystocia characterized by trouble delivering the placenta (afterbirth).

dystonia Involuntary movements and prolonged muscle contraction that result in twisting body motions, tremors, and abnormal posture. These movements may involve the entire body or only an isolated area. Dystonia can be inherited, may occur sporadically without any genetic pattern, may be associated with medications (particularly antipsychotic drugs), or may be a symptom of certain diseases (for example, a specific form of lung cancer). The genes responsible for several types of dystonia have been identified. Some types of dystonia respond to dopamine. Dystonia can sometimes also be controlled with sedative-type medications or surgery.

dystonia, cranial A form of dystonia that affects the muscles of the head, face, and neck. Meige syndrome is the combination of blepharospasm, oromandibular dystonia, and sometimes spasmodic dysphonia. Spasmodic torticollis can be classified as a type of cranial dystonia.

dystonia, dopa-responsive See *dopa-responsive dystonia.*

dystonia, focal A form of dystonia that affects only one muscle group. Common focal dystonias that affect the muscles of the hand and sometimes the forearm have been called typist's cramp, pianist's cramp, musician's cramp, golfer's cramp, and writer's cramp.

dystonia, focal, due to blepharospasm The involuntary, forcible closure of the eyelids. Focal dystonia due to blepharospasm is the second most common focal dystonia. The first symptom may be uncontrollable blinking. Only one eye may be affected initially, but eventually both eyes are usually involved. The spasms may leave the eyelids completely closed, causing functional blindness even though the eyes and vision are normal. Uncontrollable blinking may also be caused by tic disorders, including Tourette syndrome.

dystonia, focal, due to torticollis See *torticollis.*

dystonia, generalized torsion See *dystonia, idiopathic torsion.*

dystonia, idiopathic torsion A form of torsion dystonia that begins in childhood, around age 12. Symptoms typically start in one part of the body, usually in an arm or a leg, and eventually spread to the rest of the body within about 5 years. Early-onset torsion dystonia is not fatal, but it can be severely debilitating. Also known as generalized torsion dystonia. See also *dystonia, torsion.*

dystonia, laryngeal See *dysphonia, spasmodic.*

dystonia musculorum deformans See *dystonia, torsion.*

dystonia, oromandibular Dystonia that affects the muscles of the jaw, lips, and tongue. The jaw may be pulled either open or shut, and speech and swallowing can be difficult.

dystonia, Segawa   See *dopa-responsive dystonia.*

dystonia, torsion   A type of dystonia in which symptoms typically start in one part of the body, usually in an arm or a leg, and eventually spread to the rest of the body. A form that strikes in childhood is known as idiopathic torsion dystonia, early-onset torsion dystonia, and generalized torsion dystonia. See also *dystonia, idiopathic torsion.*

dystrophy, muscular   See *muscular dystrophy.*

dystrophy, myotonic   A relatively common inherited disease in which the muscles contract but have decreasing ability to relax (myotonia). Myotonic dystrophy is also characterized by the development of a mask-like, expressionless face, premature balding, cataracts, and abnormalities in heart rhythm. See *amplification; anticipation.*

dysuria   Pain during urination, or difficulty urinating. Dysuria is usually caused by inflammation of the urethra, frequently as a result of infection.

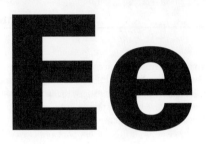

E. coli Escherichia coli, a bacterium that normally resides in the colon. E. coli has been studied intensively in genetics and in molecular and cell biology because of its availability, its small genome size, its usual lack of disease-causing ability, and its ability to be grown easily in the laboratory. Although E. coli is normally present in the colon with no harmful consequences, it can cause disease when transmitted from human to human via water, food, or feces. Infants, young children, the elderly, and people with compromised immune systems are especially at risk for E. coli infection.

E&RP Exposure and response prevention.

Eagle syndrome Inflammation of the styloid process, a spike-like growth that projects out from the base of the skull. If the styloid process is oversized or projects too far, the tissues in the throat can rub on it causing pain during the act of swallowing and pain on rotation of the neck. Diagnosis of Eagle syndrome is made by an X-ray showing an abnormally elongated styloid process. Anti-inflammatory drugs are the first line of treatment, and surgical removal of the styloid process may be necessary.

ear The hearing organ. There are three sections of the ear: outer, middle, and inner. The outer, or external, ear helps concentrate the vibrations of air created by sound onto the eardrum, causing the eardrum to vibrate. These vibrations are transmitted by a chain of little bones in the middle ear to the inner ear, where they stimulate the fibers of the auditory nerve to transmit impulses to the brain. The brain plays an essential role in hearing, because the auditory cortex of the brain interprets speech and other sounds that the ear receives as information we can use. See also *ear, inner; ear, middle; ear, outer.*

ear canal, self-cleaning A typical situation in which there is a slow and orderly migration of ear canal skin from the eardrum to the outer opening. Old earwax is constantly being transported from the deeper areas of the ear canal to the opening, where it usually dries, flakes, and falls out.

ear, cauliflower See *cauliflower ear.*

ear cleaning by a physician A necessary procedure that occurs when so much wax accumulates in the ear canal that it blocks it (and impairs hearing). To remove the blockage, a physician may have to wash the wax out, vacuum it out, or remove it with special instruments. Alternatively, a physician may prescribe eardrops designed to soften the wax.

ear cleaning by oneself A procedure in which a person cleans his or her own ears. Cleaning the deep portions of the ear canal is not recommended and could be harmful. Ear specialists state that a person should never put anything smaller than an elbow into an ear. Wax is not formed in the deep part of the ear canal near the eardrum, but only in the outer part of the canal. So when a patient has wax pushed up against the eardrum, it is often because he or she has been probing the ear with such things as cotton-tipped swabs, bobby pins, or twisted napkin corners. Such objects only serve as ramrods to push the wax deeper. Also, the skin of the ear canal and the eardrum is very thin, fragile, and easily injured. The ear canal is more prone to infection after it has been wiped clean of its wax coating. In addition, many perforated eardrums occur as a result of self-cleaning.

ear, external See *ear, outer.*

ear infection Infection of the ear by bacteria or viruses. Ear infections are the most frequent diagnosis in sick children. Ear infections occur less commonly in adults. Almost every child has one or more bouts of otitis media before age 6. The Eustachian tube is shorter in children than in adults, allowing easy entry of bacteria and viruses into the middle ear. Outer ear infection in adults is sometimes associated with excessive cotton swab irritation of the ear canal. Bottle-feeding is a risk factor for ear infections. Breast-feeding passes to the baby immunity that helps prevent ear infections. The position of the breast-feeding child is better than that of the bottle-feeding child for Eustachian tube function. If a child needs to be bottle-fed, holding the infant rather than allowing the child to lie down with the bottle is best. A child should not take the bottle to bed. Ear infections are not contagious, but the bacteria or viruses that cause them may be. A child with an ear infection can travel by airplane, but if the Eustachian tube is not functioning well, changes in pressure can cause discomfort. A child with a draining ear should not fly or swim. See also *ear infection, external.*

ear infection, external Infection of the skin covering the outer ear canal that leads in to the ear drum, usually due to bacteria such as streptococcus, staphylococcus, or pseudomonas. External ear infection is usually caused by excessive water exposure. When water pools in the ear canal (frequently trapped by wax), the skin will become soggy and serve as an inviting culture media for bacteria. The first sign of an external ear infection is a feeling of fullness and itching in the ear. Next the ear canal swells, and drainage and pain follow. With severe infection, the ear canal can swell completely shut and the side of the face can become swollen. The glands of the neck may enlarge. Moisture and irritation will prolong the course of swimmer's ear. For this reason, the ear should be kept dry. While showering or swimming, use an earplug (one that is designed to keep water out), or use cotton with Vaseline on the outside. Scratching the inside of the ear or using Q-tips should be avoided. A hearing aid should be left out. Treatment consists of antibiotic eardrops with or without an oral antibiotic. A "wick" may need to be placed in the ear canal to stent it open and serve as a conduit for the eardrops. Also known as otitis externa and swimmer's ear.

ear, inner　A highly complex structure whose essential component for hearing is the membranous labyrinth, where the fibers of the auditory nerve that connect the ear to the brain end. The membranous labyrinth is a system of communicating sacs and ducts (tubes) filled with fluid (endolymph), and it is lodged within a cavity called the bony labyrinth. At some points the membranous labyrinth is attached to the bony labyrinth, and at other points the membranous labyrinth is suspended within the bony labyrinth in a fluid called perilymph. The bony labyrinth has three parts: a central cavity called the vestibule; semicircular canals, which open into the vestibule; and a spiraling tube called the cochlea. The membranous labyrinth also has a vestibule, which consists of two sacs (the utriculus and sacculus) that are connected by a narrow tube. The larger of the two sacs, the utriculus, is the principal organ of the vestibular system, which is the system of balance. This system informs a person about the position and movement of the head. The smaller of the two sacs, the sacculus, is also connected by a membranous tube to the cochlea that contains the organ of Corti. The hair cells, which are the special sensory receptors for hearing, are found within the organ of Corti.

ear, internal　See *ear, inner.*

ear, low-set　A minor anomaly in which the ear is situated below the normal location. Technically, the ear is low-set when the helix of the ear meets the cranium at a level below that of a horizontal plane through both inner canthi (the inside corners of the eyes). The presence of two or more minor anomalies such as this one in a child increases the probability that the child has a major malformation.

ear, malrotated　See *ear, slanted.*

ear, middle　A part of the ear that consists of the eardrum (tympanic membrane) and, beyond it, a cavity (tympanum). This cavity is connected to the pharynx (nasopharynx) via a canal known as the Eustachian tube.

The middle ear cavity also contains a chain of three little bones, the ossicles (the malleus, incus, and stapes), which connect the eardrum to the internal ear. The middle ear communicates with the pharynx, equilibrates with external pressure, and transmits the eardrum vibrations to the inner ear.

ear, outer　The part of the ear that is visible along the side of the head. The outer ear looks complicated but is actually the simplest part of the ear. It consists of the pinna, or auricle (the visible projecting portion of the ear), the external acoustic meatus (the outside opening to the ear canal), and the external ear canal, which leads to the eardrum. The outer ear concentrates air vibrations on the eardrum to make the eardrum vibrate.

ear piercing　The practice of using a needle or needle gun to make holes through the ear lobe or other parts of the ear so that jewelry can be worn. When ear piercing is done under hygienic conditions, there is little danger from ear piercing, other than localized and transitory inflammation. Unhygienic conditions, handling of the new piercing with unwashed hands, or the use of irritating jewelry can result in inflammation and/or infection. Infected ear piercings should be washed and then treated with antibiotic cream. Further treatment involves either allowing the piercing to close or using only nonirritating jewelry (usually gold or hypoallergenic plastic). The likelihood of inflammation and infection is greater for piercings that go through hard cartilage, as found on the side and top of the outer ear, than for the soft bottom lobe of the ear.

ear pit　A tiny pit in front of the ear, also called a preauricular pit. This minor anomaly is of no consequence in and of itself. It is more common in blacks than in whites, and in females than males. It can recur in families. However, the presence of two or more minor anomalies such as this one in a child increases the probability that the child also has a major malformation such as a congenital heart defect.

ear puncture　Puncture of the eardrum. Ear puncture may be due to an accident, as when something is stuck into the ear. Eardrums may also be punctured due to fluid pressure in the middle ear. Today the eardrum is occasionally punctured on purpose via surgery. A tiny incision (myringotomy) is made in the eardrum to allow fluid trapped behind the eardrum, usually thickened secretions, to be removed. An ear tube may be inserted after the fluid drains.

ear ringing　See *tinnitus.*

ear, slanted　A minor anomaly in which the ear is slanted more than usual—more than 15 degrees from the perpendicular. The presence of two or more minor anomalies such as this one in a child increases the probability that the child has a major malformation. Slanted ears are a common sign of fetal alcohol syndrome and fetal alcohol effect. Both of these conditions also feature a very high rate of sensorineural hearing loss and ear infections. Also known as malrotated ear. See also *fetal alcohol effect; fetal alcohol syndrome.*

ear, swimmer's   See *ear infection, external.*

ear tag   A rudimentary tag of ear tissue, often containing a core of cartilage, usually located just in front of the ear (auricle). This minor anomaly is common and harmless. However, the presence of two or more minor anomalies such as this one in a child increases the probability that the child has a major malformation. Also known as preauricular tag.

ear tube   A small plastic tube that is inserted into the eardrum (tympanum) to keep the middle ear aerated for a prolonged period of time. To put an ear tube in place, a tiny surgical incision is made in the eardrum. Any fluid is removed. Ear tubes remain in place from 6 months to several years. Water should not be allowed to enter the ear canal while the tubes are in place. A physician may remove a tube during a routine office visit, or it may simply fall out of the ear naturally without the patient realizing it. Formally known as a tympanostomy tube.

ear tumor   A formation of benign (noncancerous) bumps on the external ear or within the external ear canal. Most of these lumps and bumps are harmless sebaceous cysts. However, some are bony overgrowths known as exostoses or osteomas. If they are large and interfere with hearing, they can be surgically removed with relative ease.

eardrum   The tympanic membrane of the ear. This membrane is the first tissue of the ear to receive the waves of the sound we hear. The sound vibrations are then passed on to the tiny bones (ossicles) of the middle ear.

earwax   A natural wax-like substance secreted by glands in the skin on the outer part of the ear canal. Earwax repels water and traps dust and sand particles. Usually small amounts of wax accumulate and then dry up and fall out of the ear canal, carrying unwanted particles. Earwax is helpful in normal amounts. The absence of earwax may result in dry, itchy ears, and in infection. There are two types of earwax: wet and dry. Most whites and blacks have the wet type, and most Asians and Native Americans have the dry type.

earthquake supplies kit   See *disaster supplies.*

Ebola virus   A virus that causes a deadly form of hemorrhagic fever that is characterized by a rise in temperature and bleeding problems. Ebola virus epidemics have occurred mainly in Sudan and Zaire. The initial symptoms are fever and headache, followed by vomiting and diarrhea, muscle pain, rash, and bloody nose (epistaxis), spitting up of blood from the lungs (hemoptysis) and stomach (hematemesis), and bloody eyes (conjunctival hemorrhages). Ebola virus is highly contagious and is transmitted by contact with blood, feces, or body fluids from an infected person. The incubation period ranges from 2 to 21 days. There is no specific treatment for the disease. Death can occur within 10 days.

EBV   Epstein-Barr virus.

ecchymosis   Nonraised skin discoloration caused by the escape of blood into the tissues from ruptured blood vessels. Ecchymoses can occur in mucous membranes (for example, in the mouth).

ecchymotic   Characterized by ecchymosis.

ECG   Electrocardiogram.

echocardiography   A diagnostic test of the heart that uses ultrasound waves to form images of the heart chambers, valves, and surrounding structures. Echocardiography can measure cardiac output, and it is a sensitive test for detecting inflammation around the heart (pericarditis). It can also be used to detect abnormal anatomy and infections of the heart valves.

echolalia   Persistent repetition (echoing) of heard speech. In response to the question, "Do you want milk?" a child with echolalia might answer, "Milk?" Echolalia is most commonly seen in children with autism, but it is also found in some with Tourette syndrome.

echovirus   A group of viruses found in the intestinal tract. The "echo" part of the name is an acronym for enteric cytopathic human orphan viruses. "Orphan" implied that these viruses were not associated with any disease. However, it is now known that echoviruses can cause a number of different diseases, including rashes, diarrhea, respiratory infections (such as the common cold, sore throat, bronchitis, and bronchiolitis), myositis (muscle inflammation), meningitis, encephalitis, and pericarditis.

eclampsia   The presence of one or more convulsions in a pregnant woman who has preeclampsia. Eclampsia is a frequent cause of maternal death in underdeveloped countries, and it is a serious problem even in developed countries. Treatment is with antispasmodic medication, notably magnesium sulfate. See also *HELLP syndrome; preeclampsia.*

ecogenetics   The interaction of genetics with the environment. The genetic disease phenylketonuria (PKU) provides an illustration of ecogenetics. Persons with PKU lack an enzyme that is needed to process the amino acid phenylalanine, and they require a special environment: a diet low in phenylalanine.

economy-class syndrome   See *deep vein thrombosis.*

ECT   Electroconvulsive therapy.

ectoderm   The outermost of the three primary germ cell layers (the other two being the mesoderm and endoderm) that make up a very young embryo. The ectoderm differentiates (specializes) to give rise to many important tissues and structures, including the outer layer of the skin and its appendages (such as the sweat glands, hair, and nails), the teeth, the lens of the eye, parts of the inner ear, the nerves, the brain, and the spinal cord. Stem cell research has shown that some cells within ectodermal structures retain their ability to differentiate into other tissues. For example, some cells in the brain (ectoderm) can become bone marrow (mesoderm). See also *differentiation; embryo; endoderm; mesoderm.*

ectodermal dysplasia   A genetic disorder in which the skin and associated structures (the hair, nails, teeth, and sweat glands) develop abnormally. The most dangerous problem occurs in cases of ectodermal dysplasia with decreased sweating due to absence of the sweat glands. Affected persons have trouble controlling temperature and being in a warm environment. The hair may also be absent or sparse. The skin tends to be thin and light in color. Problems with the inner lining of the nose predispose people with ectodermal dysplasia to chronic nasal infections. The teeth may be notably absent or develop abnormally. There are a number of different types of ectodermal dysplasia. X-linked anhidrotic (nonsweating) ectodermal dysplasia is most common; because it is an X-linked trait, it mainly affects males. There is also an autosomal dominant form that affects both males and females. The term ectodermal dysplasia refers to the abnormal development (dysplasia) of structures derived from one of the germ cell layers in the embryo (ectoderm).

-ectomy   The surgical removal of something. For example, a lumpectomy is the surgical removal of a lump, a tonsillectomy is the removal of the tonsils, and an appendectomy is removal of the appendix.

ectopia cordis   A birth defect that results in an abnormal location of the heart, usually outside the chest.

ectopic   In the wrong place, out of place. For example, an ectopic kidney is a kidney that is not in the usual location.

ectopic pregnancy   A pregnancy that occurs outside of the uterus. In 95 percent of ectopic pregnancies, a fertilized egg settles and grows in the Fallopian tube. However, ectopic pregnancies can occur in other locations, such as the ovary, cervix, and abdominal cavity. An ectopic pregnancy occurs in about 1 in 60 pregnancies. Most occur in women 35 to 44 years of age, and they are usually due to the inability of a fertilized egg to make its way through a Fallopian tube into the uterus. Risk factors include pelvic inflammatory disease (PID); adhesions from surgery on or near a Fallopian tube; endometriosis, a condition in which tissue like that normally lining the uterus is found outside the uterus; a prior ectopic pregnancy; a history of repeated induced abortions; and a history of infertility problems or use of medications to stimulate ovulation. A major concern with ectopic pregnancy is internal bleeding. Pain is usually the first symptom. The pain, which is usually sharp and stabbing, is often one-sided and may occur in the pelvis, abdomen, or even the shoulder or neck (due to blood from a ruptured ectopic pregnancy building up under the diaphragm and the pain being "referred" up to the shoulder or neck). Weakness, dizziness or lightheadedness, and a sense of passing out upon standing can result from serious internal bleeding, requiring immediate medical attention. Diagnosis is made through a pelvic exam to test for pain, tenderness, and a mass in the abdomen. The most useful laboratory test is the measurement of the hormone human chorionic gonadotropin (hCG). In a normal pregnancy, the level of hCG doubles about every 2 days during the first 10 weeks, whereas in an ectopic pregnancy, the hCG rise is usually slower and lower than normal. Ultrasound can also help determine whether a pregnancy is ectopic, as can culdocentesis, the insertion of a needle through the vagina into the space behind the uterus to see whether there is blood there from a ruptured Fallopian tube. Treatment includes surgery, often by laparoscopy, to remove the ill-fated pregnancy. A ruptured Fallopian tube usually has to be removed. If the tube has not yet burst, a physician may be able to repair it. The outlook for future pregnancies depends on the extent of the surgery. If the Fallopian tube has been spared, the chance of a successful pregnancy is usually better than 50 percent. If a Fallopian tube has been removed, an egg can be fertilized in the other tube, and the chance of a successful pregnancy drops to somewhat below 50 percent.

eczema   An inflammatory reaction of the skin in which there are tiny blister-like raised areas in the early stage followed by reddening, swelling, bumps, crusting, and thickening and scaling. Eczema characteristically causes itching and burning. Also known as atopic dermatitis. Eczema is a very common skin problem that may start in infancy, later in childhood, or in adulthood. It can be caused by allergies, diabetes, sunburn, or unknown reasons. Eczema tends not to go quickly away. It is usually treated with medications, commonly topical cortisone creams, to reduce the inflammation. There are numerous types of eczema, including atopic dermatitis, contact eczema, seborrheic eczema, nummular eczema, neurodermatitis, stasis dermatitis, and dyshidrotic eczema.

eczema, allergic contact   A red, itchy, weepy reaction that occurs where the skin has come into contact with a substance that the immune system recognizes as foreign, such as poison ivy or certain preservatives in creams and lotions. Also known as allergic contact dermatitis.

eczema, contact   A localized reaction that involves redness, itching, and burning that occurs where the skin has come into contact with an allergen (an allergy-causing substance) or an irritant such as an acid, a cleaning agent, or another chemical.

eczema, dyshidrotic   Irritation of the skin on the palms of the hands and the soles of the feet that is characterized by clear, deep blisters that itch and burn.

eczema, nummular   Coin-shaped patches of irritated skin that may be crusted, scaling, and extremely itchy. Nummular eczema appears most commonly on the arms, back, buttocks, and lower legs.

eczema, seborrheic   See *seborrhea.*

EDC   Estimated date of confinement. See *due date.*

edema   The swelling of soft tissues as a result of excess water accumulation. Edema is often most prominent in the lower legs and feet toward the end of the day because fluid pools while people maintain an upright position.

edema, hereditary angioneurotic   A genetic form of angioedema. Persons with hereditary angioneurotic edema are born lacking an inhibitor protein called C1 esterase inhibitor, which normally prevents activation of a cascade of proteins that leads to the occurrence of angioedema. Patients can develop recurrent attacks of swollen tissues, pain in the abdomen, and swelling of the voice box (larynx) that can compromise breathing. The diagnosis is suspected with a history of recurrent angioedema. It is confirmed when a physician finds abnormally low levels of C1 esterase inhibitor in the blood. Treatment options include antihistamines and male steroids (androgens), which can prevent recurrent attacks. Also known as hereditary angioedema.

edema, periorbital   Swelling around the eyes due to excess water accumulation.

Edwards syndrome   See *trisomy 18 syndrome.*

EEG   Electroencephalogram.

EFA   Essential fatty acid.

effacement   Thinning of the cervix, which occurs before and while the cervix dilates.

effect, founder   See *founder effect.*

efferent   Carrying away. For example, an artery is an efferent vessel that carries blood away from the heart, and an efferent nerve carries impulses away from the central nervous system. The opposite of efferent is afferent.

efferent nerve   A nerve that carries impulses away from the central nervous system.

efferent vessel   A vessel that carries blood away from the heart. Hence, an efferent vessel is an artery or an arteriole (a little artery).

effusion   Too much fluid, an outpouring of fluid. For example, a pleural effusion is an abnormal accumulation of fluid in the space between the lungs and the chest wall, while a knee effusion is an abnormal amount of fluid in the knee joint. A hemorrhagic effusion contains blood in the fluid.

effusion, pericardial   Too much fluid within the fibrous sac (pericardium) that surrounds the heart. The inner surface of the pericardium is lined by a layer of flat cells (mesothelial cells) that normally secrete a small amount of fluid, which acts as a lubricant to allow normal heart movement within the chest. A pericardial effusion involves the presence of an excessive amount of pericardial fluid, a pale yellow serous fluid, within the pericardium.

effusion, pleural   Excess fluid between the two membranes that envelop the lungs (the visceral and parietal pleurae) separating the lungs from the chest wall. A small quantity (about 3 to 4 teaspoons) of fluid is normally spread thinly over the visceral and parietal pleurae and acts as a lubricant between the two membranes. Any significant increase in the quantity of pleural fluid is a pleural effusion. The most common symptoms of pleural effusion are chest pain and painful breathing (pleurisy). Many pleural effusions cause no symptoms but are discovered during physical examination or seen on chest X-rays; X-ray is the most convenient way to confirm the diagnosis. Many conditions are capable of causing pleural effusion including heart failure and uremia (kidney failure), hypoalbuminemia (low levels of albumin in the blood), infections (such as TB and bacterial, fungal, and viral infections), pulmonary embolism, and malignancies (metastatic tumors, as in Hodgkin's disease and mesothelioma). Despite extensive evaluation, the causation of pleural effusion is not established in about 20 percent of cases.

EGD Esophagogastroduodenoscopy. See *endoscopy, upper.*

egg See *ovum.*

EGG See *electrogastrogram.*

egg sac See *ovary.*

Ehlers-Danlos syndrome A heritable disorder of connective tissue that is characterized by easy bruising, joint hypermobility (loose joints), skin laxity, and weakness of tissues. Abbreviated EDS. There are at least nine different types of EDS, each of which has these characteristic features. The variations of EDS are treated according to their particular manifestations. Skin protection (against injury of trauma, sun, and so on) is critical. Wounds must be tended to with great care, and infections must be treated and prevented. Suturing can be difficult because the skin can be extremely fragile. Joint injury must be avoided, and bracing may sometimes be necessary to maintain joint stability. Exercises that strengthen the muscles that support the joints can help to minimize joint injury. Contact sports and activities involving joint impact should be avoided.

Ehlers-Danlos syndrome, Tenascin-X Deficient Type A type of Ehlers-Danlos syndrome (EDS) that is characterized by joint hypermobility, hyperelastic skin, and fragile tissue. Patients with this type of EDS lack the multiple shrinking (atrophied) scars in the skin that are often seen in classic EDS. This type of EDS is inherited as an autosomal recessive trait and is due to mutation of the tenascin-X gene on chromosome 6p21.

Ehlers-Danlos syndrome, Type I The gravis form of Ehlers-Danlos syndrome (EDS), which is characterized by marked joint hypermobility, skin hyperextensibility (laxity) and fragility, joint dislocation, and scoliosis (curvature of the spine). It is inherited as an autosomal dominant trait. Cases of this disease are now known to be due to mutations in collagen genes—specifically, in the collagen alpha-1(V) gene (COL5A1), the collagen alpha-2(V) gene (COL5A2), and the collagen alpha-1(I) gene (COL1A1).

Ehlers-Danlos syndrome, Type II The "mitis" form of Ehlers-Danlos syndrome (EDS), a form of EDS that is less severe than Type I EDS and is now considered part of Type I EDS.

Ehlers-Danlos syndrome, Type III The benign hypermobility form of Ehlers-Danlos syndrome (EDS), in which joint hypermobility is the major manifestation. It is inherited as an autosomal dominant trait. Type III EDS can be due to a defect in the gene for Type III collagen (COL3A1) or mutations in other genes.

Ehlers-Danlos syndrome, Type IV The arterial or vascular form of Ehlers-Danlos syndrome (EDS), which can cause spontaneous rupture of arteries and the bowel in serious cases. Skin laxity may or may not be present. Type IV EDS is inherited as an autosomal dominant trait. A defect in the gene for Type III collagen (COL3A1) is usually—perhaps always—the cause of Type IV EDS.

Ehlers-Danlos syndrome, Type V A type of Ehlers-Danlos syndrome (EDS) that is clinically similar to Type II EDS but is X-linked (the gene responsible for it is carried on the X chromosome). If a woman is carrying the gene for Type V EDS, she does not have the disease, but each of her children has a 50 percent chance of receiving the gene. A son with the gene would be affected with the disease, and a daughter with the gene would be a carrier with no symptoms, like her mother.

Ehlers-Danlos syndrome, Type VI The ocular-scoliotic form of Ehlers-Danlos syndrome (EDS), which is characterized by a fragile globe of the eyes, significant skin and joint laxity, and severe curvature of the spine (scoliosis). Type VI EDS is inherited as an autosomal recessive trait. Molecular defects have been identified in the gene for the enzyme lysyl hydroxylase (PLOD) in some patients with EDS Type VI. Also known as the kyphoscoliosis type of EDS.

Ehlers-Danlos syndrome, Type VII A type of Ehlers-Danlos syndrome (EDS) in which patients are short in height and severely affected by joint laxity and dislocations. Skin laxity may or may not be present. Type VII EDS is inherited as an autosomal dominant trait and can be diagnosed via skin biopsy. Mutation at one of at least two collagen genes, collagen alpha-1(I) gene (COL1A1) and collagen alpha-2(I) gene (COL1A2), can cause this disease. Also known as arthrochalasis multiplex congenita.

Ehlers-Danlos syndrome, Type VIIC The dermatosparaxis type of Ehlers-Danlos syndrome (EDS), which is characterized by severely fragile skin that is soft and doughy, with sagging and folding. Type VIIC EDS is inherited as an autosomal recessive trait and can be diagnosed via skin biopsy. Mutations in the gene ADAMTS2 have been identified as causes of Type VIIC EDS.

Ehlers-Danlos syndrome, Type VIII A type of Ehlers-Danlos syndrome (EDS) in which patients have different degrees of joint hypermobility, as well as inflammation of the gums and bone adjacent to the teeth (periodontitis). Type VIII EDS is inherited as an autosomal dominant trait.

ehrlichiosis An acute tick-borne disease first reported in humans in 1986. Erlichiosis is due to infection by the rickettsial agent Ehrlichia canis, which is usually carried by the brown dog tick. Erlichiosis is similar to Rocky Mountain spotted fever, characterized by high fever, headache, malaise, and muscle pain but no rash. See also *rickettsial disease.*

eight-day measles Rubeola (measles). See also *measles.*

ejaculation Ejection of sperm and seminal fluid during an orgasm in a male.

ejection fraction The percentage of blood that is pumped out of a filled ventricle as a result of a heartbeat. The heart does not eject all the blood in the ventricle. Only about two-thirds of the blood is normally pumped out with each beat, and that fraction is referred to the ejection fraction. The ejection fraction is an indicator of the heart's health. If the heart is diseased from a heart attack or another cardiac condition, the ejection fraction may fall, for example, to one-third.

EKG Electrocardiogram.

elbow The juncture of the long bones in the middle portion of the arm. The bone of the upper arm (humerus) meets both the ulna (the inner bone of the forearm) and radius (the outer bone of the forearm) to form a hinge joint at the elbow. The radius and ulna also meet one another in the elbow to permit a small amount of rotation of the forearm. The elbow therefore functions to move the arm like a hinge (forward and backward) and in rotation (outward and inward). The biceps muscle is the major muscle that flexes the elbow hinge, and the triceps muscle is the major muscle that extends it. The primary stability of the elbow is provided by the ulnar collateral ligament, located on the medial (inner) side of the elbow. The outer bony prominence of the elbow is the lateral epicondyle, a part of the humerus bone. Tendons attached to this area can be injured, causing inflammation or tendonitis (lateral epicondylitis, or tennis elbow). The inner portion of the elbow is a bony prominence called the medial epicondyle of the humerus. Additional tendons from muscles attach here and can be injured, likewise causing inflammation or tendonitis (medial epicondylitis, or golfer's elbow).

elbow, arthritis of the Inflammation (arthritis) of the elbow joint. Arthritis of the elbow can be due to many systemic forms of arthritis, including rheumatoid arthritis, gouty arthritis, psoriatic arthritis, ankylosing spondylitis, and Reiter disease. Generally, arthritis is associated with signs of inflammation of the elbow joint, including heat, warmth, swelling, pain, tenderness, and decreased range of motion. Range of motion of the elbow, impeded by the swollen joint, is decreased.

elbow bursitis A common, aseptic form of bursitis that is also known as olecranon bursitis. At the tip of the elbow (olecranon area) is the olecranon bursa, a fluid-filled sac that functions as a gliding surface to reduce friction during motion. Because of its location, the olecranon bursa is subject to trauma, ranging from simple repetitive weight-bearing while leaning to banging in a fall. Such trauma can cause elbow bursitis in the area overlying the point of the elbow. If elbow bursitis is not caused by infection, treatment includes rest and the use of ice and medications for inflammation and pain. Infectious bursitis is treated with antibiotics, aspiration, and surgery.

elbow, cellulitis of the Inflammation of the skin around the elbow, due to infection (cellulitis). Cellulitis of the elbow commonly occurs as a result of abrasions or puncture wounds that permit bacteria on the surface of the skin to invade the deeper layers of the skin. This causes inflamed skin characterized by heat, redness, and swelling. The most bacteria that most commonly cause cellulitis are staphylococcus (staph) and streptococcus (strep). Patients may have an associated low-grade fever. Cellulitis generally requires antibiotic treatment, either orally or intravenously. Heat application can help in the healing process.

elbow, golfer's Medial epicondylitis caused by injured tendons from the muscles that attach to the bony prominence in the inner portion of the elbow called the medial epicondyle.

elbow joint See *elbow.*

elbow pain Pain in the elbow, which can have many causes, including arthritis and bursitis. The elbow joint is quite complex because it is the area of union of three long bones (humerus, ulna, and radius). Tendonitis can affect the inner or outer elbow; treatment includes rest and the use of ice and medications for inflammation and pain. Bacteria can also infect the skin of a scraped (abraded) elbow. The "funny bone" nerve can be irritated at the elbow to cause numbness and tingling of the little and ring fingers.

elbow, tennis Lateral epicondylitis caused by injured tendons from the muscles that attach to the outer bone of the elbow (called the lateral epicondyle), which is a part of the humerus bone.

elbow, tip of the The bony tip of the elbow, which is formed by the near end of the ulna, one of the two long bones in the forearm (the other is the radius). See also *olecranon.*

elder abuse   The physical, sexual, or emotional abuse of an elderly person, usually one who is disabled or frail. Like child abuse, elder abuse is a crime that all health and social services professionals are mandated to report.

elective mutism   Complete lack of speech, believed to be chosen on the part of the patient. True elective mutism may be a reaction to a traumatic event, the aftermath of damage to or pain in the mouth or throat, or a symptom of extreme shyness. In other cases, the lack of speech is eventually found not to be chosen, but rather a symptom of damage or deformity of the speech apparatus or of autism. See also *selective mutism.*

electric shock   An extreme stimulation of the nerves, muscles, and other parts of the body that is caused by contact with electrical current. Electric shock can cause burning at the site of entry of the electricity, unconsciousness, and death. If a person may be in contact with high voltage, no one else should touch the person directly or go near the area. Using a dry, nonconductive object such as a wooden stick, the switch should be switched off, to break the contact between the electrical source and the patient. Immediate emergency medical help is required. While waiting for emergency treatment, the victim must be kept warm and CPR may be necessary.

electric shock therapy   See *electroconvulsive therapy.*

electrocardiogram   A recording of the electrical activity of the heart. Abbreviated ECG and EKG. An ECG is a simple, noninvasive procedure. Electrodes are placed on the skin of the chest and connected in a specific order to a machine that, when turned on, measures electrical activity all over the heart. Output usually appears on a long scroll of paper that displays a printed graph of activity. Sometimes data is output to a computer and screen, although a printout may still be made. The initial diagnosis of heart attack is usually made through observation of a combination of clinical symptoms and characteristic ECG changes. An ECG can detect areas of muscle deprived of oxygen (muscle ischemia) and/or dead tissue in the heart. If a medication is known to sometimes adversely affect heart function, a baseline ECG may be ordered before the patient starts taking the medicine, and follow-up testing may occur at regular intervals to look for any changes.

electroconvulsive therapy   The use of controlled, measured doses of electric shock to induce convulsions. Convulsions so induced can sometimes treat clinical depression that is unresponsive to medication. Abbreviated ECT.

electrodesiccation   Use of an electric current to destroy cancerous tissue and control bleeding.

electrodiathermy   See *cauterization.*

electroencephalogram   A technique for studying the electrical currents within the brain. Electrodes are attached to the scalp. Wires attach these electrodes to a machine, which records the electrical impulses. The results are either printed out or displayed on a computer screen. Different patterns of electrical impulses can denote various forms of epilepsy. Abbreviated EEG.

electrogastrogram   A test in which the electrical current generated by the muscle of the stomach is sensed and recorded in a manner very similar to that of an electrocardiogram of the heart. Abbreviated EGG. An EGG is performed by taping electrodes to the skin on the upper abdomen over the stomach. Recordings from the muscle are stored and analyzed by a computer. An EGG is performed to diagnose motility disorders of the stomach, conditions that prevent the muscles of the stomach from working normally.

electrolarynx   A battery-operated instrument that makes a humming sound to help people who have lost their larynx talk.

electrolysis   Permanent removal of body hair, including the hair root, with an electronic device. Although electrolysis is billed as a permanent process, many people find that hair does grow back (albeit slowly) after electrolysis. Electrolysis may be done by a dermatologist, by an electrolysis technician, or by a facial technologist or esthetician.

electrolyte   A substance that dissociates into ions in solution and acquires the capacity to conduct electricity. Sodium, potassium, chloride, calcium, and phosphate are examples of electrolytes. Electrolyte replacement is needed when a patient has prolonged vomiting or diarrhea, and as a response to strenuous athletic activity. Commercial electrolyte solutions are available, particularly for sick children (solutions such as Pedialyte) and athletes (sports drinks, such as Gatorade). Electrolyte monitoring is important in treatment of anorexia and bulimia. Informally known as lytes.

electron microscope   A microscope in which an electron beam replaces light to form the image. An electron microscope permits greater magnification and resolution than an optical microscope, but the electron densities of objects are shown rather than their actual images. Abbreviated EM.

electron microscopy   See *electron microscope.*

electrophoresis   A method used in clinical and research laboratories for separating molecules according to their size and electrical charge. Electrophoresis is used to separate large molecules (such as DNA fragments or proteins) from a mixture of molecules. An electric current is passed through a medium that contains the mixture of molecules. Each kind of molecule travels through the medium at a different rate, depending on its electrical charge and molecular size. Separation of the molecules occurs based on these differences. Although many substances, including starch gels and paper, have historically served as media for electrophoresis, agarose and acrylamide gels are now the most commonly used media for electrophoresis of proteins and nucleic acids.

electroretinography   A test in which the electrical potentials generated by the retina of the eye are measured when the retina is stimulated by light. Abbreviated ERG. In an ERG, an electrode is placed on the cornea at the front of the eye. The electrode measures the electrical response of the rods and cones, the visual cells in the retina at the back of the eye. An ERG may be useful in the evaluation of hereditary and acquired disorders of the retina. A normal ERG shows the appropriate responses with increased light intensity. Abnormal ERGs are found in conditions such as arteriosclerosis of the retina, detachment of the retina, and temporal arteritis with eye involvement. The instrument used to conduct ERG is an electroretinograph, and the resultant recording is called an electroretinogram.

electroshock therapy   See *electroconvulsive therapy.*

elephant nails   See *pachyonychia congenita.*

ELISA   Enzyme-linked immunosorbent assay, a rapid immunochemical test that involves an enzyme. It also involves an antibody or antigen (immunologic molecules). ELISA method is used for measuring a wide variety of tests of body fluids. ELISA tests detect substances that have antigenic properties, primarily proteins rather than small molecules and ions, such as glucose and potassium. Some of these substances include hormones, bacterial antigens, and antibodies. There are variations of this test, but the most basic involves an antibody attached to a solid surface, such as human chorionic gonadotropin (hCG), the commonly measured protein that indicates pregnancy. A mixture of purified hCG linked to an enzyme and the test sample (blood, urine, and so on) are added to the test system. If no hCG is present in the test sample, then only the hCG and the linked enzyme bind. The more hCG present in the test sample, the less enzyme-linked hCG binds. The substance the enzyme acts on is then added, and the amount of product is measured in some way, such as by a change in color of the solution. ELISA tests are generally highly sensitive and specific, and they compare favorably with radioimmune assay (RIA) tests. They have the added advantage of not requiring the use of radioisotopes or radiation-counting apparatus.

elliptocytosis   A blood disorder characterized by elliptically shaped red blood cells with variable breakup of red cells (hemolysis) and varying degrees of anemia. Inherited as a dominant trait, elliptocytosis is due to the mutation of one of the genes that encodes proteins of the red cell membrane skeleton. There are several forms of elliptocytosis. The gene for one form of elliptocytosis, EL1, is linked to the Rh locus on chromosome 1 and encodes the erythrocyte membrane protein 4.1. The gene for another form of elliptocytosis, EL2, is not linked to Rh and is due to mutations in the alpha-spectrin gene, the beta-spectrin gene, or the band 3 gene. The elliptocytosis/ Rh linkage was one of the first autosomal linkages discovered.

EM   **1** Electron microscope. **2** Electron microscopy.

embolism   The obstruction of a blood vessel by a foreign substance or a blood clot that blocks a vessel. An embolism results from something traveling through the bloodstream, lodging in a blood vessel, and plugging the vessel. Foreign substances that can cause embolisms include air bubbles, amniotic fluid, globules of fat, clumps of bacteria, chemicals (such as talc), and drugs (mainly illegal ones). Blood clots are the most common causes of embolisms. A pulmonary embolus is a blood clot that has been carried through the blood into the pulmonary artery (the main blood vessel from the heart to the lung) or one of its branches, plugging that vessel within the lung. The term *embolus* refers to the plug that obstructs the blood vessel.

embolism, crossed   See *embolism, paradoxical.*

embolism, paradoxical   Passage of a clot (thrombus) from a vein to an artery. When clots in veins break off (embolize), they travel first to the right side of the heart and, normally, then to the lungs, where they lodge. The lungs act as a filter to prevent the clots from entering arterial circulation. However, when there is a hole in the wall between the two upper chambers of the heart (atrial septal defect), a clot can cross from the right to the left side of the heart, and then pass into the arteries as a paradoxical embolism. When a clot enters arterial circulation, it can travel to the brain, block a vessel there, and cause a stroke (cerebrovascular accident). Because of the risk of stroke from paradoxical embolism, it is usually recommended that even small atrial septal defects be repaired. Also known as crossed embolism.

embolization   The clogging of small blood vessels with a substance that blocks the flow of blood. Embolization can occur as an abnormal natural event, such as when a blood clot travels from the leg to lodge in the blood vessels of the lungs, or it can be used as a treatment method, such as when material is purposely placed in blood vessels that supply a tumor in the hopes of destroying that tumor.

embolus A blockage or plug that obstructs a blood vessel. Examples of emboli are detached blood clots, clumps of bacteria, and clumps of other foreign material, such as air.

embryo An organism in the early stages of growth and differentiation, from fertilization to the beginning of the third month of pregnancy (in humans). After that point in time, an embryo is called a fetus.

embryonal rhabdomyosarcoma See *sarcoma botryoides.*

embryonic development See *prenatal development.*

embryonic hemoglobin See *hemoglobin E.*

emergency contraceptive See *contraceptive, emergency.*

emergency medical technician A person trained in the performance of the procedures required in emergency medical care. Abbreviated EMT. EMTs generally work with mobile emergency response teams, such as ambulance or fire and rescue teams. Some EMTs are employed in emergency rooms, and some are hired to be present at sporting events, camps, or other locations where emergency response might be needed.

emergency supplies kit See *disaster supplies.*

emesis Vomiting.

emetic Something that causes vomiting. A common emetic is syrup of ipecac.

emotional child abuse See *child abuse, emotional.*

emphysema **1** A lung condition characterized by an abnormal accumulation of air in the lung's many tiny air sacs (alveoli). As air continues to collect in these sacs, they become enlarged and may break or be damaged and form scar tissue. Emphysema is strongly associated with cigarette smoking, a practice that causes lung irritation. It can also be associated with or worsened by repeated infection of the lungs, such as that seen in chronic bronchitis. The best response to the early warning signs of emphysema is prevention: smoking cessation and immediate treatment for incipient lung infections. Curing established emphysema is not yet possible. Because emphysema patients do not have an adequate amount of space in the lungs to breathe, they gasp for breath and may not be able to obtain enough oxygen. Those with

severe emphysema usually end up using oxygen machines to breathe. In some cases, medication may be helpful to ease symptoms or to treat infection in already-damaged lungs. **2** The escape of air into other body tissues, such as between layers of skin. When this occurs during surgery, it is referred to as surgical emphysema.

empiric risk The chance that a disease will occur in a family, based on experience with the diagnosis, past history, and medical records rather than theory.

empirical Based on experience and observation rather than on systematic logic. Experienced physicians often use empirical reasoning to make diagnoses, based on having seen many cases over the years. Less-experienced physicians are more likely to use diagnostic guides and manuals. In practice, both approaches (if properly applied) usually lead to the same diagnosis.

empyema Pus in the pleural space between the outer surface of the lung and the chest wall. Empyema is typically a result of a serious bacterial infection. Empyema is a type of pleural effusion, one that is grossly infected. See also *effusion, pleural; pneumonia.*

EMT Emergency medical technician.

enanthem A rash inside the body. Koplik spots within the mouth in measles constitute enanthem. By contrast, a rash on the outside of the body is called exanthem. A patient with measles can have both exanthem and enanthem. See also *exanthem; measles; rash.*

encapsulated Confined to a specific area. For example, an encapsulated tumor remains in a compact form.

encephalitis Inflammation of the brain, which may be caused by a bacterium, a virus (such as one of the human herpes viruses or the viruses that cause mumps and measles), or an allergic reaction. Some forms of viral encephalitis are contagious. For example, encephalitis occurs in 1 in 1,000 cases of measles. It may start up to 3 weeks after onset of the measles rash, and it is characterized by high fever, convulsions, and coma. Encephalitis usually runs a short course, with full recovery within a week, but encephalitis can cause brain damage and death. The form of encephalitis called encephalitis lethargica ("sleeping sickness") results in a set of Parkinson's disease–like symptoms called postencephalitic Parkinson's disease. Treatment of encephalitis must begin as early as possible to avoid potentially serious and lifelong effects. Depending on the cause of the inflammation, treatment may include use of antibiotics, antiviral medications, and anti-inflammatory drugs. If brain damage results from encephalitis, therapy (such as physical therapy or cognitive restoration therapy) may help patients regain lost functions.

encephalitis, West Nile See *West Nile virus.*

encephalomyelitis Inflammation of both the brain and the spinal cord. Encephalomyelitis can be caused by a variety of conditions, including viruses that infect the nervous system. One type of encephalomyelitis, acute disseminated encephalomyelitis, occurs most commonly after an acute viral infection, such as measles (rubeola). It is due to an autoimmune attack on the nervous system, meaning that the immune system mistakenly attacks body tissue that it believes to be the measles virus. Also known as myeloencephalitis.

encephalopathic syndrome A dangerous condition that is associated with lithium toxicity.

encephalopathy, mitochondrial See *MELAS syndrome.*

enchondroma A common benign tumor of cartilage within bone. Enchondroma most often appears as a bony nodule in the hand or foot of a patient aged 10 to 30 years. Pain may be a sign of a fracture or malignant transformation. If fracture occurs, the enchondroma may be treated with removal and bone grafting. No treatment is needed if there are no symptoms. Enchondromas rarely become malignant as chondrosarcomas.

enchondromatosis See *Ollier disease.*

encopresis The inability to control the elimination of stool. Encopresis can have a variety of causes, including inability to control the anal sphincter muscle or gastrointestinal problems, particularly chronic diarrhea and Crohn's disease. Several neurological disorders, including Tourette syndrome and obsessive-compulsive disorder, are also occasionally associated with the symptom of encopresis, particularly in children. Preventive care for encopresis includes frequent scheduled toileting and the wearing of pads or diapers to prevent embarrassing soiling. Careful cleaning is important to prevent skin breakdown. Treatment of encopresis usually involves treatment of the underlying disorder; cognitive behavioral therapy or behavior modification is also sometimes helpful. Also known as fecal incontinence.

endemic Present in a community at all times, but occurring in low frequency. For example, malaria is endemic in some areas of the world. In comparison to endemic, epidemic denotes a sudden outbreak, and pandemic denotes an epidemic that spreads across a region. See also *epidemic; pandemic.*

endemic typhus See *typhus, murine.*

endocardium The lining of the interior surface of the heart chambers. The endocardium consists of a layer of endothelial cells and an underlying layer of connective tissue.

endocervical curettage The removal of tissue from the inside of the cervix, using a spoon-shaped instrument called a curette.

endocrinology The study of the medical aspects of hormones, including diseases and conditions associated with hormonal imbalance, damage to the glands that make hormones, or the use of synthetic or natural hormonal drugs. An endocrinologist is a physician who specializes in the management of hormone conditions.

endocrinopathy A disease of an endocrine gland. The term endocrinopathy is commonly used as a medical term for a hormone problem. Common endocrinopathies include hyperthyroidism and hypothyroidism.

endoderm The innermost of the three primary germ cell layers (the other two being the mesoderm and ectoderm) that make up the very early embryo. It differentiates to give rise first to the embryonic gut and then to the linings of the respiratory and digestive tracts and the liver and pancreas. Also referred to as entoderm. See also *differentiation; ectoderm; embryo; mesoderm.*

endogenous Originating from inside an organism. For example, endogenous cholesterol is cholesterol that is made inside the body, not derived from the diet. See also *exogenous.*

endometrial biopsy A common and medically valuable procedure for sampling the lining of the uterus (the endometrium). Endometrial biopsy is usually done to learn the cause of abnormal uterine bleeding, although it may be used to determine the cause of infertility, test for uterine infections, and monitor the response to certain medications. Endometrial biopsy can be performed in a physician's office. The main problems resulting from endometrial biopsy are cramping and pain. Oral pain medications taken beforehand may help reduce cramping and pain. Vaginal bleeding, infection, and, very rarely, perforation of the uterus can also occur.

endometrial hyperplasia A condition characterized by overgrowth of the lining of the uterus.

endometriosis A noncancerous condition in which tissue that looks like endometrial tissue grows in abnormal places, most often in the abdomen. Although most women with endometriosis have no symptoms, pelvic pain during menstruation or ovulation can be a symptom of endometriosis. Endometriosis can also be suspected by a physician during a physical examination and confirmed by surgery, usually laparoscopy. Treatment options include medication for pain, hormone therapy, and laparoscopic surgery to remove the growths (hysterectomy was once done but is usually ineffective). Most women with endometriosis are completely unaware of these growths, and are not harmed by their presence. However, endometriosis can increase the risk of ectopic pregnancy, a potentially life-threatening condition that can cause infertility. See also *adenomyosis.*

endometritis   Inflammation of the endometrium, the inner layer of the uterus.

endometrium   The inner layer of the uterus.

endonuclease   An enzyme that cleaves a nucleic acid (DNA or RNA) at specific sites in the nucleotide base sequence.

endorphin   A hormonal compound that is made by the body in response to pain or extreme physical exertion. Endorphins are similar in structure and effect to opiate drugs. They are responsible for the so-called runner's high, and release of these essential compounds permits humans to endure childbirth, accidents, and strenuous everyday activities.

endoscope   A lighted optical instrument that is used to get a deep look inside the body. An endoscope, which may be rigid or flexible, can be used to examine organs, such as the throat or esophagus. Specialized endoscopes are named for where they are intended to look. Examples include the cystoscope (bladder), nephroscope (kidney), bronchoscope (bronchi), laryngoscope (larynx), otoscope (ear), arthroscope (joint), laparoscope (abdomen), and gastrointestinal endoscopes.

endoscopic gastrostomy, percutaneous   See *gastrostomy, percutaneous endoscopic.*

Endoscopic Retrograde Cholangio-Pancreatography   See *ERCP.*

endoscopy   Examination of the inside of the body by using a lighted, flexible instrument called an endoscope. In general, an endoscope is introduced into the body through a natural opening such as the mouth or anus. Although endoscopy can include examination of other organs, the most common endoscopic procedures evaluate the esophagus, stomach, and portions of the intestine.

endoscopy, upper   A procedure that enables the examiner (usually a gastroenterologist) to examine the esophagus, the stomach, and the first portion of small bowel (duodenum) by using a thin, flexible tube that can be looked through or seen through on a TV monitor. Also known as esophagogastroduodenoscopy (EGD).

endostatin   A fragment of a protein, collagen 18, that is found in all blood vessels. Endostatin is normally secreted by blood vessels in response to tumors. Endostatin appears to halt the process of developing new blood vessels (angiogenesis), which is necessary to tumor development.

endothelial   Relating to the endothelium.

endothelium   The layer of cells that lines the closed internal spaces of the body, such as inside blood vessels, lymphatic vessels, the heart, and body cavities. By contrast, the epithelium is the outside layer of cells that covers all the free, open surfaces of the body, including the skin and mucous membranes, that communicate with the outside of the body. See also *epithelium.*

endotracheal tube   A flexible plastic tube that is put in the mouth and then down into the trachea (airway). A physician inserts an endotracheal tube under direct vision, with the help of a laryngoscope, in a procedure called endotracheal intubation. The purpose of using an endotracheal tube is to ventilate the lungs.

endourologist   A urologist with special expertise in navigating inside the kidneys, ureter, and bladder, using endoscopic optical instruments and other tools. Endourologists are specialists in diagnosing and treating diseases of these organs.

engagement   The sensation that a pregnant woman feels when the presenting (lowermost) part of the fetus descends and is engaged in the mother's pelvis, an event that classically occurs 2 to 3 weeks before labor begins. Women who have had two or more prior viable pregnancies (multiparas) may not experience engagement until labor actually begins. When engagement occurs, there is a visible change in the shape of the woman's stomach because the baby drops lower in the abdomen. Engagement is also known as lightening because the pregnant woman feels lighter after this event. Most women feel more comfortable after engagement, but some may experience lower back pain as the fetus presses close to the tailbone and the sciatic nerve. Others may find movement more difficult due to the lower center of gravity caused by engagement.

ENGERIX-B   A vaccine against the hepatitis B virus. ENGERIX-B stimulates the body's immune system to produce antibodies against the virus.

engram   An enduring change in the brain that is postulated to account for the persistence of memory.

enophthalmos   Sunken eyeball. Enophthalmos can be a sign of severe dehydration.

enoxaparin   A low-molecular-weight version of heparin that acts like heparin as an anticoagulant medication. Enoxaparin is used to prevent thromboembolic complications (blood clots that travel from their site of origin through the bloodstream to clog another vessel) and in the early treatment of blood clots in the lungs (pulmonary embolisms).

ENT   Ears, nose, and throat. An ENT physician is a specialist in the diagnosis and treatment of disorders of the head and neck, particularly those of the ears, nose, and throat. ENT physicians are also known as otolaryngologists.

Entamoeba histolytica   The agent that causes amebic dysentery. Entamoeba histolytica is a single-celled parasite that is transmitted to humans via contaminated water and food. It can also infect the liver and other organs. See also *amebiasis; amebic colitis; amebic dysentery.*

enteric   Of or relating to the small intestine.

enteric-coated medication   A medication that is coated with a material that permits transit through the stomach to the small intestine before the medication is released. Aspirin, which commonly causes stomach irritation and upset, is among the medications that may have enteric coating.

enteritis, Crohn's   See *Crohn's enteritis.*

enteritis, regional   See *Crohn's disease.*

entero-   Prefix referring to the intestine, as in enteropathy (a disease of the intestine) and enterospasm (a painful, intense contraction of the intestine).

enterobiasis   See *pinworm infestation.*

enterocentesis   The use of a hollow needle inserted through the wall of the stomach or intestine to relieve pressure from gas or fluid buildup.

enterococcus   Bacteria normally found in the feces. Two types, Enterococcus fecalis and Enterococcus fecium, cause human disease, most commonly in the form of urinary tract and wound infections. Other infections, including those of the blood stream (bacteremia), heart valves (endocarditis), and the brain (meningitis) can occur in severely ill patients in hospitals. Enterococci also often colonize open wounds and skin ulcers, and are among the most common antibiotic-resistant bacteria.

enterocolitis, Crohn's   See *Crohn's enterocolitis.*

enterogenous   Carried within the intestine. For example, an enterogenous bacterial infection is a bacterial infection within the intestine.

enteropathy   A disease of the intestine.

enteropathy, gluten   See *celiac sprue.*

enteropathy, protein-losing   A condition in which an excessive amount of plasma protein is lost into the intestine. Protein-losing enteropathy can be due to diverse causes, including celiac sprue, extensive ulceration of the intestine, intestinal lymphatic blockage, and infiltration of leukemic cells into the intestinal wall.

enterospasm   A painful, intense contraction of the intestine.

enterostomal therapist   A health care specialist who is trained to help patients care for and adjust to their colostomies.

enterostomy   An operation that opens the small intestine and brings it through the abdominal wall to create a new opening (stoma) to permit intestinal draining. See also *colostomy; ostomy.*

enterovirus   A virus that comes into the body through the gastrointestinal tract and thrives there, often moving on to attack the nervous system. Enteroviruses include the polioviruses, rhinoviruses, and echoviruses. See also *polio.*

Entoderm   See *endoderm.*

enuresis   Involuntary urination, which may be caused by a variety of factors, including disorders of the kidneys, bladder, or ureter, and poor control of the muscles that control release of urine. Enuresis is also occasionally associated with neurological disorders, such as Tourette syndrome, particularly in children. Nighttime (nocturnal) enuresis may be related to any of the above, or it may be a symptom of a sleep disorder. Palliative treatment options include ensuring regularly scheduled toileting, increasing awareness of the need to urinate, performing exercises intended to strengthen the muscles that control release of urine, using pads or diapers to prevent embarrassing and uncomfortable wetness, and in some cases using special devices that alert the patient to the initial signs of wetness. Treatment of enuresis usually involves treatment of the underlying disorder. Cognitive behavioral therapy or behavior modification techniques sometimes also proves helpful. Also known as urinary incontinence. See also *bedwetting; Kegel exercises.*

environmental tobacco smoke   See *secondhand smoke.*

enzyme   A protein or protein-based molecule that speeds up a chemical reaction in a living organism. An enzyme acts as a catalyst for specific chemical reactions, converting a specific set of reactants (substrates) into specific products. Without enzymes, life as we know it would not exist. Errors in the design of enzymes are responsible for numerous diseases. Also known as pancratic juice. See also *enzyme defect.*

enzyme defect   A disorder resulting from a deficiency (or functional abnormality) of an enzyme. For example, newborns are routinely screened for certain enzyme defects, such as phenylketonuria (PKU) and galactosemia.

enzyme-linked immunosorbent assay See *ELISA.*

eosinophil A normal type of white blood cell that has coarse granules within its cytoplasm. Eosinophils are produced in the bone marrow and migrate to tissues throughout the body. When a foreign substance enters the body, other types of white blood cells (lymphcytes and neutrophils) release substances to attract eosinophils and then release toxic substances to kill the invader. The numbers of eosinophils in blood often rise when an allergic reaction is in progress. Elevated eosinophil counts are also common in some diseases, such as parasite diseases and asthma.

eosinophilic fasciitis A disease that leads to inflammation and thickening of the skin and of the lining tissue under the skin that covers the surface of underlying tissues (fascia). In eosinophilic fasciitis, the involved fascia is inflamed with the eosinophil white blood cells. Progressive thickening occurs, and often redness, warmth, and hardness of the skin surface occur as well. Also known as Shulman syndrome.

eosinophilic granuloma A disease in which histiocytes multiply and attack the tissues, forming solitary or multiple eosinophilic granulomas. Eosinophilic granuloma predominantly affects children and young adults. It is the most common type of Langerhans cell histiocytosis. In patients with eosinophilic granuloma, granulomas may develop in bone, with overlying tender and sometimes warm areas of swelling with an inability to bear weight.

ependymoma A type of brain tumor that derives from the glial cells that line the cavities within the brain's ventricles. Because cerebrospinal fluid normally flows through these ventricles, blockage due to an ependymoma can cause buildup of fluid, pressure on the brain, and hydrocephalus.

ephedrine A vasoconstricting, bronchodilating drug that is used to treat asthma and also found in over-the-counter remedies for cold and flu symptoms and in some herbal remedies (in the form of the ephedrine-containing herbs ephedra or Ma Huang). Side effects of ephedrine can include jitteriness, racing heartbeat, nausea, sleeplessness, and headache. Ephedrine misuse or abuse can be dangerous and even life-threatening, especially for people with heart conditions.

epicanthal fold A fold of skin that comes down across the inner angle of the eye. Epicanthal folds appear most frequently in persons with Down syndrome and some other multiple congenital malformation syndromes (constellations of birth defects). To the untrained eye, an epicanthal fold may look similar to the eye fold found in peoples of Asian origin, but the normal Asian eye fold is actually quite distinct, whereas an epicanthal fold is continuous with the lower edge of the upper eyelid.

epicardium See *pericardium, visceral.*

epidemic The occurrence of more cases of a disease than would be expected to occur in a community or region during a given time period. A sudden outbreak (as, for example, of cholera). See also *endemic; pandemic.*

epidemic hemorrhagic fever See *hemorrhagic fever.*

epidemic myalgia See *Bornholm disease.*

epidemic typhus See *typhus, epidemic.*

epidemiologist A person engaged in epidemiology. Epidemiologists can be people with MD, PhD, DPH (Doctor of Public Health), MPH (Master of Public Health), RN, or other degrees.

epidemiology, classical The study of populations in order to determine the frequency and distribution of diseases, and then to measure the risks of those diseases.

epidemiology, clinical Epidemiology focused specifically on patients with diseases of clinical importance.

epidermis The upper, or outer, layer of the two main layers of cells in the skin (the other being the dermis). The epidermis is mostly made up of flat, scale-like cells called squamous cells. Under the squamous cells are round cells called basal cells. The deepest part of the epidermis also contains melanocytes, cells that produce the substance melanin, which gives skin its color. See also *dermis; skin.*

epidermoid carcinoma See *carcinoma, squamous cell.*

epididymis A structure within the scrotum that is attached to the back side of the testis. The epididymis is a coiled segment of the spermatic ducts that stores spermatozoa while they mature and then transports the spermatozoa between the testis and the tube connecting the testes with the urethra (vas deferens).

epididymitis Inflammation of the epididymis. Epididymitis can be caused by sexually acquired bacteria, such as gonorrhea and chlamydia; or by bacteria that come from somewhere else, such as E. coli from the bowel. Sometimes no bacteria are found to be associated with inflammation of the epididymis. Bacterial epididymitis is treated with antibiotics. If gonorrhea or chlamydia is suspected, both ceftriaxone and doxycycline are often used. If bowel microbes are suspected, ofloxacin is used.

If no bacterial cause is detected, medications to reduce inflammation are sometimes helpful.

epidural anesthetic An anesthetic that is injected into the epidural space surrounding the fluid-filled sac (the dura) around the spine to partially numb the abdomen and legs. An epidural is used fairly commonly in childbirth, if anesthesia is requested, and during birth by caesarean section.

epidural hematoma See *hematoma, epidural.*

epigastrium The part of the abdominal wall that is above the umbilicus (belly button).

epiglottis The flap that covers the trachea during swallowing, so that food does not enter the lungs.

epilation Removal of body hair, including the hair root, by means of electrical device, tweezers, or wax. Epilation may be performed by a dermatologist but is more commonly done for cosmetic purposes by a facial technologist or esthetician. After epilation, the skin may be particularly sensitive. Also known as depilation.

epilepsy A seizure disorder. When nerve cells in the brain fire electrical impulses at a rate up to four times higher than normal, a sort of electrical storm, called a seizure, occurs in the brain. Epilepsy is characterized by a pattern of repeated seizures. Known causes of epilepsy include head injuries, brain tumors, lead poisoning, maldevelopment of the brain, and genetic and infectious illnesses. However, in half of cases, no cause can be found. Medication can control seizures for the majority of patients. In cases of epilepsy that cannot be managed with drugs, a ketogenic diet or brain surgery may be considered. See also *Aicardis syndrome; Landau-Kleffner syndrome; Lennox-Gastaut syndrome; Otahara syndrome; Ramsey Hunt syndrome; Rasmussen syndrome; Rett syndrome; seizure; seizure disorder; seizure, tonic-clonic; Sturge-Weber syndrome; Tassinari syndrome.*

epilepsy, akinetic A seizure disorder that is characterized by drop seizures, in which the patient experiences a temporary loss of consciousness and lack of movement (akinesia).

epilepsy, benign rolandic The most common type of partial seizure disorder, which is usually characterized by partial seizures during sleep. The only outward sign of benign rolandic epilepsy may be movements of the face and mouth or staring spells. Benign rolandic epilepsy begins between the ages of 2 and 13 years, and it is called benign because it remits on its own by adulthood. Diagnosis is made through observation and via sleep-deprived or 24-hour EEG. On an EEG, benign rolandic epilepsy shows blunted, high-voltage central temporal ("rolandic") spiking, followed by slow waves. The spikes tend to spread or shift from side to side. Most children diagnosed with benign rolandic epilepsy are not treated with antiseizure medications. However, 30 percent need medication due to repeated and more difficult-to-handle episodes. Also known as benign rolandic epilepsy of childhood (BREC) and benign partial epilepsy with centrotemporal spikes. See also *seizure, partial.*

epilepsy, grand mal Epilepsy that includes tonic-clonic (grand mal) seizures, which are the most obvious type of seizure. There are two parts to a tonic-clonic seizure. In the tonic phase, the body becomes rigid, and in the clonic phase, there is uncontrolled jerking. A tonic-clonic seizure may or may not be preceded by an aura, and these seizures are often followed by headache, confusion, and sleep. They may last for mere seconds or continue for several minutes. If a tonic-clonic seizure does not resolve or if such seizures follow each other in rapid succession, emergency help is needed because the patient could be in a life-threatening state known as status epilepticus. Treatment is with antiseizure medications.

epilepsy, Jacksonian A seizure disorder that is characterized by progressive spreading of abnormal sensations or movements from one local area of the body to more widespread areas. Jacksonian epilepsy is caused by the progressive spread of abnormal electrical activity in the motor cortex of the brain. Seizures of this type typically cause no change in awareness or alertness. They are transient, fleeting, and ephemeral. Jacksonian seizures are extremely varied and may involve, for example, apparently purposeful movements such as turning of the head, eye movements, smacking of the lips, mouth movements, drooling, rhythmic muscle contractions in a part of the body, abnormal numbness, tingling, and a crawling sensation over the skin. Diagnosis is made through observation and EEG. Treatment, if necessary, is with antiseizure medications. Also called Jacksonian seizure disorder. See also *seizure, partial.*

epilepsy, juvenile myoclonic A form of epilepsy that occurs in people between the ages of 8 and 26 years, most commonly in the teenage years. It is characterized by jerking (myoclonic) movements of the arms and upper torso, without loss of consciousness. Seizures are most likely to occur when a person is awakening from sleep. Many children with this disorder are sensitive to light (photosensitive) and may have myoclonic jerks or seizures when exposed to bright light. Diagnosis is made through observation and EEG. During a myoclonic seizure, polyspike-wave discharges occur over a normal EEG background. Juvenile myoclonic epilepsy appears to be an inheritable genetic disorder, with the gene located on chromosome 6. Treatment is with antiseizure medications.

epilepsy, Landau-Kleffner See *Landau-Kleffner syndrome.*

epilepsy, partial Epilepsy characterized by seizures that affects only one part of the brain. Symptoms depend on which part of the brain is affected. One part of the body, or multiple parts on one side of the body, may start to twitch uncontrollably. Partial seizures may involve head turning, eye movements, lip smacking, mouth movements, drooling, rhythmic muscle contractions in a part of the body, apparently purposeful movements, abnormal numbness, tingling, and a crawling sensation over the skin. Partial seizures can also include sensory disturbances, such as smelling or hearing things that are not there, or having a sudden flood of emotions. Although the patient may feel confused, consciousness is not lost. Also known as focal seizures and local seizures. See also *seizure; seizure disorder; seizure, partial.*

epilepsy, petit mal A form of epilepsy in which only absence (petit mal) seizures occur, with very brief, unannounced lapses in consciousness. See also *seizure, absence.*

epilepsy, temporal lobe Epilepsy that is characterized by abnormal electrical activity in the temporal lobe of the brain. This activity does not cause grand mal seizures; rather, it causes unusual behaviors and patterns of cognition. Temporal lobe epilepsy may, for example, cause sudden outbursts of unexpected aggression or agitation, or it may be characterized by aura-like phenomena. Temporal lobe epilepsy is difficult to diagnose because temporal lobe seizures may not show up on an EEG. Diagnosis may instead be made through observation of symptoms or the use of brain imaging technology. Temporal lobe epilepsy can often be treated with the same antiseizure medications that are used for other forms of epilepsy. See also *seizure; seizure disorders; temporal lobe.*

epileptic aura See *aura.*

epilepticus, status See *status epilepticus.*

epinephrine The official name for adrenaline in the British Pharmacopoeia. See also *adrenaline.*

epiphyseal plate fracture See *fracture, Salter-Harris.*

epiphysis The growth area near the end of a bone.

episcleritis Inflammation of the episclera, a thin membrane that covers the white of the eye (sclera). Episcleritis is typically benign, easily treated with topical anti-inflammatory drops, and usually quickly resolved. Episcleritis can sometimes accompany other diseases, such as rheumatoid arthritis and lupus.

episiotomy A surgical procedure for widening the outlet of the birth canal to facilitate delivery of the baby and to avoid a jagged rip of the area between the anus and the vulva (perineum). During an episiotomy, an incision is made between the vagina and the rectum. The usual cut goes straight down and does not involve the muscles around the rectum or the rectum itself. An episiotomy can decrease the amount of maternal pushing, and it may also decrease trauma to the vaginal tissues and expedite delivery of the baby when quick delivery is necessary. However, episiotomies are associated with increased incidence of extensions or tears into the muscle of the rectum or even the rectum itself. This damage is difficult to repair and painful for the mother. In fact, current obstetric opinion holds that jagged tears of the perineum that occur naturally are less likely to affect muscle and more likely to heal quickly and cleanly than surgical episiotomies. Episiotomies and natural tearing can often be avoided with the use of perineal massage during delivery. Repair of the episiotomy is by simple stitching. The typical healing time for an episiotomy is about 4 to 6 weeks, depending on the size of the incision and the type of suture material used to close the episiotomy.

epispadias A congenital malformation in which the opening of the urethra is on the top side of the penis. Hypospadias is a corresponding malformation in which the opening of the urethra is on the underside of the penis. Surgical repair is usually recommended for epispadias. See also *hypospadias.*

epistaxis See *nosebleed.*

epistaxis, treatment of See *nosebleed, treatment of.*

epithelial Relating to the epithelium.

epithelial basement corneal dystrophy See *Cogan corneal dystrophy.*

epithelial carcinoma Cancer that begins in the cells that line an organ (the epithelium). For example, epithelial carcinoma of the skin is a cancer of the skin, while epithelial carcinoma of the tongue is cancer of the cells that line the surface of the tongue.

epithelium The outside layer of cells that covers all free, open surfaces of the body, including the skin and the mucous membranes that communicate with the outside of the body. By contrast, the endothelium is the layer of cells lining the closed internal spaces of the body, such as the blood vessels and lymphatic vessels. See also *endothelium.*

EPO 1 Erythropoietin. 2 Evening primrose oil.

EPO test A test of the hormone erythropoietin (EPO) in blood. The EPO level can indicate bone marrow disorders, kidney disease, or EPO abuse. Testing EPO blood levels is of value because too little EPO might be responsible for too few red blood cells (such as in evaluating anemia); too much EPO can cause too many red blood cells (polycythemia), might be evidence of a kidney tumor, and in an athlete might suggest EPO abuse. The patient is usually asked to fast for 8 to 10 hours (overnight) before taking an EPO test and may be asked to lie quietly and relax for 20 or 30 minutes before the test. The test requires a routine sample of blood. Normal levels of EPO are 0 to 19 (some say up to 24) milliunits per milliliter (mU/ml). See also *erythropoietin*.

eponym Something named after someone. For example, a condition called Shiel syndrome might be named after (an eponym for) someone named Shiel who discovered it or who was the first to describe and clearly delineate it.

Epstein-Barr virus A double-stranded DNA virus in the herpes family that is best known as the cause of infectious mononucleosis (also called mono and glandular fever). Abbreviated EBV. EBV infection is characterized by fatigue and general malaise. It was at one time believed to be the cause of chronic fatigue syndrome, but chronic infection with this virus is actually a separate (although similar) disorder. Infection with EBV is fairly common and is normally transient and minor. However, in some individuals EBV can trigger chronic illness, including immune and lymphoproliferative syndromes. It is a particular danger to people with compromised immune systems, including those with AIDS. Treatment is with antiviral medication and rest. Also known as human herpesvirus 4 (HHV-4).

ERCP Endoscopic retrograde cholangio-pancreatography, a diagnostic procedure used to examine diseases of the liver, bile ducts, and pancreas. ERCP is usually performed under intravenous sedation rather than general anesthesia, and it has a low incidence of complications. ERCP provides important information that cannot be obtained by other means. Therapeutic measures can often be taken at the time of ERCP to remove stones in the bile ducts or to relieve obstructions of the bile ducts.

erectile dysfunction A consistent inability to sustain an erection sufficient for sexual intercourse. Commonly known as impotence. Medically, the term erectile dysfunction is used to properly to differentiate this form of impotence from other problems that interfere with sexual intercourse, such as disease, injury, drug side effects, or a disorder that impairs the nerve supply or the blood flow to the penis. Other forms of impotence include lack of sexual desire and problems with ejaculation and orgasm. Erectile dysfunction is treatable in all age groups, and treatment includes using medication (notably Viagra) and penile implants.

erection, penile The state of the penis when it is filled with blood and becomes rigid. The penis contains two chambers called the corpora cavernosa, which run the length of the organ, are filled with spongy tissue, and are surrounded by a membrane called the tunica albuginea. The spongy tissue contains smooth muscles, fibrous tissues, spaces, veins, and arteries. The urethra, which is the channel for urine and ejaculate, runs along the underside of the corpora cavernosa. Erection begins with sensory and mental stimulation. Impulses from the brain and local nerves cause the muscles of the corpora cavernosa to relax, allowing blood to flow in and fill the open spaces. The blood creates pressure in the corpora cavernosa, making the penis expand. The tunica albuginea helps to trap the blood in the corpora cavernosa, thereby sustaining erection. Erection is reversed when muscles in the penis contract, stopping the inflow of blood and opening outflow channels.

ERG 1 Electroretinography. 2 Electroretinograph, the instrument used to perform electroretinography. 3 An electroretinogram, the recording produced by an electroretinograph.

ergonomics The science of making things fit people, instead of asking people to fit things. Ergonomics uses knowledge from the fields of anatomy, mechanics, physiology, and psychology to utilize human energy most effectively. Something that is ergonomic is designed for safe, comfortable, and efficient use. For example, a computer keyboard with an ergonomic design is intended to help the user avoid carpal tunnel syndrome and wrist pain.

ergot A fungus (Claviceps purpurea) that contaminates rye and wheat and that produces substances (alkaloids) called ergotamines. Ergotamines constrict blood vessels and cause the muscle of the uterus to contract. They have been much used—and are very useful—for the treatment of migraines. They have also been used and misused as abortifacients. In excess, ergotamines can cause symptoms such as hallucinations, severe gastrointestinal upset, a type of dry gangrene, and a painful burning sensation in the limbs and extremities. Chronic ergot poisoning (ergotism) was rife during the Middle Ages due to the consumption of contaminated rye. Because of the burning pain, it was known as ignis sacer (holy fire) and ignis infernalis (hell's fire), and was one of the causes of St. Anthony's fire. A form of ergot was also the original basis for the illicit drug lysergic acid diethylamide (LSD).

erotomania The false yet persistent belief that one is loved by a person (often a famous or prominent person), or the pathologically obsessive pursuit of a disinterested object of love. Erotomania can be a symptom of schizophrenia or other psychiatric disorders that are characterized by delusional symptoms.

error, alpha See *alpha error.*

error, beta See *beta error.*

error, type I See *alpha error.*

error, type II See *beta error.*

errors of metabolism, inborn See *metabolic disease.*

ERT Estrogen replacement therapy.

erythema Redness of the skin that results from capillary congestion. Erythema can occur with inflammation, as in sunburn and allergic reactions to drugs.

erythema chronicum migrans The classic initial rash of Lyme disease. In the early phase of erythema chronicum migrans, within hours to weeks of the tick bite, the local skin develops an expanding ring of unraised redness. There may be an outer ring of brighter redness and a central area of clearing. See also *Lyme disease.*

erythema infectiosum See *fifth disease.*

erythema nodosum An inflammatory reaction that occurs deep in the skin and is characterized by the presence of tender, red, raised lumps or nodules that range in size from 1 to 5 centimeters and are most commonly located over the shins but occasionally on the arms or other areas. The causes of erythema nodosum include medications (such as sulfa-related drugs, birth control pills, estrogens, iodides, and bromides), strep throat, cat scratch fever, fungal diseases, infectious mononucleosis, sarcoidosis, Behcet's syndrome, inflammatory bowel disease (Crohn's disease and ulcerative colitis), and normal pregnancy. In many cases, no cause can be determined. Erythema nodosum may be self-limited and go away on its own in 3 to 6 weeks. If treatment is needed, the underlying condition is treated, and treatment is simultaneously directed toward the erythema nodosum itself. Treatment can include anti-inflammatory drugs and cortisone given by mouth or injection. Colchicine is sometime used effectively to reduce inflammation.

erythroblastosis See *hemolytic disease of the newborn.*

erythrocyanosis Discoloration on the legs that has a bluish or purple hue.

erythrocyte See *red blood cell.*

erythrocyte membrane protein band 4.1 See *elliptocytosis.*

erythroleukemia A form of acute myeloid leukemia (AML) that involves the cells that give rise to the erythrocytes (red blood cells). In erythroleukemia, the body produces large numbers of abnormal, immature red blood cells.

erythromycin An antibiotic that is commonly prescribed to treat bacterial infection. Erythromycin prevents bacteria from producing proteins and interferes with bacterial growth and multiplication. See also *macrolide antibiotic.*

erythroplakia An abnormal reddened patch with a velvety surface that is found in the mouth. Erythroplakia carries an increased risk for becoming a cancer in the oral cavity. Treatment methods include observation, topical ointments, and surgical techniques including laser surgery.

erythropoietin A hormone that is produced by the kidney and leads to the formation of red blood cells in the bone marrow. Abbreviated EPO. Human EPO is a glycoprotein (a protein with an attached sugar) that has a molecular weight of 34,000. The kidney cells that make EPO are specialized and are sensitive to low oxygen levels in the blood that comes into the kidney. These cells release EPO when the oxygen level is low in the kidney. EPO stimulates the bone marrow to produce more red blood cells, which in turn increases the oxygen-carrying capacity of the blood. EPO is produced not only in the kidney but also, to a lesser extent, in the liver. The amount of EPO in the blood can indicate bone marrow disorders or kidney disease. Normal levels of EPO are 0 to 19 milliunits per milliliter (mU/ml). Elevated levels can be seen in polycythemia rubra vera, a disorder characterized by an excess of red blood cells. Lower-than-normal values of EPO are seen in chronic renal failure. Using recombinant DNA technology, EPO has been synthetically produced for use in persons with anemia due to kidney failure, anemia secondary to AZT treatment of AIDS, and anemia associated with cancer. EPO has been much misused as a performance-enhancing drug in endurance athletes, reportedly including cyclists, long-distance runners, speed skaters, and cross-country skiers. When it is, EPO is thought to be especially dangerous, perhaps because dehydration can further increase the viscosity of the blood, increasing the risk for heart attacks and strokes. EPO has been banned by the Tour de France, the Olympic committee, and other sports organizations. See also *EPO test.*

eschar   **1** The scab that is formed when a wound or skin is sealed by the heat of cauterization or burning.   **2** The dark crusted ulcer (tache noire) at the site of the chigger (mite larva) bite in scrub typhus.

Escherichia coli   See *E. coli.*

esophageal   Related to the esophagus.

esophageal cancer   A malignant tumor of the esophagus. The risk of cancer of the esophagus is increased by long-term irritation of the esophagus, such as from smoking, heavy alcohol intake, and Barrett esophagitis. Very small tumors in the esophagus usually do not cause symptoms. As a tumor grows, the most common symptom is difficulty in swallowing. There may be a feeling of fullness, pressure, or burning as food goes down the esophagus. Problems with swallowing may come and go. At first, they may be noticed mainly when the person eats meat, bread, or coarse foods, such as raw vegetables. As the tumor grows larger and the pathway to the stomach becomes narrower, even liquids can be hard to swallow, and swallowing may be painful. Cancer of the esophagus can also cause indigestion, heartburn, vomiting, and frequent choking on food. Because of these problems, weight loss is common. Esophageal cancer can be diagnosed through a barium X-ray study of the esophagus and endoscopy and biopsy of the tumor. Treatment includes chemotherapy and sometimes surgery.

esophageal reflux   See *gastroesophageal reflux.*

esophageal speech   Speech produced with air that is trapped in the esophagus and forced out again.

esophageal stricture, acute   A narrowing or closure of the normal opening of the swallowing tube that leads to the stomach, usually caused by scarring from acid irritation. Acute, complete obstruction of the esophagus occurs when food (usually meat) is lodged in the esophageal stricture. Patients experience chest pain and are unable to swallow saliva. Attempts to relieve the obstruction by inducing vomiting at home are usually unsuccessful. Patients with complete esophageal obstruction can breathe and are not at risk of suffocation. Endoscopy is usually used to retrieve the obstruction and relieve the condition.

esophageal stricture, chronic   A long-standing narrowing or closure of the normal opening of the swallowing tube that leads to the stomach, usually caused by scarring from acid irritation. Chronic esophageal stricture is a common complication of chronic gastroesophageal reflux disease (GERD). Several procedures are available for stretching (dilating) the strictures without having to resort to surgery. One procedure involves placing a deflated balloon across the stricture at the time of endoscopy. The balloon is then inflated, thereby opening the narrowing caused by the stricture. Another method involves inserting tapered dilators of different sizes through the mouth and into the esophagus to dilate the stricture.

esophageal ulcer   A hole in the lining of the esophagus that is created by the corrosive acidic digestive juices secreted by the stomach cells. Ulcer formation is related to the presence of Helicobacter pylori (H. pylori) bacteria in the stomach, use of anti-inflammatory medications, and cigarette smoking. Ulcer pain may not correlate with the presence or severity of ulceration. Diagnosis is made through barium X-ray or endoscopy. Complications of ulcers include bleeding and perforation. Treatment includes using antibiotics to eradicate H. pylori, eliminating risk factors, and preventing complications.

esophagectomy   An operation to remove a portion of the esophagus.

esophagitis   Inflammation of the esophagus.

esophagogastric tamponade   See *balloon tamponade.*

esophagogastroduodenoscopy   See *endoscopy, upper.*

esophagoscopy   Examination of the esophagus by using a thin, lighted instrument.

esophagram   A series of X-rays of the esophagus. The X-ray pictures are taken after the patient drinks a barium solution that coats and outlines the walls of the esophagus. See also *barium swallow.*

esophagus   The tube that connects the throat with the stomach. The esophagus lies between the trachea (windpipe) and the spine. In an adult, the esophagus is about 25 centimeters (10 inches) long. When a person swallows, the muscular walls of the esophagus contract to push food down into the stomach. Glands in the lining of the esophagus produce mucus, which keeps the passageway moist and facilitates swallowing. Also known as gullet.

esotropia   A condition in which a person is cross-eyed or, in medical terms, has convergent or internal strabismus.

essential   In medicine, of unknown cause, as in essential hypertension (hypertension of unknown cause). Also known as idiopathic.

essential fatty acid   An unsaturated fatty acid that is essential to human health but cannot be manufactured in the body. Abbreviated EFA. There are three types of EFAs: arachnoidic acid, linoleic acid, and linolenic acid. When linoleic acid is obtained in the diet, it can be converted to both arachnoidic and linolenic acid. Linoleic acid is commonly found in cold-pressed oils, especially oils extracted from cold-water fish and certain seeds. Supplementation with EFAs appears to be useful as a treatment for certain neurological disorders. However, arachnoidic acid may lower the seizure threshold. For that reason, it is important to consult a knowledgeable physician before starting a program of EFA supplementation.

essential oil   An oil derived from a natural substance, usually either for its healing properties or as a perfume. Some pharmaceuticals, and many over-the-counter or "holistic" remedies, are based on or contain essential oils. For example, products containing camphor or eucalyptus essential oils can help relieve congestive coughs, and many essential oils are used in the practice of aromatherapy.

estimated date of confinement   See *due date*.

estrogen   A female steroid hormone that is produced by the ovaries and, in lesser amounts, by the adrenal cortex, placenta, and male testes. Estrogen helps control and guide sexual development, including the physical changes associated with puberty. It also influences the course of ovulation in the monthly menstrual cycle, lactation after pregnancy, aspects of mood, and the aging process. Production of estrogen changes naturally over the female lifespan, reaching adult levels with the onset of puberty (menarche) and decreasing in middle age until the onset of menopause. Estrogen deficiency can lead to lack of menstruation (amenorrhea), persistent difficulties associated with menopause (such as mood swings and vaginal dryness), and osteoporosis in older age. In cases of estrogen deficiency, natural and synthetic estrogen preparations may be prescribed, including estradiol (brand names: Climara, Estrace, Estroderm), estrafied estrogens (brand names: Estratab, Memest), estropipate (brand name: Ogen), and conjugated estrogens (brand name: Premarin). Estrogen is also a component of many oral contraceptives. An overabundance of estrogen in men causes development of female secondary sexual characteristics (feminization), such as enlargement of breast tissue.

estrogen-associated blood clots   See *estrogen-associated hypercoagulability*.

estrogen-associated hypercoagulability   Hypercoagulability (a supranormal tendency for blood to clot) occurs as an occasional but serious side effect of estrogen therapy. The blood clots in this situation are dose-related; that is, they occur more frequently with higher doses of estrogen. All estrogen therapy preparations carry this risk. Cigarette smokers on estrogen therapy are at a higher risk for blood clots than nonsmokers. Therefore, patients requiring estrogen therapy are strongly encouraged not to smoke.

estrogen, designer   See *designer estrogen*.

estrogen replacement therapy   The use of natural or synthetic estrogen to treat changes associated with menopause, such as hot flashes, disturbed sleep, and vaginal dryness, that are associated with decreased estrogen levels. Abbreviated ERT. ERT can also prevent osteoporosis, which can be a consequence of decreased estrogen levels. Vaginal ERT products help with vaginal dryness, more severe vaginal changes, and bladder effects. The use of unopposed ERT (that is, ERT alone) is associated with an increase in the risk of endometrial cancer (cancer of the lining of the uterus). However, taking the hormone progestogen along with estrogen reduces the risk of endometrial cancer substantially. See also *hormone replacement therapy*.

ESWL   Extracorporeal shock wave lithotripsy.

etiology   The study of causes, as in the causes of a disease. The form *aetiology* is generally used in the UK.

eugenics   A pseudoscience with the stated aim of improving the genetic constitution of the human species by selective breeding. Eugenics is from a Greek word meaning "normal genes." The use of Albert Einstein's sperm to conceive a child by artificial insemination would represent an attempt at positive eugenics. The Nazis notoriously engaged in negative eugenics by genocide. The practice of eugenics was once legally mandated in the US state of Indiana, resulting in the forcible sterilization, incarceration, and occasionally euthanasia of the mentally or physically handicapped, the mentally ill, and ethnic minorities (particularly people of mixed racial heritage), and the adopting out of their children to nondisabled Caucasian parents. Similar programs spread widely in the early part of the 20th century and they still exist in some parts of the world. It is important to note that no experiment in eugenics has ever been shown to result in measurable improvements in human health. In fact, in the best-known attempt at positive eugenics, the Nazi Lebensborn program, there was a higher-than-normal level of birth defects in resulting offspring.

eukaryote   An organism that consists of one or more cells with a nucleus and other well-developed compartments. Eukaryotes include all organisms except bacteria, viruses, and blue-green algae, which are prokaryotes, so people are eukaryotes. See also *prokaryote*.

euphenics   A discipline that aims to improve the outcome of a genetic disease by altering the environment. The term euphenics is from a Greek word meaning "normal appearing." For example, people with phenylketonuria (PKU) can avoid the expression of their disease by staying on a low-phenylalanine diet and avoiding major sources of phenylalanine such as diet softdrinks sweetened with aspartame.

euphoria Elevated mood. Euphoria is a desirable and natural occurrence when it results from happy or exciting events. An excessive degree of euphoria that is not linked to events is characteristic of hypomania and mania, which are abnormal mood states associated with bipolar disorders. See also *bipolar disorder.*

euploid The normal number of chromosomes for a species. In humans, the euploid number of chromosomes is 46; with the notable exception of the unfertilized egg and sperm, in which it is 23.

Eustachian tube The tube that runs from the middle ear to the pharynx. The function of the Eustachian tube is to protect, aerate, and drain the middle ear and mastoid. The Eustachian tube permits the gas pressure in the middle ear cavity to adjust to external air pressure. When you are descending in an airplane, the Eustachian tube opens when your ears "pop." It is harder to get air into the middle ear than get it out, which is why we have more trouble with our ears when a plane is descending than when it takes off. Occlusion of the Eustachian tube can lead to the development of middle ear infection (otitis media). The Eustachian tube opens into the nasopharynx. The Eustachian tube measures only 17 to 18 mm, and it is horizontal at birth. As it grows to double that length, it grows to be positioned at an incline of 45 degrees in adulthood. For this reason the nasopharyngeal opening in an adult is significantly below the tympanic opening, found in the middle ear near the eardrum. The shorter length and the horizontal orientation of the Eustachian tube in infancy protects the middle ear poorly, makes for poor drainage of fluid from the middle ear, and predisposes infants and young children to middle-ear infection. The greater length and particularly the slope of the tube as it grows serve more effectively to protect, aerate, and drain the middle ear. The Eustachian tube in the adult is opened by two muscles, the tensor palati and the levator palati, but the anatomy of children permits only the tensor palati to work. Also known as otopharyngeal tube because it connects the ear to the pharynx and auditory tube.

euthanasia The hastening of death for a terminally ill patient. Euthanasia is from the Greek for "dying well." See also *active euthanasia; assisted suicide; eugenics.*

euthyroid The state of having normal thyroid gland function. See also *hyperthyroid; hypothyroid.*

evacuation supplies kit See *disaster supplies.*

evening primrose oil A natural source of essential fatty acids (EFOs).

event, adverse In pharmacology, an unexpected or dangerous reaction to a drug.

evolution The continuing process of change.

evolution, biologic See *biologic evolution.*

evolution, cultural See *cultural evolution.*

evolutionarily conserved gene A gene that has remained essentially unchanged throughout evolution. Conservation of a gene indicates that it is unique and essential: There is not an extra copy of that gene with which evolution can tinker, and changes in the gene are likely to be lethal.

evolutionarily conserved sequence A base sequence in a DNA molecule (or an amino acid sequence in a protein) that has remained essentially unchanged throughout evolution.

Ewing sarcoma See *sarcoma, Ewing.*

exaggerated startle disease See *hyperexplexia.*

exam, pelvic See *pelvic exam.*

exam, rectal See *digital rectal exam.*

exanthem A rash on the outside of the body. By contrast, a rash on the inside of the body (for example, inside the mouth) is called enanthem. A patient with measles can have both exanthem and enanthem. See also *enanthem; measles; rash.*

exanthem subitum A sudden rash. See also *measles.*

excess iron An overload of iron that can damage the heart, liver, gonads, and other organs. See also *iron excess.*

exclamation point hair A short, broken-off hair that is found in an area of hair loss and is narrower closer to the scalp than at the other end (and therefore looks like an exclamation point). Exclamation point hair is a key diagnostic finding in a disorder called alopecia areata. See also *alopecia areata.*

exercise, aerobic See *aerobic exercise.*

exercise-induced asthma See *asthma, exercise-induced.*

exercise-induced bronchospasm See *asthma, exercise-induced.*

exercise treadmill A machine used to obtain a continuous electrocardiogram recording of the heart as a patient performs increasing levels of exercise. An exercise treadmill permits the detection of abnormal heart rhythms (arrhythmias) and provides a screening test for the presence of narrowed arteries to the heart (coronary arteries). Narrowing of these arteries can limit the supply of oxygenated blood to the heart muscle during exercise.

exfoliate **1** To peel off scaly skin spontaneously. The skin exfoliates from the palms and soles in Kawasaki disease and Reiter syndrome. **2** To deliberately wear away the top layer of skin, as may be done gently by a facial technologist who is applying a topical skin treatment for cosmetic purposes or more severely by a dermatologist treating acne. In the latter case, the most common exfoliating methods are sanding and chemical peels.

exogenous Originating from outside an organism. For example, insulin taken by a diabetic is exogenous insulin. See also *endogenous.*

exon A region of DNA in a gene that is transcribed (read) into mature messenger RNA. An exon is the protein-coding part of a gene. See also *intron.*

exonuclease An enzyme that cleaves nucleotide bases sequentially from the free ends of a nucleic acid (DNA or RNA).

exophthalmos A condition in which the patient has protruding eyeballs, as in hyperthyroidism and Graves disease.

exotropia Divergent gaze. Also known as external strabismus and, pejoratively, walleye.

exposure In cognitive behavioral therapy, the process of exposing oneself to an event or a place that causes anxiety or panic. The intention of controlled exposure is to gradually lower the level of stress and anxiety associated with the stimulus, to eventually prevent panic attacks, obsessive-compulsive behaviors, and other unwanted reactions. See also *cognitive behavior therapy.*

exposure and response prevention A cognitive behavior therapy technique that uses planned exposures and exercises to reduce unwanted responses. Abbreviated E&RP. See also *cognitive behavior therapy; exposure.*

expression, gene See *gene expression.*

expressivity The consistency of a genetic disease. For example, Marfan syndrome shows variable expressivity. Some persons with Marfan syndrome merely have long fingers and toes, and others have the full-blown disease, with dislocation of the lens and dissecting aneurysm of the aorta.

expulsion, stage of The second and final stage of labor, lasting from the full dilation of the cervix until the baby is completely out of the birth canal.

extension The process of straightening or the state of being straight. For example, extension of the hip and knee joints is necessary to stand up from a sitting position.

external ear See *ear, outer.*

external jugular vein The more superficial of the two jugular veins in the neck that drain blood from the head, brain, face, and neck and convey blood toward the heart. The external jugular vein collects most of the blood from the outside of the skull and the deep parts of the face. It lies outside the sternocleidomastoid muscle, passes down the neck, and joins the subclavian vein. See also *internal jugular vein.*

external radiation therapy See *radiation therapy, external.*

extracorporeal shock wave lithotripsy See *lithotripsy, extracorporeal shock wave.*

extrapyramidal side effects Physical symptoms, including tremor, slurred speech, akathesia, dystonia, anxiety, distress, paranoia, and bradyphrenia, that are primarily associated with improper dosing of or unusual reactions to neuroleptic (antipsychotic) medications.

extrapyramidal system The part of the nervous system that regulates muscle reflexes.

extrauterine pregnancy See *ectopic pregnancy.*

extremity An uttermost part of the body, such as a hand or a foot.

eye The organ of sight. The eye has a number of components, including the cornea, iris, pupil, lens, retina, macula, optic nerve, and vitreous humor. The cornea is the clear front window of the eye that transmits and focuses light into the eye. The iris is the colored part of the eye, and it helps regulate the amount of light that enters the eye. The pupil is the dark aperture in the iris that determines how much light is let into the eye. The lens is the transparent structure inside the eye that focuses light rays onto the retina. The retina is the nerve layer that lines the back of the eye, senses light, and creates impulses that travel through the optic nerve to the brain. The macula is a small area in the retina that contains special light-sensitive cells and allows people to see fine details clearly. The optic nerve is the nerve that connects the eye to the brain. It carries the impulses formed by the retina to the visual cortex of the brain. The vitreous humor is a clear, jelly-like substance that fills the middle of the eye.

eye chart test   A test that measures how well you see at various distances. An eye chart is imprinted with block letters that line-by-line decrease in size, corresponding to the distance at which each line of letters is normally visible. See also *chart, Snellen.*

eyedrop test   A test that involves putting eyedrops into the eye. There are many types of eyedrops and many types of eyedrop tests. One of the most common eyedrop tests is pupil dilation. See also *dilation, pupil.*

eyelids, adult ptosis of the   Drooping of the upper eyelids in adults, most commonly due to separation of the tendon of the lid-lifting (levator) muscle from the eyelid. This may occur with age, after cataract or other eye surgery, or due to an injury, an eye tumor, or a complication of another disease that involves the levator muscle or its nerve supply, such as diabetes. If treatment is necessary, it is usually surgical. Sometimes a small tuck in the lifting muscle and eyelid can raise the lid sufficiently. More severe ptosis requires reattachment and strengthening of the levator muscle.

eyelids, congenital ptosis of the   Drooping of the upper eyelids at birth. The lids may droop only slightly, or they may cover the pupils and restrict or even block vision. Moderate or severe ptosis calls for surgical treatment to permit normal vision development. If moderate or severe ptosis is not corrected, amblyopia ("lazy eye") may develop, which can lead to permanently poor vision. Congenital ptosis is often caused by poor development of the levator muscle that lifts the eyelid. Children with ptosis may tip their heads back into a chin-up position to see underneath the eyelids or raise their eyebrows in an attempt to lift up the lids. Congenital ptosis rarely improves with time. Mild or moderate ptosis usually does not require surgery early in life. Treatment is usually surgery to tighten the levators. If the levator is very weak, the lid can be attached or suspended from under the eyebrow so that the forehead muscles can do the lifting. Even after surgery, focusing problems can develop as the eyes grow and change shape. All children with ptosis, whether they have had surgery or not, should therefore regularly visit ophthalmologists.

eyes, flashing lights in the   Spontaneous flashing-light sensations in the eyes that can be caused by a number of factors. A sensation of flashing lights can be caused when the vitreous humor (the clear, jelly-like substance that fills the middle of the eye) shrinks and tugs on the retina. These flashes of light can appear off and on for several weeks or months. With age, flashes become increasingly common. Flashes usually do not reflect a serious problem. However, if one notices the sudden appearance of light flashes or a sudden increase in flashing lights, one should see an ophthalmologist immediately to see whether the retina has been torn or whether there is another cause. Flashes of light that appear as jagged lines or "heat waves" in both eyes, often lasting 10 to 20 minutes, are different from these benign flashes. They are usually caused by migraine, a spasm of blood vessels in the brain. These jagged lines can also occur without a headache, in which case they are termed ophthalmic migraine or migraine without headache. Treatment may or may not be necessary depending on the cause.

eyes, spots in front of the   The spontaneous appearance of spots in the eyes. Also known as "floaters," spots are usually images formed by deposits of protein drifting about in the vitreous humor (the clear, jelly-like substance that fills the middle of the eye). The appearance of permanent or recurring white or black spots in the same area of the field of vision may be an early warning sign of cataracts or other serious problems.

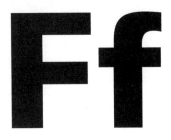

Ff

F **1** Chemical symbol for the element flourine. **2** Abbreviation for Fahrenheit. **3** The symbol for the coefficient of inbreeding. See also *coefficient of inbreeding.*

Fabry disease A genetic disease that causes a deficiency of the enzyme alpha-galactosidase A. This enzyme is essential to the metabolism of molecules known as glycosphingolipids. Without alpha-galactosidase A, glycosphingolipids accumulate in the kidneys, heart, nerves, and throughout the body, impairing function. Males with Fabry disease are more severely affected than females with it because the gene for Fabry disease is on the X chromosome. Males have only one X, whereas females have a second X and therefore some enzyme activity. Females with partial enzyme activity may not show any symptoms, or symptoms may not emerge until late in life. Diagnosis is made by determining the level of alpha-galactosidase A in blood plasma or through genetic testing to detect the abnormal gene. Symptoms may include blood vessel-filled skin lesions over the hips, buttocks, thighs, and lower belly with fever accompanying attacks of pain in the fingers and toes. The pain in the hands and feet usually responds to medications such as carbamazepine (brand name: Tegretol) and dilantin. Gastrointestinal hyperactivity may be treated with metoclopramide. Enzyme replacement therapy has been done in clinical trials. Gene therapy may make this a curable disease. Also known as Anderson-Fabry disease and angiokeratoma corporis diffusum universale.

face, masklike An expressionless face with little or no sense of animation; a face that is more like a mask than a normal face. Masklike face is seen in a number of disorders, including Parkinson's disease and myotonic dystrophy. Also known as masklike facies.

facelift A surgical procedure that is designed to make the face appear younger by pulling loose facial skin taut. Recovery time is usually 1 week, and the results last approximately 10 years. Additional procedures to supplement a facelift—including necklift, blepharoplasty (eyelid surgery), liposuction, autologous fat injection, removal of buccal (cheek) fat pads, forehead lift, and browlift; chemical or laser peel; and malar (cheek), submalar, or chin implants—may be necessary to achieve the desired results. Although they are infrequent, risks and complications of facelift surgery include bleeding; hematoma; bruising; infection; neurological dysfunction (loss of muscle function or sensation), which is usually temporary; widened or thickened scars; loss of hair around the incision site; asymmetry (unevenness between two sides); and skin necrosis (loss of skin due to tissue death).

facial canal introitus The entrance to the facial canal, a passage in the temporal bone of the skull through which the facial nerve (the seventh cranial nerve) travels. In anatomy, an introitus is an entrance that goes into a canal or hollow organ.

facial nerve The seventh cranial nerve, a nerve that has fibers both going out and coming in (both efferent and afferent fibers). The facial nerve supplies the muscles of facial expression. See also *facial nerve paralysis.*

facial nerve paralysis Loss of voluntary movement of the muscles of one side of the face due to abnormal function of the facial nerve. Paralysis of the facial nerve causes a characteristic drooping of one side of the face, inability to wrinkle the forehead, inability to whistle, inability to close an eye, and deviation of the mouth toward the other side of the face. Paralysis of the facial nerve is called Bell's palsy. The cause of facial-nerve paralysis is not known, but it is thought to be related to a virus (or to various viruses). The disease typically starts suddenly and causes paralysis of the muscles of the side of the face on which the facial nerve is affected. Treatment is directed toward protecting the eye on the affected side from dryness during sleep. Massage of affected muscles can reduce soreness. Sometimes corticosteroid medication is given to reduce inflammation during the first weeks of illness. The prognosis is generally good, with about 80 percent of patients recovering within weeks to months.

facies Face.

facio-genito-popliteal syndrome See *popliteal pterygium syndrome.*

factor VIII A coagulation (clotting) factor. Classic hemophilia (hemophilia A) is due to a deficiency in factor VIII activity. Also known as antihemophiliac factor (AHF) or antihemophiliac globulin (AHG). See also *hemophilia A.*

factor, rheumatoid An antibody that is measurable in the blood. Rheumatoid factor is commonly used as a blood test for the diagnosis of rheumatoid arthritis. Rheumatoid factor is present in about 80 percent of adults (and a much lower proportion of children) with rheumatoid arthritis. It is also present in patients with other connective tissue diseases, such as systemic lupus erythematosus, and in some with infectious diseases, including infectious hepatitis.

FAE Fetal alcohol effect.

Fahr syndrome A progressive brain disorder that is characterized clinically by involuntary movements, prolonged muscle contractions, and dementia. It is characterized by abnormal deposits of calcium in the basal ganglia of the brain. The gene that is responsible for Fahr syndrome has been mapped to chromosome 14. There is no cure for Fahr syndrome. Also called idiopathic basal ganglia calcification. Treatment is directed toward relieving symptoms.

failure, heart See *congestive heart failure*.

failure to thrive The inability of a child to physically grow as quickly and as much as his or her peers. Abbreviated FTT. There is no official consensus as to what constitutes FTT. It usually refers to a child whose growth is below the 3rd or 5th percentiles for his or her age or whose growth has fallen off precipitously and crossed two major growth quartiles (for example, from above the 75th percentile to below the 25th percentile). FTT in early infancy sometimes results in death, and in older infancy or childhood it is an important disease marker. FTT has many causes, including chronic kidney disease, unrecognized food allergies that lead to refusal of food and vomiting, undiagnosed metabolic disorders, and other diseases. A specific type of FTT is sometimes seen in abandoned or institutionalized infants who seem to become listless and unwilling to nurse. It is assumed that this phenomenon is emotional in nature, although other factors may also be at work. Treatment of FTT requires discovery and treatment of the underlying causes. In the interim, IV feeding is necessary in some cases, and in others, supplemental high-calorie feedings can help.

fainting See *syncope*.

falciparum malaria The most dangerous type of malaria.

FALDH deficiency See *Sjogren-Larsson syndrome*.

fallopian tube One of the two tubes that transport eggs from the ovary to the uterus. The Fallopian tubes have small hair-like projections called cilia on the cells of the lining. These tubal cilia are essential to the movement of the egg through the tube and into the uterus. If the tubal cilia are damaged by infection, an egg may not be pushed along normally but may stay in the tube. Infection can also cause partial or complete blockage of the tube with scar tissue, physically preventing eggs from getting to the uterus. Infection, endometriosis, tumors, scar tissue in the pelvis (pelvic adhesions), and any other process that damages a Fallopian tube or narrows its diameter increase the chance of an ectopic pregnancy.

false negative A result that appears negative when it should not. An example of a false negative would be if a particular test designed to detect cancer returns a negative result but the person actually does have cancer.

false positive A result that is erroneously positive when a situation is normal. An example of a false positive would be if a particular test designed to detect cancer returns a positive result but the person does not have cancer.

false rib One of the last five pairs of ribs. A rib is said to be false if it does not attach to the sternum (the breastbone). The upper three false ribs connect to the costal cartilages of the ribs just above them. The last two false ribs usually have no ventral attachment to anchor them in front and so are called floating, fluctuating, or vertebral ribs.

familial A condition that tends to occur more often in family members than is expected by chance alone. A familial disease may be genetic (such as cystic fibrosis) or environmental (such as tuberculosis).

familial adenomatous polyposis A genetic disease characterized by the presence of numerous precancerous polyps in the colon and rectum. The polyps usually begin to form at puberty, and colon cancer occurs 10 to 15 years later. Abbreviated FAP. FAP is inherited as an autosomal dominant trait. A person who has it has a 50 percent chance of passing the gene for the disease on to each of his or her children. Most people who receive the gene manifest the disease, although the expression of FAP can vary markedly from person to person. The gene that is mutated in FAP is the APC (adenomatous polyposis coli gene, which maps to chromosome 5 in region 5q21–5q22. The polyps can be prevented by regular ingestion of Cox-2 antiinflammatory drugs, such as celecoxib (brand name: Celebrex). Also known as familial polyposis.

familial breast cancer See *breast cancer, familial*.

familial cancer Cancer or a predisposition (tendency) to it that runs in families.

familial hypercholesterolemia The most common inherited type of hyperlipidemia (high lipid levels in the blood). Familial hypercholesterolemia is recognizable in childhood and is due to genetic defects in the receptor (target) for low-density lipoprotein (LDL). Familial hypercholesterolemia predisposes a person to premature arteriosclerosis, including coronary artery disease, and can lead to heart attacks at an unusually young age. Persons with familial hypercholesterolemia can reduce their risk of heart attack by adhering to a very low-cholesterol diet under a physician's supervision; they may also need to take cholesterol-lowering medications.

familial Mediterranean fever　A genetic disorder that is characterized by recurrent attacks of inflammation, with fever and pain in the abdomen, chest, and/or joints. Abbreviated FMF. FMF attacks last 2 to 3 days. The symptoms may differ from patient to patient, even in the same family. Protein deposits, called amyloid, can accumulate in tissues (amyloidosis). When this injures the kidneys it can lead to kidney failure. There is a form of FMF in which the first clinical sign is amyloidosis. Colchicine prevents the attacks of pain and the deposition of amyloid. FMF is inherited as an autosomal recessive trait. When both parents are carriers of a gene for FMF, each of their children is at 25 percent risk for developing the disease. Molecular testing for the MEFV gene (on chromosome 16) confirms the diagnosis. Molecular genetic testing can also detect carriers and the prenatal presence of FMF.

familial mental retardation 1　See *FMR1*.

familial neurovisceral lipidosis　See *GM1-gangliosidosis*.

familial polyposis　See *familial adenomatous polyposis*.

family planning　See *birth control*.

family tree　See *pedigree*.

Fanconi anemia　An inherited disease that adversely affects all the elements of bone marrow and is associated with malformations of the heart, kidney, and limbs, as well as pigmentary changes of the skin. Fanconi anemia predisposes a person to cancer, particularly to a disturbance of bone marrow growth called myelodysplasia and to acute myeloid leukemia. Patients also tend to develop cancers in areas of the body where cells normally reproduce rapidly, such as the mouth, the esophagus, the intestinal and urinary tracts, and the reproductive organs. Fanconi anemia is particularly common in Ashkenazi Jews. At least five different genes can cause the disease, which is inherited as an autosomal recessive trait.

FAO deficiency　See *Sjogren-Larsson syndrome*.

FAP　Familial adenomatous polyposis.

Farber lipogranulomatosis　A deadly genetic disease that is characterized by the onset, in the first few weeks of life, of swollen, painful joints; nodules under the skin; profound motor and developmental delay; cherry-red spots in the retina; and respiratory problems. Respiratory insufficiency usually causes death before age 2. The disease is inherited as an autosomal recessive trait and is due to a deficiency of the enzyme acid ceramidase. Farber lipogranulomatosis is one of the sphingolipidoses, a group of genetic diseases that involve overproduction or accumulation of fatty substances called sphingolipids in the brain and nervous system. See also *sphingolipidosis*.

farsightedness　An error of refraction in the human eye that causes light rays to focus behind the retina instead of on it. A person who is farsighted has normal vision at a distance but has trouble focusing on nearby objects. Farsightedness can be corrected with refractive lenses—either glasses or contact lenses—and in some cases by surgery. Also known as hyperopia.

fart　See *flatulence*.

FAS　Fetal alcohol syndrome.

fascia　A flat band of tissue below the skin that covers underlying tissues and separates different layers of tissue. Fascia also encloses muscles.

fasciitis　Inflammation of the fascia.

fasciitis, eosinophilic　See *eosinophilic fasciitis*.

fasciitis, plantar　Inflammation of the plantar fascia, the bowstring-like tissue that stretches from the heel underneath the sole. Plantar fasciitis is often due to calcaneal spurs, which typically cause localized tenderness and pain that is made worse by stepping down on the heel. Plantar fasciitis and calcaneal spurs may occur on their own or may be related to underlying diseases that cause arthritis, such as Reiter disease, ankylosing spondylitis, and diffuse idiopathic skeletal hyperostosis. Treatment is designed to decrease inflammation and avoid reinjury. Icing reduces pain and inflammation. Anti-inflammatory agents, such as ibuprofen and injections of cortisone, can help. Infrequently, surgery is done on chronically inflamed spurs. A donut-shaped shoe insert can take pressure off a calcaneal spur and lessen plantar fasciitis.

fasting blood glucose　A test to determine how much glucose (sugar) is in a blood sample after an overnight fast. The fasting blood glucose test is commonly used to detect diabetes mellitus. A blood sample is taken in a lab, physician's office, or hospital. The test is done in the morning, before the person has eaten. The normal range for blood glucose is 70 to 110 mg/dl, depending on the type of blood being tested. If the level is over 140 mg/dl, the person probably has diabetes, although newborns and some pregnant women may have higher glucose levels without having diabetes.

fasting blood sugar See *fasting blood glucose.*

fat 1 Along with proteins and carbohydrates, one of the three nutrients used as energy sources by the body. The energy produced by fats is 9 calories per gram. Proteins and carbohydrates each provide 4 calories per gram. 2 Total fat; the sum of saturated, monounsaturated, and polyunsaturated fats. Intake of monounsaturated and polyunsaturated fats can help reduce blood cholesterol when substituted for saturated fats in the diet. 3 A slang term for obese or adipose. 4 In chemistry, a compound formed from chemicals called fatty acids. These fats are greasy, solid materials found in animal tissues and in some plants. Fats are the major component of the flabby material of a body, commonly known as blubber.

fat, trans See *trans fatty acid.*

fatty acid, trans See *trans fatty acid.*

fatty liver of pregnancy, acute See *acute fatty liver of pregnancy.*

fauces Throat.

fava bean A broad bean to which many people react adversely. Fava beans look like large, tan lima beans. They are popular in Mediterranean and Middle Eastern cuisines, are eaten raw when very young, can be cooked in soups and many other dishes, or may be made into fava brittle candy. Fava beans are the main commercial source of the drug L-dopa. See also *favism.*

favism A condition characterized by hemolytic anemia (breakup of red blood cells) that occurs after a person eats fava beans or is exposed to the pollen of the fava plant. This dangerous reaction occurs exclusively in people with a deficiency of the enzyme glucose-6-phosphate dehydrogenase (G6PD), an X-linked genetic trait. However, not all G6PD-deficient families appear to be at risk for favism; this indicates that an additional single autosomal (not X-linked) gene is needed in order to create susceptibility to favism. The active hemolytic principle in fava beans is likely dopa-quinone. Differences in susceptibility to favism may be related to differences in the enzymatic system that converts L-dopa to dopa-quinone. See also *deficiency, G6PD.*

FDA Food and Drug Administration.

febrile Feverish.

febrile headache See *headache, febrile.*

febrile seizure See *seizure, febrile.*

fecal incontinence See *encopresis.*

fecal occult blood test A test to check for hidden blood in the stool.

feces The excrement discharged from the intestines.

fecund See *fertile.*

fecundity See *fertility.*

feedback A process in which the factors that produce a result are themselves modified, corrected, and strengthened by that result. Many biologic processes are controlled by feedback, just as the temperature in a home (from a furnace or air conditioner) can be regulated by a thermostat. This principle is the basis for the practice of biofeedback. See also *biofeedback.*

feeding, breast See *breastfeeding.*

feet As a measure of length, the plural of foot.

female An individual of the sex that bears young or that produces ova or eggs, or a person who has a particular physical appearance, chromosome constitution, or gender identification. See also *female chromosome complement.*

female chromosome complement The whole set of chromosomes for a female. The large majority of females have a 46, XX chromosome complement (46 chromosomes, including 2 X chromosomes). A minority of females have other chromosome complements, such as 45, X (45 chromosomes, including 1 X chromosome) or 47, XXX (47 chromosomes, including 3 X chromosomes).

female external genitalia The external genital structures of the female, including the labia minora, labia majora, and the clitoris.

female genital mutilation See *circumcision, female.*

female gonad See *ovary.*

female internal genitalia The internal genital structures of the female, which include the ovaries, the Fallopian tubes, the uterus, the uterine cervix, and the vagina. These are, collectively, the female organs of reproduction.

female organs of reproduction The ovaries, which produce eggs (ova) and female hormones; the Fallopian tubes, which transport the egg from the ovaries to the uterus; the uterus, which receives the egg for fertilization and provides a growth environment for the developing embryo and fetus; the cervix, the lower, narrow part of the uterus that opens into the vagina; and the vagina, the muscular canal that extends from the cervix to the outside of the body and enables sperm to enter the female reproductive tract.

female pelvis   The lower part of the abdomen that is located between the hip bones in a female. The female pelvis is usually more delicate than, wider than, and not as high as the male pelvis. The angle of the female pubic arch is wide and round. The female sacrum is wider than the male's, and the iliac bone is flatter. The pelvic basin of the female is more spacious and less funnel-shaped than the male's. From a purely anatomic viewpoint, the female pelvis is better suited than the male pelvis to accommodate a fetus during pregnancy and permit the baby to be born.

female urethral meatus   See *female urethral opening.*

female urethral opening   The transport tube that leads from the bladder to discharge urine outside the body in a female. The urethra in a female is shorter than the urethra in the male. The meatus (opening) of the female urethra is below the clitoris and just above the opening of the vagina.

femoral   Having to do with the femur.

femoral vein   The large vein in the groin that passes with the femoral artery under the inguinal ligament to enter the abdomen, at which point it becomes the external iliac vein. The femoral vein is a continuation of the popliteal vein, and it carries blood back to the heart from the lower extremities.

femur   The single bone in the thigh, which is the largest bone in the human body. Also known as the thighbone.

fenestration   The creation of a new opening. From the Latin for "the making of a window."

ferritin   The major protein concerned with iron storage. Blood ferritin level serves as an indicator of the amount of iron stored in the body, and it can become elevated due to the presence of conditions featuring significant inflammation.

fertile   Able to conceive and bear offspring. Also known as fecund.

fertility   The ability to have children, usually many of them, with ease. Also known as fecundity.

fertilization   The process of combining the male gamete, or sperm, with the female gamete, or ovum. The product of fertilization is a cell called a zygote.

fetal alcohol effect   A condition in which a child has some signs of fetal alcohol syndrome (FAS) but does not meet all of the necessary criteria for FAS and there is a history of alcohol exposure before birth. Abbreviated FAE.

Although FAE is considered a "softer" diagnosis than FAS, it can still have severe and lifelong consequences for the child, including mental retardation and facial malformation. Frequent ear infections and hearing loss are also present in nearly half of all children with FAE.

fetal alcohol syndrome   A syndrome of damage that occurs to a child before birth as a result of the mother drinking alcohol during pregnancy. Abbreviated FAS. FAS always involves brain damage, impaired growth, and head and face abnormalities. Most children with FAS also have frequent ear infections and some degree of hearing loss. FAS is one of the leading causes of mental retardation in the US. FAS is an irreversible, lifelong condition that affects every aspect of a child's life. However, FAS is 100 percent preventable if a woman does not drink alcohol while she is pregnant. If a pregnant woman drinks alcohol, but her child does not have all the symptoms of FAS, it is possible that her child may be born with alcohol-related neurodevelopmental disabilities (ARND). Children with ARND may demonstrate learning and behavioral problems caused by prenatal exposure to alcohol. Besides education of women and surgery on children with FAS to correct major physical defects, there is no treatment for FAS. No amount of alcohol has been proven safe during pregnancy. Women who are or may become pregnant are advised to avoid alcohol. If a pregnant woman does drink, it is never too late for her to stop. The sooner a pregnant woman stops drinking, the better for both her and her baby. To establish the diagnosis of FAS, the following signs must be present: small size and weight before and after birth (pre- and postnatal growth retardation); evidence of brain delay in development, intellectual impairment, or neurologic abnormalities; and specific appearance of the head and face. At least two of the following groups of signs must be present: small head size (microcephaly); small eyes (microphthalmia) and/or short eye openings (palpebral fissures); and underdevelopment of the upper lip, indistinct groove between the lip and nose (the philtrum), and flattened cheekbones.

fetal circulation   See circulation, fetal.

fetal development   See prenatal development.

fetal distress   Compromise of a fetus during the antepartum period (before labor) or intrapartum period (during the birth process). The term fetal distress is commonly used to describe fetal hypoxia (low oxygen levels in the fetus). The concern with fetal hypoxia is that it may result in fetal damage or death if it is not reversed or if the fetus is not promptly delivered. Fetal distress can be detected via abnormal slowing of labor, the presence of meconium (dark green fecal material from the fetus) or other abnormal substances in the amniotic fluid, or fetal monitoring with an electronic device that shows a fetal scalp pH of less than 7.2.

fetal dystocia   See *dystocia, fetal.*

fetal hemoglobin   See *hemoglobin F.*

fetal mortality rate   The number of fetal deaths divided by the sum of all births in that year. In the US, the fetal mortality rate plummeted from 19.2 per 1,000 births in 1950 to 6.7 per 1,000 births in 1999. However, the fetal mortality rate is higher than this in certain ethnic groups and among mothers with health problems during pregnancy, especially if the mother does not receive adequate personal and prenatal health care. The fetal mortality rate is considered a good measure of the quality of health care in a country or a medical facility.

fetal movement   Movement of the fetus in the womb. The first fetal movements felt by the mother usually occur between 18 and 22 weeks of pregnancy. Also known as quickening.

fetoprotein, alpha-   See *alpha-fetoprotein.*

fetoscope   A device used to look at a fetus within the uterus. There are two types of fetoscopes: A fiberoptic scope for looking directly at the fetus within the uterus and a stethoscope designed for listening to the fetal heart beat.

fetoscopy   A technique for look at a fetus within the uterus by using a fetoscope.

fetus   An unborn offspring, from the embryo stage (the end of the eighth week after conception, when the major structures have formed) until birth.

fever   Technically, any body temperature above the normal oral measurement of 37°C (98.6°F) or the normal rectal temperature of 99°F. However, fever is not considered medically significant until the temperature is above 38°C (100.4°F). Fever is part of the body's own disease-fighting arsenal: Rising body temperatures are apparently capable of killing many disease-producing organisms. For that reason, low fevers should normally go untreated, unless they are accompanied by any other troubling symptoms. As fevers range to 40°C (104°F) and above, however, there can be unwanted consequences, such as delirium and convulsions, particularly for children. A fever of this sort demands immediate home treatment and then medical attention. Home treatment possibilities include the use of aspirin or, in children, nonaspirin pain killers such as acetaminophen, cool baths, or sponging to reduce the fever. Fever may occur with almost any type of infection or illness. Also called pyrexia.

fever blister   See *canker sore.*

fever, breakbone   See *dengue fever.*

fever, cat scratch   See *cat scratch fever.*

fever, dengue   See *dengue fever.*

fever, Ebola virus   See *Ebola virus.*

fever, epidemic hemorrhagic   See *hemorrhagic fever with renal syndrome.*

fever, five-day   See *trench fever.*

fever, intermittent   A type of fever that rises and falls, often becoming worst at night and being accompanied by drenching sweats.

fever, Lassa   An acute viral infection found in the tropics, especially in West Africa. Lassa fever is caused by a single-stranded RNA virus that is animal borne (zoonotic). Lassa fever is a grave health concern because it can cause a potentially fatal illness, is highly contagious, and can rapidly spread. The number of Lassa virus infections per year in West Africa has been estimated at 100,000 to 300,000, with at least 5,000 deaths yearly. The virus has been found in a rodent known as the "multi-mammate rat." People can become infected by eating this infected rat or by eating food contaminated by the rat's excretions. Person-to-person transmission also occurs via direct contact, contamination of skin breaks with infected blood, and aerosol spreads (virus particles moving through the air). The first symptoms typically occur 1 to 3 weeks after the patient comes into contact with the virus and may include high fever, sore throat, cough, eye inflammation (conjunctivitis), facial swelling, pain behind the breastbone, back pain, abdominal pain, vomiting, diarrhea, and general weakness that lasts for several days. The most common complication of Lassa fever is deafness. If a person has traveled to West Africa and has a severe fever within 3 weeks after returning, the illness should be reported to a physician. The key agent for treatment is ribavirin, an antiviral drug, which is most effective when given early in the course of the disease. Patients are also given supportive care with fluid balance, oxygen as needed, and treatment of any other complicating infections. Medical isolation procedures should be followed for those with Lassa fever, due to the highly contagious nature of the disease. Patients may excrete the virus weeks after recovery. Patients' bodily fluids should therefore be monitored for the virus before they leave the hospital.

fever, Mediterranean   See *familial Mediterranean fever.*

fever, Q   See *Q fever.*

fever, remittent A type of fever that gradually decreases in intensity over time.

fever, Rocky Mountain spotted See *Rocky Mountain spotted fever.*

fever, scarlet See *scarlet fever.*

fever, spotted See *Rocky Mountain spotted fever.*

fever therapy A treatment in which abnormal elevations in body temperature are used to treat disease. Fever therapy was done in the past but is rarely, if ever, used today. Sometimes if a patient has a very high fever due to infection, upon recovery from the infection, the patient enters into a seemingly impossible remission from an unrelated disease or is even cured of it.

fever, tick See *Rocky Mountain spotted fever.*

fever, trench See *trench fever.*

fever, undulant See *Brucellosis.*

fever with renal syndrome, hemorrhagic See *hemorrhagic fever with renal syndrome.*

FGFR2 Fibroblast growth factor receptor 2.

fiber The parts of fruits and vegetables that cannot be digested. Fiber is of vital importance to digestion; it helps the body move food through the digestive tract, reduces serum cholesterol, and contributes to disease protection. Also known as bulk and roughage.

fiber, bowel disorders and Intestinal conditions that respond to diets that are high in fiber. For example, high-fiber diets help delay the progression of diverticulosis and, at least, reduce the number of bouts of diverticulitis. In many cases, fiber helps reduce the symptoms of irritable bowel syndrome and constipation.

fiber, cancer and Cancer of the colon is felt to be influenced by fiber intake. It is generally accepted that a diet that is high in fiber is protective of the colon or at least reduces the incidence of colon polyps and colon cancer.

fiber, cholesterol and Cholesterol blood levels can be influenced by intake of fiber. Soluble fiber substances are effective in helping reduce the level of blood cholesterol. This is especially true with oat bran, fruits, psyllium, and legumes. Diets that are high in soluble fiber may lower cholesterol and low-density lipoproteins by 8 to 15 percent.

fiber, constipation and Constipation can be influenced by intake of fiber. Insoluble fiber retains water in the colon, resulting in softer and larger stool. Fiber is used effectively in treating constipation that results from poor dietary habits. Bran is particularly rich in insoluble fiber.

fiber, diabetes and Diabetes can be influenced by intake of fiber. Soluble fibers found in oat bran, apples, citrus fruits, pears, peas and beans, psyllium, and other foods slow down the digestion of carbohydrates (sugars), which results in improved glucose metabolism. Some patients with adult-onset diabetes may be successfully treated with a high-fiber diet alone, and those on insulin can often reduce their insulin requirements by adhering to a high-fiber diet.

fiber, insoluble Fiber that cannot be digested within the gastrointestinal tract. Insoluble fiber is found in wheat bran, cabbage, peas and beans, and other foods. Both are important diet components for optimal health. See also *fiber, soluble.*

fiber, soluble Fiber that can be digested within the gastrointestinal tract. Soluble fiber is found in oat bran, apples, citrus, pears, peas and beans, psyllium, and other foods. Both soluble and insoluble fiber are important diet components for optimal health. See also *fiber, insoluble.*

fibrates Cholesterol-lowering drugs that are effective in lowering triglycerides and, to a lesser extent, in increasing HDL cholesterol levels. Gemfibrozil (brand name: Lopid), the fibrate most widely used in the US, can be effective for patients with high triglyceride levels, but it is not very effective for lowering LDL cholesterol. As a result, it is used less often than other drugs for patients with heart disease for whom LDL cholesterol lowering is the main goal of treatment. Fibrates are generally well tolerated by most patients. Gastrointestinal complaints are the most common side effect, and fibrates appear to increase a patient's likelihood of developing cholesterol gallstones. Fibrates can increase the effects of medications that thin the blood.

fibril A small fiber, a fine thread.

fibrillation In cardiology, an abnormal and erratic twitching of the heart muscle.

fibrillation, atrial An abnormal and irregular heart rhythm in which electrical signals are generated chaotically throughout the upper chambers (atria) of the heart. Many people with atrial fibrillation have no symptoms. Among those who do, the most common symptom is an uncomfortable awareness of the rapid and irregular heartbeat (palpitations). Atrial fibrillation can promote the formation of blood clots that travel from the heart to the brain, resulting in stroke. Treatment of atrial fibrillation involves risk-factor control, use of medications to slow the heart rate and/or convert the heart to normal rhythm, and prevention of blood clots. Also known as auricular fibrillation.

fibrillation, auricular See *fibrillation, atrial.*

fibrillation, ventricular An abnormal and irregular heart rhythm in which there are rapid uncoordinated fluttering contractions of the lower chambers (ventricles) of the heart. Ventricular fibrillation disrupts the synchrony between the heartbeat and the pulse beat. Ventricular fibrillation is commonly associated with heart attacks and scarring of the heart muscle from previous heart attacks. Ventricular fibrillation is life threatening.

fibrin The protein that is formed during normal blood clotting and that is the essence of the clot.

fibrinogen The protein from which fibrin is formed in normal blood clotting.

fibroblast growth factor receptor 2 A gene on chromosome 10. Mutations in FGFR2 cause the best-known type of acrocephalosyndactyly, Apert syndrome. Different mutations in FGFR2 are responsible for other genetic diseases, including Pfeiffer syndrome (a type of acrocephalosyndactyly) and Crouzon syndrome (a craniofacial disorder with no hand or foot problems). All these disorders are inherited as autosomal dominant traits. See also *acrocephalosyndactyly; Apert syndrome; Crouzon syndrome; Pfeiffer syndrome.*

fibroid A common benign tumor of the uterus. Fibroids can be present without symptoms. However, in about 25 percent of women, fibroids cause symptoms such as prolonged or heavy menstrual bleeding, pelvic pressure or pain, and, in rare cases, reproductive dysfunction. Both the economic cost of fibroids and their effect on quality of life are substantial. Drugs that manipulate the levels of steroid hormones are effective in treating fibroids, but side effects limit their long-term use. Fibroids may be removed if they cause discomfort or if they are associated with uterine bleeding. In addition to hysterectomy and abdominal myomectomy, various minimally invasive procedures have been developed to remove fibroids. Also known as leiomyoma and myoma of the uterus.

fibroma A mass of interlacing fibrous cells that has a spindle shape.

fibroma, cemento-ossifying A lesion that continues to grow, sometimes to very large size, unless treated. Abbreviated COF. A COF has a hard, fibrous consistency. COFs are most frequently seen in the jaw or mouth area,

sometimes in connection with fracture or injury. Treatment is surgery. Also known as ossifying fibroma.

fibroma, collagenous See *fibroma, desmoplastic.*

fibroma, desmoplastic A rare type of primary bone tumor that is characteristically composed of well-differentiated cells that produce collagen. Desmoplastic fibromas are discovered most often in the first three decades of life, in the mandible (the femur and pelvis are also favored sites). Although benign, these tumors infiltrate locally and may cause pain and swelling or fluid accumulation. Treatment is surgical removal, but desmoplastic fibromas may recur. Also known as collagenous fibroma.

fibroma, ossifying See *fibroma, cemento-ossifying.*

fibromatosis A condition characterized by multiple fibromas. See also *fibroma.*

fibromyalgia A syndrome characterized by chronic pain, stiffness, and tenderness of muscles, tendons, and joints, without detectable inflammation. Fibromyalgia does not cause body damage or deformity. However, undue fatigue plagues 90 percent of patients with fibromyalgia. Sleep disorder is also common in patients with fibromyalgia. Fibromyalgia can be associated with other rheumatic conditions, and irritable bowel syndrome (IBS) can occur with fibromyalgia. There is no definitive medical test for the diagnosis of fibromyalgia, so diagnosis is made by eliminating other possible causes of the symptoms. The most effective treatment is a combination of education, stress reduction, exercise, and medication. Also known as fibrositis.

fibrosarcoma A malignant tumor that begins in fibrous connective tissue at the ends of the arm or leg bones and may spread to surrounding soft tissue. Fibrosarcoma is the most common soft tissue sarcoma found in children under 1 year of age. It presents as a rapidly growing mass at birth or during early infancy. Fibrosarcoma can also occur in older children and adults. The symptoms may include a lump, soreness, pain, or a limp (if the tumor is in the leg).

fibrosis, radiation Scarring of the lungs from radiation. Radiation fibrosis occurs following radiation pneumonitis (inflammation of the lungs due to radiation), as from radiation therapy. Radiation pneumonitis typically occurs after radiation treatments for cancer within the chest or breast, and it usually manifests 2 weeks to 6 months after completion of radiation therapy. Symptoms include shortness of breath upon activity, cough, and fever. Radiation pneumonitis is frequently discovered as an incidental finding on chest X-ray in patients who have no symptoms. Radiation fibrosis typically occurs 1 year after the completion of radiation treatments. Whereas radiation pneumonitis is often reversible with medications that reduce inflammation, such as cortisone drugs (prednisone), radiation fibrosis is usually irreversible and permanent.

fibrositis   See *fibromyalgia.*

fibrous dysplasia, monostotic   See *monostotic fibrous dysplasia.*

fibrous dysplasia, polyostotic   See *polyostotic fibrous dysplasia.*

fibula   The smaller of the two bones in the lower leg.

fièvre boutonneuse   See *typhus, African tick.*

fifth disease   A disease that is caused by a virus called parvovirus B-19. The characteristic symptoms of fifth disease include low-grade fever, fatigue, a "slapped cheeks" rash, and a rash over the whole body. Although fifth disease is not serious in most children, some children with immunodeficiency (such as those with AIDS or leukemia) or with certain blood disorders (such as sickle cell anemia or hemolytic anemia) may become seriously ill with fifth disease. Parvovirus B-19 can temporarily decrease or halt the body's production of red blood cells, causing anemia. About 80 percent of adults with fifth disease have joint aches and pains (arthritis), which may become long term, with stiffness in the morning and redness and swelling of the same joints on both sides of the body (a "symmetrical" arthritis), most commonly involving the knees, fingers, and wrists. Pregnant women who have not previously had fifth disease should avoid contact with patients who have it because parvovirus B-19 can infect a fetus prior to birth. Although no birth defects have been reported as a result of fifth disease, it can cause the death of an unborn fetus. The risk of fetal death is 5 to 10 percent if the mother becomes infected. The odd name, fifth disease, comes from the prevaccination era, when this disease was often the fifth disease that a child contracted. Also known as erythema infectiosum.

film   Slang shortening of X-ray film.

film, AP   An X-ray picture in which the beams pass from front to back (anteroposterior). See also *film, PA.*

film, lateral   An X-ray picture taken from the side.

film, PA   An X-ray picture in which the beams pass from back to front (posteroanterior). See also *film, AP.*

filovirus   A virus in the virus family filoviridae that causes hemorrhagic fever. Filoviruses have single-stranded RNA as their genetic material. Ebola virus and the Marburg virus are both filoviruses.

fine needle aspiration   The use of a thin needle to withdraw material from the body. For example, when a nodule is felt in the thyroid, fine needle aspiration may be done to determine whether the nodule is benign or malignant. A fine-gauge needle is placed into the nodule, and it removes a drop of fluid. The cells are studied under the microscope by a pathologist.

fingernail   A covering for the tip of the finger that is produced by living skin cells in the finger. A fingernail consists of several parts, including the nail plate (the visible part of the nail), the nail bed (the skin beneath the nail plate), the cuticle (the tissue that overlaps the plate and rims the base of the nail), the nail folds (the skin folds that frame and support the nail on three sides), the lunula (the whitish half-moon at the base of the nail), and the matrix (the hidden part of the nail unit under the cuticle). A fingernail grows from the matrix. It is composed largely of keratin, a hardened protein that is also found in skin and hair. As new cells grow in the matrix, the older cells are pushed out and compacted, taking on the familiar flattened, hardened form of the fingernail. The average growth rate for fingernails is 0.1 mm each day (or 1 cm in 100 days). The exact rate of nail growth depends on numerous factors, including the age and sex of the individual and the time of year. Fingernails generally grow fastest in young people, in males, and in the summer. Fingernails grow faster than toenails. The fingernails on the right hand of a right-handed person grow faster than those on the person's left hand, and vice versa. See also *nail; nail care.*

fingers, six   See *hexadactyly.*

fire ant   Originally from South America, and now in 13 states in the US, a red or yellowish ant of small to medium size that has a severe sting that burns like fire. Fire ants normally feed on small insects, but they may also eat seeds and seedling plants, damage grain and vegetable crops, invade kitchens, and attack newly hatched poultry and the young of ground-nesting wild birds. Fire ants can kill newborn domestic and wild animals. Each fire ant colony is composed of a queen, winged males and females, and three kinds of workers. A nest averages about 25,000 workers, but far larger populations are common. Fire ants' semipermanent nests are large mounds of excavated soil with openings for ventilation. Because nests may number 50 or more in a heavily infested field, cultivating becomes difficult or impossible. Fire ants belong to the genus Solenopsis and are also called thief ants. The severe sting of a fire ant causes a pustule to form with 24 hours, and the pustule takes 10 to 14 days to resolve. Fire ant toxin can trigger an allergic reaction, particularly in people allergic to bee, wasp, and yellowjacket stings. Avoidance and prompt treatment are essential.

fire, St. Anthony's   An intensely painful burning sensation in the limbs and extremities that is caused by ergot, which is the consequence of a fungus (Claviceps purpurea) that contaminates rye and wheat. See also *ergot*.

fire supplies kit   See *disaster supplies*.

first do no harm   A classic slogan that is used in medicine, often in the Latin wording primum non nocere, that is attributed to Hippocrates.

first stage of labor   The part of labor when the cervix dilates fully, to approximately 10 centimeters in diameter. Also known as the stage of dilatation.

FISH   Fluorescent in situ hybridization, an important molecular cytogenetic technique that vividly paints chromosomes with fluorescent molecules. FISH is useful for identifying chromosomes and parts of chromosomes, deciphering chromosome rearrangements, detecting chromosome abnormalities, and mapping genes. For example, a FISH probe to chromosome 21 permits one to look for cells with trisomy 21 (an extra chromosome 21, which is the cause of Down syndrome).

fishbowl granuloma   See *granuloma, fishbowl*.

Fisher's exact test   A statistical test of independence that is much used in medical research. It tests the independence of rows and columns in a 2×2 contingency table (a table with two horizontal rows crossing two vertical columns, creating four places for data) based on the exact sampling distribution of the observed frequencies. Hence it is an "exact" test.

fish-odor syndrome   An inborn error of metabolism that is associated with an offensive body odor whose scent is similar to the smell of rotting fish. Fish-odor syndrome is due to the excessive excretion of trimethylaminuria (TMA) in urine, sweat, and breath. Persons with this syndrome may experience fast heart rate and severe high blood pressure after eating cheese (which contains tyramine, as does red wine and some other foods) and after using nasal sprays that contain epinephrine. This syndrome is caused by a mutation in the gene for the enzyme flavin-containing monooxygenase-3 (FMO3). Fish-odor syndrome is associated with various psychosocial reactions, including social isolation, clinical depression, and attempted suicide. Also known as trimethylaminuria.

fistula   An abnormal passageway. For example, an anal fistula is an opening in the skin near the anus: This opening may lead to a tunnel into the rectal canal or to a passage that ends in a blind pouch.

five-day fever   See *trench fever.*

flail chest   A condition that occurs when enough ribs are broken (usually from a crush injury) to compromise the rigidity of the chest wall. On inspiration, the chest wall moves inward instead of outward, and it does the opposite on expiration.

flat feet   Absence of an arch in the sole of the foot that causes the foot to lie flat when the person is standing. All babies have flat feet because their arches are not yet built up (and their feet tend to be plump). This condition may persist into adulthood, or an arch may form as the child grows. Flat feet can also be acquired, as in jobs that require a great deal of walking and carrying of heavy objects. People with flat feet sometimes experience clumsiness and fatigue from prolonged walking or running. Wearing shoes with built-in arch supports can help. People with weakness in the ankle as well as flat feet may have their feet turn in or roll toward the middle, damaging shoes and causing discomfort. Exercises may also be useful in reducing discomfort. Also called pes planus.

flatulence   The passing of gas from the intestinal tract. What constitutes excess gas is difficult to define because symptom-free individuals have recorded approximately 14 passages of gas per 24 hours. Also commonly known as farting. See also *flatus.*

flatus   Gas in the intestinal tract or gas passed through the anus. The intestinal gases are hydrogen, nitrogen, carbon dioxide, and methane, all of which are odorless. The occasional unpleasant smell of flatus is the result of trace gases, such as indole, skatole, and, most commonly, hydrogen sulfide.

flavin-containing monooxygenase-3   FMO3.

flavivirus   One of a family of viruses that cause hemorrhagic fever and are transmitted by mosquitoes and ticks. Flaviviruses have single-stranded RNA as their genetic material. The virus of yellow fever, for example, is a flavivirus.

flexion   The process of bending, or the state of being bent. For example, flexion of the fingers results in a clenched fist.

Flexner Report   A report whose full name is "Medical Education in the United States and Canada," quite possibly the most important written document in the history of

US and Canadian medical education. The 1910 report is named for its author, professional educator Abraham Flexner, who researched and wrote this report for the Carnegie Foundation. At the time that the report was written, many medical schools were proprietary schools operated more for profit than for education. In their stead, Flexner proposed medical schools in the German tradition of strong biomedical sciences, together with hands-on clinical training. The Flexner Report caused many medical schools to close, and most of the remaining schools were reformed to conform to the Flexnerian model.

floaters Spots due to deposits of protein drifting about in the vitreous humor (the clear jelly-like substance that fills the middle of the eye). Also known as spots in front of the eyes.

floating rib The last two false ribs, which usually have no ventral attachment to anchor them in front. Also known as fluctuating or vertebral rib. See also *false rib*.

flood supplies kit See *disaster supplies*.

floppy baby syndrome An abnormal condition of newborns and infants manifested by inadequate tone of the muscles. Floppy baby syndrome can be due to a multitude of neurologic and muscle problems. See also *hypotonia*.

flow cytometry Analysis of biological material via detection of the light-absorbing or fluorescing properties of cells, or of subcellular fractions such as chromosomes, as they pass in a narrow stream through a laser beam. Flow cytometry can be used with automated sorting devices to sort successive droplets of a stream into different fractions, depending on the fluorescence emitted by each droplet.

flow karyotyping Use of flow cytometry to analyze and/or separate chromosomes on the basis of their DNA content.

flu See *influenza*.

flu shot See *influenza vaccine*.

flu, stomach A gastrointestinal illness caused by a microorganism. Stomach flu actually has nothing to do with the influenza (flu) virus.

flu vaccine See *influenza vaccine*.

fluctuating rib See *floating rib*.

fluid, cerebrospinal See *cerebrospinal fluid*.

fluorescent in situ hybridization FISH.

fluorescent microscope A microscope that is equipped to examine material that fluoresces under ultraviolet (UV) light.

fluoroscopy An X-ray procedure that makes it possible to see internal organs in motion. Fluoroscopy uses X-rays to produce real-time video images. Instead of using film, fluoroscopy captures X-rays with a device called an image intensifier and converts the X-rays into light. The light is then captured by a TV camera and displayed on a video monitor.

fluorouracil An anticancer drug whose chemical name is 5-fluorouracil (5-FU).

flush **1** A redness of the skin, typically over the cheeks or neck. A flush is usually temporary and brought on by excitement, exercise, fever, or embarrassment. Flushing is an involuntary (uncontrollable) response of the nervous system that leads to widening of the capillaries of the involved skin. Also referred to as a blush (or, as a verb). Flushing may also be caused by medications or other substances that cause widening of the capillaries, such as niacin. **2** To wash out a wound, body area, or medical device.

fluvastin A cholesterol-lowering drug (brand name: Lescol) that is prescribed to prevent medical problems associated with high cholesterol levels, such as atherosclerosis and heart disease. Fluvastin is also used to treat inherited lipid disorders and similar disorders caused by liver or kidney disease.

FMF Familial Mediterranean fever.

FMO3 Flavin-containing monooxygenase-3, an enzyme that is encoded on chromosome 1 and normally metabolizes tyramine. See also *fish-odor syndrome*.

FMR1 Familial mental retardation 1, the gene that is responsible for the production of the protein familial mental retardation protein (FMRP). See also *fragile X syndrome*.

FMRP Familial mental retardation protein, a protein whose lack results in fragile X syndrome, the most common inherited cause of mental retardation. See also *FMR1; fragile X syndrome*.

focused H and P A medical history (H) and physical examination (P) that focuses on the patient's present problem. For example, if a patient is complaining of an earache, the physician concentrates on the ear rather than doing a complete clinical exam.

folate See *folic acid*.

Foley catheter   See *catheter, Foley.*

folic acid   A B vitamin that is an important factor in nucleic acid synthesis. A deficiency of folic acid causes megaloblastic anemia. Lack of folic acid during pregnancy can lead to neural tube birth defects, including spina bifida and anencephaly. In order for folic acid to be effective in preventing these birth defects, it must be consumed every day, beginning before conception and continuing through the first 3 months of pregnancy. An adequate intake of folic acid reduces the risks for a remarkably broad range of birth defects and appears to be important to the health of arteries, reducing the risk of second heart attacks and strokes. See Appendix C, "Vitamins."

follicle   A shaft in the skin through which hair grows. Inflammation of the follicle is referred to as folliculitis.

follicle-stimulating hormone   A hormone produced by the pituitary gland that controls estrogen production by the ovaries. Abbreviated FSH. See also *gonadotropin.*

follicular cyst of the ovary   See *cyst of the ovary, follicular.*

Fondation Jean Dausset   The Centre d'Etudes du Polymorphisme Humain (CEPH), an internationally renowned research laboratory created in Paris in 1984 by Professor Jean Dausset to provide the scientific community with resources for human genome mapping.

Fong disease   See *nail-patella syndrome.*

fontanel   A soft spot of the skull of a newborn infant where the cartilage has not yet hardened into bone between the skull bones. There are normally two fontanels, both in the midline of the skull. The anterior fontanel is well in front of the posterior fontanel. The posterior fontanel closes first, at latest by the age of 8 weeks in a full-term baby. The anterior fontanel closes at around 18 months of age, but it can close normally as early as 9 months. The fontanels closing too early or too late might be a sign of a problem. Also known as fontanelle.

food   Any substance that is eaten to provide nutritional support for the body.

Food and Drug Administration   An agency within the US Public Health Service that provides a number of health-related services. Abbreviated FDA. The FDA's services include inspecting food and food-processing facilities to ensure wholesomeness and safety; scrutinizing food and drugs for pets and farm animals; ensuring that cosmetics will not cause harm; monitoring the health of the nation's blood supply; ensuring that medicines, medical devices, and biologicals (such as insulin and vaccines) are safe and effective; and testing radiation-emitting products such as microwave ovens to protect the public. The FDA also oversees health and safety labeling of these products. All new prescription and over-the-counter drugs are subject to FDA approval. The FDA must determine that a new drug produces the benefits it's supposed to produce, without causing side effects that would outweigh the benefits. It does so by looking at the results of clinical trials done outside the FDA. When serious adverse effects from a medication are reported, the FDA has the power to force the manufacturer to make changes in the drug, change its safety labeling or marketing practices, or remove the medication from the market.

food, functional   Food that is potentially healthful, including any modified food or ingredient that may provide a health benefit beyond the traditional nutrients it contains. Functional foods include such items as cereals, breads, beverages that are fortified with vitamins, some herbs, and nutraceuticals.

food poisoning   Disease caused by food-borne infectious organisms, such as the Clostridium botulinum bacteria that produces deadly botulism toxin. Food poisoning is a major public health threat that causes thousands of people to become seriously ill each year and kills many. Symptoms may include stomach upset, nausea, vomiting, and weakness, depending on the organism involved. Improper food storage and preparation increase the risk of food poisoning. Food poisoning is most dangerous to children, the elderly, and people with impaired immune systems. The most prominent causes of food poisoning are Norwalk and Norwalk-like viruses (often from shellfish and salads), Campylobacter jejuni (the leading cause of bacterial food poisoning, often from undercooked poultry), Salmonella (often from raw or undercooked eggs), Listeria monocytogenes (often from unpasteurized milk and cheese), Vibrio vulnificus (through raw or inadequately cooked seafood), and E. coli 0157:H7 (often from undercooked hamburger). See also *botulism; E. coli; listeriosis; salmonellosis.*

food, "super"   Food with alleged healing or health-promoting capabilities. The healing power of foods is a popular concept. Medicinal or nutritionally high-powered foods have been part and parcel of the natural products industry for a long time and, through emerging scientific research and particularly through growing public interest, they have reached the mainstream. Not all items advertised as "super" foods or healing foods have been proven to promote health, however, and some may be contraindicated for people with certain health conditions.

foot   **1** The extremity at the end of the leg, with which a person stands and walks. The foot is a particularly complex structure, made up of dozens of bones that work together with muscles and tendons to execute precise movements. The bones of the foot include the 10 metatarsals and the 28 phalanges (toe bones). **2** As a measurement, 12 inches, or one-third of a yard. The foot was originally the length of a man's foot, and it served as a measurement of land. Abbreviated ft.

foot, athlete's See *athlete's foot.*

foot drop brace See *ankle-foot orthosis.*

foot fungus See *athlete's foot.*

footling birth A foot- or feet-first birth. A footling birth is called single-footling or double-footling, depending on whether the presenting part of the baby at delivery is just one foot or both feet. Also known as footling presentation.

footling presentation See *footling birth.*

foramen A natural opening. Although a foramen is usually through bone, it can be an opening through other types of tissue, as with the foramen ovale in the heart. The plural of foramen is foramina.

foramen, interventricular An opening between the lateral and third ventricles in the brain.

foramen magnum The large hole at the base of the skull that allows passage of the spinal cord.

foramen of Magendie An opening from the fourth ventricle in the brain to the central canal of the upper end of the spinal cord.

foramen ovale An oval opening between the two upper chambers of the heart (the atria) that is a normal feature of fetal and newborn circulation. The foramen ovale normally closes by 3 months of age.

foramina of Luschka A pair of openings from the fourth ventricle of the brain to the central canal of the upper end of the spinal cord.

forceps An instrument that has two blades and a handle and is used for handling, grasping, or compressing.

forceps, obstetrical A forceps designed as an aid in the vaginal delivery of a baby. Forceps may be used to ease delivery or to cope with problems of fetal distress or fetal position. The decision to use forceps must be made by an obstetrician.

forearm The portion of the upper limb from the elbow to the wrist. The forearm has two bones: the radius and ulna.

foreign body airway obstruction Partial or complete blockage of the breathing tubes to the lungs due to the presence of a foreign body, such as food, a bead, or a toy. See also *airway obstruction.*

foreskin The fold of skin that covers the head (glans) of the penis. The inside of the foreskin has preputial glands, a special type of sebaceous (oil) glands that secrete an oily lubricant known as smegma. Smegma probably has protective qualities, as does the foreskin itself. However, uncircumcised men must retract the foreskin periodically to remove buildup smegma. Only about 1 in every 20 boys is born with a retractable foreskin because the tissue development of the foreskin is usually not complete at birth. The foreskin is thus not fully separable from the glans in most newborn boys. By 1 year of age, the foreskin can be retracted in 50 percent of boys, and by 3 years of age, the foreskin can be retracted in 80 percent to 90 percent of uncircumcised boys. The foreskin is often surgically removed via circumcision. Also known as prepuce. See also *circumcision, male.*

foreskin and glans, inflammation of the See *balanoposthitis.*

foreskin, inflammation of the See *posthitis.*

foreskin, tight See *phimosis.*

Forestier disease See *diffuse idiopathic skeletal hyperostosis.*

formula A prepared substitute for breast milk that may be based on cow's milk, goat's milk, soy milk, or another food product. Formula does not contain the special immunity factors found in breast milk that help the baby to fight off infections, and it may not include all the vitamins, minerals, and enzymes found in human breast milk. For that reason, experts in infant nutrition agree that breastfeeding is best, particularly in families with a history of allergies.

formula feeding Feeding an infant or toddler prepared formula instead of or in addition to breastfeeding. Formula feeding is indicated when the mother has an illness that could be passed on to the baby through breast milk or through the close physical proximity required for breastfeeding. Otherwise, experts in infant nutrition agree that breastfeeding is best.

fornices Plural of fornix.

fornix In anatomy, any vaultlike or arched structure, such as the fornix cerebri (an arching fibrous band in the brain).

fornix cerebri   One of two arching fibrous bands in the brain that connect the two lobes of the cerebrum. Each of the two fornices in the brain is an arched tract of nerves.

fornix conjunctivae   The loose arching folds that connect the conjunctival membrane lining the inside of the eyelid with the conjunctival membrane covering the eyeball.

fornix uteri   The anterior (front) and posterior (back) recesses into which the upper vagina is divided. These vaultlike recesses are formed by protrusion of the cervix into the vagina. The fornix uteri is also known as the fornix vaginae (or the vaginal fornices) and the uterine fornices.

fornix vaginae   See *fornix uteri.*

founder effect   The positive effect on gene frequency when a population (colony) has only a small number of original settlers, one or more of whom had that gene. For example, the gene for Huntington's disease was introduced into the Lake Maracaibo region in Venezuela early in the 19th century. There are now more than 100 persons with Huntington's disease and at least 900 persons at risk for that disease in that region, the largest known aggregation of the Huntington's gene in the world.

fourth stage of labor   The hour or two after delivery when the tone of the uterus is reestablished as the uterus contracts again, expelling any remaining contents. These contractions are hastened by breastfeeding, which stimulates production of the hormone oxytocin.

fourth ventricle   One cavity in a system of four communicating cavities within the brain, which are continuous with the central canal of the spinal cord. The fourth ventricle is the most inferior (lowest) of these. It extends from the aqueduct of the midbrain to the central canal of the upper end of the spinal cord, with which it communicates via the foramina of Luschka and the foramen of Magendie. It is filled with cerebrospinal fluid that is formed by structures called choroid plexuses located in the walls and roofs of the ventricle.

fraction, ejection   See *ejection fraction.*

fracture   A break in bone or cartilage. Although usually a result of trauma, a fracture can be the result of an acquired disease of bone, such as osteoporosis, or of abnormal formation of bone in a congenital disease of bone, such as osteogenesis imperfecta ("brittle bone disease"). Fractures are classified according to their character and location (for example, greenstick fracture of the radius).

fracture, buckle   See *fracture, torus.*

fracture, clay-shoveler's   An uncommon breakage of the spine, of the vertebrae from the lower neck or upper back, that results from stress. Clay-shoveler's fracture usually occurs in laborers who rapidly lift heavy weights with their arms extended. Examples of such activities include shoveling soil, rubble, or snow up and back over the head; using a pickax or scythe; and pulling out roots. The force of the trapezius and rhomboid muscles pulling on the spine at the base of the neck tears off the bone of the spine. Symptoms of clay-shoveler's fracture include burning, knife-like pain at the level of the fractured spine, between the upper shoulder blades. The pain can sharply increase with repeated activity that strains the muscles of the upper back. The broken spine and nearby muscles are exquisitely tender. Clay-shoveler's fracture is diagnosed via X-ray examination of the spine. Although the intense pain of a clay-shoveler's fracture gradually subsides in days to weeks, the area can intermittently develop burning pain with certain activities that involve prolonged extension of the arms, such as computer work. Most patients require no treatment other than rest and avoidance of activities that stress the area of the fracture. Pain medications, physical therapy, and massage can be helpful. Occasionally surgical removal of the tip of the broken spine is performed for those with long-standing pain.

fracture, comminuted   A fracture in which a bone is broken, splintered, or crushed into a number of pieces.

fracture, compound   A fracture in which a bone is sticking through the skin. Also known as an open fracture.

fracture, compression   A fracture caused by compression, the act of pressing together. Compression fractures of the vertebrae are especially common in elderly people.

fracture, greenstick   A fracture in which one side of a bone is broken and the other is bent (like a green stick).

fracture, open   See *fracture, compound.*

fracture, Salter-Harris   A traumatic fracture of the physeal and/or epiphyseal growth plate. Salter-Harris fractures occur in the extremities of children at the point where new bone is being formed as the bones grow.

fracture, spiral   See *fracture, torsion.*

fracture, stress   A fracture caused by repetitive stress, as may occur in sports, strenuous exercise, or heavy physical labor. Stress fractures are especially common in the metatarsal bones of the foot, particularly in runners. Osteoporosis increases the possibility of stress fractures. Treatment includes rest, disuse, and sometimes splinting or casting to prevent reinjury during healing.

fracture, supracondylar-intercondylar A fracture of a bone within a moving joint, such as the knee or elbow.

fracture, toddler's A torsion fracture of the tibia that occurs without bone displacement. This fracture is called toddler's fracture because it occurs in infants who are early on in their walking, causing a stress breakage of bone in the large bone of the leg below the knee.

fracture, torsion A fracture in which a bone has been twisted apart. Also called a spiral fracture. See also *fracture, toddler's.*

fracture, torus A fracture in which one side of a bone bends but does not actually break. Torus fractures normally heal on their own within a month, with rest and disuse, although they can cause soreness and discomfort.

fracture, transverse A fracture in which the break is across a bone, at a right angle to the long axis of the bone.

fracture, Y A fracture with a Y-like shape that occurs at the end of a bone.

fragile site A point on a chromosome where gaps and breaks tend to occur, which can be passed on from one generation to another.

fragile X chromosome An X chromosome that has a fragile site and is associated with a common form of mental retardation. Fragile X chromosome is due to a trinucleotide repeat (a recurring motif of three bases) in the DNA at that spot. Not all people who inherit the fragile site have the fragile X syndrome, and it is not yet known what genetic or environmental factors cause the breaks or deletions at this fragile site. Also known as FRAXA (as is fragile X syndrome). See also *fragile X syndrome.*

fragile X syndrome The most common heritable form of mental retardation, which occurs in about 1 in 2,000 males and a smaller percentage of females. Characteristics of fragile X syndrome in boys include prominent or long ears, a long face, delayed speech, large testes (macroorchidism), hyperactivity, tactile defensiveness, gross motor delays, and autistic-like behaviors. Much less is known about girls with fragile X syndrome than about boys with it. Only about half of all females who carry the genetic mutation for fragile X syndrome have symptoms themselves. Of those, half are of normal intelligence and only one-fourth have an IQ below 70. Few girls with fragile X syndrome have autistic symptoms, although they tend to be shy and quiet. Fragile X syndrome is due to a dynamic mutation (a trinucleotide repeat) at an inherited fragile site on the X chromosome; therefore, it is an X-linked disorder. Because the mutation is dynamic, it can change in length and hence in severity from generation to generation, from person to person, and even within a given individual. The diagnosis of the syndrome is confirmed by molecular genetic testing that defines an increased number of CGG trinucleotide repeats (more than 230) in the FMR1 gene, usually with aberrant methylation of the FMR1 gene. Also known as FRAXA (as is the fragile X chromosome itself) and Martin-Bell syndrome.

frambesia See *yaws.*

FRAXA See *fragile X chromosome.*

free radical An unstable compound whose behavior is characterized by rapid reactions. Free radicals are often blamed for such physical phenomena as cell degeneration and malfunction. Their full role in physical health is not understood.

frenulum A physical structure that has a restraining function. For example, the lingual frenulum attaches the tongue to the floor of the mouth and appears to restrain it.

Freudian Pertaining to Sigmund Freud, the neurologist, psychiatrist, and founder of psychoanalysis, or to the theory and practice of psychoanalysis and psychotherapy developed by Freud. Freudian psychoanalysis concentrates on finding the roots of adult behavior in childhood conflicts. The term Freudian also refers to interpretations of behavior based on Freud's precepts.

Frey syndrome Sweating on one side of the forehead, face, scalp, and neck that occurs soon after ingestion of food, as a result of damage to a nerve that goes to the large saliva gland in the cheek (the parotid gland). Frey syndrome is the most common cause of sweating after eating (gustatory sweating). Gustatory sweating is also a rare complication of diabetes mellitus, in which case the sweating is on both sides of the head, and the severity of the sweating may be mild or substantial. Frey syndrome can be difficult to treat. Treatment used includes the use of oxybutynin chloride, propantheline bromide, and clonidine (brand name: Catapres). Some success has been reported with topical applications of glycopyrrolate lotion that is applied to the skin of the forehead and face, sparing the eyes and mouth.

frostbite Damage to tissues that results from exposure to extreme cold. The tissues become injured from blood clotting and ice-crystal formation. Severe frostbite can result in death of the tissues (gangrene). The best way to prevent frostbite is to dress warmly and move indoors if the fingers or toes begin to feel cold. Hands and feet should be kept dry, and ears should be covered. The best way to warm a frozen part is to put it into a tub of hot water at 40°C to 42°C (104°F to 108°F). The extremity should not be thawed if there is a risk of it refreezing, which could further damage tissue. Warming over a fire or next to a heater should be avoided. These methods have a high risk of burns and tend to dry out the injured tissue. The extremity should not be rubbed with snow because any rubbing may aggravate the injury. The injured tissue can be fragile and must be handled gently. There may be considerable pain when the frostbitten area is rewarmed. Acetaminophen (brand name: Tylenol), aspirin, naproxen (brand name: Aleve), or ibuprofen (brand name: Advil) may be used to ease the pain. See also *cold injury*.

frozen shoulder Permanent severe limitation of the range of motion of the shoulder due to scarring around the shoulder joint (adhesive capsulitis). Frozen shoulder is an unwanted consequence of rotator cuff disease: damage to the rotator cuff, the set of four tendons that stabilize the shoulder joint and help move the shoulder in diverse directions. See also *rotator cuff; rotator cuff disease*.

FSH Follicle-stimulating hormone.

ft. Abbreviation for foot, a measure of length.

FTT Failure to thrive.

fucosidosis An inherited lysosomal storage disease characterized by lack of the enzyme fucosidase. Without fucosidase, there is accumulation of fucose in the tissues. Fucosidosis is an autosomal recessive disorder. The gene that is responsible for fucosidosis, FUCA1, is on chromosome 1. Fucosidosis in its most severe form can cause neurologic deterioration, growth retardation, visceromegaly (enlargement of the internal organs), and seizures.

fugue state An altered state of consciousness in which a person may move about purposely and even speak but is not fully aware. A fugue state is usually a type of complex partial seizure. See also *seizure, complex partial*.

functional food See *food, functional*.

functional gene test A test for a specific protein which indicates not only that the corresponding gene is present but also that it is active.

fundus In medicine, the bottom or base of an organ. For example, the fundus of the eye is the retina. However, the fundus of the stomach is inexplicably the upper portion. From the Latin for "the bottom."

fungal nail infection See *onychomycosis*.

fungiform Mushroom-shaped.

fungiform papillae Broad, flat structures that house taste buds in the central portion of the dorsum (back) of the tongue. Fungiform papillae were once thought to resemble little mushrooms.

fungus A plantlike organism that feeds on organic matter. An example of a common fungus is the yeast organism that causes thrush and diaper rash (diaper dermatitis).

fungus, foot See *athlete's foot*.

funnel chest "Caved-in" chest. Usually an unimportant isolated finding first evident at birth, funnel chest can occasionally be part of a connective-tissue disorder such as Marfan syndrome. Also known as pectus excavatum.

funny bone A sensation, rather than an actual bone, that one gets when the elbow is bumped and the ulnar nerve that runs past the elbow is stimulated and produces a strange, almost painful, sensation.

furosemide A diuretic medication (brand name: Lasix) that is prescribed to rid the body of excess fluid. Furosemide may be recommended to treat fluid accumulation as a result of kidney trouble, fluid in the lungs, congestive heart failure, high blood pressure, and other conditions. See also *diuretic, loop*.

furuncle See *boil*.

fusiform Formed like a spindle: wider in the middle and tapering toward the ends. For example, a fusiform aneurysm is a vascular outpouching that is shaped like a spindle.

fusiform aneurysm An outpouching or widening of an artery or a vein that is shaped like a spindle.

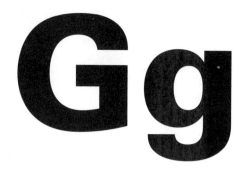

G In genetics, guanine, a member of the G-C (guanine-cytosine) base pair in DNA. See also *DNA; guanine; RNA*.

G protein A molecule that has been described as a "biological traffic light." Located inside a cell, G protein is able to respond to signals outside the cell—light, smell, or hormones—and translate (transduce) these signals into action within the cell.

G6PD Glucose-6-phosphate dehydrogenase, an enzyme that red blood cells rely heavily on because it protects the cells against oxidative stresses. See also *deficiency, G6PD*.

GAG Glycosaminoglycan.

gait A manner of walking. Observation of gait can provide early diagnostic clues for a number of disorders, including cerebral palsy, Parkinson's disease, and Rett syndrome.

galactose A sugar found in milk. Galactose is a disaccharide that is made up of two sugars, galactose and glucose, that are bound together.

galactosemia An inherited disorder of galactose metabolism that occurs in newborns and can result in dire problems, including failure to thrive, liver failure, and bloodstream infection (sepsis). The symptoms of galactosemia resolve if a diet that restricts the intake of galactose and lactose is started during the first 10 days of life. Despite prompt treatment, there remains an increased risk of developmental delay as well as speech and motor problems; females are at increased risk for premature ovarian failure. Perhaps someday gene replacement therapy will be available. Galactosemia is inherited as an autosomal recessive trait; therefore, a couple that has an affected child has a 25 percent risk of having another child with galactosemia with each pregnancy. Galactosemia is due to deficient activity of the enzyme galactose-phosphate uridyltransferase (GALT). Molecular testing for the gene that produces GALT permits carrier detection, genetic counseling, and prenatal diagnosis.

galactosylceramidosis See *Krabbe disease*.

gallbladder A pear-shaped organ located below the liver that stores the bile secreted by the liver. During and after a fatty meal, the gallbladder contracts, delivering the bile through the bile ducts into the intestines to help with digestion.

gallbladder absence See *agenesis of the gallbladder*.

gallium A rare metal with the atomic weight 69. There are several isotopic forms of gallium that differ from it in atomic weight. One is gallium-68, which is produced by cyclotrons and emits gamma rays. The citrate form of gallium-68 is used as a radiotracer to locate sites of inflammation and tumor tissue within the body.

gallop rhythm An abnormal heart rhythm that pounds in the chest resembling the gallop of a horse when heard during examination with a stethoscope.

gallstone A stone that forms when substances in bile harden. A gallstone can be as small as a grain of sand or as large as a golf ball. There can be just one large stone, hundreds of tiny stones, or any combination and number. Gallstones can block the normal flow of bile if they lodge in any of the ducts that carry bile from the liver to the small intestine, including the hepatic ducts, which carry bile out of the liver; the cystic duct, which takes bile to and from the gallbladder; and the common bile duct, which takes bile from the cystic and hepatic ducts to the small intestine. Bile trapped in these ducts can cause inflammation in the gallbladder, the ducts, or, rarely, the liver. Other ducts open into the common bile duct, including the pancreatic duct, which carries digestive enzymes out of the pancreas. If a gallstone blocks the opening to that duct, digestive enzymes can become trapped in the pancreas and cause extremely painful inflammation called gallstone pancreatitis. Gallstone attacks often occur after a meal, especially a fatty one. Symptoms can include pain for up to several hours in the upper back or under the right shoulder, together with nausea, vomiting, abdominal bloating, or indigestion. There are two types of gallstones: cholesterol stones and pigment stones. Gallstones are most common among women, Native Americans, Mexican Americans, and people who are overweight. Laparoscopic surgery to remove the gallbladder is the most common treatment. Also known as cholelithiasis.

gallstone, microscopic See *biliary sand*.

gamete Germ cell.

gamma knife A tool that uses highly focused radiation to perform neurosurgery without making an incision. A gamma knife is used to treat many types of brain tumors as well as arteriovenous malformations in the brain. It is being used experimentally to treat Parkinson's disease, chronic pain, and other disorders. See also *radiation therapy, stereotactic*.

ganglion **1** An aggregation of nerve cell bodies. **2** A tendon cyst, commonly near the wrist.

gangliosidosis, GM1 See *GM1-gangliosidosis.*

gangliosidosis, GM2 See *Sandhoff diseasee.*

gangrene Tissue death due to loss of adequate blood supply. Sometimes bacteria invade such tissue and accelerate its decay. Dry gangrene is the death of tissue due to vascular insufficiency without bacterial invasion. The tissue dies, loses sensation and simply dries up, blackens, and shrivels. Dry gangrene eventually requires amputation. Gas gangrene occurs when body tissue is invaded by bacteria that thrive in areas of low oxygen content. These bacteria are called anaerobic bacteria and include the Clostridium family of bacteria. The bacteria generate gas and pus and the tissues swells and can become painful. Wet gangrene requires urgent antibiotic treatment and sometimes surgical drainage.

Gareis-Mason syndrome See *MASA syndrome.*

gargoylism See *Hurler syndrome.*

gas chromatography See *chromatography, gas.*

gas, intestinal See *flatulence; flatus.*

gas, laughing See *nitrous oxide.*

gastrectomy Surgery to remove part or all of the stomach.

gastric Having to do with the stomach.

gastric atrophy A condition in which the stomach muscles shrink and become weak. Gastric atrophy results in a lack of digestive juices.

gastric cancer See *cancer, gastric.*

gastric emptying study A test that evaluates the process of emptying food from the stomach. For a gastric emptying study, a patient eats a meal in which the food or beverage is mixed with a small amount of radioactive material. A scanner that acts like a Geiger counter is placed over the stomach to monitor the amount of radioactivity in the stomach for several hours after the test meal. In patients with abnormal emptying of the stomach, the food and radioactive material stay in the stomach longer than normal (usually for hours) before emptying into the small intestine.

gastric stapling A surgical procedure that converts the upper part of the stomach into a very small pouch, forcing the patient to eat only tiny portions yet still feel full.

Gastric stapling is normally done only in severe cases of obesity and in combination with diet and exercise. As the name suggests, surgical staples are used in this procedure. A similar operation is called gastric banding. Both operations have the potential for serious side effects.

gastric ulcer A hole in the lining of the stomach that is caused by the acidic digestive juices secreted by the stomach cells. Ulcer formation is related to infection with H. pylori bacteria in the stomach, the use of anti-inflammatory medications, and the smoking of cigarettes. Ulcer pain may not correlate with the presence or severity of ulceration. Diagnosis is made via barium X-ray endoscopy.

gastritis Inflammation of the stomach.

gastroenteritis Inflammation of the stomach and the intestines. Gastroenteritis can cause nausea, vomiting, and diarrhea. Gastroenteritis has numerous causes, including infections (viruses, bacteria, and so on), food poisoning, and stress.

gastroenterologist A physician who specializes in the diagnosis and treatment of diseases of the digestive system.

gastroesophageal reflux disease A condition in which the stomach contents return back up into the esophagus. Abbreviated GERD. GERD frequently causes heartburn because of irritation of the esophagus by stomach acid. GERD can lead to scarring and stricture of the esophagus, which requires stretching (dilating) of the esophagus. Ten percent of patients with GERD develop Barrett esophagus, which increases the risk of cancer of the esophagus. Eighty percent of patients with GERD also have hiatal hernias.

gastrointestinal tract The stomach and intestines. Abbreviated GI tract.

gastroparesis A disease of the muscles of the stomach or the nerves controlling the muscles that causes the muscles to stop working. Gastroparesis results in inadequate grinding of food by the stomach and poor emptying of food from the stomach into the intestine. The primary symptoms of gastroparesis are nausea and vomiting. Gastroparesis may be associated with paralysis of the small intestine and colon. The most common underlying cause is diabetes mellitus. Gastroparesis is diagnosed via gastric emptying study. It is usually treated with medications that stimulate the stomach muscle to contract.

gastroscope A flexible, lighted instrument that is put through the mouth and esophagus to view the stomach. Tissue from the stomach can be removed through a gastroscope.

gastrostomy A surgical opening into the stomach. A gastrostomy may be used for feeding, usually via a feeding tube called a gastrostomy tube. Feeding can also be done through a percutaneous endoscopic gastrostomy (PEG) tube.

gastrostomy, percutaneous endoscopic A surgical procedure for placing a feeding tube without having to perform an open laparotomy operation on the abdomen. Abbreviated PEG. The aim of PEG is to feed those who cannot swallow. PEG may be done by a surgeon, an oto-laryngologist, or a gastroenterologist. It is done in a hospital or an outpatient surgical facility. Local anesthesia (usually lidocaine or another spray) is used to anesthetize the throat. An endoscope is passed through the mouth, throat, and esophagus to the stomach. The surgeon then makes a small incision in the skin of the abdomen, pushes an IV tube through the skin into the stomach, and then sutures (ties) the tube in place. The patient can usually go home the same day or the next morning. Possible complications include wound infection and dislodging or malfunction of the tube. PEG takes less time, carries less risk, and costs less than a classic surgical gastrostomy, which requires opening the abdomen. PEG is used for feeding as well as administering medications.

Gaucher disease A series of five disorders that are due to deficient activity of the enzyme glucocerebrosidase, which leads to accumulation of glucocerebroside in tissues of the body. The five types of Gaucher disease encompass a continuum of clinical findings from a lethal form that occurs before or just after birth to a form so mild that it may not be diagnosed until old age. All five types of Gaucher disease are inherited in an autosomal recessive manner.

Gaucher disease, type 1 The most common and best-known form of Gaucher disease, which affects the spleen, liver, and bone marrow but spares the brain. The symptoms of type 1 Gaucher disease include enlargement of the spleen (usually the first sign), anemia, low blood platelet level, increased skin pigmentation, and a yellow fatty spot on the white of the eye (pinguecula). Severe bone involvement can lead to pain and collapse of the bones of the hips, shoulders, and spine. This type of Gaucher disease is the most common genetic disease among Jews in the US.

Gaucher disease, types 2 through 5 Relatively uncommon forms of Gaucher disease. Types 2 and 3 are characterized by primary neurologic disease. The onset of types 2 and 3 occurs before age 2, with death by age 2 to 4 in type 2 and a more slowly progressive course with survival into the third or fourth decade in type 3. Type 4 is lethal in the perinatal period and is marked by glossy skin

and excessive fluid in the fetal tissues. Type 5 is a cardiovascular form of Gaucher disease, with calcification of the aortic and mitral valves, mild spleen enlargement, and eye involvement.

gene 1 In classical genetics, a unit of inheritance. 2 In molecular genetics, a sequence of chromosomal DNA that is required to make a functional product.

gene, breast cancer susceptibility See *breast cancer susceptibility gene.*

gene deletion The total loss or absence of a gene. Gene deletion plays a role in birth defects and in the development of cancer.

gene duplication An extra copy of a gene. Gene duplication is a key mechanism in evolution. After a gene is duplicated, the once-identical genes can undergo changes and diverge to create two different genes.

gene, evolutionarily conserved A gene that has remained essentially unchanged throughout evolution. Conservation of a gene indicates that it is unique and essential. There is not an extra copy of that gene with which evolution can tinker. Changes in the gene are likely to be lethal.

gene expression The translation of information encoded in a gene into protein or RNA structures that are present and operating in the cell. Expressed genes include genes that are transcribed into messenger RNA (mRNA) and then translated into protein, as well as genes that are transcribed into RNA, such as transfer and ribosomal RNAs, but not translated into protein.

gene family A group of genes that are related in structure and often in function. The genes in a gene family are descended from an ancestral gene. For example, the hemoglobin genes belong to one gene family that was created by gene duplication and divergence.

gene mapping The charting of the positions of genes on a DNA molecule or chromosome and the distance, in linkage units or physical units, between genes. Although the human genome has been sequenced, many human genes have still not yet been mapped.

gene marker A detectable genetic trait or distinctive segment of DNA that serves as a landmark for a target gene. Markers are on the same chromosome as the target gene. They must be near enough to the target gene to be genetically linked to it and to be inherited, usually together with that gene, and thereby serve as signposts to it.

gene product The RNA or protein that results from the expression of a gene. The amount of gene product is a measure of the degree of gene activity.

gene, target The primary gene of concern. See also *gene, marker.*

gene testing The testing of a sample of blood (or another fluid or tissue) for evidence of a gene. The aim of gene testing is usually to learn whether a gene for a disease is present or absent.

gene therapy The treatment of disease by replacing, altering, or supplementing a gene that is absent or abnormal and that is responsible for the disease. In studies of gene therapy for cancer, researchers are trying to bolster the body's natural capacity to combat cancer and make the cancer more sensitive to other kinds of therapy. Gene therapy, still in its early stages, holds great promise for the treatment of many diseases. The first gene therapy was done successfully in humans in 1990.

gene, zygotic lethal A gene that is fatal for the zygote, the cell formed by the union of a sperm and an egg. The zygote would normally develop into an embryo, as instructed by the genetic material within the unified cell. However, a zygotic lethal gene kills prenatal development at its earliest point. A zygotic lethal gene is a mutated version of a normal gene that is essential to the survival of the zygote. The extent of the mutation can range from a change in a single base in the DNA to deletion of the entire gene.

general paresis Progressive dementia and generalized paralysis due to chronic inflammation of the covering and substance of the brain (meningoencephalitis). General paresis is a part of late (tertiary) syphilis, occurring a decade or more after the initial infection.

genetic Having to do with genes and genetic information.

genetic code See *code, genetic.*

genetic counseling An educational counseling process for individuals and families who have a genetic disease or may be at risk for a disease. Genetic counseling is designed to provide patients and their families with information about their condition, to permit them to make informed decisions. Genetic counseling is, by design, nondirectional. Decisions are made by the patient.

genetic counselor A health professional who has a graduate degree, most commonly a master's degree, and training in the areas of genetics and genetic counseling.

genetic infantile agranulocytosis See *severe congenital neutropenia.*

genetic screening Testing of a population to identify individuals who are at risk for a genetic disease or for transmitting a gene for a genetic disease. For example, newborns may be screened for phenylketonuria (PKU) and galactosemia, Jews may be screened for the Tay-Sachs disease gene, and African-Americans may be tested for the sickle cell gene.

genetic transport disease Within the body, many molecules are able to pass across the membranes that surround cells. The molecules can accomplish this feat because of specific transport systems that include special receptors on the membrane of the cell and because of special carrier proteins. The receptor recognizes the molecule and receives it on the cell membrane, and the molecule then hitches a ride through the cell membrane on the back of a carrier protein. With such remarkable specificity, it is little wonder that sometimes there are defects in transport systems. Several dozen diseases are known to be due to transport defects. An example of a transport disease is cystinuria, the most common defect known in the transport of an amino acid (namely, cystine) and a significant cause of kidney stones.

genital Pertaining to the external and/or internal organs of reproduction.

genital herpes A viral infection that is transmitted through intimate contact with the moist mucous linings of the genitals. This contact can involve the mouth, the vagina, or the genital skin. The herpes simplex type 2 virus enters the mucous membranes through microscopic tears. Once it is inside, the virus travels to nerve roots near the spinal cord and settles there permanently. When an infected person has a herpes outbreak, the virus travels down the nerve fibers to the site of the original infection; when it reaches the skin, redness and blisters occur. The outbreak of herpes is closely related to the functioning of the immune system. Women who have suppressed immune systems, either through stress, disease, or medications, have more frequent and longer-lasting outbreaks than those with normal immunity. Commonly called herpes.

genital warts Warts confined primarily to the moist skin of the genitals or around the anus. Genital warts are due to viruses belonging to the human papillomavirus (HPV) family, which are transmitted through sexual contact. The virus can also be transmitted from mother to baby during childbirth. Also known as condyloma acuminatum, condylomata, and venereal warts. See also *HPV.*

genitalia The male or female reproductive organs. The genitalia include internal and external structures. The female internal genitalia are the ovaries, Fallopian tubes, uterus, cervix, and vagina. The female external genitalia are the labia minora and majora (the vulva) and the clitoris. The male internal genitalia are the testes, epididymis, and vas deferens. The male external genitalia are the penis and scrotum.

genitourinary Pertaining to the genital and urinary systems.

genome All the genetic information possessed by any organism (for example, the human genome, the elephant genome, the mouse genome, the yeast genome, and the genome of a bacterium). Humans and many other higher animals actually have two genomes—a chromosomal genome and a mitochondrial genome—that together make up their genome.

genome, chromosomal All the genetic information in the chromosomes of an organism. For humans, the chromosomal genome is all the DNA contained in the normal complement of 46 rod-like chromosomes in virtually every cell in the body. (Mature red blood cells, for one exception, have no nucleus and, therefore, no chromosomes.) Together with the mitochondrial genome, the chromosomal genome constitutes the genome of the human being. Also known as nuclear genome.

genome, human All the genetic information in a person. Humanity's DNA is the treasury of human inheritance. The human genome is made up of the DNA in chromosomes as well as in the DNA in mitochondria. The human genome includes every gene as well as all the junk DNA in humans.

genome, mitochondrial The sum of the genetic information contained in the chromosome of the mitochondrion, a structure located in the cytoplasm outside the nucleus of the cell. The mitochondrial genome is composed of mitochondrial DNA (mDNA), a double-stranded circular molecule that contains a limited number of genes. During fertilization, mDNA is transmitted only by the mother. Together, the mitochondrial genome and the chromosomal genome constitute the entire human genome.

genome, nuclear See *genome, chromosomal.*

genomic library A collection of clones that is made from a set of randomly generated overlapping DNA fragments and that represents the entire genome of an organism. Also known as clone bank.

genotype The genetic constitution (genome) of a cell, an individual, or an organism. The genotype is distinct from the expressed features, or phenotype, of the cell, individual, or organism. The genotype of a person is that person's genetic makeup. It can pertain to all genes or to a specific gene.

genu The Latin word for knee, as in genu recurvatum (hyperextension of the knee), genu valgum (knock knee), and genu varum (bowleg). See *knee.*

GERD Gastroesophageal reflux disease.

germ cell Either the egg or the sperm cell; a reproductive cell. Each mature germ cell is haploid, meaning that it has a single set of 23 chromosomes containing half the usual amount of DNA and half the usual number of genes. Except for the egg and the sperm, most cells in the human body contain the entire human genome. Also known as a gamete.

germ cell tumor A tumor that arises from a germ cell. A germ cell tumor may arise within the gonads (in the ovary or testis). Most testicular tumors, in fact, are germ cell tumors. Germ cell tumors also may arise in extragonadal sites, reflecting the fact that germ cells travel to diverse areas of the body, such as the chest, abdomen, and brain.

German measles See *rubella.*

German measles immunization See *MMR.*

germinoma A rare cancer of the germ cells (the tissue that normally differentiates to become the eggs or sperm cells). For example, a teratoma of the testis is a type of germinoma.

gestalt therapy An older psychotherapeutic concept that stresses understanding mental processes as holistic entities (gestalts) rather than as discrete steps. Gestalt therapy often uses group therapy techniques to help patients gain this type of insight. For example, gestalt therapy would come to an understanding that the chicken crossed the road to get to the other side, as opposed to analyzing how the chicken stepped off of the curb, then walked across the road, then stepped up onto the opposite curb. See also *group therapy.*

gestation From conception to birth.

gestational diabetes See *diabetes, gestational.*

GI tract See *gastrointestinal tract.*

giant cell arteritis See *arteritis, cranial.*

giant cell pneumonia See *pneumonia, giant cell.*

giant platelet syndrome See *Bernard-Soulier syndrome.*

gigantism **1** Extreme growth in height. Gigantism is usually associated with disorders of the pituitary gland, which secretes human growth hormone (somatotrophin) during childhood, before the bones fuse. **2** Extreme growth of specific body parts. See also *gigantism, focal.*

gigantism, eunuchoid   Extremely tall stature due to the delayed onset of puberty that permits the continued growth of the long bones before their growing ends (epiphyses) fuse and growth stops.

gigantism, focal   Extreme growth of specific body parts, such as one arm, the tongue, or a combination of parts, as seen in Beckwith-Wiedemann syndrome or acromegaly. Focal gigantism may occur before or after the bones fuse. If it occurs afterward, it causes disfigurement. Surgery for mass reduction can help improve function, and other treatments may be available for specific conditions.

gigantism, pituitary   Extreme growth in height caused by oversecretion of growth hormone (somatotrophin) by the anterior pituitary gland. Other features of pituitary gigantism include thickening of the skin, enlargement of the bones, and elongation of the jaw and other areas. Pituitary gigantism may be caused by an adenoma of the pituitary gland, a benign tumor of the pituitary gland, or other causes. Treatment is usually possible with hormones, surgery, or both. See also *acromegaly.*

Gilbert syndrome   A common but harmless genetic condition in which UDP-glucuronosyltransferase, a liver enzyme that is essential to the disposal of bilirubin, is abnormal. This enzyme abnormality causes mild elevations of bilirubin pigment in the blood, and the elevated bilirubin pigment can sometimes cause mild yellowing (jaundice) of the eyes. People with Gilbert syndrome otherwise have no other signs or symptoms. There is no need for treatment of Gilbert syndrome, and the prognosis is excellent. It is usually detected by accident in the course of routine blood screening. Gilbert syndrome is caused by mutation in the UDP-glucuronosyltransferase gene. Gilbert syndrome is inherited as an autosomal dominant trait. A person who has Gilbert syndrome has a 50 percent chance of transmitting the UDP-glucuronosyltransferase gene for Gilbert syndrome to each of his or her children. Mutations in the same gene cause the Crigler-Najjar syndrome, which is a more severe and dangerous form of hyperbilirubinemia (high bilirubin in the blood). Also known as hyperbilirubinemia type 1.

gingiva   The gums.

gingivitis   Gum disease with inflammation of the gums. On inspection, the gums appear red and puffy, and they usually bleed during tooth-brushing or dental examination. Treatment involves improved cleaning, with more frequent and longer-duration brushing and flossing, and/or the use of electronic tooth-cleaning equipment.

Antiseptic mouthwashes may also be recommended. See also *acute membranous gingivitis; gum disease.*

gland   **1** A group of cells that secrete a substance for use in the body. For example, the thyroid gland. **2** A group of cells that remove materials from the circulation. For example, a lymph gland.

gland, mammary   One of the glands within the breast that secretes milk when prompted to do so by special hormones. During menstruation and pregnancy, the mammary glands become tender to the touch. They also become enlarged when they are engorged with milk. See also *mastitis.*

gland, Meibomian   One of the little glands in the eyelids that make a lubricant called sebum that is discharged through tiny openings in the edges of the lids. The Meibomian glands can become inflamed, a condition termed meibomianitis or meibomitis. Chronic inflammation leads to cysts of the Meibomian glands, called chalazions. Also known as the palpebral gland, tarsal gland, and tarsoconjunctival gland. See also *cyst, Meibomian; sebum.*

gland, palpebral   See *gland, Meibomian.*

gland, parotid   See *parotid gland.*

gland, prostate   A gland in the male reproductive system that is located just below the bladder. The prostate gland surrounds part of the urethra, the canal that empties the bladder. The prostate is actually not 1 gland; it is 30 to 50 glands. Between these glands is tissue that contains bundles of smooth muscle. The prostate gland secretes a milky fluid that is discharged into the urethra at the time of ejaculation of semen and is part of semen. See also *prostate enlargement; prostatitis.*

gland, sebaceous   One of the skin glands that empty an oily secretion called sebum into the hair follicles near the surface of the skin. Sebum helps to keep skin moist and protected. See also *cyst, sebaceous.*

gland, sudoriferous   See *gland, sweat.*

gland, sweat   A small tubular gland that is situated in the subcutaneous tissue within and under the skin. Sweat glands discharge sweat through tiny openings in the surface of the skin. The sweat itself is a transparent, colorless, acidic fluid that contains some fatty acids and mineral matter. Also known as sudoriferous gland.

gland, tarsal   See *gland, Meibomian.*

gland, thyroid   A gland that makes and stores hormones that help regulate heart rate, blood pressure, body temperature, and the rate at which food is converted into energy. Thyroid hormones are essential for the function of every cell in the body. They help regulate growth and the rate of chemical reactions (metabolism) in the body. Thyroid hormones also help children grow and develop. The thyroid gland is located in the lower part of the neck, below the Adam's apple, wrapped around the windpipe (the trachea). It has the shape of a butterfly: two wings (lobes) attached to one another by a middle part. The thyroid uses iodine, a mineral found in some foods and in iodized salt, to make its hormones. The two most important thyroid hormones are thyroxine (T4) and triiodothyronine (T3). Thyroid stimulating hormone (TSH), which is produced by the pituitary gland, acts to stimulate hormone production by the thyroid gland. The thyroid gland also makes the hormone calcitonin, which is involved in calcium metabolism and stimulating bone cells to add calcium to bone. See also *calcitonin; hyperthyroid; hypothyroidism; thyroxine; triiodothyronine.*

glandular fever   Infectious mononucleosis. See also *mononucleosis.*

glans   1 The glans penis, the rounded head of the penis. 2 The rounded head of the clitoris.

glans and foreskin, inflammation of the   See *balanoposthitis.*

glans penis, inflammation of the   See *balanitis.*

glaucoma   A common eye condition in which the fluid pressure inside the eye rises because of slowed fluid drainage from the eye. If untreated, glaucoma may damage the optic nerve and other parts of the eye, causing the loss of vision or even blindness. There are no symptoms in the early stages of glaucoma. Vision stays normal, and there is no pain. As the disease progresses, however, a person with glaucoma may notice that side vision is gradually failing; objects in front may still be seen clearly, but objects to the side may be missed. As the disease worsens, the field of vision narrows, and blindness may result. Glaucoma has been called "the sneak thief of sight." By the time someone notices the loss of vision, glaucoma can only be halted, not reversed. There are several types of glaucoma, including open-angle glaucoma and acute angle-closure glaucoma. Open-angle glaucoma is the common adult-onset type of glaucoma. Acute angle-closure glaucoma is a less common form of glaucoma, but one that can rapidly impair vision. Glaucoma treatment may include medication, surgery, or laser surgery. Eyedrops or pills alone can usually control glaucoma, although they can't cure it. Some drugs are designed to reduce pressure by slowing the flow of fluid into the eye, and others help to improve fluid drainage. Surgery to help fluid escape from the eye was once extensively used, but except for laser surgery, surgery is now reserved for the most difficult cases. In laser surgery for glaucoma, a laser beam of light is focused on the part of the anterior chamber where the fluid leaves the eye. This results in a series of small changes, making it easier for fluid to exit. Over time, the effect of laser surgery may wear off.

glaucoma, angle-closure   See *angle-closure glaucoma.*

glaucoma detection   The common "air puff" test to measure eye pressure during routine eye examinations. This screening test alone cannot detect glaucoma. Glaucoma is found most often during eye examinations after drops have been put into the eyes to dilate (enlarge) the pupils. This allows the eye-care professional to see more of the inside of the eye and to check for physical signs of glaucoma such as changes of the optic nerve of the retina. The eye pressure can then be accurately diagnosed using a pressure measuring device called a tonometer.

glaucoma, risk factors   Factors that predispose individuals to being at risk for glaucoma, including family history of glaucoma, being over age 60, and being African-American and over age 40. Glaucoma is five times more likely to occur and about four times more likely to cause blindness in African-Americans than in whites. People of Asian or Eskimo ancestry are at particularly high risk for developing angle-closure glaucoma. People belonging to a high-risk group for glaucoma should have their eyes examined through pupil dilation by an eye-care professional every 2 years.

gliaden   A protein found in wheat and some other grains that is part of wheat gluten. People with celiac sprue, Crohn's disease, and related conditions may be sensitive to gliaden in the diet. See also *celiac sprue; Crohn's disease; dermatitis herpetiformis.*

glial cell   A supportive cell in the central nervous system. Unlike neurons, glial cells do not conduct electrical impulses. The glial cells surround neurons and provide support for and insulation between them. Glial cells are the most abundant cell types in the central nervous system. There are three types of glial cells: astrocytes, oligodendrocytes, and microglia. Astrocytes are concerned with neurotransmission and neuronal metabolism. Oligodendrocytes are involved in the production of myelin, the insulating material around neurons. Microglia are part of the immune system.

glioblastoma multiforme   A highly malignant type of brain tumor that arises from glial cells in the brain. Glioblastoma multiforme is highly malignant, grows very quickly, and has cells that look quite different from normal glial cells. Early symptoms may include sleepiness, headache, and vomiting. Also called a grade IV astrocytoma. Treatment can involve surgery and radiation treatment.

glioma A brain tumor that begins in a glial cell in the brain or spinal cord. Malignant gliomas are the most common primary tumors of the central nervous system. They are often resistant to treatment and carry a poor prognosis. See also *glioma, optic.*

glioma, optic A benign tumor on the optic nerve or the optic chiasm (the crossing of the two optic nerves). Optic gliomas cause pressure and destruction of normal optic nerve tissue. They may result in proptosis (protrusion of the eye) and progressive loss of vision. Optic gliomas are associated with neurofibromatosis (NF1).

globus The sensation of having a lump in the throat when nothing is really there. Although this symptom can be all in the patient's imagination, globus can also be a symptom of disease, such as reflux laryngitis. Also known as globus hystericus.

globus hystericus See *globus.*

globus major The head of the epididymis, the structure just behind the testis.

globus minor The tail of the epididymis, a cordlike structure just behind the testis.

globus pallidus A comparatively pale-looking, spherical area in the brain. The globus pallidus is specifically part of the lentiform nucleus, which in turn is part of the striate body, a component of the basal ganglia. Also called pale globe, palladum, and paleostriatum.

glossitis Inflammation of the tongue. There are many possible causes of glossitis, including vitamin B12 deficiency, Sjogren's syndrome, and side effects of medications or chemotherapy.

glossolalia **1** A condition in which a person makes nonsensical sounds that mimic the rhythms and inflections of actual speech. Glossolalia may be seen in deep sleep or in trance states. **2** The scientific term for the religious phenomenon known as "speaking in tongues."

glossopharyngeal nerve The ninth cranial nerve, which supplies the tongue, throat, and one of the salivary glands (the parotid gland). Problems with the glossopharyngeal nerve result in trouble tasting and swallowing.

glottis The middle part of the larynx, where the vocal cords are located.

glucocerebrosidase deficiency An enzyme deficiency that causes Gaucher disease. See also *Gaucher disease; Gaucher disease, type 1; Gaucher disease, types 2 through 5.*

glucocorticoid See *corticosteroid.*

glucosamine A molecule derived from the sugar glucose by the addition of an amino group. Glucosamine is a component of a number of structures, including the blood group substances and cartilage. Glucosamine is currently in use as a nutritional supplement (often in combination with chondroitin) and is touted as a remedy for arthritic symptoms.

glucose The simple sugar that is the chief source of energy. Glucose is found in the blood and is the main sugar that the body manufactures. The body makes glucose from all three elements of food—protein, fats, and carbohydrates—but the largest amount of glucose derives from carbohydrates. Glucose serves as the major source of energy for living cells. It is carried to each cell through the bloodstream. However, cells cannot use glucose without the help of insulin. Also known as dextrose.

glucose, fasting blood See *fasting blood glucose.*

glucose tolerance test A test of carbohydrate metabolism that is used in the diagnosis of diabetes, among other disorders. Abbreviated GTT. After the patient has fasted overnight, but before breakfast, a specific amount (100 grams) of glucose is given by mouth, and the blood levels of this sugar are measured every hour. Normally, the blood glucose should return to normal within 2 to 2½ hours. The GTT result depends on a number of factors, including the ability of the intestines to absorb glucose, the power of the liver to take up and store glucose, the capacity of the pancreas to produce insulin, and the amount of "active" insulin.

glucose-6-phosphate dehydrogenase See *G6PD.*

glucosylceramidosis See *Gaucher disease.*

glucuronosyltransferase, UDP- A liver enzyme that is essential to the disposal of bilirubin. An abnormality of UDP-glucuronosyltransferase results in a condition called Gilbert syndrome. See also *Gilbert syndrome.*

gluteal Pertaining to the buttocks region, which is formed by the gluteus maximus, gluteus medius, and gluteus minimus muscles.

gluten A protein that is found in wheat and related grains. Gluten can be found in a large variety of processed foods, including soups, salad dressings, and natural flavorings. Unidentified starches, hydrolyzed proteins, and binders and fillers used in medications or vitamins can be unsuspected sources of gluten. People with celiac sprue, Crohn's disease, or related disorders may need to avoid gluten products. See also *gliaden*.

gluten enteropathy   See *celiac sprue*.

glycosaminoglycan   A negatively charged chain of polysaccharides (modified sugars) that is composed of repeating disaccharide units. Abbreviated GAG. Important GAGs in the human body include chondroitin sulfate, dermatan sulfate, heparan sulfate, heparin, hyaluronate, and keratan sulfate. GAGs are involved as lubricants and components of bone, cartilage, blood vessels, and certain types of cells. Also known as mucopolysaccharides.

GM1-gangliosidosis   A genetic lipid storage disorder that is similar to Hurler syndrome and Tay-Sachs disease but that affects both the brain and the viscera. Symptoms include skeletal deformities and severe effects on the brain and organs. Death occurs by age 2 in most cases. The mutation that is responsible for the disease is located on chromosome 3 in band 3p21. There is no treatment for GM1-gangliosidosis. Also known as familial neurovisceral lipidosis and Landing disease. See also *Hurler syndrome; sphingolipidosis; Tay-Sachs disease*.

GM2-gangliosidosis   A genetic lipid storage disorder that affects the brain. The two GM2 gangliosidoses are Tay-Sachs disease (due to hexosaminidase A deficiency) and Sandhoff disease (due to hexosaminidase B deficiency). See also *Sandhoff disease; Tay-Sachs disease*.

goiter   A noncancerous enlargement of the thyroid gland. With a goiter, the levels of thyroid hormones may be normal (euthyroid), elevated (hyperthyroidism), or decreased (hypothyroidism).

goiter, diffuse toxic   See *Graves disease*.

goiter, exophthalmic   See *Graves disease*.

goiter, iodide   A goiter caused by prolonged intake of too much iodine and abnormally low thyroid activity (hypothyroidism). Certain foods and medications contain large amounts of iodine. Examples include seaweed; iodine-rich expectorants (Brand names: SSKI and Lugol solution) used in the treatment of cough, asthma, and chronic pulmonary disease; and amiodarone (brand name: Cardorone), an iodine-rich medication used in the control of abnormal heart rhythms.

goiter, toxic multinodular   A condition in which the thyroid gland contains multiple lumps (nodules) that are overactive and that produce excess thyroid hormones. Also known as Parry disease and Plummer disease.

goiter-deafness syndrome   See *Pendred syndrome*.

golfer's cramp   A dystonia that affects the muscles of the hand and sometimes the forearm and that occurs only when a person is playing golf. Similar focal dystonias have also been called typist's cramp, pianist's cramp, musician's cramp, and writer's cramp.

golfer's elbow   See *elbow, golfer's*.

gonad   A reproductive gland that produces germ cells (gametes): an ovary or testis.

gonad, female   See *ovary*.

gonad, indifferent   A gonad in an embryo that has not differentiated into a definitive testis or ovary. An indifferent gonad becomes a testis if the embryo has a Y chromosome, but if the embryo has no Y chromosome, the indifferent gonad becomes an ovary. Thus, an XY chromosome complement leads to testes, and an XX chromosome complement leads to ovaries. People with just one X chromosome and no Y are females with Turner syndrome, and are infertile. The absence of a Y chromosome permits the indifferent gonad to become an ovary, but both X chromosomes are needed for the ovary to function normally.

gonad, male   See *testis*.

gonadotropin   One of the hormones that are secreted by the pituitary gland and that affect the function of the male or female gonads. See also *follicle-stimulating hormone; human chorionic gonadotropin; luteinizing hormone*.

gonadotropin, human chorionic   See *human chorionic gonadotropin*.

gonorrhea   A bacterial infection that is transmitted by sexual contact. Gonorrhea is one of the oldest known sexually transmitted diseases (STDs), and it is caused by the Neisseria gonorrhoeae bacteria. Gonorrhea cannot be transmitted via toilet seats or other inanimate objects. Men with gonorrhea may have a yellowish discharge from the penis, accompanied by itching and burning. More than half of women with gonorrhea do not have any symptoms. If symptoms occur, they may include burning or frequent urination, yellowish vaginal discharge, redness and swelling of the genitals, and a burning or itching of the vaginal area. If untreated, gonorrhea can lead to severe pelvic infections and even sterility. Complications in later life can include inflammation of the heart valves, arthritis, and eye infections. Gonorrhea can also cause eye infections in babies born of infected mothers. Gonorrhea is treated with antibiotics.

goose bumps A temporary local change in the skin that starts with a stimulus, such as cold or fear. That stimulus causes a nerve discharge from the sympathetic nervous system, which is part of the autonomic nervous system. The nerve discharge causes contraction of the hair erector muscle (arrectores pilorum), elevating the hair follicles above the rest of the skin. These tiny elevations are what we perceive as goose bumps. Some biologists believe that goose bumps evolved as part of the fight-or-flight reaction. A similar phenomenon, bristling, makes fur-covered animals look larger and more frightening than they are. Also called cutis anserina, goose flesh, and horripilation.

goose flesh See *goose bumps*.

Gottron sign A scaly, patchy redness over the knuckles that is seen in patients with dermatomyositis, an inflammatory muscle disorder. See also *polymyositis*.

gout A condition that is characterized by abnormally elevated levels of uric acid in the blood, recurring attacks of joint inflammation (arthritis), deposits of hard lumps of uric acid in and around the joints, and decreased kidney function and kidney stones. Uric acid is a breakdown product of purines, which are part of many foods we eat. The tendency to develop gout and elevated blood levels of uric acid (hyperuricemia) is often inherited, and it can be promoted by obesity, weight gain, alcohol intake, high blood pressure, abnormal kidney function, and certain drugs. The most reliable diagnostic test for gout is the identification of crystals in joints, body fluids, and tissues. The treatment of an attack of gouty arthritis includes taking measures to reduce inflammation such as ice applications, resting the inflamed joint, and antiinflammatory medications. See also *gout, tophaceous; gouty arthritis; hyperuricemia*.

gout, tophaceous A form of chronic gout that is characterized by the deposit of nodular masses of uric acid crystals (tophi) in different soft tissue areas of the body. Even though tophi are most commonly found as hard nodules around the fingers, at the tips of the elbows, and around the big toe, tophi nodules can appear anywhere in the body. They have been reported in unexpected areas, such as in the ears, in the vocal cords, or around the spinal cord. See also *gout*.

gouty arthritis An attack of joint inflammation that is due to deposits of uric acid crystals in the joint fluid (synovial fluid) and joint lining (synovial lining). Gouty arthritis attacks can be precipitated by dehydration, injury, fever, heavy eating, heavy drinking of alcohol, and recent surgery. Intense joint inflammation occurs when white blood cells engulf the uric acid crystals, causing pain, heat, and redness of the joint tissues. The term gout is

commonly used to refer to these painful arthritis attacks, but gouty arthritis is only one manifestation of gout. See also *gout*.

Gower syndrome See *syncope, situational*.

graft Healthy skin, bone, kidney, liver, or other tissue that is taken from one part of the body to replace diseased or injured tissue removed from another part of the body. For example, skin grafts can be used to cover areas of skin that have been burned.

graft-versus-host disease A complication of bone marrow transplants in which the donor bone marrow attacks the host's organs and tissues. Abbreviated GVHD. GVHD is seen most often in cases where the blood marrow donor is unrelated to the patient or when the donor is related to the patient, but is not a perfect match. There are two forms of GVHD: acute GVHD and chronic GVHD. Acute GVHD typically occurs within the first 3 months after a transplant and can affect the skin, liver, stomach, and/or intestines. The earliest sign is usually a rash on the hand, feet, and face that may spread and look like a sunburn. Severe problems with acute GVHD may include blisters on the skin, watery or bloody diarrhea with cramping, and jaundice (yellowing of the skin and eyes) due to liver involvement. Chronic GVHD typically occurs 2 to 3 months after the transplant and causes symptoms similar to those of autoimmune disorders such as lupus and scleroderma. Patients develop a dry, itchy rash that is raised and like alligator skin. There may also be hair loss, decrease in sweating in the skin, and premature graying of the hair. Mouth dryness is a common symptom, and it may progress to sensitivity to spicy and acidic foods. The eyes may also be dry, irritated, and red. Almost any organ can be affected by chronic GVHD. Prevention of severe GVHD includes elutriation (T-cell depletion), a technique in which the donor bone marrow is largely depleted of the T-cells that cause GVHD. Most patients also receive immunosuppressive drugs such as cyclosporine and methotrexate. Severe GVHD is usually treated with steroids and sometimes a drug called antithymocyte globulin.

grand mal seizure See *seizure, tonic-clonic*.

granulation That part of the healing process in which lumpy, pink tissue containing new connective tissue and capillaries forms around the edges of a wound. Granulation of a wound is normal and desirable.

granulocyte A type of white blood cell that is filled with microscopic granules, little sacs containing enzymes that digest microorganisms. Granulocytes are part of the innate immune system, and they have somewhat nonspecific, broad-based activity. They do not respond exclusively to specific antigens, as do B-cells and T-cells. Neutrophils, eosinophils, and basophils are all types of granulocytes, and their names are derived from the staining features of their granules in the laboratory: Neutrophils have subtle "neutral" granules, eosinophils have prominent granules that stain with the acid dye eosin, and basophils have prominent granules that stain with basic (alkaline) dyes. This naming scheme dates back to a time when certain structures could be identified in cells by histochemistry, but the functions of these intracellular structures were still not known. These old classifications are still widely used.

granulocytopenia   A marked decrease in the number of granulocytes that results in a syndrome of frequent chronic bacterial infections of the skin, lungs, throat, and other tissues. Granulocytopenia can be inherited, or it can be acquired. For example, it may be acquired as an aspect of leukemia. Granulocytopenia can more specifically be neutropenia (shortage of neutrophils), eosinopenia (shortage of eosinophils), and/or basopenia (shortage of basophils). The term neutropenia is sometimes used interchangeably with granulocytopenia. See also *agranulocytosis; agranulocytosis, infantile genetic; neutropenia; severe congenital neutropenia.*

granuloma   One of several forms of localized, nodular inflammation found in tissues. Granulomas have a typical pattern when examined under a microscope. They can be caused by a variety of biologic, chemical, and physical irritants of tissue. See also *granuloma, calcified; granuloma, fishbowl.*

granuloma, calcified   A granuloma that contains calcium deposits. Because it usually takes time for calcium to be deposited in a granuloma, a calcified granuloma is generally assumed to be an old granuloma.

granuloma, fishbowl   Localized nodular skin inflammation (small, reddish, raised areas of skin) that is caused by the bacterium Mycobacterium marinum (M. marinum). Fishbowl granuloma is typically acquired by occupational or recreational exposure to salt or fresh water; often it is the result of scratches or scrapes of the skin during the care of aquariums. The diagnosis is suggested by the history of exposure and confirmed through a culture of tissue specimens that yield M. marinum. The infection can be treated with a variety of antibiotics, including doxycycline, minocycline, clarithromycin, rifampin, and trimethoprim-sulfamethoxazole. Also known as swimming pool granuloma.

granuloma, swimming pool   See *granuloma, fishbowl.*

granuloma tropicum   See *yaws.*

granulomatosis, allergic   See *Churg-Strauss syndrome.*

granulomatosis, Wegener   An inflammatory disease of small arteries and veins (vasculitis) that classically involves vessels supplying the tissues of the lungs, nasal passages (sinuses), and kidneys. Symptoms include fatigue, weight loss, fever, shortness of breath, bloody sputum, joint pains, and sinus inflammation, sometimes with nasal ulcerations and bloody nasal discharge. Wegener granulomatosis most commonly affects young or middle-aged adults. The diagnosis of Wegener granulomatosis is confirmed by finding evidence of vasculitis and granulomas on biopsy of tissue that is inflamed. Wegener granulomatosis is a serious disease. Without treatment, it can be fatal within months. Treatment is directed toward stopping the inflammation process by suppressing the immune system.

granulomatous colitis   See *colitis, Crohn's.*

Graves disease   General overactivity (toxicity) of the thyroid gland, which becomes enlarged into a goiter. Graves disease is the most common disease that causes an excess of thyroid hormone (hyperthyroidism). There are three components to Graves disease: hyperthyroidism, protrusion of the eyes (ophthalmopathy), and skin lesions (dermopathy). Ophthalmopathy can cause sensitivity to light and a "sandy" feeling in the eyes. With further protrusion of the eyes, double vision and vision loss may occur. Ophthalmopathy tends to worsen with smoking. Dermopathy is a rare, painless, reddish lumpy skin rash that occurs on the front of the leg. The tendency to develop Graves disease can be inherited. Factors that can trigger Graves disease include stress, smoking, radiation to the neck, medications (such as interleukin-2 and interferon-alpha), and infectious organisms such as viruses. Graves disease can be diagnosed via a typical thyroid scan (diffuse increase uptake); by finding the characteristic triad of ophthalmopathy, dermopathy, and hyperthyroidism; or by testing the blood for thyroid-stimulating immunoglobulin (TSI) and finding abnormally high levels. Treatment includes antithyroid medications, removal of thyroid tissue via surgery (subtotal thyroidectomy), and radioiodine (RAI). Also known as diffuse toxic goiter.

gravid   Pregnant.

gray matter   The cortex of the brain, which contains nerve cell bodies. The gray matter is so named because it is darker than the white matter, the part of the brain that contains myelinated nerve fibers.

Gray's Anatomy   A book that was originally titled *Anatomy Descriptive and Surgical*, by Henry Gray, that appeared in 1858. Little could Dr. Gray have suspected that his textbook of human anatomy would still be in print today, and perhaps the best known of all medical books.

Known as *Gray's Anatomy* to generations of medical students, the book is a scientific and artistic masterpiece. Gray let the natural beauty and grace of the body's interconnected systems and structures shine forth. The illustrations are superb, and the text is clear (and, some might say, dull). It is one of the great reference works of all time, used by physicians, students, artists, and anyone interested in human anatomy.

Great Plague The typhus outbreak that swept London in 1665. See also *bubonic plague; typhus, epidemic.*

great saphenous vein The larger of the two saphenous veins, the principal veins that run up the leg near the surface. The great saphenous vein goes from the foot all the way up to the saphenous opening, an oval aperture in the broad fascia of the thigh. The vein then passes through this fibrous membrane. Also known as large saphenous vein.

greenstick fracture See *fracture, greenstick.*

groin The area where the thigh meets the hip.

gross anatomy See *anatomy, gross.*

gross hematuria See *hematuria, gross.*

Group A strep See *streptococcus pyogenes.*

Group B strep See *streptococcus, group B.*

group therapy 1 A type of psychiatric care in which several patients meet with one or more therapists at the same time. Patients form a support group for each other, and they receive expert care and advice. The group therapy model is particularly appropriate for psychiatric illnesses that are support intensive, such as anxiety disorders, but is not well suited for treatment of some other psychiatric disorders, such as schizophrenia. 2 A type of psychoanalysis in which patients analyze each other, with the assistance of one or more psychotherapists, as in an "encounter group." See also *gestalt therapy.*

growing pains Mysterious pains in growing children, usually in the legs. These pains are similar to what weekend gardeners suffer from on Monday: an overuse problem. If children exceed their regular threshold in playing, they are sore, just as adults are sore after overexerting themselves. Growing pains are typically somewhat diffuse, and they are not associated with physical changes of the area, such as swelling or redness. The pains are usually easily relieved by massage, acetaminophen, or rest. If pain persists for over a week or there are physical changes, the child should be seen by a physician.

gtt. Abbreviation for drops, as of a liquid medication. See also Appendix A, "Prescription Abbreviations."

guanine A member of the G-C (guanine-cytosine) pair of bases in DNA.

guarding, abdominal See *abdominal guarding.*

guided imagery An alternative medicine technique in which patients use their imagination to visualize improved health, or to "attack" a disease, such as a tumor. Some studies indicate that this positive thinking can have an effect on disease outcome, so guided imagery is now utilized as complementary medicine in some oncology centers and other medical facilities.

Guillain-Barre syndrome A disorder that is characterized by progressive symmetrical paralysis and loss of reflexes, usually beginning in the legs. In most cases of Guillain-Barre syndrome, the patient has a complete or nearly complete recovery. The paralysis characteristically involves more than one limb (most commonly the legs), is progressive, and usually proceeds from the end of an extremity toward the torso. Areflexia (loss of reflexes) or hyporeflexia (diminution of reflexes) may occur in the legs and arms. Guillain-Barre syndrome is not associated with fever. It usually occurs after a respiratory infection, and it is apparently caused by a misdirected immune response that results in the direct destruction of the myelin sheath surrounding the peripheral nerves or of the axon of the nerve itself. The syndrome sometimes follows other triggering events, including vaccinations. Among the vaccines reportedly associated with Guillain-Barre syndrome are the 1976–1977 swine flu vaccine, oral poliovirus vaccine, and tetanus toxoid. Aside from vaccinations, infection with the bacteria Campylobacter jejuni and viral infections can trigger Guillain-Barre syndrome. Other conditions that may mimic Guillain-Barre need to be ruled out before diagnosis is made. Treatment includes plasmapheresis and intravenous gamma globulin (IVIG). See also *demyelination; Landry ascending paralysis.*

gum disease Inflammation of the soft tissue (gingiva) and abnormal loss of bone that surrounds the teeth and holds the teeth in place. Gum disease is caused by toxins secreted by bacteria in the plaque that accumulates over time along the gum line. Plaque is a mixture of food, saliva, and bacteria. Early symptoms of gum disease include gum bleeding without pain. Pain is a symptom of more advanced gum disease, as the loss of bone around the teeth leads to the formation of gum pockets. Bacteria in these pockets cause gum infection, swelling, pain, and further bone destruction. Advanced gum disease can cause loss of otherwise healthy teeth. See also *acute membranous gingivitis; gingivitis.*

gustatory sweating See *sweating, gustatory.*

Guthrie test A blood test to screen for phenylketonuria (PKU) and the original impetus for the screening of newborns for metabolic diseases. See *phenylalanine; phenylalanine hydroxylase deficiency; PKU; PKU, maternal.*

gutta percha   A natural material derived from tree sap that can be formed to various shapes under heat. Because gutta percha does not cause allergic reactions, it is often used to pack the empty spaces left when a root canal is performed.

GVHD   Graft-versus-host disease.

gyn   Short for gynecology and gynecologist.

gynecoid   Like a woman; womanly, female.

gynecoid obesity   Overweight with a fat distribution generally characteristic of a woman, with the largest accumulation around the hips.

gynecoid pelvis   A pelvis that is generally characteristic of a woman in its bone structure and therefore its shape. A gynecoid pelvis is more delicate, wider, and not as high as a male pelvis. The angle of the female pubic arch is wide and round. The female sacrum is wider than the male's, and the iliac bone is flatter. The pelvic basin of the female is more spacious and less funnel shaped. From a purely anatomic viewpoint, the female pelvis is better suited to accommodate the fetus during pregnancy and to permit the baby to be born.

gynecologic oncologist   A physician who specializes in treating cancers of the female reproductive organs.

gynecologist   A physician who specializes in treating diseases of the female reproductive organs and providing well-woman health care that focuses primarily on the reproductive organs. In some health plans and health maintenance organizations (HMOs), women may choose to see a gynecologist as their primary care physician, in which case he or she also provides routine medical care or referrals.

gynecology   The branch of medicine that is particularly concerned with the health of the female organs of reproduction.

gynecomastia   Excessive development of the male breasts. Temporary enlargement of the breasts is not unusual or abnormal in boys during adolescence or during recovery from malnutrition. Gynecomastia may be abnormal, as, for example, in Klinefelter syndrome.

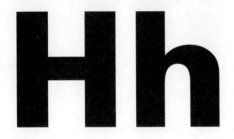

stimulates the baby's immature immune cells to produce antibodies to the HIB sugars, protecting the child against HIB infection.

hair, exclamation point   See *exclamation point hair.*

hair follicle   See *follicle.*

hair, lanugal   See *lanugo.*

hairball   A wad of swallowed hair. Hairballs sometimes cause blockage of the digestive system, especially at the exit of the stomach. Interestingly, in some Asian cultures hairballs are felt to have medicinal properties. Also called trichobezoar.

hairy cell leukemia   See *leukemia, hairy cell.*

hallux   The big toe.

hallux valgus   A condition in which the big toe (hallux) is bent outward (valgus) so that it overlaps the second toe. Hallux valgus may be accompanied by a bunion (localized painful swelling) and is frequently associated with inflammation. It can be related to inflammation of the nearby bursa (bursitis) or degenerative joint disease (osteoarthritis).

hallux varus   A condition in which the joint of the big toe is bent inward (varus).

Halstead mastectomy   See *mastectomy, radical.*

hammer toe   A condition in which the toe is flexed (curly), but with no abnormal rotation of the toe. Hammer toe may require surgical correction.

hamstring   One of the prominent tendons at the back of the knee. The hamstrings are the side walls of the hollow behind the knee (popliteal space). Both hamstrings connect to muscles that flex the knee. A pulled hamstring is a common athletic injury.

hand-foot-and-mouth disease   A viral syndrome that features a rash on the hands and feet and in the mouth. The internal rash (enanthem) consists of blisters and little ulcers. These may involve not only the lining of the mouth but also the gums, palate, and tongue. The external rash on the body (exanthem) typically affects the hands, the feet, and sometimes the buttocks. There may also be sore throat, irritability, decreased appetite, and fever. Hand-foot-and-mouth disease is caused by various viruses, including several types of coxsackievirus: most often Coxsackievirus A16, but also Coxsackieviruses A5, A9, A10, B1, or B3, and enterovirus 71. The incubation period is short, usually 4 to 6 days. The disease occurs most frequently in summer and fall. The rate of clinical expression in hand-foot-and-mouth disease is high, with the enanthem-exanthem pattern evident in nearly 100 percent of preschoolers, nearly 40 percent of school-age children, and about 10 percent of adults. The illness is

H and H   Common shorthand for hemoglobin and hematocrit, two very common and important blood tests. Sometimes written as H & H.

H and P   Medical shorthand for history and physical, the initial clinical evaluation and examination of the patient.

H. flu   Haemophilus influenzae type B.

H. flu immunization   Haemophilus influenzae type B immunization.

H. heilmannii   Helicobacter heilmannii.

H. pylori   Helicobacter pylori.

Haemophilus influenzae type B   A bacterium that is capable of causing a range of diseases, including ear infections, soft tissue infection (cellulitis), upper respiratory infections, and pneumonia; as well as such serious, invasive infections as meningitis with potential brain damage and epiglottitis with airway obstruction. Abbreviated HIB. HIB spreads by droplet through coughs and sneezing. Half the cases of HIB present as meningitis with fever, headache, and stiff neck. The remainder present as cellulitis, arthritis, or sepsis (bloodstream infection). About 5 percent of cases are fatal. Up to 20 percent of survivors of HIB have permanent hearing loss. More than 90 percent of all HIB infections occur in children 5 years or younger—the peak attack rate is at 6 to 12 months of age. See also *Haemophilus influenzae type B immunization.*

Haemophilus influenzae type B immunization   An immunization designed to prevent diseases caused by Haemophilus influenzae type B (HIB). In the US, the HIB vaccine is usually given at 2, 4, and 6 months of age, with a final booster at 12 to 15 months of age. The HIB vaccine rarely causes severe reactions, and it has almost eradicated HIB-related diseases in children. Before the vaccine, some 20,000 cases of HIB invasive disease in preschool children were reported every year in the US, compared to fewer than 300 cases after the advent of the vaccine. The HIB vaccine joins (conjugates) sugars from the HIB bacteria with a protein from another bacteria that characteristically mild and self-limited, and it is usually over and done within a week when due to Coxsackievirus A16. In outbreaks due to enterovirus 71, the illness may be more severe, with such complications as viral meningitis, encephalitis, and paralytic disease. Also known as hand-foot-and-mouth syndrome and hand, foot, and mouth disease or syndrome.

Hand-Schuller-Christian disease　A disease in which histiocytes start to multiply and attack the tissues or organs of the patient. The disease usually affects children aged 2 to 5, and it less often affects older children and adults. The most frequent sites of bony involvement are the flat bones of the skull, ribs, pelvis, and scapula (wing bone). Chronic otitis media due to involvement of the mastoid and the temporal bone is common. Diabetes insipidus affects some patients, mainly children who have systemic disease. Up to 40 percent of children with Hand-Schuller-Christian disease have short stature. Hand-Schuller-Christian disease is a form of Langerhans cell histiocytosis.

Hansen's disease　See *leprosy.*

hantavirus　A group of viruses that cause hemorrhagic fever and pneumonia. The hantaviruses include the hantaan virus that causes Korean (and Manchurian) hemorrhagic fever. Hantaviruses are transmitted to humans by direct or indirect contact with the saliva and excreta of rodents, such as deer mice, field mice, and ground voles.

hantavirus pulmonary syndrome　A severe lung condition caused by hantavirus infection. Abbreviated HPS. In 1993, HPS struck the Four Corners area (where the states of Arizona, New Mexico, Nevada, and Utah meet) with devastating, frequently fatal consequences. As the name indicates, HPS is due to a hantavirus. The HPS outbreak in Four Corners followed 2 years of more rain, more foliage, and more deer mice than usual.

haploid　A set of chromosomes that contains only one member of each chromosome pair. The sperm and egg are haploid and, in humans, each has 23 chromosomes.

hard measles　See *measles.*

hard palate　The first section of the bony part of the roof of the mouth, located in front of the soft palate.

Hardy-Weinberg law　A basic concept in population genetics that relates the gene frequency to the genotype frequency. The Hardy-Weinberg law can be used, for example, to determine allele frequency and heterozygote frequency when the incidence of a genetic disorder is known.

Hashimoto disease　A progressive disease of the thyroid gland characterized by the presence of antibodies directed against the thyroid and by infiltration of the thyroid gland by lymphocytes (white blood cells activated by the immune system). Hashimoto disease is the most common cause of hypothyroidism in North America and Europe. In Hashimoto disease, the thyroid gland is usually enlarged (goiter) and has a decreased ability to make thyroid hormones. Hashimoto disease predominantly affects women, and it can be inherited. Also known as autoimmune thyroiditis and Hashimoto thyroiditis.

HAV　Hepatitis A virus. See *hepatitis A.*

Havrix　A vaccine that is made from killed hepatitis A virus (HAV) and is intended to stimulate the body's immune system to produce antibodies against HAV.

hay fever　See *allergic rhinitis.*

Hb　Hemoglobin.

HBIG　Hepatitis B immune globulin, which contains antibodies to hepatitis B virus (HBV). HBIG offers prompt but short-lived protection against infection with HBV. HBIG may be given in cases of accidents that carry a transmission risk, as when health care workers get needle sticks.

HBO　Hyperbaric oxygen. See *hyperbaric oxygen therapy.*

HBV　Hepatitis B virus. See *hepatitis B.*

HCFA　Health Care Financing Administration. See *CMS.*

hCG　Human chorionic gonadotropin.

HCM　Hypertrophic cardiomyopathy. See *cardiomyopathy, hypertrophic.*

Hct　Hematocrit.

HCV　Hepatitis C virus. See *hepatitis C.*

HDL　High density lipoprotein. See *HDL cholesterol.*

HDL cholesterol　High density lipoprotein cholesterol. Lipoproteins, which are combinations of fats (lipids) and proteins, are the form in which lipids are transported in the blood. HDLs transport cholesterol from the tissues of the body to the liver, so the cholesterol can be gotten rid of in the bile. HDL cholesterol is therefore considered the "good" cholesterol: The higher the HDL cholesterol level, the lower the risk of coronary artery disease. Even small increases in HDL cholesterol reduce the risk of heart attack. Although there are no formal guidelines, proposed treatment goals for patients with low HDL cholesterol are to increase HDL cholesterol to above 35 mg/dl in men and to above 45 mg/dl in women with a family history of coronary heart disease; and to increase HDL cholesterol to approach 45 mg/dl in men and 55 mg/dl in women with known coronary heart disease. The first step in increasing HDL cholesterol levels is lifestyle modification. Regular aerobic exercise, loss of excess weight (fat), and cessation of cigarette smoking increase HDL cholesterol levels. Moderate alcohol consumption (such as one drink per day) also raises HDL cholesterol. When lifestyle modifications are insufficient, medications can be used. Medications that are effective in increasing HDL cholesterol include nicotinic acid (niacin), gemfibrozil (Lopid), estrogen, and, to a lesser extent, the statin drugs.

HDV   Hepatitis D virus. See *hepatitis D.*

head bones   See *bones of the head.*

head lice   Pediculus humanus capitis, parasitic insects found on the heads of people. Head lice are most commonly found on the scalp behind the ears and near the neckline at the back of the neck. Head lice hold on to hair with hook-like claws at the ends of their six legs. Head lice are rarely found on the body, eyelashes, or eyebrows. These insects lay their sticky white eggs on the hair shaft close to the root, and hatched lice stay mostly on the scalp. Head lice infection is very common and easily acquired by coming in close contact with someone who has head lice, infested clothing, or infested belongings. Preschool and elementary school children and their families are infested most often. Symptoms of head lice infestation include a tickling feeling of something moving in the hair, itching caused by an allergic reaction to the bites, irritability, and sores on the head caused by scratching. Although lice are very small, they can be seen on the scalp when they move. The eggs (nits) are easily seen on hair shafts. Treatment involves a combination of topical insecticidal medication and manual removal of all nits with a lice comb or the fingers. Both medication and complete nit removal are necessary to prevent reinfestation. All clothing, bedding, and furniture surfaces must also be washed or sprayed with insecticide. Note that pyrethin-based medications such as 1 percent lindane solution (brand name: Qwell) contain benzene, which can be toxic to brain tissue and has been linked to childhood leukemia. For this reason these medications are no longer generally recommended for use as a treatment for head lice.

headache   A pain in the head, with the pain being above the eyes or the ears, behind the head (occipital), or in the back of the upper neck. Headache has many causes. All headaches are classified as primary or secondary headaches. Primary headaches are not associated with other diseases. Examples of primary headaches are migraine headaches, tension headaches, and cluster headaches. Secondary headaches are caused by other diseases, and the associated diseases can be minor or major. Tension headaches are the most common type of primary headache. As many as 90 percent of adults have tension headaches. Migraine headaches are the second most common type of primary headache. An estimated 28 million people in the US have migraine headaches. Cluster headaches are a rare but important type of primary headache, affecting mainly men. Secondary headaches may result from innumerable conditions, ranging from life-threatening ones such as brain tumors, strokes, meningitis, lupus, and subarachnoid hemorrhages to less serious but common conditions such as withdrawal from caffeine and discontinuation of analgesics (pain-killing medications). Many people suffer from "mixed" headache disorders, in which tension headaches or secondary headaches may trigger migraines. The treatment of the headache depends on the type and severity of the headache and on other factors, such as the age of the patient. Treatment options include short-term and long-term medications. Also known as cephalgia. See also *cluster headache; headache, tension; hematoma, epidural; hematoma, subdural; hemorrhage, subarachnoid; migraine headache; subarachnoid hemorrhage.*

headache, cervicogenic   A headache that has its origins in the muscles, tendons, and nerves of the neck. It may be a simple tension headache, or it may result from damage to neck joints, ligaments, muscles, tendons, or the trigeminal nerve. Treatment for chronic cervicogenic headaches includes massage, physical therapy, analgesic medication, and in some extreme cases injected nerve-block medication or surgery. See also *headache, tension.*

headache, cluster   See *cluster headache.*

headache, febrile   A headache associated with fever. Because febrile headache can sometimes indicate serious conditions such as inflammation of the brain (encephalitis), a person who is suffering from a febrile headache should immediately seek medical attention.

headache, migraine   See *migraine headache.*

headache, muscle tension   See *headache, tension.*

headache, rebound   A headache experienced by someone who has taken ergotamine or analgesic medications for migraines or other health conditions and has built up a tolerance for these medications. Often a rebound headache occurs right after the medication wears off. Treatment involves using the medication less frequently or switching to a different pain reliever. Some patients with acute rebound headaches find relief with injected phenothiazine or long-acting steroid medication.

headache, sinus A headache caused by pressure within the sinus cavities of the head, usually in connection with sinus infection. The sufferer has pain and tenderness in the sinus area, discharge from the nose, and sometimes a swollen face. Vascular headaches are often mistaken for sinus headaches. Treatment involves treating the underlying condition, which is often an allergy, and using nasal vasoconstrictors and analgesic medications, such as aspirin (in adults only), acetaminophen, ibuprofen, or naproxen sodium.

headache, stress See *headache, tension.*

headache, tension A headache caused by contraction of the muscles in the back of the neck, on the scalp, and sometimes in the jaw. Tension headaches are usually related to stress. Treatment includes stress reduction, massage, and use of analgesic medication, such as aspirin (in adults only), acetaminophen, ibuprofen, or naproxen sodium. For chronic tension headaches, some physicians recommend tricyclic antidepressants, such as amitriptyline, which work to defuse stress and to lessen pain. Also known as muscle tension headache and stress headache.

headache, thunderclap A sudden and excruciatingly painful headache. Some physicians feel that in the absence of a known headache disorder, such as migraines, a thunderclap headache may sometimes signal a ruptured aneurysm in the brain. A person who experiences this type of headache should immediately seek medical attention.

headache, vascular One of a group of headaches felt to involve abnormal sensitivity of the blood vessels (arteries) in the brain to various triggers, resulting in rapid changes in the artery size due to spasm (constriction). Other arteries in the brain and scalp then open (dilate), and throbbing pain is perceived in the head. Migraine headache is the most common type of vascular headache. See also *migraine headache.*

health As officially defined by the World Health Organization, a state of complete physical, mental, and social well-being, not merely the absence of disease or infirmity.

Health and Human Services, Department of See *HHS.*

Health Care Financing Administration See *CMS.*

health care proxy An advance medical directive in the form of a legal document that designates another person (a proxy) to make health care decisions in case a person is rendered incapable of making his or her wishes known. The health care proxy has, in essence, the same rights to request or refuse treatment that the person would have if he or she were capable of making and communicating decisions.

health, child See *child health.*

health outcomes research Research that measures the value of a particular course of therapy.

heart The muscle that pumps blood received from veins into arteries throughout the body. The heart is positioned in the chest behind the sternum (breastbone); in front of the trachea, esophagus, and aorta; and above the diaphragm. A normal heart is about the size of a closed fist and weighs about 298 grams or 10.5 ounces. It is cone-shaped, with the point of the cone pointing down to the left. Two-thirds of the heart lies in the left side of the chest, with the balance in the right side of the chest. The heart is composed of specialized cardiac muscle, and it is four-chambered, with a right atrium and ventricle, and an anatomically separate left atrium and ventricle. The blood flows from the systemic veins into the right atrium, thence to the right ventricle, from which it is pumped to the lungs and then returned into the left atrium, thence to the left ventricle, from which it is driven into the systemic arteries. The heart is thus functionally composed of two hearts: the right heart and the left heart. The right heart consists of the right atrium, which receives deoxygenated blood from the body, and the right ventricle, which pumps the deoxygenated blood to the lungs under low pressure; and the left heart, which consists of the left atrium, which receives oxygenated blood from the lung, and the left ventricle, which pumps the oxygenated blood out to the body under high pressure.

heart, artificial A human-made heart that is used to replace a diseased or malfunctioning heart when a donor organ is not available.

heart attack A sudden blockage of a coronary artery. Not infrequently, this leads to the death of part of the heart muscle due to its loss of blood supply. Typically, the loss of blood supply is caused by a complete blockage of a coronary artery by a blood clot. The interruption of blood flow is usually caused by arteriosclerosis, with narrowing of the coronary arteries, the culminating event being a thrombosis (clot). Death of the heart muscle often causes chest pain and electrical instability of the heart muscle tissue. Electrical instability of the heart causes ventricular fibrillation (chaotic electrical disturbance). Orderly transmission of electrical signals in the heart is important for the regular beating (pumping) of the heart. A heart undergoing ventricular fibrillation simply quivers and cannot pump or deliver oxygenated blood to the brain. Permanent brain damage and death can result from heart attack unless oxygenated blood flow is restored within 5 minutes. Many heart attack deaths are due to ventricular fibrillation of the heart that occurs before the victim can reach any medical assistance. Approximately 90 percent to 95 percent of heart attack victims who reach the hospital survive. The 5 percent to 10 percent who later die are those who have suffered major heart muscle damage or who suffer an "extension," or enlargement, of their heart attack. Heart attack deaths can be avoided if a bystander starts CPR (cardiopulmonary resuscitation) within 5 minutes of the onset of ventricular fibrillation. When paramedics arrive, medications and/or electrical shock (cardioversion) to the heart can be administered to convert ventricular fibrillation to a normal heart rhythm. Therefore, prompt CPR and rapid paramedic response can improve the survival chances after a heart attack. Also known as a myocardial infarction (MI). See also *cardiac arrest.*

heart block   A blockage in the conduction of the normal electrical impulses in the heart. Heart block is not uncommon and is detected with an electrocardiogram. Heart block occurs from degeneration or scarring of the electrical pathways in the heart muscle, either naturally or as a result of disease. Heart block typically requires no treatment, but can be a factor in the decision of whether or not to put a pacemaker in a heart that is failing or irregularly beating.

heart conduction system   See *cardiac conduction system.*

heart failure   See *congestive heart failure.*

heart, left   The left atrium and left ventricle.

heart murmur   An unusual, "whooshing" heart sound that may be innocent or may reflect disease or malformation. A heart murmur is created by blood flow through a heart valve, by blood flow through a narrowed chamber, or by an unusual connection between the chambers, as seen with congenital heart disease. Sometimes a heart murmur does not represent any disease or condition and is, therefore, referred to as functional heart murmur. There are many forms of heart murmurs representing a variety of heart conditions. Each type of murmur is characterized by its location, timing, duration, as well as the intensity and quality of the sound it makes. A heart murmur is usually heard by a physician while he or she listens to the chest with a stethoscope. While the heart murmur itself is never treated, sometime the condition it represents may require treatment.

heart rate   The number of heartbeats per unit of time, usually per minute. The heart rate is based on the number of contractions of the ventricles (the lower chambers of the heart). The heart rate may be too fast (tachycardia) or too slow (bradycardia). The pulse is a bulge of an artery

from waves of blood that course through the blood vessels each time the heart beats. The pulse is often taken at the wrist to estimate the heart rate.

heart, right   The right atrium and right ventricle.

heart septum   The dividing wall between the right and left sides of the heart. That portion of the septum that separates the right and left atria of the heart is termed the atrial, or interatrial, septum, whereas the portion of the septum that lies between the right and left ventricles of the heart is called the ventricular, or interventricular, septum.

heart transplant   An operation in which a diseased or malfunctioning heart is replaced with a healthy donor heart taken from a deceased person. See also *transplant.*

heart valve   One of the four heart valves. All four heart valves are one-way valves, permitting forward and avoiding backward flow of blood. Blood entering the heart first passes through the tricuspid valve, and then the pulmonary valve. After returning from the lungs, the blood passes through the mitral (bicuspid) valve and leaves the heart via the aortic valve to pass through the aorta.

heart ventricle   One of the two lower chambers of the heart. The right ventricle receives blood from the right atrium and pumps it into the lungs via the pulmonary artery, and the left ventricle receives blood from the left atrium and pumps it into the circulation system via the aorta.

heartburn   An uncomfortable feeling of burning and warmth that occurs in waves, rising up behind the breastbone (sternum) and moving toward the neck. Heartburn has nothing to do with the heart. It is usually due to gastroesophageal reflux, the return of stomach acid into the esophagus.

heart-lung machine   A machine that does the work both of the heart and of the lungs: pumping and oxygenating blood. Blood returning to the heart is diverted through a heart-lung machine before being returned to arterial circulation. Such machines may be used during open-heart surgery. Also known as pump-oxygenator.

heat prostration   See *hyperthermia.*

heatstroke   See *hyperthermia.*

Heberden's disease   1 Angina.   2 Osteoarthritis of the small joints with bony enlargement (Heberden's nodes) of joint at the end of the finger. See also *angina pectoris.*

Heberden's node   A small fixed bony enlargement of the joint at the end of the finger. A Heberden's node is a calcified spur of the bone of that joint (distal interphalangeal joint) and is associated with osteoarthritis.

Hecht syndrome   An inherited disorder that is transmitted as an autosomal dominant trait, in which short, tight muscles make it impossible to open the mouth fully or keep the fingers straight when the hand is flexed back. The small mouth creates feeding problems. The hands may be so tightly fisted that infants with Hecht syndrome crawl on their knuckles. Also known as trismus pseudo-camptodactyly syndrome.

Hecht's pneumonia   See *pneumonia, giant cell.*

heel bone   See *bone, heel.*

heel spur   See *calcaneal spur.*

Heimlich maneuver   An emergency treatment for obstruction of the airway in adults. The Heimlich maneuver may be needed when someone chokes on a piece of food that has "gone down the wrong way." To perform the Heimlich maneuver, a rescuer stands behind the victim, wraps his or her arms around the victim's waist, makes a fist with one hand, and holds the fist with the thumb side just below the breast bone at the top of the abdomen. The rescuer places his or her other hand over the fist and uses it to pull sharply into the top of the victim's stomach and forcefully press up into the victim's diaphragm to expel the obstruction (most commonly food). The Heimlich maneuver should be repeated as necessary. If the Heimlich maneuver is unsuccessful, an emergency tracheostomy may be necessary to prevent suffocation. Named for the US surgeon Henry Heimlich, who noted that food and other objects that caused choking by blocking the airway from the mouth to the lungs were not expelled by giving sharp blows to the back. See also *airway obstruction; tracheostomy.*

helical CAT scan   See *spiral CAT scan.*

Helicobacter heilmannii   A bacterium that infects most cats, dogs, and pigs and causes them stomach inflammation (gastritis). H. heilmannii is not usually transmitted from animals to people, but people who have been infected by H. heilmannii are known to have developed gastric and duodenal ulcers. Antibiotics can cure H. heilmannii infections. H. heilmannii is closely related to H. pylori.

Helicobacter pylori   A bacterium that causes stomach inflammation (gastritis) and ulcers in the stomach and duodenum. This bacterium is the most common cause of ulcers worldwide. H. pylori infection may be acquired from contaminated food and water or through person-to-person contact. It is common in people who live in crowded conditions with poor sanitation. In the US, 30 percent of the adult population is infected. One out of six patients with H. pylori infection develops ulcers of the duodenum or the stomach. This bacterium is also

believed to be associated with stomach cancer (gastric adenocarcinoma) and a rare type of lymphoid tumor called gastric MALT lymphoma. Infected persons usually carry H. pylori indefinitely, often without symptoms, unless treated with antibiotics to eradicate the bacterium. Also known as ulcer bug.

HELLP syndrome   A combination of the breakdown of red blood cells (hemolysis; the *H* in the acronym), elevated liver enzymes (*EL*), and low platelet count (*LP*). HELLP syndrome is a recognized complication of preeclampsia and eclampsia (toxemia) of pregnancy, occurring in 25 percent of these pregnancies. Common symptoms include a general sense of feeling unwell (malaise), nausea and/or vomiting, and pain in the upper abdomen. Increased fluid in the tissues (edema) is also common. Protein is often found in the urine. Blood pressure may be elevated. Occasionally, coma can result from seriously low blood sugar (hypoglycemia). The first order of treatment is the management of blood clotting. Urgent delivery is required if the health of the fetus is compromised by HELLP syndrome in the pregnant mother. Delivery is also performed if the syndrome develops after 34 weeks' gestation, if the fetus' lungs are mature, or if the mother's health is in jeopardy. HELLP syndrome can be complicated by liver rupture, anemia, bleeding, and death. HELLP syndrome can also develop during the early period after delivery of a baby. Women with a history of HELLP syndrome are considered at increased risk for complications in future pregnancies.

helper T cell   See *T-4 cell.*

helper/supressor ratio   The ratio of T-helper (T-4) cells to supressor (T-8) cells in the bloodstream. Results of testing for each type of cells are compared to gauge the progress of HIV infection (AIDS). Both types of cells are helpful to the immune response so, as levels of both decline, the prognosis worsens.

hemangioma   A benign tumor formed by a collection of excess blood vessels. A hemangioma may be visible through the skin as a birthmark, known colloquially as a "strawberry mark." Most hemangiomas that occur at birth disappear after a few months or years.

hemangioma, capillary   A type of hemangioma that is composed almost entirely of tiny capillary vessels. Capillary hemangiomas may appear anywhere on the body but are most common on the face, scalp, back, and chest. They may be evident at birth or become noticeable several weeks later. They usually grow quickly and then remain fixed in size and, with time, spontaneously subside. The vast majority are gone by the time the patient is age 10. No treatment is needed. Capillary hemangiomas include strawberry hemangiomas, strawberry marks, and salmon patches. See also *salmon patch.*

hemangioma, cavernous A type of hemangioma composed of blood-filled "lakes" and channels. A cavernous henangioma is raised and red or purplish. It may diminish in size following trauma, bleeding or ulceration, but it rarely disappears on its own. Small cavernous hemangiomas on the surface of the body may be removed or treated by electrocoagulation. Surgery is sometimes needed.

hemarthrosis Blood in a joint.

hematemesis Bloody vomit.

hematocrit The proportion of the blood that consists of red blood cells. Abbreviated Hct. Hct is expressed as a percentage. For example, an Hct of 25 percent means that there are 25 milliliters of red blood cells in 100 milliliters of blood: one-fourth of the blood consists of red cells. The normal ranges for Hct depend on the age and, after adolescence, the sex of the patient. The normal ranges are 55 to 68 percent for newborns, 47 to 65 percent at 1 week of age, 37 to 49 percent at 1 month of age, 30 to 36 percent at 3 months of age, 29 to 41 percent at 1 year of age, 36 to 40 percent at 10 years of age, 42 to 54 percent in adult males, and 38 to 46 percent in adult females. The values returned on Hct tests may vary slightly between laboratories. An abnormally low level of Hct is referred to as anemia and can come from bleeding, iron deficiency, breakage of red blood cells (hemolysis), and many other causes. An abnormally high level of Hct is referred to as polycythemia and can be a result of chronic lung disease, polycythemia rubra vera, and other causes.

hematologist A physician who specializes in diagnosing and treating diseases of the blood.

hematoma A localized swelling that is filled with blood caused by a break in the wall of a blood vessel. The breakage may be spontaneous, as in the case of an aneurysm, or caused by trauma. The blood is usually clotted or partially clotted, and it exists within an organ or in a soft tissue space, such as muscle. Treatment depends on the location and size of the hematoma but usually involves draining the accumulated blood. A hematoma in or near the brain is particularly dangerous.

hematoma, epidural A hematoma between the skull and the brain's tissue-like covering, which is known as the dura. Epidural hematoma is usually caused by a full-on blow to the head and is often associated with skull fracture. Diagnosis is usually made via MRI or CAT scan. Treatment is trepanation: drilling through the skull to drain the excess blood.

hematoma, intracerebral A hematoma within the brain itself. Diagnosis is usually made by CAT or MRI scan. Treatment involves surgery.

hematoma, intracranial A hematoma within the brain cavity (cranium). The hematoma may or may not be within the brain itself. Treatment can require surgical drainage and depends on the location, size, and duration of the hematoma. See also *hematoma, epidural; hematoma, intracerebral; hematoma, subdural.*

hematoma, subcutaneous A hematoma beneath the skin.

hematoma, subdural A hematoma between the brain and its covering, the dura. If the hematoma causes increased pressure on the brain, neurological abnormalities including slurred speech, impaired gait, and dizziness may result and progress to coma and even death. Subdural hematomas can be caused by minor accidents to the head, major trauma, or the spontaneous bursting of a blood vessel in the brain (aneurysm). Acute subdural hematomas are usually due to severe head trauma. Chronic subdural hematomas may be very insidious. They usually go unnoticed, sometimes for 2 to 4 weeks: When they do cause problems, the incident that caused the bleeding is often long past. Symptoms include increasing daily headache, fluctuating drowsiness or confusion, and mild weakness on one side of the body. In infants, subdural hematomas can cause the fontanel to bulge and the head circumference to enlarge. Diagnosis is usually made by MRI or CAT scan. Treatment is trepanation: drilling through the skull to drain the excess blood.

hematopoiesis The production of all types of blood cells. Hematopoiesis is a remarkable self-regulated system that is responsive to the demands put on it. All types of blood cells are derived from primitive cells (stem cells) in the bone marrow. The production of blood cells is largely controlled by feedback. When the demand for production of cells of a particular type increases or the levels of the cells fall in blood, stimulatory substances called cytokines are released, and the cytokines stimulate the stem cells to generate new mature blood cells. This occurs in the few days required for blood cell maturation. When hematopoiesis is disturbed, the first cells to drop are usually the neutrophils (which have a life span in the blood of only 6 to 8 hours) followed by platelets (with a 10-day life span). Anemia develops more slowly, over a much longer span of time (because the red blood cells have a 120-day life span).

hematuria See *blood in the urine.*

hematuria, gross Blood in the urine that can be seen with the naked eye. Hematuria may or may not be accompanied by pain, but it is always abnormal and should be further investigated.

hemiparesis Weakness on one side of the body.

hemiplegia   Paralysis on one side of the body.

hemizygous   Having only a single copy of a gene instead of the customary two copies. All the genes on the single X chromosome in the male are hemizygous.

hemochromatosis   An inherited disorder characterized by abnormally high absorption of iron by the intestinal tract, resulting in excessive storage of iron, particularly in the liver, skin, pancreas, heart, joints, and testes. Common early symptoms include abdominal pain, weakness, lethargy, and weight loss. The onset of symptoms is between 40 and 60 years of age in males and after menopause in females. The excess iron gives the skin a bronze color and damages the liver, causing liver scarring (fibrosis) or cirrhosis, usually after age 40. Diabetes also occurs due to damage to the pancreas. Other findings include congestive heart failure or arrhythmias, arthritis, and hypogonadism. Treatment is removal of excess iron by periodic phlebotomy (removal of blood) to deplete the body iron. Early diagnosis and treatment before symptoms develop prevents all the complications of the disease. Because hemochromatosis is inherited in an autosomal recessive manner, all brothers and sisters of a patient need to be screened for the disorder. Also known as bronze diabetes and hereditary hemochromatosis.

hemodialysis   See *dialysis.*

hemoglobin   The oxygen-carrying protein pigment in the blood, specifically in the red blood cells. Abbreviated Hb. Hb is usually measured as total Hb expressed as the amount of Hb in grams (gm) per deciliter (dl) of whole blood. The normal ranges for hemoglobin depend on the age and, beginning in adolescence, the sex of the person. The normal ranges are 17 to 22 gm/dl for newborns, 15 to 20 gm/dl at 1 week of age, 11 to 15 gm/dl at 1 month of age, 11 to 13 gm/dl in children, 14 to 18 gm/dl for adult men, 12 to 16 gm/dl for adult women, 12.4 to 14.9 gm/dl for men after middle age, and 11.7 to 13.8 gm/dl for women after middle age. Values returned on Hb tests may vary slightly between laboratories, as some laboratories do not differentiate between "adult" and "after middle age" Hb values.

hemoglobin A   Normal adult hemoglobin, the main type of hemoglobin found after infancy. The *A* stands for adult.

hemoglobin E   Normal embryonic hemoglobin, the main type of hemoglobin found in the human embryo. The *E* stands for embryonic and also for epsilon, a chain that is unique to embryonic hemoglobin. Originally known as Gower-2.

hemoglobin F   Normal fetal hemoglobin, the main type of hemoglobin found in the fetus and newborn baby. The *F* stands for fetal.

hemoglobin S   The most common type of abnormal hemoglobin, which is found in people with sickle cell trait and sickle cell anemia. It differs from hemoglobin A only by a single amino acid substitution. The *S* stands for sickle. See also *anemia, sickle cell; sickle cell trait.*

hemoglobinuria   The presence of free hemoglobin in the urine, which may make the urine look dark. Normally, there is no hemoglobin in the urine. Hemoglobinuria is a sign of a number of abnormal conditions, such as bleeding and paroxysmal nocturnal hemoglobinuria.

hemolysis   Breakage of red blood cells. This occurs to a minor degree normally as red blood cells age. However, excessive hemolysis is very abnormal and leads to hemolytic anemia. See also *hemolytic anemia.*

hemolytic anemia   Anemia due to the destruction, rather than underproduction, of red blood cells. Hemolytic anemia can result from a medication reaction, from the immune system attacking the red blood cells (autoimmune hemolytic anemia), from destruction of blood cells passing through diseased heart valves, and other causes.

hemolytic disease of the newborn   Abnormal breakup of red blood cells in a fetus or newborn. Hemolytic disease of the newborn is usually due to antibodies made by the mother that are directed against the baby's red blood cells. It is typically caused by Rh incompatibility (a difference between the Rh blood groups of mother and baby). Severe hemolytic disease can cause anemia and heart failure. Less severe cases feature jaundice and can lead to brain damage if left untreated. Also known as erythroblastosis.

hemolytic jaundice, congenital   See *spherocytosis, hereditary.*

hemolytic-uremic syndrome   A condition (abbreviated HUS) involving the breakup of red blood cells and kidney failure. The platelets (the blood cells responsible for clotting) clump within the kidney's small blood vessels with a resultant reduced blood flow that leads to kidney failure. The partial blockage of the blood vessels also leads to the destruction of red blood cells (hemolysis). Platelets are also decreased, which can cause bleeding problems. There are many causes for HUS, including shigella bacteria, drugs, tumors, pregnancy, and systemic lupus erythematosus. One of the most prominent causes of HUS today is a strain of the E. coli bacteria called E. coli 0157:H7, usually acquired from eating raw or undercooked ground beef (hamburger), or from drinking raw milk or contaminated water. HUS is the most common cause of acute kidney failure in infants and young children.

hemophagocytic lymphohistiocytosis A rare, cancer-like disorder in which both histiocytes and lymphocytes start to proliferate and attack body tissues or organs. Hemophagocytic lymphohistiocytosis can be an inherited condition, or it can occur as a result of immunosuppression (as in organ transplants) or infection. Most patients are young children. Treatment involves chemotherapy and in some cases bone-marrow transplantation. See also *histiocytosis.*

hemophilia An inherited disorder in which the ability of blood to clot normally is impaired. There are two types of hemophilia: hemophilia A and hemophilia B.

hemophilia A Classic hemophilia, which is due to a profound deficiency in the activity of clotting factor VIII. Affected individuals suffer hemorrhage into joints and muscles, easy bruising, and prolonged bleeding from wounds. The disease is inherited as an X-linked trait, so males are affected and females carry the gene. Females carry the gene, and each of their sons stands a 50 percent chance of receiving the gene and having hemophilia. Treatment involves administration of blood products that introduce clotting factor VIII and replace lost blood. Use of contaminated blood products exposed many people with hemophilia to HIV infection in the 1980s and 1990s. Hemophilia A has affected the Russian royal house and the descendants of Queen Victoria.

hemophilia B Hemophilia due to deficiency of coagulation factor IX in the blood, which results in prolonged oozing after minor and major injuries, tooth extractions, or surgery. There is renewed bleeding after the initial bleeding has stopped. The gene for hemophilia B is on the X chromosome, so males are affected and females carry the gene. About 10 percent of carrier females are at risk for bleeding. Treatment involves administration of blood products that introduce clotting factor IX and replace lost blood. Also called Christmas disease (named for the first patient with the disease to be studied in detail).

hemoptysis Spitting up blood or blood-tinged sputum from the respiratory tract. Hemoptysis occurs when tiny blood vessels that line the lungs airways are broken. Hemoptysis can be harmless such as from irritated bronchial tubes with bronchitis, or be serious such as from cancer of the lung.

hemorrhage Abnormal bleeding. A hemorrhage can be internal, and therefore invisible, or external, and therefore visible on the body. For example, bleeding into the spleen or liver is internal hemorrhage, and bleeding from a cut on the face is an external hemorrhage. See also *bleeding.*

hemorrhagic fever, epidemic See *hemorrhagic fever with renal syndrome.*

hemorrhagic fever with renal syndrome A set of diseases characterized by the abrupt onset of high fever and chills, headache, cold and cough, and pain in the muscles, joints, and abdomen, with nausea and vomiting. These symptoms are followed by bleeding into the kidney (renal syndrome) and elsewhere. Some victims have bleeding from the eyes, mouth, nose, and/or pores of the skin. Viruses known to cause hemorrhagic fever with renal syndrome include the arboviruses, the hantaviruses, and the Ebola virus. One thing these three types of viruses have in common is transmission from animal or insect host to humans. See also *arbovirus; Ebola virus; hantavirus.*

hemorrhoids Dilated (enlarged) veins in the walls of the anus and sometimes around the rectum, usually caused by untreated constipation but occasionally associated with chronic diarrhea. Symptoms start with bleeding after defecation. If untreated, hemorrhoids can worsen, protruding from the anus. In their worst stage, they must be returned manually to the anal cavity. Fissures can develop and may cause intense discomfort. Treatment involves changing the diet to prevent constipation and avoid further irritation, the use of topical medication, and sometimes surgery. Also known as piles.

Henoch-Schonlein purpura See *anaphylactoid purpura.*

heparin One of several glycosaminoglycans (GAGs), an anticlotting agent produced naturally by the liver and some other cells in the body. Heparin may also be purified or synthesized for use as a medication. As a drug, heparin is useful in preventing blood clots that travel from their site of origin through the bloodstream to clog another vessel (thromboembolic complications); it is used also in the early treatment of blood clots in the lungs (pulmonary embolisms) and clotting-related heart conditions. See also *glycosaminoglycans; heparin, low-weight.*

heparin, low-weight A relatively new form of the drug heparin (brand names: Loverox and Fragmin) that has a lower molecular weight than normal heparin. Fewer blood tests are needed for monitoring when low-weight heparin is given, as opposed to traditional unfractionated heparin. Low-weight heparin may be superior to regular (unfractionated) heparin in cases of unstable angina and other cardiac diseases. See also *heparin.*

hepatic Having to do with the liver.

hepatic ductular hypoplasia, syndromatic See *Alagille syndrome.*

hepatitis Inflammation of the liver, irrespective of the cause. Hepatitis is caused by a number of conditions, including drug toxicity, immune diseases, and viruses such as hepatitis A, B, C, D, E, F, and G.

hepatitis A   Inflammation of the liver caused by the hepatitis A virus (HAV), which is usually transmitted by food or drink that has been handled by an infected person whose hygiene is poor. Symptoms include nausea, fever, and jaundice (yellowing of the skin and/or eyes), although some patients have no symptoms at all. Hepatitis A does not lead to chronic disease. Diagnosis is made by blood test. When immediate protection against hepatitis A infection is needed, immunoglobulin (gamma globulin) is used. Immunoglobulin is effective only if given within 2 weeks of exposure, and it lasts only 2 to 4 months. Immunoglobulin can be used to protect people who have contact with someone with acute viral hepatitis and by travelers who must depart for regions with poor sanitation and high hepatitis A rates before vaccines can take effect. Patients can receive immunoglobulin and hepatitis A vaccine simultaneously. Also called infectious hepatitis and epidemic jaundice. See also *hepatitis A immunization.*

hepatitis A immunization   A vaccine that may be considered for individuals in high-risk settings, including frequent world travelers, sexually active individuals with multiple partners, homosexual men, IV drug users, employees of daycare centers, certain health care workers, and sewage workers. Two hepatitis A vaccines (brand names: Havrix and Vaqta) are commercially available in the US. Both are highly effective and provide protection even after one dose. Two doses are recommended for adults, and three doses are recommended for children under 18 years of age to provide prolonged protection.

hepatitis B   Inflammation of the liver due to the hepatitis B virus (HBV), once thought to be passed only through blood products. It is now known that hepatitis B can also be transmitted via needle sticks, body piercing and tattooing with unsterilized instruments, the dialysis process, sexual and even less intimate close contact, and childbirth. Symptoms include fatigue, jaundice, nausea, vomiting, dark urine, and light stools. Diagnosis is made by blood test. Treatment includes administration of antiviral drugs and/or hepatitis B immune globulin (HBIG). Chronic hepatitis B may be treated with interferon. Health care workers accidentally exposed to materials infected with hepatitis B and individuals with known sexual contact with hepatitis B patients are usually given both HBIG and the hepatitis B vaccine to provide both immediate and long-term protection. HBV infection can be prevented with the hepatitis B vaccine and through avoidance of activities that could lead to getting the virus. Also known as serum hepatitis. See also *hepatitis B immunization.*

Hepatitis B immune globulin   HBIG.

hepatitis B immunization   A vaccine that protects against both hepatitis B and hepatitis D. It gives prolonged protection, but three shots over 6 months are usually required. Adults in high-risk situations, including health care workers, dentists, intimate and household contacts of patients with chronic hepatitis B infection, male homosexuals, individuals with multiple sexual partners, dialysis patients, IV drug users, and recipients of repeated transfusions, may also want to get this vaccine.

hepatitis C   Inflammation of the liver due to the hepatitis C virus (HCV), which is usually spread via blood transfusion, hemodialysis, and needle sticks. HCV causes most transfusion-associated hepatitis, and the damage it does to the liver can lead to cirrhosis and cancer. Transmission of the virus by sexual contact is rare. At least half of HCV patients develop chronic hepatitis C infection. Diagnosis is made by blood test. Treatment is via antiviral drugs. Chronic hepatitis C may be treated with interferon, sometimes in combination with antivirals. There is no vaccine for hepatitis C. Previously known as non-A, non-B hepatitis.

hepatitis D   Liver inflammation due to the hepatitis D virus (HDV), which causes disease only in patients who already have the hepatitis B virus. Transmission occurs via infected blood, needles, or sexual contact with an infected person. Symptoms are identical to those of hepatitis B. Chronic infection with HDV is currently treated with interferon, although this treatment is not very successful. HDV infection can be prevented with the hepatitis B vaccine and through avoidance of activities that could lead to getting the virus.

hepatitis E   A rare form of liver inflammation caused by infection with the hepatitis E virus (HEV). It is transmitted via food or drink handled by an infected person or through infected water supplies in areas where fecal matter may get into the water. There is no vaccine or treatment for hepatitis E, although antiviral drugs may be tried.

hepatitis F   A rare form of liver inflammation caused by infection with the hepatitis F virus (HFV), which may be a mutation of hepatitis B. There is no vaccine or treatment for hepatitis F, although antiviral drugs may be tried.

hepatitis G   A rare form of liver inflammation caused by infection with the hepatitis G virus (HGV), which may be a mutation of hepatitis B. There is no vaccine or treatment for hepatitis G, although antiviral drugs may be tried.

hepatitis, infectious   An infectious form of hepatitis, such as hepatitis A.

hepatitis, non-A, non-B   The old name for hepatitis C, before the causative virus was identified.

hepatitis, viral   Liver inflammation caused by a virus. Specific hepatitis viruses have been labeled A, B, C, D, E, F, and G. Some other viruses, such as the Epstein-Barr virus and cytomegalovirus, can also cause hepatitis, but the liver is not their primary target.

hepatomegaly An abnormally enlarged liver. Hepatomegaly can be caused by heart failure, blockage of blood vessels from the liver, or be a sign of chronic liver disease.

hepatosplenomegaly Abnormal enlargement of the liver and spleen. Hepatosplenomegaly is typically associated with chronic liver diseases.

hepatotoxic Being injurious to the liver. For example, alcoholic beverages and acetaminophen (brand name: Tylenol) can be hepatotoxic.

herbal remedy A medication prepared from plants, including most of the world's traditional remedies for disease. Most people think of herbal remedies as products sold over the counter as "supplements," such as saw palmetto extract and goldenseal ointment. However, many over-the-counter and prescription drugs, including aspirin and digoxin, are based on ingredients originally derived from plants. Lab tests have shown that some herbal remedies are indeed effective against illness. One should use these drugs as carefully as prescription medicines, taking care to avoid overdose, interactions with other medications, and misuse. See also *dietary supplement; herbalism.*

herbalism The practice of making or prescribing herbal remedies for medical conditions. Practitioners of herbalism may be licensed or unlicensed. See also *herbalist.*

herbalist One versed in herbal lore and, in regard to therapy; an herb physician. Herbalists may be licensed MDs, naturopaths, or osteopaths. They may also be unlicensed. People who are interested in herbalism should seek out knowledgeable, and preferably licensed, herbalists. See also *herbalism.*

hereditary angioneurotic edema See *angioedema, hereditary.*

hereditary hemorrhagic telangiectasia A genetic disease characterized by the presence of multiple direct connections between arteries and veins called arteriovenous malformations (AVMs). Small AVMs, or telangiectases, close to the surface of skin and mucous membranes often rupture and bleed after slight trauma. Abbreviated HHT. The most common manifestations of HHT are recurrent nosebleeds beginning at about 12 years of age. About one-fourth of individuals with HHT have gastrointestinal bleeding, which typically begins after age 50 years. Large AVMs may also bleed in the brain, lung, or other sites.

HHT is inherited as an autosomal dominant trait. Most patients have a parent with HHT. Each child of a person with HHT has a 50 percent risk of inheriting the condition. HHT is unusual in that it can be caused by a mutation in one of two different genes: the endoglin gene on chromosome 9 or the activin receptor gene on chromosome 12. Also known as Osler-Rendu-Weber syndrome and Rendu-Osler-Weber syndrome.

hereditary multiple exostoses See *osteochondromatosis.*

hereditary mutation A gene change that occurs in a germ cell (an egg or a sperm) and is then incorporated into every cell in the developing body of the new organism. Hereditary mutations play a role in cancer, as, for example, in the eye tumor retinoblastoma and Wilms' tumor of the kidney. Also known as germline mutation.

hereditary spherocytosis See *spherocytosis, hereditary.*

heredity The genetic transmission of characteristics from parent to child.

heritability The degree to which something is inherited.

heritable Capable of being transmitted from parent to child.

Hermansky-Pudlak syndrome A genetic disease characterized by a deficiency of pigment in the skin and eye, a bleeding tendency resulting from a platelet storage pool deficiency, and fibrosis of the lungs. Abbreviated HPS. Albinism that occurs in the eyes results in significant reduction in visual acuity. The patient's hair color ranges from white to brown, and the skin color is usually a shade lighter than that of other family members. The bleeding tendency results in easy bruising, frequent nosebleeds, and excessive bleeding with menstrual periods, childbirth, tooth extraction, circumcision, and other surgeries. Pulmonary fibrosis typically causes symptoms in the early 30s and progresses to death within a decade. Granulomatous colitis, a common finding, is severe in about one-sixth of patients. The disease is inherited as an autosomal recessive trait and can be due to mutation in the HPS1 gene on chromosome 10 or the ADTB3A gene on chromosome 5. Diagnosis is made by examining blood platelets under an electron microscope. There is currently no treatment for HPS. Also known as albinism with hemorrhagic diathesis, pigmented reticuloendithelial cells, and delta-storage pool disease.

hernia A general term referring to a protrusion of a tissue through the wall of the cavity in which it is normally contained. Also known as rupture.

hernia, hiatus   Protrusion of the stomach up into the opening that is normally occupied by the esophagus in the diaphragm, the muscle that separates the chest cavity from the abdomen. A hiatus hernia can be congenital, or it can be acquired through strenuous physical activity. Symptoms usually start with a tingling or burning sensation, and the patient may be able to see a bulge where the hernia is located. If the patient feels extreme pain, emergency surgery may be needed. Treatment is via conventional or laproscopic (minimally invasive) surgery. Also known as hiatal hernia.

hernia, Velpeau   A protrusion of tissue in front of the femoral blood vessels in the groin. Treatment is via surgery.

herniated disk   A disk, situated between two vertebrae, that protrudes and tends to press on a nerve root, causing radiating pain. A herniated disk may cause sciatica (pain in the lower back, leg, and behind the knee). Treatment options include use of anti-inflammatory medications, local injection of steroids, and surgical procedures. Also known as herniated disc, slipped disk or disc, prolapsed disk or disc, and ruptured disc or disk.

herniation   Abnormal protrusion of tissue through an opening.

heroin   A semisynthetic drug derived from, but more potent than, morphine. In 1898, heroin was introduced commercially as a painkiller. It is still used in this capacity in Europe, but it is not used medically in the US. Heroin is now better known as a drug of abuse than for its medical uses. Heroin may be injected into a vein, injected under the skin, snorted, or smoked. It is highly addictive, and overdose is an ever-present possibility due to the varying purity of street drugs. Physical addiction to heroin is often found with concurrent use of other opiates when heroin itself is not available. Treatment is by withdrawal, either gradual or sudden. Medication may be used to ease the physical effects of withdrawal, which include cramping, nausea, and intense craving. Opiate-blocker drugs, such as reboxetine (brand name: ReVia), may be used to speed up the withdrawal process and help the addict maintain compliance. Counseling, 12-step groups such as Narcotics Anonymous, nutritional support, and often antidepressant medication to help reregulate the nervous system are helpful adjunct treatments. Another method of treating heroin addiction is to prescribe methadone, a synthetic opioid liquid, as a substitute for heroin. In some European countries heroin itself is prescribed for addicts.

herpes   **1** Infection with one of the human herpes viruses, particularly herpes simplex 1 or 2.   **2** The family of herpesviruses.

herpes, genital   See *genital herpes.*

herpes simplex type 1   A herpesvirus that causes cold sores and fever blisters in and around the mouth. In rare cases, as when a patient's immune system is severely compromised, this virus can cause infection of the brain (encephalitis). Also known as human herpesvirus 1 (HHV-1). Treatments include topical ointments and antibiotic creams. See also *fever blister.*

herpes simplex type 2   A herpes virus that causes genital herpes, which is characterized by sores in the genital area. In rare cases, as when a patient's immune system is severely compromised, this virus can cause infection of the brain (encephalitis). Treatment involves use of topical or oral antiviral medication. Also known as human herpesvirus 2 (HHV-2). See also *genital herpes.*

herpes zoster   The herpes virus that causes chickenpox (varicella). Herpes zoster and chickenpox are usually contracted in childhood, at which time the virus infects nerves (namely, the dorsal root ganglia). It remains latent for years but can later be reactivated to cause shingles (blisters over the distribution of the affected nerve). Shingles is often accompanied by intense pain and itching. Also known as shingles, zona, zoster, and human herpesvirus 3 (HHV-3). See also *chickenpox; chickenpox immunization; shingles.*

herpesvirus   One of a family of viruses that contain DNA and that cause infections in humans (human herpesviruses) or animals. Herpesviruses are common and often live in the host's tissue for years or even decades without causing symptoms.

herpetiform virus   A virus with the characteristic shape and behavior of a virus in the herpes family. Not all members of the herpes virus family have been identified. Some herpatiform viruses may eventually be called herpesviruses, and others are merely similar to herpesviruses. See also *herpesvirus.*

hetero-   Prefix meaning different, as in heteromorphism (something that is different in form) and heterozygous (possessing two different forms of a particular gene). The opposite of hetero- is homo-.

heterochromatin   A genetically inactive part of the genome. Heterochromatin was so named because its chromosomal material (chromatin) stains more darkly throughout the cell cycle than most chromosomal material (euchromatin). There are two types of heterochromatin: constituitive heterochromatin and facultative heterochromatin.

heterochromia iridis   A difference in color between the iris of one eye and the iris of the other eye. A person with one brown eye and one blue eye has heterochromia iridis.

heterochromia iridis, sectoral A difference in color within an iris. A person with both brown and blue in the same eye has sectoral heterochromia iridis.

heterokaryon A cell with two separate nuclei formed by the experimental fusion of two genetically different cells. For example, heterokaryons composed of nuclei from Hurler syndrome and Hunter syndrome, both diseases of mucopolysaccharide metabolism, have normal mucopolysaccharide metabolism. This proves that the two syndromes affect different proteins and so can correct each other in the heterokaryon.

heteromorphism Something that is different in form. Chromosome heteromorphisms are normal variations in the appearance of chromosomes.

heteroploid A different chromosome number than the normal number of chromosomes. Abnormal numbers of chromosomes are associated with a number of disorders. For example, Down syndrome is the result of having three instead of two chromosome 21s.

heterosexual **1** A person who is sexually attracted to persons of the opposite sex. Colloquially known as straight. **2** The act or habit of opposite-sex attraction.

heterosexuality Sexuality directed toward someone of the opposite sex.

heterozygote An individual who has two different forms of a particular gene, one inherited from each parent. A heterozygote with cystic fibrosis (CF) has the CF gene on one chromosome 7 and the normal paired gene on the other chromosome 7. Also known as carrier.

heterozygous Possessing two different forms of a particular gene, one inherited from each parent.

HEV Hepatitis E virus. See *hepatitis E.*

hex-A deficiency Hexosaminidase A deficiency. See *Tay-Sachs disease.*

hexadactyly The presence of an extra digit: a sixth finger or toe. Hexadactyly is a very common birth defect. The sixth digit can be located in three different locations: on either side of the extremity or somewhere in between. With the hand, for example, the extra finger can be out beyond the little finger (ulnar hexadactyly), out beyond the thumb (radial hexadactyly), or between two of the normally expected fingers (intercalary hexadactyly). Hexadactyly can be absolutely harmless and is easily remedied. For example, ulnar hexadactyly with just a rudimentary tag of a sixth digit can be very simply treated

by being tied off with one suture. However, hexadactyly can also signal one of a number of congenital malformations. In such a case, treatment of hexadactyly may not be so simple, and the prognostic outlook may not be as good. See also *polydactyly.*

hexoseaminidase A An enzyme whose deficiency causes Tay-Sachs disease. See also *Tay-Sachs disease.*

HFV Hepatitis F virus. See *hepatitis F.*

HGV Hepatitis G virus. See *hepatitis G.*

HHS The Department of Health and Human Services of the US government, which has jurisdiction over public health, welfare, and civil rights issues and is the highest-level US government body with such jurisdiction. Agencies under HHS include the Public Health Service (PHS) and the Social Security Administration (SSA).

HHV Human herpesvirus. HHV-1 is herpes simplex type 1. HHV-2 is herpes simplex type 2. HHV-3 is herpes zoster, the cause of shingles. HHV-4 is the Epstein-Barr virus, the cause of infectious mononucleosis. HHV-5 is cytomegalovirus. See also *human herpesvirus 6; human herpesvirus 7; human herpesvirus 8.*

hiatus hernia See *hernia, hiatus.*

HIB Haemophilus influenzae type B.

HIB immunization See *Haemophilus influenzae type B immunization.*

hibernation reaction See *seasonal affective disorder.*

hiccough See *hiccup.*

hiccup An extraordinary type of breathing movement that involves a sudden intake of air (inspiration) due to a sudden involuntary contraction of the diaphragm, accompanied by closure of the glottis in the larynx. Closure of the glottis then halts the incoming air. The column of air strikes the closed glottis to produce the characteristic sound of a hiccup. Hiccups are often rhythmic. If self-limited, they are just a minor nuisance, but prolonged hiccups can become a major medical problem and be a sign of underlying disease (such as lung cancer or tumors in or around the diaphragm). Intractable hiccups can be painful and require medication to cause them to stop. In some patients with tic disorders, hiccups can be a tic. Also known as a singultus and hiccough.

hidradenitis suppurativa An illness characterized by multiple abscesses that form under the armpits and in the groin area. The cause is not known. Hydradenitis suppurativa is generally treated by surgical resection of the involved skin.

high altitude An altitude of 2,438 meters (8,000 feet) or more, at which altitude sickness commonly occurs. Most people can go up to 2,438 meters (8,000 feet) with minimal effects.

high blood pressure A repeatedly elevated blood pressure exceeding 140 over 90 mmHg. Chronic high blood pressure can stealthily cause blood vessel changes in the back of the eye (retina), abnormal thickening of the heart muscle, kidney failure, and brain damage. No specific cause for high blood pressure is found in 95 percent of patients. Treatment for high blood pressure involves salt restriction, regular aerobic exercise, and medication. There are many types of medications used to treat high blood pressure including diuretics, beta-blockers, blood vessel dilators, and others. Also known as hypertension.

high colonics See *irrigation of the colon.*

hip bursitis See *bursitis, hip.*

hip pointer A bruise of the upper edge of the ilium, one of the hip bones. Also known as iliac crest contusion.

hippocampus An area deep in the forebrain that helps regulate emotion and memory.

Hippocratic Oath One of the oldest binding documents in history, the Oath written by *Hippocrates* is still held sacred by physicians: to treat the ill to the best of one's ability, to preserve a patient's privacy, to teach the secrets of medicine to the next generation, and so on. See also *Daily Prayer of a Physician.*

Hirschsprung's disease An abnormal condition that is present at birth and is due to absence of the normal nerves (ganglia) in the bowel wall. Nerves can be missing starting at the anus and extending up a variable distance of the bowel. This results in enlargement of the bowel above the point of the missing nerve, as the nerves normally assist in the natural movement of the muscles in the lining of the bowels to move bowel contents through. Hirschsprung's disease is the most common cause of lower intestinal blockage in newborns, and it may later cause chronic constipation or diarrhea. The symptoms are vomiting, constipation, distention of the abdomen, and intestinal obstruction. Hirschsprung's disease is a feature of a number of syndromes, including chromosome abnormalities such as Down syndrome and genetic diseases such as neurofibromatosis. Hirschsprung's disease can also occur in isolation due to a mutation in the RET oncogene or in the EDNRB gene (endothelin receptor type B). Also known as congenital aganglionic megacolon.

hirsute Having an overabundance of hair.

hirsutism Having excessive facial and bodily hair. Hirsutism can be a side effect of certain medications (such as prednisone) or reflect an underlying hormonal imbalance.

hirudin An anticlotting agent that prevents blood clots from traveling through the bloodstream to clog up a vessel (thromboembolic complications). Hirudin is the main chemical in the secretion of leeches that allows them to suck out blood freely from the body after they attach to the skin. Desirudin and lepirudin (brand name: Refludan) are genetically engineered recombinant forms of hirudin.

His disease See *trench fever.*

histamine A substance that plays a major role in many allergic reactions, dilating blood vessels and making the vessel walls abnormally permeable. Histamine is part of the body's natural allergic response to substances such as pollens. Antihistamines work by preventing the release of histamine from certain cells (mast cells) thereby blocking the allergic reaction.

histamine cephalalgia See *cluster headache.*

histiocyte A type of white blood cell, also called a macrophage, that is created by bone marrow. Histiocytes usually stay in place, but when they are stimulated by infection or inflammation, they become active, attacking bacteria and other foreign matter in the body. See also *histiocytosis.*

histiocytosis A disorder in which histiocytes start to multiply and attack the person's own tissues or organs. The result can be tissue damage, pain, the development of tumor-like lumps called granulomas, fatigue, and other symptoms. If histiocytosis affects the pituitary gland, diabetes insipidus may also develop. Treatment includes radiation and chemotherapy, although for reasons unknown, some cases of histiocytosis go into remission without treatment.

histiocytosis, Langerhans cell See *Langerhans cell histiocytosis.*

histiocytosis, lipid See *Niemann-Pick disease.*

histiocytosis, sinus A type of histiocytosis in which the lymph nodes are the main site of histiocyte proliferation. The sinuses of the lymph nodes become filled with and distended by masses of histiocytes.

histiocytosis X See *Langerhans cell histiocytosis.*

histocompatible Literally, tissue compatible, meaning that the tissue can exist together with tissue of another organism without the immune system rejecting it. If a tissue donor and tissue recipient are histocompatible, a transplant is expected to be easily accepted.

histology The study of the form of structures as seen under a microscope. Also known as microscopic anatomy, as opposed to gross anatomy.

histone A protein around which DNA coils to form chromatin. Without histones, DNA could not organize into chromosomes, and life as we know it would not exist.

Histoplasma capsulatum A fungus that is found worldwide. In the US, it is so common in the Midwest and South that in parts of Kentucky and Tennessee nearly 90 percent of adults have a positive histoplasma skin test. It is carried in bird and bat droppings, and it is deposited in the soil. Although people can contract histoplasma from their environment, it cannot be passed from person to person. While most persons exposed to H. capsulatum do not become ill, some people develop a disease that predominantly affects the lungs called histoplasmosis. See also *histoplasmosis*.

histoplasmosis A disease caused by the fungus Histoplasma capsulatum. Most people with histoplasmosis have no symptoms. However, it can cause acute or chronic lung disease and progressive disseminated histoplasmosis, which affects a number of organs. Infants, young children, and older persons—particularly those with chronic lung disease — are at increased risk for severe disease. Disseminated histoplasmosis is most frequently seen in people with cancer or AIDS. The acute respiratory disease of histoplasmosis is characterized by respiratory symptoms, a general ill feeling, fever, chest pains, and a dry or nonproductive cough. Distinct patterns may be seen on a chest x-ray. Chronic lung disease related to histoplasmosis resembles tuberculosis and can worsen over months or years. The disseminated form is fatal unless treated. Mild cases resolve without treatment. Severe cases of acute histoplasmosis and all cases of chronic and disseminated histoplasmosis are treated with antifungal medications, usually for life in those with compromised immune systems.

history See *history, medical*.

history, developmental An account of how and when a child passed developmental milestones, such as walking and talking. For adults, information on social-emotional development may be included. A developmental history is used primarily in the diagnosis of developmental disorders.

history, family An account of past and current family structure and relationships within the family, including medical information about family members. The information may be recorded in pedigree form.

Illnesses, hospitalizations, causes of death, miscarriages, abortions, congenital malformations, and any other important features are noted. A family history is essential for genetic counseling.

history, medical A complete account of all past and present medical events and problems a person has experienced, including psychiatric illness. A medical history is especially helpful when differential diagnosis is needed. The medical history may contain helpful clues to prevent health problems in the future.

history, social An account of a patient that puts his or her illness or behavior in context. A social history may include aspects of the patient's developmental, family, and medical history, as well as relevant information about life events, social class, race, religion, and occupation. A social history is useful for designing treatment plans, especially for psychiatric or neurological illness.

His-Werner disease See *trench fever*.

HIV Human immunodeficiency virus, the cause of AIDS. HIV is a retrovirus: It has an RNA genome and a reverse transcriptase enzyme. Using the reverse transcriptase, the virus uses its RNA as a template for making complementary DNA. This DNA can then integrate itself into the DNA of the host organism. Also known as the AIDS virus, human lymphotropic virus type III, lymphadenopathy-associated virus, and lymphadenopathy virus. See also *AIDS*.

HIV infection, acute The body's initial reaction to infection by human immunodeficiency virus (HIV), a flu-like syndrome that occurs immediately after a person contracts HIV. Symptoms include fever, sore throat, headache, skin rash, and swollen glands (lymphadenopathy). This syndrome precedes the development of detectable antibodies to HIV in the blood (seroconversion), which normally takes weeks or months. When antibodies to HIV appear in the blood, a person tests positive in the standard ELISA test for HIV. See also *AIDS; AIDS-related complex*.

HIV infection, primary The stage of infection by human immunodeficiency virus (HIV), in which detectable antibodies to HIV appear in the blood (seroconversion). It normally takes from several weeks to several months for antibodies to the virus to develop after HIV transmission. When antibodies to HIV appear in the blood, a person tests positive in the standard ELISA test for HIV. Primary HIV infection may or may not include the symptoms of acute HIV. See also *AIDS; HIV infection, acute*.

hive A raised, itchy area of skin that is usually a sign of an allergic reaction. A hive can be rounded or flat topped but is always elevated above the surrounding skin. It reflects circumscribed dermal edema (local swelling of the skin). Hives are usually well circumscribed but may be coalescent, and they blanch with pressure. They typically last less than 4 hours but they may stay for days or weeks. Approximately 20 percent of the population has experienced hives. Treatment is administration of antihistamines. Also known as urticaria and welt.

HLA Human leukocyte antigen, the major human histocompatibility system. HLA typing is done before transplantation to determine the degree of tissue compatibility between donor and recipient.

Hodgkin's disease A type of lymphoma, a cancer that develops in the lymph system, part of the body's immune system. Because there is lymph tissue in many parts of the body, Hodgkin's disease can start in almost any part of the body. The cancer can spread to almost any organ or tissue in the body, including the liver, bone marrow, and spleen. Hodgkin's disease most commonly affects young adults in their 20s and 30s, as well as people older than 55 years. Symptoms include painless swelling of the lymph nodes in the neck, underarm, or groin; fever; night sweats; tiredness; weight loss; and itchy skin. If there are symptoms, a physician should carefully check for swelling or lumps in the neck, armpits, and groin. If the lymph nodes do not feel normal, a biopsy may be done. The chance of recovery (prognosis) and choice of treatment depend on a number of factors, including the stage of the cancer and whether it is in just one area or has spread throughout the body. Treatment includes radiation and/or chemotherapy. Hodgkin's disease is lifethreatening if untreated, but it has a very high cure rate. Also called Hodgkin's lymphoma.

Hodgkin's lymphoma See *Hodgkin's disease.*

holandric inheritance Inheritance of genes on the Y chromosome. Because only males normally have Y chromosomes, Y-linked genes can only be transmitted from father to son.

hole, macular See *macular hole.*

Holter monitor A type of portable heart monitor that is a small electrocardiogram (EKG) device worn in a pouch around the neck or waist. A Holter monitor keeps a record of the heart rhythm, typically over a 24-hour period, and the patient keeps a diary of activities and symptoms. The EKG recording is then correlated with the person's activities and symptoms. This type of test is useful for identifying heart disturbances that are sporadic and not readily identified with a resting EKG.

homeobox A short stretch of nucleotides (DNA or RNA) with an almost identical base sequence in all the genes that contain that stretch. Homeoboxes occur in many organisms and appear to determine when particular groups of genes are expressed during development. For example, homeoboxes play a role in making certain cells within the embryo develop into heart muscle, or into brain tissue, etc.

homeopath A person who practices homeopathy.

homeopathy Founded in the 19th century, a practice that is based on the concept that disease can be treated with minute doses of drugs thought capable of producing in healthy people the same symptoms as those of the disease being treated. This principle is similar to the concept behind exposure therapy for allergies, but the amounts of active medication used in homeopathy are so small as to be almost undetectable. Scientific studies of homeopathy have returned mixed results. It is a mainstream medical practice in the UK but considered alternative medicine in the US.

homo- Prefix meaning same, as in homology (similarity in DNA or protein sequences between individuals or between species) and homosexual (a person who is sexually attracted to persons of the same sex). The opposite of homo- is hetero-. For example, heterogeneous and homogeneous, heterosexual and homosexual, and so on.

homocysteine An amino acid that is produced by the human body, usually as a byproduct of consuming meat. Homocysteine is normally converted into other amino acids. An abnormal accumulation of homocysteine, which can be measured in the blood, can be a marker for the development of heart disease. Elevated levels of homocysteine in the blood appear to increase the risk of heart attack, stroke, peripheral vascular disease, and venous thromboembolism (blood clots in the veins). Homocysteine can damage blood vessels in several ways. It injures the cells that line arteries and stimulates the growth of smooth muscle cells. Homocysteine can also disrupt normal blood clotting mechanisms, increasing the risk of clots that can bring on heart attack or stroke. Elevated levels of homocysteine also appear to increase the risk of Alzheimer's disease. The ways to lower homocysteine are to eat less meat and take supplements of the B vitamins folic acid (folate), B6, and B12 that are needed by the enzymes that process homocysteine.

homocystinuria A genetic disease that is due to an enzyme deficiency that permits a buildup of the amino acid homocysteine. Progressive mental retardation is common in untreated cases of homocystinuria. The finding of vascular disease and premature arteriosclerosis in persons with homocystinuria led to the theory that homocysteine may be a factor in heart disease. Homocystinuria is inherited in an autosomal recessive manner and is one of the diseases commonly included among the diseases for which newborns are screened. Treatments include special diets and vitamin B6.

homolog One chromosome of a pair. Also spelled homologue.

homology Similarity in DNA or protein sequences between individuals or between species.

homologous The relationship between two chromosomes that are paired and so are homologs of each other.

homologous chromosomes A pair of chromosomes that contain the same gene sequences, each derived from one parent.

homosexual **1** A person who is sexually attracted to persons of the same sex. Colloquially known as gay. **2** The act or habit of same-sex attraction.

homosexuality Sexuality directed toward someone of the same sex.

hookworm An intestinal parasite that infests a billion people, mainly in tropical and subtropical areas. Infection is from contact with soil contaminated by hookworm larvae. First signs are itching and rash at the site where the larvae penetrate the skin. This is followed by diarrhea, intestinal cramps, pain, anorexia, weight loss, and anemia. Loss of iron and protein due to hookworm can retard the growth and mental development of children, sometimes irreversibly. The infection can be fatal, particularly for infants, pregnant women, and persons who are malnourished. See also *Necator americanus.*

horizontal Parallel to the floor. A person lying on a bed is considered to be in a horizontal position. See also Appendix B, "Anatomic Orientation Terms."

hormone A chemical substance produced in the body that controls and regulates the activity of certain cells or organs. Many hormones are secreted by special glands, such as thyroid hormone produced by the thyroid gland. Hormones are essential for every activity of life, including the processes of digestion, metabolism, growth, reproduction, and mood control. Many hormones, such as neurotransmitters, are active in more than one physical process.

hormone, androgenic Any hormone that promotes the development and maintenance of male sex characteristics. Testosterone is an androgenic hormone.

hormone, follicle-stimulating See *follicle-stimulating hormone.*

hormone, mineralocorticoid A group of hormones, the most important of which is aldosterone, that regulates the balance of water and electrolytes (ions such as sodium and potassium) in the body. The mineralocorticoid hormones act specifically on the tubules of the kidney. See also *corticosteroid.*

hormone replacement therapy The use of medications containing both estrogen and progestogen to reduce or stop short-term changes associated with menopause, such as hot flashes, disturbed sleep, and vaginal dryness. Abbreviated HRT. HRT can ease the symptoms of menopause and protect against osteoporosis and hip fractures.

hormone therapy Treatment of disease or symptoms with synthetic or naturally derived hormones. Hormone therapy may be used to treat some forms of cancer, taking advantage of the fact that certain cancers depend on hormones to grow. It may also be used for thyroid disorders, problems associated with menopause, and illnesses associated with hormone production or use. Hormone therapy may include giving hormones to the patient or using medications that decrease the level of hormones in the body.

hormone, thyroid A chemical substance that is made by the thyroid gland, which is located in the front of the neck. The two most important thyroid hormones are thyroxine (T4) and triiodothyronine (T3). See also *thyroxine; triiodothyronine.*

hormone, thyroid stimulating See *thyroid stimulating hormone.*

hormone, thyrotropin See *thyroid stimulating hormone.*

Horner ptosis See *Horner syndrome.*

Horner syndrome A complex of abnormal findings, including the sinking in of one eyeball, the drooping of the upper eyelid on the same side (ipsilateral ptosis), and the constriction of the pupil of that eye (miosis), together with lack of sweating (anhidrosis) and flushing of the affected side of the face. Horner syndrome is due to paralysis of cervical sympathetic nerves. Also known as Horner-Bernard syndrome, Bernard syndrome, Bernard-Horner syndrome, and Horner ptosis.

hornet sting A sting from a hornet, which can trigger an allergic reaction of varying severity. Avoidance and prompt treatment are essential. For those with severe reactions, injectable adrenaline should always be kept on hand. In selected cases, allergy injection therapy is highly effective.

horripilation See *goose bumps.*

hospital A place for receiving medical or surgical care, usually as an inpatient (resident). An ill person in the US may be put "in the hospital," and his ailing UK counterpart would say he is "in hospital."

hospitalist A hospital-based general physician. Hospitalists assume the care of hospitalized patients in the place of patients' primary care physicians. In the most prevalent US model of hospitalist care, several physicians practice together as a group and work full time to care for inpatients.

hot flash A sudden wave of mild or intense body heat caused by a rush of hormones. Hot flashes result from blood vessels opening and constricting, an action that is triggered by hormonal changes caused by decreased levels of estrogen. They can occur at any time and may last from a few seconds to a half hour. Hot flashes are a symptom of menopause.

housemaid's knee See *patellofemoral syndrome.*

HPS 1 Hantavirus pulmonary syndrome. 2 Hermansky-Pudlak syndrome.

HPV Human papilloma virus.

HRT Hormone replacement therapy.

HS Hereditary spherocytosis. See *spherocytosis, hereditary.*

ht 1 Abbreviation for height. 2 Abbreviation for heart.

HUGO Human Genome Organization, the international organization concerned with researching and mapping the human genes.

human chorionic gonadotropin A hormone that is made by chorionic cells in the fetal part of the placenta. Abbreviated hCG. hCG is directed at and stimulates the gonads. hCG becomes detectable within days of fertilization, and it forms the foundation of most common pregnancy tests. The level of hCG in maternal serum is also one component in the double and triple screens used during pregnancy to assign risks of Down syndrome and other fetal disorders. See also *gonadotropin.*

human gene therapy See *gene therapy.*

human genome See *genome, human.*

Human Genome Organization See *HUGO.*

Human Genome Project Begun formally in 1990, the US Human Genome Project was an international effort coordinated by the US. Its goals included the identification and sequencing (ordering) of all the bases in the human genome. US participation in this monumental undertaking was supported by funds from the National Institutes of Health (NIH) and the Department of Energy (DOE). The project was successful.

human herpesvirus 1 through 5 See *HHV.*

human herpesvirus 6 A herpes virus that apparently lies dormant in many people, and is most likely to cause problems when the immune system is compromised by disease, as in AIDS patients, or by deliberate immune suppression, as in organ transplant patients. Abbreviated HHV-6. There are two forms of HHV-6: A and B. A is rare and is acquired in adulthood. B is relatively common, is usually acquired in childhood, and is associated with roseola. Both HHV-6 A and B can reactivate at a later date and are believed to contribute to diseases of the bone marrow and/or central nervous system in some patients, including fatal encephalitis, chronic fatigue syndrome, and possibly multiple sclerosis. Diagnosis is made via rapid blood culture or other blood test. Treatment is experimental at this time, but antiviral drugs or beta interferon may be tried.

human herpesvirus 7 A herpes virus that causes seizures and other central nervous system symptoms in children. Abbreviated HHV-7. Closely related to HHV-6, HHV-7 has also been linked to roseola. Diagnosis is made via rapid blood culture or other blood test. Treatment is experimental at this time, but antiviral drugs or beta interferon may be tried.

human herpesvirus 8 A herpesvirus that may contribute to Kaposi sarcoma, a rare form of cancer that is sometimes seen in AIDS patients, and to some B-cell lymphomas. Abbreviated HHV-8. Diagnosis is made via rapid blood culture or other blood test. Treatment is experimental at this time, but antiviral drugs or beta interferon may be tried. Also known as Kaposi sarcoma-associated herpesvirus (KSHV).

human immunodeficiency virus See *HIV.*

human leukocyte antigen See *HLA.*

human papilloma virus A family of more than 60 viruses that are responsible for causing warts. Abbreviated HPV. The majority of HPVs produce warts on the hands, fingers, or face. Most of these warts are innocuous, causing nothing more than cosmetic concerns. Several types of HPV are confined primarily to the moist skin of the genitals, producing genital warts and elevating the risk for cancer of the cervix. The HPVs that cause wartlike growths on the genitals are sexually transmitted.

humerus The long bone in the upper arm that extends from the shoulder to the elbow.

humidifier A machine that puts moisture into the air. Humidified air makes it easier to breathe for persons with certain conditions, such as cystic fibrosis, Sjogren's syndrome, and others.

humor In medicine, a fluid or semifluid substance. For example, the aqueous humor is the fluid normally present in the front and rear chambers of the eye.

humor, aqueous The fluid that is normally present in the front and rear chambers of the eye.

humoral Pertaining to elements in the blood or other body fluids.

humoralism An ancient theory holding that health came from balance between the bodily liquids termed humors. Disease arose when imbalance occurred between the humors. The humors were phlegm (water), blood, gall (black bile, thought to be secreted by the kidneys and spleen), and choler (yellow bile secreted by the liver). The humoral theory was devised well before Hippocrates, and it was not definitively demolished until 1858. Physicians now know that health rests on a cellular and molecular foundation, although the word *humor* lives on as a medical term for liquid or semiliquid substances in the body and as a euphemism for mood (such as being "in good humor"). Also known as humorism.

humorism See *humoralism.*

Hunter syndrome A genetic metabolic disorder that arises from deficiency of the enzyme iduronate sulfatase, resulting in tissue deposits of molecules called mucopolysaccharides. The characteristic features of Hunter syndrome include dwarfism, bone deformities, a thickened, coarse face, hepatosplenomegaly (enlargement of the liver and spleen) from mucopolysaccharide deposits, cardiovascular disorders from mucopolysaccharide deposits, and deafness. There are two forms of Hunter syndrome: a severe form that causes progressive mental retardation, physical disability, and death before age 15 in most cases; and a mild form in which patients survive to adulthood, are able to reproduce, and have intellect that is impaired minimally, if at all. The gene for the enzyme iduronate sulfatase (deficient in Hunter's syndrome) is on the X chromosome (in band Xq28). Also known as mucopolysaccharidosis II.

Huntington's chorea See *Huntington's disease.*

Huntington's disease A genetic disorder characterized by progressive mental and physical deterioration that leads to death. Abbreviated HD. Although HD is usually an adult-onset disorder, it can affect children as well. The average survival time is 15 to 18 years after the onset of symptoms. Mood disturbance is usually the first symptom seen, with bipolar disorder–like mood swings that may include mania, depression, extreme irritability or angry outbursts, and psychosis. Other symptoms include chorea (restless, wiggling, turning movements), muscle stiffness and slowness of movement, and difficulties with memory and other cognitive processes. HD is inherited in an autosomal dominant manner. Children of an individual with the HD gene have a 50 percent chance of inheriting the disease-causing gene. The HD gene is on chromosome 4 (in band 4p16). Diagnosis is made via molecular genetic testing. At this time there is no cure for HD, although medication may be used to control symptoms of the illness, such as mood swings and chorea. See also *chorea.*

Hurler syndrome An inherited error of metabolism characterized by deficiency of the enzyme alpha-L-iduronidase, which normally breaks down molecules called mucopolysaccharides. Without the activity of this enzyme, mucopolysaccharides accumulate abnormally in the tissues of the body. There are two clinical subtypes of disease due to deficiency of alpha-L-iduronidase: Hurler syndrome and Scheie syndrome. Hurler syndrome patients have progressive mental degeneration, gross facial features, enlarged and deformed skull, small stature, corneal opacities, hepatosplenomegaly (enlargement of the liver and spleen), valvular heart defects, thick skin, joint contractures, and hernias. Hurler syndrome is inherited in an autosomal recessive manner. The gene that codes for alpha-L-iduronidase is on chromosome 4 (in band 4p16.3). Bone marrow transplantation may slow the progression of Hurler syndrome, but it is not yet known whether it will be an effective treatment. Attempts at enzyme replacement therapy have not been successful to date. Also known as mucopolysaccharidosis type I.

hurricane supplies See *disaster supplies.*

Hutchinson-Gilford progeria syndrome See *progeria.*

hybrid The result of a cross between genetically unlike parents. A hybrid is therefore the offspring of parents who differ in regard to the particular gene in question.

hybridoma A cell hybrid resulting from the fusion of a cancer cell and a normal lymphocyte (a type of white blood cell). The hybridoma is immortal in the laboratory and can be used to produce a specific antibody indefinitely.

hydatid mole See *hydatidiform mole.*

hydatidiform mole A tumor that forms in the uterus as a mass of cysts resembling a bunch of grapes. Hydatidiform moles occur during the childbearing years, and they do not spread outside the uterus. However, a malignancy called choriocarcinoma may start from a hydatidiform mole. In its early stages, a hydatidiform mole may look like a normal pregnancy. Diagnosis is based on a history of lack of fetal movement, a pelvic examination, an ultrasound, and a blood test to look for high levels of a hormone called beta human chorionic gonadotropin (hCG). hCG in the blood of a woman who is not pregnant can be a sign of a hydatidiform mole. Treatment includes removal of the mole by dilation and curettage (D & C) and suction evacuation and surgery to remove the uterus (hysterectomy). After surgery, regular blood tests are done to make sure the level of beta hCG in the blood falls to normal levels. If the blood levels of beta hCG do not go down to normal or increase, more tests are needed to see whether the mole has persisted or if there is choriocarcinoma. Also known as a molar pregnancy.

hydro- Prefix meaning related to water.

hydrocele Accumulation of fluid in the coat around the testis. Small hydroceles tend to disappear by 1 year of age. Larger hydroceles may persist and warrant surgery.

hydrocephalus An abnormal buildup of cerebrospinal fluid (CSF) in the ventricles and/or subarachnoid space of the brain. The fluid often increases intracranial pressure, which can compress and damage the brain. This increased pressure is most commonly caused by obstruction of the flow of CSF, but it may also be due to overproduction of CSF, a condition known as choroid plexus papilloma, or failure of the brain to reabsorb CSF. Hydrocephalus can arise before birth or at any time afterward. Causes include birth defects (particularly spina bifida), hemorrhage into the brain, infection, meningitis, tumor, and head injury. Most forms of hydrocephalus are the result of obstructed CSF flow in the ventricular system. Symptoms depend on the person's age. In infants, the most obvious sign is usually an abnormally large head; other symptoms may include vomiting, sleepiness, irritability, an inability to look upward, and seizures. In older children and adults, there is no head enlargement from hydrocephalus, but symptoms may include headache, nausea, vomiting, and sometimes blurred vision. Patients may have problems with balance, delayed development in walking or talking, and poor coordination. Irritability, fatigue, seizures, and personality changes (such as an inability to concentrate or remember things) may also develop. Drowsiness and double vision are common symptoms as hydrocephalus progresses. Treatment involves insertion of a shunt to let the excess fluid exit, thereby relieving the pressure on the brain. The shunt is inserted into the ventricular system of the brain to divert the flow of CSF into another area of the body, where the CSF can drain and be absorbed into the bloodstream. The outlook with hydrocephalus depends on the cause and on the timing of the diagnosis and treatment. Many children treated for hydrocephalus are able to lead normal lives with few, if any, limitations. In some cases, cognitive impairments in language and nonlanguage functions may occur. Problems with shunts, such as infection or malfunction, require revision of the shunt. Also known as water on the brain and hydrocephaly. See also *hydrocephalus, acquired; hydrocephalus, congenital.*

hydrocephalus, acquired Hydrocephalus that is due to a postnatal cause, something that happened sometime after birth. See also *hydrocephalus.*

hydrocephalus, communicating Hydrocephalus in which there is no obstruction to the flow of the cerebrospinal fluid (CSF). Specifically, there is no obstruction within the ventricular system of the brain or where the CSF passes into the spinal canal. Communicating hydrocephalus is due to overproduction of CSF or failure of the brain to reabsorb CSF normally.

hydrocephalus, congenital Hydrocephalus that is present at birth. See also *hydrocephalus.*

hydrocephalus ex-vacuo Hydrocephalus that occurs when there is damage to the brain caused by stroke or injury, in which there may be an actual shrinkage of brain substance. The CSF pressure itself is normal. In elderly persons or persons with Alzheimer's disease, the entire brain may shrink, enabling the CSF to fill up the space created by the shrinkage. This is not due to hydrocephalus. See also *hydrocephalus; hydrocephalus, normal pressure.*

hydrocephalus, normal pressure Hydrocephalus that occurs because of a gradual blockage of CSF drainage pathways in the brain. Although the ventricles enlarge, intracranial pressure remains within normal range. Abbreviated NPH. NPH can occur as a complication of brain infection or bleeding (hemorrhage). In some patients, no predisposing cause can be identified. NPH is characterized by memory loss (dementia), gait disorder (ataxia), urinary incontinence, and a general slowing of activity. See also *hydrocephalus; hydrocephalus ex-vacuo.*

hydrocephaly See *hydrocephalus.*

hydronephrosis Distention of the kidney with urine. Hydronephrosis is caused by obstruction of urine outflow (for example, by a stone blocking the ureter).

hydrops fetalis Gross edema (swelling), usually with anemia, that affects a fetus. Hydrops fetalis can be due to Rh blood group incompatibility, in which antibodies crossing the placenta from the mother destroy the red blood cells of the fetus. It can also be caused by alpha thalassemia, a lethal form of the genetic disorder thalassemia, in which alpha-chain polypeptides that are needed to make fetal or adult hemoglobin are not produced. See also *Rh incompatibility; thalassemia, alpha.*

hydroxyapatite An essential ingredient of normal bone and teeth that makes up bone mineral and the matrix of teeth and gives them their rigidity. See also *hydroxyapatite crystal disease.*

hydroxyapatite crystal disease Inflammation caused by hydroxyapatite crystals. Hydroxyapatite molecules can group together (crystallize) to form microscopic clumps. If the tiny crystals of hydroxyapatite are deposited by mistake in or around joints, they may cause inflammation of the joints and nearby tissues, such as tendons and ligaments. Hydroxyapatite crystal disease is sometimes the cause of rotator cuff problems in the shoulder.

hygiene The science of preventive medicine and the preservation of health. Also commonly used as a euphemism for cleanliness and proper sanitation.

hymen A thin membrane that may completely or partially cover the vaginal opening before first sexual intercourse but that usually disappears before puberty.

hyoglossus The muscle that permits the tongue to be held on the floor of the mouth.

hyper- Prefix meaning high, beyond, excessive, or above normal, as in hyperglycemia (high sugar in the blood) and hypercalcemia (high calcium in the blood). The opposite of hyper- is hypo-.

hyperactivity A higher-than-normal level of activity. An organ can be described as hyperactive if it is more active than is usual. Behavior can also be described as hyperactive. See also *attention deficit hyperactivity disorder.*

hyperadrenocorticism See *Cushing syndrome.*

hyperaldosteronism See *aldosteronism.*

hyperbaric oxygen chamber A pressurized chamber in which a patient receives pure oxygen, either directly or through a mask, tent, or tube. The oxygen is delivered at high pressure, more than 1.4 times normal atmospheric pressure. See also *hyperbaric oxygen therapy.*

hyperbaric oxygen therapy The use of a hyperbaric oxygen (HBO) chamber to treat any of a number of conditions, notably carbon monoxide poisoning, decompression sickness ("the bends"), smoke inhalation, and gas gangrene. HBO therapy also helps to heal skin grafts and major burn injuries. The patient is enclosed in the chamber and receives appropriately pressurized pure oxygen for a specified length of time. HBO therapy activates white blood cells, and so it is sometimes used in cases of antibiotic-resistant or severe infection, such as for necrotizing fasciitis.

hyperbilirubinemia An elevated level of the pigment bilirubin in the blood. A sufficient elevation of bilirubin produces jaundice. Some degree of hyperbilirubinemia is very common right after birth, especially in premature babies. Treatment of hyperbilirubinemia in the newborn involves exposure of the skin to special lights and removal of serum from the blood and replacing with solutions free of bilirubin (exchange transfusion).

hyperbilirubinemia type 1 See *Gilbert syndrome.*

hypercalcemia A higher-than-normal level of calcium in the blood. Hypercalcemia can cause a number of non-specific symptoms, including loss of appetite, nausea, thirst, fatigue, muscle weakness, restlessness, and confusion. Excessive intake of calcium may cause muscle weakness and constipation, affect the conduction of electrical impulses in the heart (heart block), lead to calcium stones (nephrocalcinosis) in the urinary tract, impair kidney function, and interfere with the absorption of iron, predisposing the person to iron deficiency. According to the National Academy of Sciences, adequate intake of calcium is 1 g daily for both men and women. The upper limit for calcium intake is 2.5 g daily.

hypercholesterolemia High blood cholesterol. See also *familial hypercholesterolemia.*

hypercoagulable state A condition in which there is an abnormally increased tendency toward blood clotting (coagulation). There are numerous hypercoagulable states. Each has different causes, and each increases a person's chances of developing blood clots, such as those associated with thrombophlebitis (inflammation due to a clot in the veins). These causes include medications (particularly female hormones and birth control pills), surgery (especially hip, knee, and urinary system procedures), pregnancy, phospholipid antibodies in blood (anticardiolipin antibodies, lupus anticoagulant), cancer (although most patients with hypercoagulable states do not have cancer), elevated blood homocysteine levels, and inherited protein deficiencies, such as deficiencies of antithrombin III, factor V Leiden, protein S, and protein C. Treatment involves avoidance of the triggering mechanism and sometimes use of blood-thinning medication. See also *antiphospholipid syndrome; estrogen-associated hypercoagulability.*

hyperemesis gravidarum Excessive vomiting in early pregnancy. By definition, hyperemesis gravidarum leads to the loss of 5 percent or more of the woman's body weight. It affects about 1 in every 300 pregnant women and is most common in young women, in first pregnancies, and in women carrying multiple fetuses. Hyperemesis gravidarum usually stops on its own and is of little clinical consequence. Sometimes, however, hyperemesis can keep the mother from getting necessary fluids and nutrition. Some women with hyperemesis gravidarum have high concentrations of the hormones human chorionic gonadotropin (hCG), estrogen, or thyroid hormone in their blood. A few also have clinical manifestations of hyperthyroidism (overactive thyroid state). Treatment of mild hyperemesis gravidarum usually involves dietary measures, rest, and use of antacids. Very severe hyperemesis gravidarum may call for the use of intravenous fluids and nutrition.

hyperexplexia A genetic disorder in which babies have an exaggerated startle reflex. Symptoms at birth may include muscle stiffness (hypertonia), an exaggerated response to being startled, and strong brain stem reflexes (especially head-retraction reflex). Hypertonia is apparent when the limbs move, disappears during sleep, and diminishes over the first year of life. The startle reflex is sometimes accompanied by sudden stiffness (acute generalized hypertonia), which can cause the affected person to fall to the ground like a log. Additional findings include a tendency to umbilical and inguinal hernias (presumably due to increased pressure within the abdomen) and congenital dislocation of the hip. The exaggerated startle response persists throughout life. The gene that is responsible for hyperexplexia has been found on chromosome number 5, in bands 5q33.2–q33.3. Treatment is via medications. The neurological features can usually be controlled with clonazepam (brand name: Klonopin). In some cases, antispasmodic medications or tranquilizers have also been found useful. Also known as exaggerated startle disease, hyperekplexia, Kok disease, startle disease, and stiff baby syndrome.

hyperglycemia Elevated blood glucose (sugar). Hyperglycemia is often found in diabetes mellitus. See also *diabetes mellitus.*

hyperkalemia Elevated potassium in the blood. Hyperkalemia can be caused by taking excessive amounts of potassium, by medications, and by diseases such as kidney failure.

hyperlipidemia Elevated lipid (fat) levels in the blood. Hyperlipidemia can be inherited and increases the risk of disease of the blood vessels leading to stroke and heart disease.

hypermagnesemia Excess magnesium in the blood. Persons with impaired kidney function should be especially careful about their magnesium intake because they can accumulate magnesium, which is a dangerous (and sometimes fatal) situation. According to the National Academy of Sciences, the recommended dietary allowance of magnesium is 420 mg per day for men and 320 mg per day for women. The upper limit for magnesium supplements is 350 mg daily, in addition to the magnesium taken in through food and water.

hypermobility syndrome A common, mostly harmless childhood condition in which joints can move beyond the normal range of motion. Symptoms of hypermobility syndrome can include pains in knees, fingers, hips, and elbows, and the affected joints may sprain or dislocate. Scoliosis (curvature of the spine) is a common symptom. Hypermobility syndrome usually disappears on its own by adulthood. Also known as joint hypermobility syndrome. See also *Ehlers-Danlos syndrome.*

hypernatremia Elevated sodium in the blood. Hypernatremia can be caused by medications or conditions, such as dehydration. See also *sodium.*

hyperopia See *farsightedness.*

hyperostosis Overgrowth of bone. Also known as exostosis.

hyperphenylalaninemia Elevated levels of the amino acid phenylalanine in the blood. See also *phenylalanine; phenylalanine hydroxylase deficiency; PKU; PKU, maternal.*

hyperphosphatemia An elevated level of phosphate in the blood. Phosphate molecules are particularly important as part of larger molecules in cell energy cycles. Higher-than-normal levels can be caused by ingestion of phosphate-rich foods, such as dairy products, or by kidney failure.

hyperpigmentation Dark spots on the skin. Hyperpigmentation is primarily a cosmetic concern that can be covered with makeup, although in some cases (such as the cafe au lait spots associated with neurofibromatosis) it can be a sign of an underlying medical problem. If treatment of hyperpigmentation is desired, a dermatologist may be able to use dermabrasion, laser treatments, or bleaching agents to effect change.

hyperplasia An increase in the number of normal cells in a tissue or an organ. Hyperplasia can represent a precancerous condition.

hyperplasia, benign prostatic See *benign prostatic hyperplasia.*

hyperplasia, endometrial A condition characterized by overgrowth of the lining of the uterus. This is considered a precancerous condition.

hypertension See *high blood pressure.*

hypertension, benign intracranial See *pseudotumor cerebri.*

hypertension, pulmonary High blood pressure in the pulmonary arteries. The pressure in the pulmonary arteries is normally low compared to that in the aorta. Pulmonary hypertension can irrevocably damage the lungs.

hyperthermia Overheating of the body, possibly due to extreme weather conditions. Unrelieved hyperthermia can lead to collapse and death, particularly in the elderly. Hyperthermia can be prevented through use of air conditioning and ventilation, as well as by ensuring that vulnerable persons drink extra water. In emergency cases of hyperthermia, injections of saline solution and rapid cooling of the body may be necessary. Also known as heatstroke and heat prostration.

hyperthermia, malignant A series of potentially fatal problems that can occur during surgery, caused by a reaction to anesthesia such as halothane or muscle relaxants such as succinyl choline chloride. With malignant hyperthermia, the body's metabolism rises suddenly, causing a sudden jump in body temperature and muscle rigidity. The result can be damage to tissues and organs (including the brain) or death. The propensity to malignant hyperthermia is inherited in an autosomal dominant manner. Malignant hyperthermia is produced by mutation of the ryanodine receptor gene (RYR1). The RYR1 gene encodes the calcium-ion-release channel of the sarcoplasmic reticulum. There are at least five other genetic forms of malignant hyperthermia. Treatment involves administration of dantrolene sodium (brand name: Dantrium) and rapid cooling of the patient.

hyperthyroid Excessive thyroid hormone resulting from an overactive thyroid gland or from taking too much thyroid hormone. Symptoms of hyperthyroid can include increased heart rate, weight loss, depression, and cognitive slowing. Treatment includes medication use, the use of radioactive iodine, thyroid surgery, and reduction in the dose of thyroid hormone.

hypertonia Increased tightness of muscle tone. Untreated hypertonia can lead to loss of function and deformity. Treatment includes physical and/or occupational therapy and in some cases use of muscle-relaxant medication. Injections of botulism toxin (botox) are a recent treatment for chronic hypertonia in cerebral palsy and other disorders. Also known as spasticity.

hypertonic solution A solution that contains more salt than is found in normal cells and blood. For example, hypertonic solutions are used for soaking wounds.

hypertrophic cardiomyopathy See *cardiomyopathy, hypertrophic.*

hypertrophy, benign prostatic See *benign prostatic hyperplasia.*

hyperuricemia Abnormally elevated uric acid in the blood. Uric acid is a breakdown product of purines, which are part of many foods. Hyperuricemia may indicate an increased risk of gout, but many patients with hyperuricemia do not develop gout, and some patients with repeated gout attacks have normal or low blood uric acid levels. Hyperuricemia can also lead to kidney stones and hard deposits of uric acid (tophi) in the skin. People with hyperuricemia should avoid taking aspirin. Treatment includes dietary change, and for those without gout or kidney problems, use of medications that lower uric acid level.

hyperventilation Overbreathing. Hyperventilation causes dizziness, lightheadedness, a sense of unsteadiness, and tingling around the mouth and fingertips. Hyperventilation can be severe enough to mimic the early warning symptoms of a heart attack, and is therefore a common cause of emergency room visits in the US. Hyperventilation is common and normal after aerobic exercise. Hyperventilation can be caused by serious diseases of metabolism and anxiety. Relief for hyperventilation caused by anxiety can be had by breathing in and out of a paper bag to increase the level of carbon dioxide in the blood.

hypo- Prefix meaning low, under, beneath, down, or below normal, as in hypoglycemia (low blood sugar) and hyposensitivity (undersensitivity). The opposite of hypo- is hyper-.

hypocalcemia Lower-than-normal level of calcium in the blood, which makes the nervous system highly irritable, as evidenced by tetany (spasms of the hands and feet, muscle cramps, abdominal cramps, and overly active reflexes). Chronic hypocalcemia contributes to poor mineralization of bones, soft bones (osteomalacia), and osteoporosis. In children, hypocalcemia leads to rickets and impaired growth. Treatment involves increased dietary intake of calcium or calcium supplementation. Food sources of calcium include dairy foods, some leafy green vegetables, canned salmon, clams, oysters, calcium-fortified foods, and tofu. According to the National Academy of Sciences, adequate intake of calcium is 1 g daily for both men and women. The upper limit for calcium intake is 2.5 g daily.

hypochondria The condition of being obsessed with imaginary medical complaints. A person with hypochondria tends to misinterpret minor physical changes as symptoms of major illness. It is closely related to, and may be a subtype of, obsessive-compulsive disorder. Treatment with antidepressant medication and/or cognitive behavioral therapy is often successful. See also *obsessive-compulsive disorder.*

hypochondroplasia A type of short-limb dwarfism, with shortening especially of the ends of the limbs. A child with hypochondroplasia usually has a prominent forehead, mildly shortened extremities and digits, limited range of motion at the elbows, and inward curvature of the lower back. Diagnosis is made through physical examination and X-rays. Hypochondroplasia is inherited in an autosomal dominant manner, so each child born to a person with hypochondroplasia has a 50 percent chance of inheriting the condition. Hypochondroplasia can also occur spontaneously. The gene for hypochondroplasia is the same gene that causes achondroplastic dwarfism: the fibroblast growth factor receptor 3 (FGFR3). However, the two forms of dwarfism are caused by different mutations in FGFR3.

hypoglossal nerve   The twelfth cranial nerve, which supplies the muscles of the tongue.

hypoglossal neuropathy   Disease of the hypoglossal nerve. Paralysis of the hypoglossal nerve affects the tongue, making speech sound thick and causing the tongue to deviate toward the paralyzed side. In time, the tongue diminishes in size (atrophies).

hypoglycemia   Low blood sugar (glucose). When symptoms of hypoglycemia occur together with a documented blood glucose under 45 mg/dl, and the symptoms promptly resolve with the administration of glucose, the diagnosis of hypoglycemia can be made with some certainty. Hypoglycemia is significant only when it is associated with symptoms such as anxiety, sweating, tremor, palpitations, nausea, and pallor. Hypoglycemia also starves the brain of glucose energy, which is essential for proper brain function. Lack of glucose energy to the brain can cause symptoms ranging from headache, mild confusion, abnormal behavior, loss of consciousness, seizure, and coma. Severe hypoglycemia can cause death. The causes of hypoglycemia include use of drugs (such as insulin), liver disease, surgical absence of the stomach, tumors that release excess amounts of insulin, and prediabetes. In some patients, symptoms of hypoglycemia occur during fasting (fasting hypoglycemia). In others, symptoms of hypoglycemia occur after meals (reactive hypoglycemia). Immediate treatment of severe hypoglycemia consists of administering large amounts of glucose and repeating this treatment at intervals if the symptoms persist. Treatment must also be directed at the underlying cause. Treatment of reactive hypoglycemia involves changing the diet, including eating fewer concentrated sweets and ingesting multiple small meals throughout the day.

hypokalemia   Low potassium in the blood. Hypokalemia is commonly caused by conditions that lead to vomiting and by medications, such as diuretics.

hypomagnesemia   Low magnesium in the blood, which can occur due to inadequate intake or impaired intestinal absorption of magnesium. Hypomagnesemia is often associated with low calcium (hypocalcemia) and low potassium (hypokalemia). It causes increased irritability of the nervous system with tetany (spasms of the hands and feet, muscular twitching and cramps, spasm of the larynx, and overly active reflexes). According to the National Academy of Sciences, the recommended dietary allowance of magnesium is 420 mg per day for men and 320 mg per day for women. The upper limit of magnesium supplements is 350 mg daily, in addition to the magnesium taken in through food and water.

hyponatremia   Low sodium in the blood. Hyponatremia can be caused by many conditions and when severe can lead to confusion and seizures.

hypophosphatemia   A lower-than-normal level of phosphate in the blood. Phosphate molecules are particularly important as part of larger molecules in cell energy cycles. Hypophosphatemia can be associated with a number of conditions including bone diseases and hormone conditions.

hypopigmentation   Lack of color in the skin or eyes. Hypopigmentation is characteristic of the various forms of albinism and of several genetic diseases. See *albinism; Hermansky-Pudlak syndrome.*

hypoplasia   Underdevelopment or incomplete development of a tissue or an organ. For example, hypoplasia of the enamel of the teeth indicates that the enamel coating is thinner than normal or missing in some but not all areas. Hypoplasia is less drastic than aplasia, where there is no development of a tissue or an organ at all.

hypoplasia of the thymus and parathyroids   See *DiGeorge syndrome.*

hypoplastic left heart syndrome   A form of congenital heart disease in which the whole left half of the heart—including the aorta, aortic valve, left ventricle, and mitral valve—is underdeveloped (hypoplastic). Blood returning from the lungs has to flow through an opening in the wall between the upper chambers of the heart (an atrial septal defect). The right ventricle pumps blood into the pulmonary artery, and blood reaches the aorta through a shunt (the ductus arteriosus). A child with hypoplastic left heart syndrome may seem normal at birth but has trouble within a few days of when the ductus arteriosus closes. The infant becomes ashen, has rapid and difficult breathing, and has problems feeding. This heart defect is usually fatal within the first days or months of life without a sequence of surgeries or a heart transplant. See also *atrial septal defect; ductus arteriosus.*

hypospadias   A birth defect in which the urethra opens on the underside of the penis or below the penis. In first-degree hypospadias, the urethral opening is below the tip, but nearby and on the glans. In second-degree hypospadias, the urethra opens closer to the body, on the underside of the shaft of the penis. In third-degree or perineal hypospadias, the urethral opening is below the penis on the skin. Males with first- or second-degree hypospadias can simply sit to urinate. If hypospadias is more significant, treatment involves surgery to repair and reconstruct the urethra.

hypotension Blood pressure that is below the normal expected for an individual in a given environment. Blood pressure normally varies greatly with activity, age, medications, and underlying medical conditions. Hypotension can result from conditions of the nervous system, conditions that do not begin in the nervous system, and drugs. Neurological conditions that can lead to low blood pressure include changing position from lying to a more vertical position (postural hypotension), stroke, shock, lightheadedness after urinating or defecating, Parkinson's disease, neuropathy, and fright. Nonneurological conditions that can cause low blood pressure include bleeding, infections, dehydration, heart disease, adrenal insufficiency, pregnancy, prolonged bed rest, poisoning, toxic shock syndrome, and blood transfusion reactions. Treatment is not usually necessary, although people with mildly low blood pressure may need to be careful about their activities, and if necessary, medication is available. Hypotensive drugs include blood pressure drugs; diuretics (water pills); heart medications, especially calcium antagonists such as nifedipine (brand name: Procardia); beta blockers, such as propranolol (brand name: Inderal); antidepressants, such as amitriptylene (brand name: Elavil); and alcohol. Hypotension is the opposite of hypertension (abnormally high blood pressure). See also *hypotension, orthostatic.*

hypotension, orthostatic A temporary lowering of blood pressure, usually related to suddenly standing up. Healthy people may experience orthostatic hypotension if they rise quickly from a seated position, especially after a meal. Orthostatic hypotension occurs most commonly in older people. The change in position causes a temporary reduction in blood flow and therefore a shortage of oxygen to the brain. This leads to lightheadedness and, sometimes, a temporary loss of consciousness. Symptoms include dizziness, feeling as though one is about to black out, and tunnel vision. The symptoms are typically worse when standing, and they improve with lying down. Tilt-table testing can be used to confirm a diagnosis of orthostatic hypotension. Tilt-table testing involves placing the patient on a table with a foot support. The table is tilted upward, and blood pressure and pulse are measured while symptoms are recorded in various positions. If someone with orthostatic hypotension faints, he or she regains consciousness by simply sitting or lying down. The person is thereafter advised to exercise caution and slow the process of changing positions from lying to sitting to standing. This simple technique can allow the body to correct for the more vertical position by a gradual adjustment of the circulation of the legs, and it can be especially important in older people. Also known as postural hypotension.

hypotension, postural See *hypotension, orthostatic.*

hypothalamus The area of the brain that controls body temperature, hunger, and thirst.

hypothermia Abnormally low body temperature. Someone who falls asleep in a cold temperature may become hypothermic, and the condition can be fatal. Hypothermia is intentionally produced to slow the metabolism during some types of surgery. Severe hypothermia can be fatal. Those with mild or moderate hypothermia (are alert and conscious, and have not lost the shivering reflex) will usually simply require removing them from the cold environment and providing them with additional insulation. Treatment of severe hypothermia involves slow heating of the body using blankets or other ways of increasing body warmth. Body temperature should increase by no more than a couple of degrees per hour.

hypothyroid Deficiency of thyroid hormone. The hypothyroid state (hypothyroidism) is characterized by fatigue, weight gain, and constipation. Severe, longstanding hypothyroidism can lead to swelling of the extremities, coma, and death.

hypothyroidism, congenital See *cretinism.*

hypothyroidism, infantile Underactivity of the thyroid gland that starts after birth in infancy or early childhood, as manifested by delays in growth and development, and by myxedema (a dry, waxy type of swelling, often including swollen lips and nose). Treatment involves use of thyroid hormone medication. Also known as Brissaud infantilism and infantile myxedema.

hypotonia Decreased muscle tone and strength that results in floppiness. Hypotonia is a common finding with cerebral palsy and other neuromuscular disorders. Untreated hypotonia can lead to hip dislocation and other problems. Treatment is via physical therapy. In some cases, braces may be needed to permit a full range of movement in patients with hypotonia.

hypotonic solution A solution that contains less salt than is found in normal cells and blood. Hypotonic solutions are commonly used to give fluids intravenously to hospitalized patients in order to treat or avoid dehydration.

hypovolemia Abnormal decrease in the volume of blood plasma. Hypovolemia occurs with dehydration or bleeding.

hypovolemic shock   See *shock, hypovolemic.*

hypoxia   A lower-than-normal concentration of oxygen in arterial blood, as opposed to anoxia, a complete lack of blood oxygen. Hypoxia will occur with any interruption of normal respiration.

hypoxia-ischemia   Blood flow to cells and organs that is not sufficient to maintain their normal function, combined with a lower-than-normal concentration of oxygen in arterial blood.

hysterectomy   An operation to remove the uterus, and sometimes also the cervix. Hysterectomies are performed to remove fibroids, cancer or severe dysplasia of the uterus, and for dysfunctional uterine bleeding.

hysterectomy, abdominal   Surgical removal of the uterus through an incision made in the abdominal wall, as opposed to a vaginal hysterectomy. See also *hysterectomy, vaginal.*

hysterectomy, complete   See *hysterectomy, total.*

hysterectomy, partial   Surgical removal of the uterus but not the cervix. Also known as subtotal hysterectomy.

hysterectomy, subtotal   See *hysterectomy, partial.*

hysterectomy, total   Complete surgical removal of the uterus and cervix. Also known as complete hysterectomy.

hysterectomy, vaginal   Removal of the uterus through a surgical incision within the vagina, as opposed to abdominal hysterectomy. With a vaginal hysterectomy, the scar is not outwardly visible. See also *hysterectomy, abdominal.*

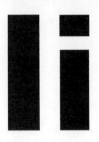

iatr- Prefix indicating something related to a physician or medicine, as in iatromisia (an intense dislike of doctors).

iatrapistic Having a lack of faith in doctors.

iatrogenic Due to the activity of a physician or therapy. For example, an iatrogenic illness is an illness that is caused by a medication or physician.

iatromelia An ineffective or negligent medical treatment.

iatromisia An intense dislike of doctors.

IBD Inflammatory bowel disease. See *bowel disease, inflammatory.*

IBS Irritable bowel syndrome.

ibuprofen A nonsteroidal anti-inflammatory drug (NSAID) that is commonly used to treat pain, swelling, and fever. Common brand names of ibuprofen include Advil, Motrin, and Nuprin.

I-cell disease A severe genetic disorder of the lysosomes (organelles within a cell that contain enzymes that can lyse, or digest, substances). In children born with I-cell disease, lysosomal enzymes are made, but they are dumped outside the cell instead of being sent to the lysosomes. Various cellular nutrients thus cannot be digested and so pile up in dark lumps, called inclusion bodies, within the lysosomes. I-cell disease affects the kidneys, heart, and nervous system, and children with it usually die of heart failure or pneumonia before reaching puberty. I-cell disease is inherited in an autosomal recessive manner. There is no known treatment for I-cell disease. Also known as mucolipidosis II.

ichthyosis simplex See *ichthyosis vulgaris.*

ichthyosis, spasticity, oligophrenia syndrome See *Sjogren-Larsson syndrome.*

ichthyosis vulgaris A genetic skin disease characterized by scaly areas of skin that usually appear after 3 months of age. The palms and soles are often affected. Areas that tend to be spared include the armpits, the insides of the elbows, and the skin behind the knee. Many people with ichthyosis vulgaris also have asthma, eczema, or hay fever. The gene responsible for this disease has been mapped to chromosome band 1q21. Also known as ichthyosis simplex.

ichthyosis-keratitis-deafness syndrome See *keratitis-ichthyosis-deafness syndrome.*

ICSH interstitial-cell-stimulating hormone (ICSH) See *luteinizing hormone.*

ICSI Intracytoplasmic sperm injection.

icterus See *jaundice.*

ICU Intensive care unit. The intensive care unit is a designated area of a hospital facility that is dedicated to the care of patients who are seriously ill.

ICU psychosis A disorder in which patients in an intensive care unit (ICU) or a similar hospital setting experience anxiety, become paranoid, hear voices, see things that are not there, become severely disoriented in time and place, become very agitated, or even become violent. One-third of patients who spend more than 5 days in an ICU experience some form of psychotic reaction, according to current estimates. ICU psychosis is a form of acute brain failure (delirium). Organic factors, including dehydration, low blood oxygen (hypoxia), heart failure, infection, and drugs can cause or contribute to delirium. Other factors that are believed to play into ICU psychosis are sensory deprivation, sensory overload, pain (particularly if poorly controlled), sleep deprivation, disruption of the normal day–night rhythm, and the loss of control over their lives that patients often feel in an ICU. ICU psychosis often goes away with the coming of morning or sleep. Although it may linger through the day, severe agitation usually occurs only at night. (This phenomenon, also known as sundowning, is common in nursing homes as well.) Treatment of ICU psychosis depends on the cause. Family members, familiar objects, and calm words may help. A dehydrated patient needs fluids. A patient with heart failure needs treatment with digitalis. Infections must be diagnosed and treated. Sedation with antipsychotics may help. To prevent ICU psychosis, many critical care units have taken such steps as instituting visiting hours, minimizing shift changes in the nursing staff caring for a patient, and coordinating lighting with the normal day–night cycle. ICU psychosis usually goes away when the patient leaves the ICU.

ID Intradermal.

IDDM Insulin-dependent diabetes mellitus. See *diabetes, type 1.*

idiocy, amaurotic familial See *Tay-Sachs disease.*

idiopathic See *essential.*

idiopathic hypertrophic subaortic stenosis Narrowing of the left ventricle of the heart just below the aortic valve through which blood must pass on its way up into the aorta. The narrowing cuts the flow of blood and is due to hypertrophic cardiomyopathy (HCM), a genetic disorder of the heart that is inherited in an autosomal dominant manner. HCM is the leading cause of sudden cardiac death in preadolescent and adolescent children. The hallmark of the HCM is abnormal enlargement of the left ventricle of the heart but frequently involves the interventricular septum, which results in an obstruction of flow through the left ventricular outflow tract. Treatment options include drugs and surgery. Abbreviated IHSS. See also *subaortic stenosis.*

idiopathic sclerosing cholangitis See *primary sclerosing cholangitis.*

idiopathic torsion dystonia See *dystonia, idiopathic torsion.*

IgE Immunoglobulin E.

IHSS Idiopathic hypertrophic subaortic stenosis.

IL Interleukin.

ileitis, Crohn's See *Crohn's ileitis.*

ileitis, terminal Inflammation of the end of the small intestine (terminal ileum) due to Crohn's disease. See also *Crohn's disease.*

ileocolitis, Crohn's See *Crohn's ileocolitis.*

ileum Part of the small intestine beyond the jejunum and before the large intestine (colon).

ileus Obstruction of the intestine due to its being paralyzed. The paralysis does not need to be complete to cause ileus, but the intestine must be so inactive that food cannot pass through it, which leads to blockage of the intestine. Ileus commonly follows some types of surgery. It can also result from certain drugs, injuries, and illnesses. Regardless of the cause, ileus causes constipation and bloating. When one listens to the abdomen with a stethoscope, no bowel sounds are heard because the bowel is inactive. Also known as paralytic ileus.

ileus, meconium Obstruction of the intestine due to overly thick meconium, a dark, sticky substance that is normally present in the intestine at birth. Meconium is passed in the feces after birth, after trypsin and other enzymes from the pancreas have acted on it. Meconium ileus occurs when the infant has a deficiency of trypsin and other digestive enzymes from the pancreas, as in cystic fibrosis. Treatment is with enemas and can require surgical procedures.

ileus, paralytic See *ileus.*

iliac Pertaining to the ilium.

iliac horns A horn-like malformation on the crest of each of the iliac bones of the pelvis, a characteristic finding in nail-patella syndrome. See also *nail-patella syndrome.*

ilium The upper part of the pelvis, which forms the receptacle of the hip.

illness, acute An illness with an abrupt onset and usually a short course.

illness, altitude See *altitude sickness.*

illness, chronic An illness that has persisted for a long period of time. Chronic illness is a continuing disease process.

IM Intramuscular.

imagery 1 A mental process that involves thoughts representing sensory qualities. 2 A wide variety of procedures used in therapy to encourage changes in attitudes, behavior, or physiological reactions. Imagery includes all the senses, including visual, aural, tactile, olfactory, proprioceptive, and kinesthetic. Imagery has been successfully used and tested as a strategy for alleviating nausea and vomiting associated with chemotherapy in cancer patients, for relieving stress, and for facilitating weight gain in cancer patients. It has been successfully used and tested for pain control in a variety of settings; as adjunctive therapy for several diseases, including diabetes; and with geriatric patients to enhance immunity.

immune Protected against infection, usually by the presence of antibodies.

immune response Any reaction by the immune system. For example, poison ivy can cause an immune response in the skin characterized by inflammation with tiny blisters, and itching. Also, a flu shot is designed to produce an immune response by stimulating the production of antibodies against the flu virus.

immune system A complex system that is responsible for distinguishing a person from everything foreign to him or her and for protecting his or her body against infections and foreign substances.

immunity The condition of being immune. Immunity can be innate—for example, humans are innately immune to canine distemper—or conferred by a previous infection or immunization.

immunization A vaccination that works by stimulating the immune system of the body to fight disease. A healthy immune system is able to recognize invading bacteria and viruses, and it produces antibodies to destroy or disable them. Immunizations prepare the immune system to ward off a disease. To immunize against viral diseases, the virus used in the vaccine has been weakened or killed. To immunize against bacterial diseases, it is generally possible to use only a small portion of the dead bacteria to stimulate antibodies against the whole bacteria. The effectiveness of immunizations can be improved by periodic repeat injections, called boosters. For information about specific immunizations, see the name of the disease (for examples, DTP immunization, hepatitis B immunization, polio immunization).

immunization, children's See *children's immunizations.*

immunization, flu See *influenza vaccine.*

immunization, German measles See *MMR.*

immunization, H. flu See *Haemophilus influenzae type B immunization.*

immunization, HIB See *Haemophilus influenzae type B immunization.*

immunization, infectious hepatitis See *hepatitis A immunization.*

immunization, measles See *MMR.*

immunization, mumps See *MMR.*

immunization, serum hepatitis See *hepatitis B immunization.*

immunization, varicella See *chickenpox immunization.*

immunocompetent Able to develop an immune response. An immunocompetent body is able to recognize antigens and act against them. Immunocompetent is the opposite of immunodeficient.

immunocompromised Having an immune system that has been impaired by disease or treatment.

immunodeficiency The inability to form a normal immune response. Immunodeficiency can be due to a genetic disease or it can be acquired, as in AIDS.

immunodeficient Lacking immunity, and so being susceptible to infection. Immunodeficient is the opposite of immunocompetent.

immunodepression See *immunosuppression.*

immunogenetics The genetics (inheritance) of the immune response. For example, immunogenetics includes the study of Rh, ABO, and other blood groups.

immunoglobulin E A class of immunoglobulins that includes the antibodies that are important in an allergic response. Abbreviated IgE. A person who has an allergy often has elevated blood levels of IgE. IgE antibodies attack and engage the invading army of allergens.

immunologist A physician or another degreed professional who is knowledgeable about immunology.

immunology The study of all aspects of the immune system, including its structure and function, disorders of the immune system, blood banking, immunization, and organ transplantation.

immunosuppression Suppression of the immune system and its ability to fight infection. Immunosuppression may result from certain diseases, such as AIDS or lymphoma, or from certain drugs, such as some of those used to treat cancer. Immunosuppression may also be deliberately induced with drugs, as in preparation for bone marrow or other organ transplantation, to prevent the rejection of a transplant. Also known as immunodepression.

immunosuppressive agent A medication that depresses or halts immune system activity. For example, immunosuppressive agents may be given to prevent the body from forming an immune response to an organ transplant or to treat a disease that is caused by an overactive immune system, such as rheumatoid arthritis.

immunotherapy See *biological therapy.*

immunotherapy, allergy Stimulation of the immune system with gradually increasing doses of the substances to which a person is allergic. The aim of allergy immunotherapy is to modify or stop the allergy by reducing the strength of the IgE response. This form of treatment is very effective for allergies to pollen, mites, animal dander, and especially, stinging insects. Allergy immunotherapy usually takes 6 months to 1 year to become effective, and injections are typically required for 3 to 5 years.

impact To lodge firmly or wedge in. For example, a molar tooth that is growing up and against an adjacent tooth is impacting the tooth next to it.

impaction, dental See *dental impaction.*

imperforate anus See *anus, imperforate.*

impetigo A skin infection caused by the staphylococcus or, less often, by the streptococcus bacterium. The first sign of impetigo is a patch of red, itchy skin. Pustules develop on this area, soon forming crusty, yellow-brown sores that can spread to cover entire areas of the face, arms, and other body parts. Most patients are children. Because impetigo is caused by a bacterium that is transmitted onto the skin, it is contagious and easily contracted by persons who might touch the affected person. Treatment involves use of topical antibiotics.

implant, cochlear   See *cochlear implant.*

implantable cardiac defibrillator   See *cardiac defibrillator, implantable.*

implantable pacemaker   See *pacemaker, internal.*

impotence   See *erectile dysfunction.*

imprinting, psychological   A remarkable phenomenon that occurs in animals, and theoretically in humans, in the first hours of life. The newborn creature bonds to the type of animals it meets at birth and begins to pattern its behavior after them. In humans, this is often called bonding, and it usually refers to the relationship between the newborn and its parents.

in.   Abbreviation for inch.

in situ   In the normal location. An in situ tumor is one that is confined to its site of origin and has not invaded neighboring tissue or gone elsewhere in the body. For example, squamous cell carcinoma in situ is an early stage of skin cancer.

in situ, carcinoma   See *carcinoma in situ.*

in situ hybridization   The use of a DNA or RNA probe to detect the complementary DNA sequence. In situ hybridization involves hybridizing a labeled nucleic acid to suitably prepared cells on microscope slides or to tissue sections in situ (in their normal location).

in vitro   In glass, as in a test tube. An in vitro test is one that is done in glass or plastic vessels in the laboratory. In vitro is the opposite of in vivo.

in vitro fertilization   A laboratory procedure in which sperm are put in a special dish with unfertilized eggs to achieve fertilization. The embryos that result can be transferred into the uterus or frozen (cryopreserved) for future use. In vitro fertilization was devised to permit women with damaged or absent fallopian tubes to become pregnant. Abbreviated IVF.

in vivo   In the living organism. For example, an experiment that is done in vivo is done in the body of a living organism as opposed to in a laboratory method that does not use the living organism as the host of the test. In vivo is the opposite of in vitro.

inactivated polio vaccine   See *polio immunization; polio vaccine, inactivated.*

inappropriate ADH secretion   See *ADH secretion, inappropriate.*

inborn error of metabolism   A heritable disorder of the biochemistry of the body. Examples of inborn error of metabolism include albinism and phenylketonuria (PKU). The term *inborn error of metabolism* was coined in 1908 by the British physician Sir Archibald Garrod, who described four inborn errors of metabolism: albinism, alkaptonuria, pentosuria, and cystinuria. There are now hundreds of known inborn errors of metabolism. See also *albinism; cystinuria; phenylketonuria.*

inbreeding   See *consanguinity.*

inbreeding, coefficient of   See *coefficient of inbreeding.*

incest   Sexual activity between individuals so closely related that marriage is legally prohibited. Incest involving a child is a form of child abuse.

inch   A length equivalent to one-twelfth of a foot, one-thirty-sixth of a yard, or 2.54 cm. Abbreviated in.

incidence   The frequency with which something, such as a disease or trait, appears in a particular population or area.

incision   A cut that is purposely made. When making an incision, a surgeon is making a cut.

incompetent cervix   See *cervix, incompetent.*

incontinence   The inability to control excretions, to hold urine in the bladder, or to keep feces in the rectum.

incontinence, fecal   See *encopresis.*

incontinence, urinary   See *enuresis.*

incontinent   Unable to control excretions, to hold urine in the bladder, or to keep feces in the rectum.

incontinentia pigmenti   A genetic disease that begins soon after birth and features the development of blisters on the trunk and limbs. These blisters then heal but leave dark hyperpigmented streaks and marble-like whorls on the skin. Abbreviated IP. Other key features of IP include dental and nail abnormalities, bald patches, and, in about one-third of cases, mental retardation. IP is inherited as an X-linked dominant trait. The gene for IP is called IKBKG. A girl with IP has inherited the IKBKG mutation from a parent or has a new IKBKG mutation. IP is lethal in most, but not all, males. Mothers with IP have an equal chance of having a normal son, a normal daughter, and an IP daughter. Females with IP have nonrandom X-chromosome inactivation. Normally, one X chromosome in each cell of a female is randomly inactivated. In females with IP and certain other X-linked conditions, the X chromosome with the mutant allele is preferentially inactivated; this phenomenon is termed nonrandom (or skewed) X-chromosome inactivation. Also known as Bloch-Sulzberger syndrome.

index case A person who first draws attention to his or her family because of a medical condition. For example, if an eye doctor discovers a person has glaucoma, and subsequently other cases of glaucoma are found in the person's family, that person is the index case. Also known as propositus (if male) or proposita (if female).

indifferent gonad See *gonad, indifferent.*

induced menopause See *menopause, induced.*

induction therapy The first in a series of therapeutic measures taken to treat a disease, typically a cancer. The induction therapy, for example, in acute leukemia is the initial chemotherapy designed to bring about a remission.

infant A young child, from birth to 24 months of age.

infant mortality rate The number of children dying at less than 1 year of age, divided by the number of live births that year. The infant mortality rate in the US, which was 9.2 per 1,000 live births in 1990, fell to 7.0 per 1,000 live births in 1999.

infantile genetic agranulocytosis See *agranulocytosis, infantile genetic.*

infantile hip dislocation See *congenital hip dislocation.*

infantile hypothyroidism See *hypothyroidism, infantile.*

infantile myxedema See *hypothyroidism, infantile.*

infantile paralysis See *polio.*

infarct An area of tissue death that is due to a local lack of oxygen.

infarction The formation of an infarct, an area of tissue death, due to a local lack of oxygen.

infarction, acute myocardial See *heart attack.*

infection The invasion and multiplication of microorganisms such as bacteria, viruses, and parasites that are not normally present within the body. An infection may cause no symptoms and be subclinical, or it may cause symptoms and be clinically apparent. An infection may remain localized, or it may spread through the blood or lymphatic vessels to become systemic (bodywide). Microorganisms that live naturally in the body are not considered infections. For example, bacteria that normally live within the mouth and intestine are not infections.

infection, ear See also *ear infection.*

infection, group B strep See *streptococcus, group B.*

infection, middle ear See *acute otitis media.*

infection, opportunistic An infection that grasps the opportunity to cause disease, which is presented when a person's immune system is weak. These opportunistic microorganisms may be dormant in the body or may cause few problems for healthy individuals. Opportunistic infections are a particular problem for organ transplant patients and those with diseases that affect the immune system, particularly AIDS. Toxoplasmosis and cytomegalovirus are examples of opportunistic infections.

infection, pinworm See *pinworm infestation.*

infection, primary HIV See *HIV infection, primary.*

infection, rotavirus See *rotavirus.*

infection, urinary tract See *urinary tract infection.*

infection, Vincent See *acute membranous gingivitis.*

infectious hepatitis See *hepatitis A.*

infectious hepatitis immunization See *hepatitis A, immunization.*

infectious mononucleosis See *mononucleosis.*

inferior In medicine, below, downward, or toward the feet, as opposed to superior. For example, the liver is inferior to the lungs. See also Appendix B, "Anatomic Orientation Terms."

infertile Unable to conceive despite regular intercourse without contraception. Infertility can be due to many causes. Infertility is often caused by the inadequate ability of the male partner's sperm to move. Some cases of infertility are due to physical problems or malformations of the female reproductive system. Most types of infertility are treatable. In some cases, in vitro fertilization and other lab procedures may be used to ensure fertilization, and special medical care or medication may be required to enable the pregnancy to come to term. See also *conception; infertility.*

infertility   Diminished or absent ability to conceive and bear offspring. Infertility can have many causes. In most cases of possible female infertility, the problem is found to originate with the male partner's sperm motility. Some cases are due to physical problems or malformations of the female reproductive system. Others are due to genetic difficulties, such as Rh incompatibility between mother and fetus. Most types of infertility are treatable. In some cases, in vitro fertilization and other lab procedures may be used to ensure fertilization, and special medical care or medication may be required to enable the pregnancy to come to term.

infiltrate   To penetrate. For example, if an IV infiltrates, the IV fluid penetrates the surrounding tissue.

infiltrating ductal carcinoma of the breast   See *breast, infiltrating ductal carcinoma of the.*

infiltrating lobular carcinoma of the breast   See *breast, infiltrating lobular carcinoma of the.*

inflammation   A localized redness, warmth, swelling, and pain as a result of infection, irritation, or injury. Inflammation can be external or internal.

inflammatory bowel disease   See *bowel disease, inflammatory.*

influenza   An illness caused by viruses that infect the respiratory tract. These viruses are divided into three types, designated A, B, and C. Symptoms of influenza include fever, appetite loss, an achy feeling throughout the body, and weakness. Most people who get influenza recover completely in 1 to 2 weeks, but some people develop serious and potentially life-threatening medical complications, such as pneumonia. Much of the illness and death caused by influenza can be prevented by annual influenza vaccinations. Commonly known as flu.

influenza vaccine   A vaccine recommended for persons at high risk for serious complications from influenza virus infection, including everyone age 50 or older; residents of nursing homes and other long-term care facilities that house persons of any age who have long-term illnesses; adults and children over 6 months of age who have chronic heart or lung conditions, including asthma; adults and children over 6 months of age who need regular medical care or had to be in a hospital because of metabolic diseases (such as diabetes), chronic kidney disease, or weakened immune system (including immune system problems caused by medicine or by infection with HIV/AIDS); children from 6 months to 18 years of age who are on long-term aspirin therapy and therefore could develop Reye's syndrome after the flu; women who will be more than 3 months pregnant during the flu season; and

people in close or frequent contact with anyone at high risk, including: physicians, nurses, and other employees in hospitals and physicians' offices, including emergency response workers; employees of nursing homes and long-term care facilities who have contact with patients or residents; employees of assisted living and other residences for people in high-risk groups; people who provide home care to those in high-risk groups; and household members (including children) of people in high-risk groups. The following groups of people should *not* get a flu shot before talking with their physicians: people who have a severe allergy to hens' eggs, people who have had a severe reaction to a flu shot in the past, and people who previously developed Guillain-Barré syndrome (GBS) in the 6 weeks after getting a flu shot

informatics   The application of computers and statistics to the management of information. For example, in the Human Genome Project, informatics permitted the development and use of methods to search databases quickly, analyze DNA sequence information, and predict protein sequence and structure from DNA sequence data.

infraspinatus muscle   A muscle that assists the lifting of the arm while turning the arm outward (external rotation). The tendon of the infraspinatus muscle is one of four tendons that stabilize the shoulder joint and constitute the rotator cuff.

inguinal   Having to do with the groin.

inguinal canal   A passage in the lower anterior abdominal wall that in the male allows passage of the spermatic cord and in the female contains the round ligament. Because of the weakness the inguinal canal creates in the abdominal wall, it is the most frequent site for a hernia.

inguinal orchiectomy   Surgery to remove a testicle, with the incision made through the groin.

inheritance   The transmission of a gene from parent to child. The pattern of inheritance is the manner in which a gene is transmitted. For example, the pattern of inheritance may be as an autosomal dominant trait that is transmitted from father or mother to son or daughter.

inheritance, holandric   See *inheritance, Y-linked.*

inheritance, mitochondrial   The inheritance of a trait encoded in the mitochondrial genome. Mitochondrial inheritance does not obey the classic rules of genetics. Persons with a mitochondrial disease may be male or female but are always related in the maternal line, and no male with the disease can transmit it to his children. The mitochondria are structures in the cell's cytoplasm, located outside the nucleus, and are responsible for energy production (metabolism). Mitochondrial disorders are therefore primarily disorders of metabolism. See also *mitochondria; mitochondrial diseases.*

inheritance, multifactorial A type of hereditary pattern seen when there is more than one genetic factor and, sometimes, environmental influence. Many common traits and many common diseases are multifactorial. Skin color, for example, is multifactorially determined, as is intelligence. Type 2 diabetes is multifactorial because it is due to inherited (genetic) factors but usually requires environmental factors, such as obesity, to develop.

inheritance, Y-linked Inheritance of genes on the Y chromosome. Because normally only males have Y chromosomes, Y-linked genes can be transmitted only from father to son. Also known as holandric inheritance.

inhibitor, protease See *protease inhibitor.*

injury, cold See *cold injury.*

inner ear See *ear, inner.*

INR International normalized ratio.

insect sting A sting from a large stinging insect, such as a bee, hornet, yellow jacket, or wasp, that can trigger allergic reactions. These reactions vary greatly in severity. Avoidance and prompt treatment are essential. In selected cases, allergy injection therapy is highly effective.

insemination The deposition of semen in the female reproductive tract. Under normal circumstances, the deposit is made within the vagina or the cervix. By artificial means, such as intrauterine insemination, the deposit can be made directly into the uterus.

insemination, artificial See *artificial insemination.*

insemination, heterologous See *artificial insemination by donor.*

insemination, homologous See *artificial insemination by husband.*

insemination, intrauterine See *artificial insemination.*

insertion A chromosome abnormality that is due to insertion of a segment from one chromosome into another chromosome.

insomnia The perception or complaint of inadequate or poor-quality sleep due to a number of factors, such as difficulty falling asleep, waking up frequently during the night with difficulty returning to sleep, waking up too early in the morning, or unrefreshing sleep. Insomnia is not defined by the number of hours of sleep a person gets or how long it takes to fall asleep; it is a measure of satisfaction with sleep. Individuals vary normally in their need for and their satisfaction with sleep. Insomnia may cause problems during the day, such as tiredness, a lack of energy, difficulty concentrating, and irritability.

insufficiency, pancreatic See *pancreatic insufficiency.*

insulin A hormone that is made by the beta cells in the islets of Langerhans of the pancreas and that controls the amount of sugar (glucose) in the blood. Insulin helps the body use glucose for energy. Cells cannot utilize glucose without insulin. If the beta cells that make insulin degenerate, preventing the body from making enough insulin on its own, type 1 (insulin-dependent) diabetes mellitus results. A person with this type of diabetes must inject insulin from other sources, such as synthetic insulin. See also *diabetes mellitus; diabetic shock.*

insulin reaction See *diabetic shock.*

insulin shock See *diabetic shock.*

insulin-dependent diabetes mellitus See *diabetes, type 1.*

intelligence, nonverbal The innate or learned ability to understand and carry out motor tasks, such as solving physical puzzles. Also known as performance IQ.

intelligence quotient See *IQ.*

intelligence test A questionnaire or series of exercises designed to measure intelligence. It is generally understood that intelligence tests are less a measure of innate ability to learn than they are a measure of what the person tested has already learned. There are many types of intelligence tests, and they may measure learning and/or ability in a wide variety of areas and skills. Scores may be presented as an IQ (intelligence quotient), as a mental age, or on a scale.

intelligence, verbal The innate or learned ability to understand and answer questions given in writing or verbally.

intensive care unit psychosis See *ICU psychosis.*

inter- Prefix indicating between.

interatrial septum The partition that separates the upper chambers (atria) of the heart.

intercostal muscle The muscle tissue between any two ribs.

interferon A naturally occurring substance that interferes with the ability of viruses to reproduce. Interferon also boosts the immune system. There are a number of different interferons, and they fall into three main classes: alpha, beta, and gamma. All interferons are proteins (lymphokines) normally produced by the body in response to infection. Interferons have been synthesized by using recombinant DNA technology. See also *interferon therapy*.

interferon therapy The use of interferon to eradicate a virus from an infected person. Using interferon to eradicate the hepatitis B virus in an individual may, for example, prevent the patient's future development of cirrhosis and cancer of the liver. This may require months and even years of interferon treatment, and it may not be effective in many patients. In therapeutic doses, interferon can be hard to tolerate. Side effects include flu-like symptoms (fatigue, headache, and aches) and, less regularly, low thyroid activity, arthritis, low platelet count, and severe depression. Some of these side effects, particularly depression, can be successfully treated with additional medications.

interleukin One of several similar protein substances that may be used in biological therapy to stimulate the growth and activities of certain kinds of white blood cells that are involved in immune response. Abbreviated IL. ILs can be thought of as chemical messengers that give orders to the immune system.

interleukin-1 A protein that is produced by various cells, including macrophages, and that raises body temperature, spurs the production of interferon, and stimulates growth of disease-fighting cells, among other functions. Abbreviated IL-1.

interleukin-2 A protein that can improve the body's response to disease and that stimulates division of a ctivated T cells. Abbreviated IL-2.

interleukin-3 A protein that stimulates the immune system to develop mast cells and bone marrow cells. Abbreviated IL-3.

interleukin-4 A protein that stimulates the immune system to develop mast cells, resting T cells, and activated B cells. Abbreviated IL-4.

intermittent claudication See *claudication, intermittent.*

intern In medicine, a physician who has completed medical school and is engaged in a year of additional training at a hospital before residency. An intern may, for example, be in pediatrics, surgery, or internal medicine. The internship year is often quite rigorous.

internal cardiac defibrillator See *cardiac defibrillator, implantable.*

internal ear See *ear, inner.*

internal genitalia, female See *genitalia, female internal.*

internal jugular vein The deeper of the two jugular veins in the neck that drain blood from the head, brain, face, and neck, and then convey it toward the heart. The internal jugular vein collects blood from the brain, the outside of the face, and the neck. It runs down the inside the neck, outside the internal and common carotid arteries, and unites with the subclavian vein to form the innominate vein. See also *jugular vein.*

internal medicine The medical specialty dedicated to the diagnosis and medical treatment of adults. A physician who specializes in internal medicine is referred to as an internist. Subspecialties of internal medicine include allergy and immunology, cardiology (heart), endocrinology (hormone disorders), hematology (blood disorders), infectious diseases, gastroenterology (diseases of the gut), nephrology (kidney diseases), oncology (cancer), pulmonology (lung disorders), and rheumatology (arthritis and musculoskeletal disorders).

internal pacemaker See *pacemaker, internal.*

internal radiation therapy See *radiation therapy, internal.*

international normalized ratio A system established by the World Health Organization (WHO) and the International Committee on Thrombosis and Hemostasis for reporting the results of blood coagulation (clotting) tests. Abbreviated INR. Under the INR system, all results are standardized. For example, a person taking the anticoagulant warfarin (brand name: Coumadin) would regularly have blood tested to measure the INR. The INR permits patients on anticoagulants to travel and obtain comparable test results wherever they are.

internist A physician who practices internal medicine and specializes in the diagnosis and medical treatment of adults. An internist spends a minimum of 7 years in medical school and postgraduate training, focused on learning the prevention, diagnosis, and treatment of diseases of adults. See also *internal medicine.*

interobserver variation The amount of variation between the results obtained by two or more observers examining the same material.

interphase The interval in the cell cycle between two cell divisions, during which the individual chromosomes cannot be distinguished. Interphase was once thought to be a resting phase, but it is actually the time when DNA is replicated in the cell nucleus.

interstitial Pertaining to being between things, especially between things that are normally closely spaced. The word *interstitial* is much used in medicine and has specific meaning, depending on the context. For instance, interstitial cystitis is a specific type of inflammation of the bladder wall. Interstitial radiation involves placing radioactive material directly into a tumor. Interstitial pneumonia is inflammation of the lung that involves the mesh of lung tissue (alveolar septa) rather than the air spaces (alveoli).

interstitial cystitis See *cystitis, interstitial.*

interstitial radiation See *radiation therapy, interstitial.*

interstitial-cell-stimulating hormone (ICSH) See *luteinizing hormone.*

intervening sequence See *intron.*

interventional radiology See *radiology, interventional.*

interventricular foramen An opening between the lateral and third ventricles in the system of four communicating cavities within the brain that are continuous with the central canal of the spinal cord.

interventricular septum The stout wall that separates the lower chambers (the ventricles) of the heart from one another. A hole in the interventricular septum is termed a ventricular septal defect (VSD).

intestinal gas See *flatus.*

intestinal malrotation See *malrotation of the intestine.*

intestinal obstruction Blockage of the intestine by infolding (intussusception), malformation, tumor, digestive problems, a foreign body, or inflammation. Symptoms of intestinal obstruction can include crampy abdominal pain, lack of ability to normally eliminate feces, and eventually shock. On examining the abdomen, the physician may feel a mass. Abdominal X-rays may suggest intestinal obstruction, but a barium enema may be needed to show the actual cause. Treatment depends on the cause of the obstruction. Treatments include avoiding oral ingestion of foods or drinking fluids, nasogastric suction, and surgical procedures. See also *intussusception.*

intestinal pseudo-obstruction A condition in which the patient has symptoms of intestinal obstruction with no sign of actual physical obstruction. This condition may be due to problems with the nerves that control intestinal muscles or to other causes. Treatment depends on the cause.

intestine The long, tubelike organ in the abdomen that completes the process of digestion. It consists of the small and large intestines and extends from the stomach to the anus. See also *intestine, large; intestine, small.*

intestine, large The tubelike organ that completes the process of digestion, receiving material from the small intestine. It has four parts: the caecum, the appendix (vermiform appendix), the colon, and the rectum. After the products of digestion enter the caecum through the ileocecal valve, they move rapidly past the appendix, which juts out from the intestine near the caecum. The colon absorbs any remaining water and forms the stool, which is sent to the rectum for elimination. The walls of the large intestine are muscular and contract to move material along its length. See also *intestine; intestine, small.*

intestine, small The tubelike organ that receives the products of digestion from the stomach. It has three parts: the duodenum, the jejunum, and the ileum. The duodenum is rich in glands that produce digestive enzymes, and it also receives bile from the liver. Digested material moves from the duodenum to the ileum through the jejunum. The ileum ends with the ileocecal valve, which prevents food passed into the large intestine from traveling back into the small intestine. The walls of the small intestine are muscular and contract to move digested food along its length. The intestinal tube is lined with a mucuslike tissue that sends forth tiny, finger-like projections called villi. The villi increase the surface available for absorbing nutrients from digested food. See also *intestine; intestine, large.*

intolerance, food Difficulty in digesting a food. Common offenders include milk products, wheat and other grains that contain gluten, and foods that tend to cause intestinal gas, such as cabbage and beans. Food intolerance is often mistaken for food allergy, but it does not involve a histamine response against the food. Treatments include avoiding the offending food and taking supplemental products that allow that food to be adequately digested.

intolerance, lactose See *lactose intolerance.*

intra- Prefix indicating within.

intra-arterial pressure See *arterial tension.*

intracranial hemorrhage Bleeding inside the head. Intracranial hemorrhage can be caused by many conditions including head injury, rupture aneurysm, and stroke.

intractable Unstoppable. For example, intractable diarrhea is diarrhea that can't be stopped, even with medication, and intractable pain is pain that can't be stopped, even with medication.

intracytoplasmic sperm injection A laboratory procedure in which a single sperm is injected directly into a single egg cell to achieve fertilization. Abbreviated ICSI. The ICSI procedure is used when sperm motility is the primary bar to fertility.

intradermal In the skin. For example, an intradermal injection is given into the skin. Abbreviated ID.

intradermal test A type of skin test in which an agent (often a protein) is injected into the skin to test the reaction to the agent. Intradermal tests are often used to diagnose allergies and to test cellular immunity.

intraductal papilloma A benign, wart-like growth that occurs in breast ducts.

intraepithelial Within the layer of cells that forms the surface or lining of an organ. For example, a blister forms fluid in the intraepithelial layer of the skin.

intrahepatic Within the liver. For example, a liver tumor is an intrahepatic growth.

intramuscular Into the muscle. For example, an intramuscular medication is given by needle into the muscle. Abbreviated IM.

intraobserver variation The amount of variation one observer experiences when observing the same material more than once.

intraocular In the eye. For example, intraocular pressure is the pressure within the eye.

intraocular lens An artificial lens made of plastic, silicone, acrylic or other material that is implanted in the eye during cataract surgery. Abbreviated IOL. Removal of the cataract and insertion of an IOL typically takes about an hour and does not require hospitalization.

intraocular pressure The pressure created by the continual renewal of fluids within the eye. Intraocular pressure is increased in glaucoma. In acute angle-closure glaucoma, intraocular pressure rises because the canal into which the fluid in the front part of the eye normally drains is suddenly blocked. In chronic glaucoma, there is a gradual imbalance between the production and removal (resorption) of the fluid in the back part of the eye, causing the supply of fluid to exceed demand. See also *glaucoma.*

intraoperative During surgery.

intraoperative blood salvage The recovery of blood lost into a body cavity during surgery or because of trauma. The blood is recovered in a sterile fashion and stored in a collection bag. This blood can then be reintroduced into the patient's circulation by an intravenous infusion, reducing the need for donor blood transfusion.

intraoperative radiation therapy Radiation treatment given during surgery. Abbreviated IORT. See also *radiation therapy.*

intraperitoneal Within the peritoneal cavity, the area that contains the abdominal organs.

intraperitoneal chemotherapy Treatment in which anticancer drugs are put directly into the abdomen through a thin tube. See also *chemotherapy.*

intrastromal corneal ring A plastic ring that is designed to be implanted in the cornea, the transparent structure at the front of the eye, to flatten the cornea and thereby reduce the degree of nearsightedness (myopia). The ring is placed in the corneal stroma, the middle of the five layers of the cornea.

intrathecal chemotherapy Treatment with drugs that are injected into the cerebrospinal fluid, which surrounds the brain and spinal cord, to kill cancer cells. For example, intrathecal chemotherapy is used to treat cancer that has spread to the spinal cord. See also *chemotherapy.*

intrauterine In the uterus.

intrauterine device A contraceptive device that is inserted into the uterus to prevent conception or pregnancy. Abbreviated IUD. An IUD can be a coil, loop, triangle, or T shape, and it can be plastic or metal. It is not yet known how intrauterine devices prevent pregnancy. IUDs have one of the lowest failure rates of any contraceptive method.

intrauterine growth retardation Abnormally slow growth of a fetus. When the baby is born, it appears small for its actual age. Intrauterine growth retardation is associated with an increased risk of illness and death in the newborn period.

intrauterine ultrasound A technology for creating an image of the developing fetus within the uterus by means of measuring the vibrations returned when a device emits high-frequency sound waves. Ultrasound imaging during pregnancy has proved to be a very useful and effective diagnostic tool when there are concerns about fetal development or gestational age. Intrauterine ultrasound is believed to be a safe practice.

intravenous 1 Into a vein. For example, intravenous antibiotics are antibiotics in a solution that is administered directly into the venous circulation via a syringe or an intravenous catheter (tube). Abbreviated IV. 2 A solution that is administered intravenously. 3 The device that is used to administer an IV solution, such as the familiar IV drip that is used to slowly drip a bag of electrolyte solution into a dehydrated patient through a tiny plastic tube inserted directly into a vein.

intravenous gamma globulin See *intravenous immunoglobulin.*

intravenous immunoglobulin A sterile solution of concentrated antibodies extracted from healthy people that is administered directly into a vein. Abbreviated IVIG. IVIG is used to treat disorders of the immune system or to boost the immune response to serious illness. Also known as intravenous gamma globulin (IGG).

intravenous pyelogram An X-ray of the kidneys and urinary tract. Abbreviated IVP. Structures are made visible on an IVP by the injection of a substance that blocks X-rays.

intravenous tension The pressure of the blood within a vein. Also known as venous pressure.

intraventricular In the ventricle of the heart or the brain.

introitus An entrance that goes into a canal or hollow organ.

introitus, facial canal The entrance to the facial canal, a passage in the temporal bone of the skull through which the facial nerve travels.

introitus, vaginal The vaginal opening.

intron Part of a gene that is initially transcribed into the primary RNA transcript but is later removed from it when the exxon sequences on either side of it are spliced together. Also known as intervening sequence.

intubate To put a tube in. For example, as a life-saving measure, an emergency room physician might intubate a patient who is not breathing adequately so that the lungs can be ventilated.

intussusception Infolding (prolapse) of a portion of the intestine within another immediately adjacent portion of intestine, which generally affects children. Intussusception decreases the supply of blood to the affected part of the intestine and frequently leads to intestinal obstruction. The pressure created by the two walls of the intestine pressing together causes inflammation and swelling, and

it reduces the blood flow. Death of bowel tissue can occur, with significant bleeding, perforation, abdominal infection, and shock occurring very rapidly. Most cases of intussusception occur in children between 5 months and 1 year of age. Symptoms begin with sudden, loud crying in an infant, with the baby drawing the knees up to the chest while crying. This reaction is caused by abdominal cramping. The pain and crying are intermittent but recur frequently and increase in intensity and duration. Fever is common. As the condition progresses, the infant becomes weak and then shows signs of shock, including pale color, lethargy, and sweating. About half of afflicted infants pass a bloody, mucousy ("currant jelly") stool. The cause of intussusception is not known, although viral infections of the intestine may contribute to intussusception in infancy. In older children or adults, the presence of polyps or a tumor may trigger intussusception. Early diagnosis is very important. On examining the abdomen, a physician may feel a mass. Abdominal X-rays may suggest intestinal obstruction, but a barium enema is needed to show the charactcristic telescoping of the bowel. In some cases, the intestinal obstruction can be reduced with a barium enema. If the obstruction cannot be reduced by a barium enema, surgery is needed to reduce the intussusception, relieve the obstruction, and remove any dead tissue. Intravenous feeding and fluid are continued until a normal bowel movement has passed.

invasive cervical cancer Cancer that has spread from the surface of the cervix to tissue deeper in the cervix or to other parts of the body. See also *cancer, cervical.*

inversion, chromosome See *chromosome inversion.*

invest In medicine, to envelop, cover, or embed. For example, a dentist might invest a patient's teeth with a wax material in order to form a mold of it.

involution A retrograde change. After treatment, a tumor may involute; with advancing age, there may be physical and emotional involution.

iodide The form to which iodine in the diet is reduced before being absorbed through the intestinal wall into the bloodstream and carried to the thyroid gland. See also *iodine.*

iodide goiter See *iodine excess.*

iodine An element in the diet that is essential for the manufacture of hormones by the thyroid gland. The thyroid gland uses iodine to make thyroxine (T4), which has four iodine molecules attached to its structure, and triiodothyronine (T3), which has three iodine molecules attached. Iodine is found in seafood, bread, iodized salt, and seaweed.

iodine deficiency A lack of sufficient iodine in the diet, which can lead to inadequate production of thyroid hormone (hypothyroidism) and enlargement of the thyroid gland (goiter). Since the addition of iodine to table salt became common, iodine deficiency has rarely been seen in the US.

iodine excess Prolonged intake of too much iodine that leads to swelling of the thyroid gland (goiter) and abnormally low thyroid activity (hypothyroidism). Certain foods and medications contain large amounts of iodine, including seaweed; iodine-rich expectorants such as SSKI and Lugol's solution that are used to treat cough, asthma, and chronic pulmonary disease; and amiodarone (brand name: Cardorone), an iodine-rich medication used to control abnormal heart rhythms.

IOL Intraocular lens.

IORT Intraoperative radiation therapy.

IP Incontinentia pigmenti.

ipecac, syrup of A solution that contains a naturally occurring substance that can cause vomiting (emesis). Ipecac is derived from dried roots of a Brazilian bush, Uragoga ipecacuanha. Syrup of ipecac is used to treat a few types of poisoning. It is important to consult with the local poison control center before administering syrup of ipecac because many poisons cause additional harm if vomited.

ipsilateral On the same side, as opposed to contralateral. For example, a tumor involving the right side of the brain may affect vision ipsilaterally—that is, in the right eye.

IPV Inactivated polio vaccine. See *polio immunization*.

IQ Intelligence quotient, an attempt to measure the intelligence of an individual. The IQ score is usually based on the results of a written test. To calculate the IQ, the person's mental age as determined by a test is divided by chronological age, and the result is multiplied by 100. See also *intelligence test; intelligence, nonverbal; intelligence, verbal.*

iridectomy The process of making a hole in the iris. Iridectomy is a treatment for glaucoma.

iridology The practice of diagnosing disease by examining the iris of the eye. Although some diseases affect the eye, iridology is not considered scientific medicine.

iris The circular, colored curtain of the eye. The opening of the iris forms the pupil. The iris helps regulate the amount of light that enters the eye.

iris, speckled See *Brushfield spot.*

iritis Inflammation of the iris. Iritis can occur by itself and be inherited, such as in association with the gene marker HLA-B27. It can also occur as a feature of an underlying disease, such as reactive arthritis, inflammatory bowel disease, sarcoidosis, rheumatoid arthritis, and lupus.

iron A mineral that is necessary for the transport of oxygen via hemoglobin in red blood cells and for oxidation by cells via cytochrome. Food sources of iron include meat, poultry, eggs, vegetables, and cereals, especially those fortified with iron. According to the National Academy of Sciences, the recommended dietary allowance of iron is 15 mg per day for women and 10 mg per day for men. See also *deficiency, iron; excess iron; iron poisoning.*

iron deficiency See *deficiency, iron.*

iron excess See *excess iron.*

iron poisoning An abnormally excessive ingestion of iron resulting in injury to body tissues. Iron supplements meant for adults, such as pregnant women, are a major cause of poisoning in children. Children should never be given supplements or multivitamins containing iron unless they have been prescribed by a physician, and iron preparations for adults should be kept away from children.

irrigate To wash out. For example, one can irrigate a wound to clean it.

irrigation of the colon The use of liquid solutions given by enema to remove material from the rectum or colon, ostensibly to eliminate toxins from the bowel. Unless ordered by a physician, irrigation of the colon is rarely advisable. Irrigation of the colon carries a number of risks, including interference with the normal digestive process and perforation. Also known as colonic irrigation and high colonics.

irritable bowel syndrome A functional intestinal disorder of the bowels and their nerves. Irritable bowel syndrome (IBS) may be caused by either abnormal motility (abnormal contractions) of the intestinal muscles or abnormally sensitive nerves in the intestines (visceral hyper-sensitivity). IBS is characterized by abdominal pain, bloating, mucus in stools, and irregular bowel habits, with alternating diarrhea and constipation. These symptoms tend to be chronic, and they wax and wane over the years. Although IBS can cause chronic and recurrent discomfort, it does not normally lead to any serious organ problems. Diagnosis usually involves excluding other illnesses. Treatment is directed toward relief of symptoms and includes high-fiber diet; exercise; relaxation techniques;

avoidance of caffeine, milk products, and sweeteners; and medications. Also known as spastic colitis, mucus colitis, and nervous colon syndrome.

ischemia   Inadequate blood supply to a local area due to blockage of blood vessels leading to that area. Treatment is directed toward increasing the circulation to the affected body area.

ischial bursitis   See *weaver's bottom.*

ischiopubic bar   See *ischium.*

ischiopubic synchondrosis   The central point of the ischium, which does not close until after the toddler years. See also *ischium.*

ischium   The bone that makes up the lower-rear part of the pelvis. Also known as ischiopubic bar and ischiopubic bone.

islet of Langerhans   A group of specialized cells in the pancreas that make and secrete hormones, including insulin. These cells sit in groups (islets), with five types of cells in an islet: alpha cells that make glucagon, which raises the level of glucose (sugar) in the blood; beta cells that make insulin; delta cells that make somatostatin, which inhibits the release of numerous other hormones in the body; and PP cells and D1 cells, about which little is known. Degeneration of the insulin-producing beta cells is the main cause of type 1 (insulin-dependent) diabetes mellitus.

isochromosome   An abnormal chromosome that has two identical arms due to duplication of one arm and loss of the other. Isochromosomes are found in tumors and in some girls with Turner syndrome.

isodisomy   A remarkable situation in which both chromosomes in a pair are from one parent only. Isodisomy causes some birth defects and is suspected to play a role in cancer. Also known as uniparental disomy.

isolate   A group (for example, the Amish) in which mating is always between members of the group.

isotonic solution   A solution that has the same salt concentration as cells and blood. Isotonic solutions are commonly used as intravenously infused fluids in hospitalized patients.

isotope   A form of a chemical element that has a different-from-normal atomic mass. Isotopes are used in a number of medical tests because they can produce images of tissues that can be used to detect diseases or conditions.

itching   An uncomfortable sensation in the skin that feels as if something is crawling on the skin and makes the person want to scratch the affected area. Itching is medically known as pruritis; something that is itchy is pruritic.

itching, anal   See *anal itching.*

-itis   Suffix meaning inflammation. For example, colitis is inflammation of the colon.

ITP   Idiopathic thrombocytopenic purpura. A condition characterized by the sudden, abnormal lowering of the platelet count. The cause is unknown, but the immune system seems to play a major role in the process by eliminating the platelets. ITP can lead to dangerously low platelet counts that can be associated with spontaneous bleeding. ITP requires treatments directed at suppressing the immune system.

IUD   Intrauterine device.

IUGR   Intrauterine growth retardation. Inadequate growth of the baby in the womb of the mother according to standards for the particular age.

IV   Intravenous.

IVF   In vitro fertilization.

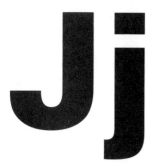

Jacksonian seizure   See *seizure, partial.*

Jadassohn-Lewandowski syndrome   See *pachyonychia congenita.*

jail fever   See *typhus, epidemic.*

Jakob-Creutzfeldt disease   See *Creutzfeldt-Jakob disease.*

JAMA   The *Journal of the American Medical Association,* one of the two leading general medical journals published in the US. JAMA is published by the American Medical Association (AMA). It carries original, generally well-documented, peer-reviewed medical articles on many clinical and research topics in medicine.

jamais vu   The illusion that the familiar does not seem familiar. See also *déjà vu; seizure disorders.*

jaundice   A yellowish staining of the skin and whites of the eyes (sclerae) with bilirubin, the pigment found in bile. Jaundice can be an indicator of liver or gallbladder disease, or it may result from the rupture of red blood cells (hemolysis). In newborn babies it is usually, but not always, a normal condition. Also known as icterus. See also *jaundice, hemolytic; jaundice, hepatocellular; jaundice, neonatal; jaundice, obstructive; kernicterus; spherocytosis, hereditary.*

jaundice, congenital hemolytic   See *spherocytosis, hereditary.*

jaundice, hemolytic   Jaundice caused by destruction of red blood cells. Hemolytic jaundice can be an inborn condition (as in hereditary spherocytosis) or it can be caused by a blood transfusion from a different blood group, infection in the bloodstream (sepsis), or some type of poisoning. See also *spherocytosis, hereditary.*

jaundice, hepatocellular   Jaundice caused by liver disease, as by hepatitis. See also *hepatitis.*

jaundice, neonatal   Jaundice in newborn babies. Neonatal jaundice is usually due to the breakdown of red blood cells, which release bilirubin that the immature liver cannot metabolize and prepare for excretion into the urine. This type of neonatal jaundice typically appears between the second and fifth days of life and clears with time, as the liver matures. Diagnosis is made through observation and measurement of the blood bilirubin level. Treatment usually involves timed exposure of the skin to special lights, sometimes through a device called a bilirubin blanket. Severe jaundice is treated by removing serum from the body and replacing with solutions without bilirubin (exchange transfusion). Jaundice that appears during the first day of life may be due to a biliary disorder and is likely to require medical treatment. See also *jaundice; kernicterus; spherocytosis, hereditary.*

jaundice, obstructive   Jaundice caused by obstruction of the bile ducts, as with gallstones. Symptoms of obstructive jaundice include the typical yellowing of jaundice as well as dark urine, pale feces, and itching, although there is no pain. Sometimes the cause of obstructive jaundice is cancer (malignant obstructive jaundice), in which case treatment is by chemotherapy, radiation, and/or biliary drainage (surgery is rarely used).

jaundice, physiologic   See *physiologic jaundice.*

jaw   The movable junction of the bones below the mouth (the mandible) and the bone just above the mouth (the maxilla).

jejunal   Having to do with the jejunum.

jejunum   The middle portion of the small intestine. The jejunum is about 2.4 meters (8 feet) in length and located halfway between the duodenum and the ileum. The jejunum is responsible for much of the absorption of the fluids and calcium that we ingest. See also *intestine; intestine, small.*

jellyfish sting   The injection into the skin of venom from the stinging unit (nematocyst) of the jellyfish. The jellyfish tentacles can extend for several feet and are lined with venom-filled cells (nematocysts). One tentacle may fire thousands of nematocysts into the skin on contact. On contact, each cell fires a barbed thread that penetrates the victim's skin. The pain can be severe, particularly in the first hours after an attack, and itching is common. The victim may have weakness, nausea, headache, muscle pain and spasms, tearing and nasal discharge, increased perspiration, changes in pulse rate, and chest pain. Welting may persist for weeks at the site, and scarring may remain. Even dead jellyfish are capable of leaving a painful mark, so they should be avoided. Sting wounds should be treated with vinegar for box jellyfish and with baking soda in a 50:50 mix with ocean water for sea nettles and the Portuguese man-of-war. Water alone may cause additional stinging cells to fire off. Aspirin or another pain reliever should be administered immediately to relieve the pain of minor stings. Narcotics may be needed for severe pain. Those who get serious stings may require oxygen or cardiorespiratory assistance. IV fluids and epinephrine may be needed if shock develops. There is no antivenom for the stings of North American jellyfish, but there is antivenom for the stings of some Australian species.

jet lag A temporary disorder that features fatigue and insomnia and that is caused when the body's natural rhythms are interrupted by rapid travel across time zones. Other symptoms of jet lag include anxiety, constipation, diarrhea, confusion, dehydration, headache, irritability, nausea, sweating, coordination problems, and even memory loss. See also *circadian clock.*

jogger's nails Very common, small, semicircular white spots on the toenails. These spots result from injury to the base (matrix) of the nail, a structure under the visible nail where the cells that make up the visible nail are produced. The injury responsible for these white spots on the nails can be due to athletic activity or poorly fitting shoes; jogging in poorly fitting shoes causes the condition so often as to coin the term jogger's nails. These spots are not a cause for concern. They eventually grow out with the nail.

joint The area where two bones are attached for the purpose of permitting body parts to move. A joint is usually formed of fibrous connective tissue and cartilage. Joints are grouped according to their motion: ball-and-socket joint; hinge joint; condyloid joint, which permits all forms of angular movement except axial rotation; pivot joint; gliding joint; or saddle joint. Joints can move in only four ways: gliding, in which one bony surface glides on another, without angular or rotatory movement; angular, a movement that occurs only between long bones, increasing or decreasing the angle between the bones; circumduction, which occurs in joints composed of the head of a bone and an articular cavity, with the long bone describing a series of circles and the whole forming a cone; and rotation, in which a bone moves about a central axis without moving from this axis. Also known as articulation and arthrosis.

joint, AC Acromioclavicular joint.

joint, acetabular The hip joint. The acetabulum is the cup-shaped socket of the hip joint, and it is a key feature of the pelvic anatomy. The upper end of the femur (thighbone) fits right into the acetabulum, articulates with it, and thereby forms the largest ball-and-socket joint in the human body.

joint, acromioclavicular See *acromioclavicular joint.*

joint, ankle See *ankle joint.*

joint aspiration See *arthrocentesis.*

joint, atlas and axis See *atlantoaxial joint.*

joint, ball-and-socket See *ball-and-socket joint.*

joint, calcaneocuboid See *calcaneocuboid joint.*

joint, elbow See *elbow.*

joint hypermobility syndrome See *hypermobility syndrome.*

joint, knee See *knee.*

joint, patellofemoral See *patellofemoral joint.*

joint, shoulder See *shoulder joint.*

joint, temporomandibular See *temporomandibular joint.*

joint, TM See *temporomandibular joint.*

joints of the body, principal The principal joints of the human body include the following:

  acromioclavicular

  ankle (tibia-fibula and talus)

  atlantoaxial

  atlantooccipital

  calcaneocuboid

  carpometacarpal

  elbow (humerus, radius, and ulna)

  femur and tibia

  hip bone and femur

  intercarpal (proximal carpal, distal carpal, and the two rows of carpal bones with each other)

  intermetacarpals

  intermetatarsals

  interphalangeal

  intervertebral joints

  knee (femur, tibia, and patella)

  manubristernal

  metacarpophalangeal

  metatarsophalangeal

  radioulnar

  ribs, heads of

  ribs, tubercles and necks of

  sacrococcygeal

sacroiliac

shoulder (humerus and scapula)

sternoclavicular

sternocostal

subtalar

symphysis

talus and calcaneus

talus and navicular

tarsometatarsal

temporomandibular

tibiofibular

ulnohumeral

wrist (radius, ulna, and carpals)

Journal of the American Medical Association See
JAMA.

jugular See *jugular vein.*

jugular vein One of the veins in the neck that drain
blood from the head, brain, face, and neck, and then convey it toward the heart. There are an external jugular vein
and an internal jugular vein on each side of the neck. The
jugular veins are particularly prominent during congestive heart failure. When the patient is sitting or in a semi-
recumbent position, the height of the jugular veins and
their pulsations provide an estimate of the central venous
pressure, as well as important information about whether
the heart is keeping up with the demands on it. See also
jugular vein, external; jugular vein, internal.

jugular vein, external The more superficial of the
two jugular veins on each side of the neck. The external
jugular vein collects most of the blood from the outside of
the skull and the deep parts of the face. It lies outside the
sternocleidomastoid muscle, passes down the neck, and
joins the subclavian vein. See also *jugular vein.*

jugular vein, internal The deeper of the two jugular
veins on each side of the neck. The internal jugular vein
collects blood from the brain, the outside of the face, and
the neck. It runs down the inside of the neck, outside the

internal and common carotid arteries, and unites with the
subclavian vein to form the innominate vein. See also
jugular vein.

June cold See *allergic rhinitis.*

juvenile Between infantile and adult. Used in medicine
to indicate onset in childhood, as in juvenile rheumatoid
arthritis.

juvenile chronic arthritis, systemic-onset See
arthritis, systemic-onset juvenile rheumatoid.

juvenile laryngeal papillomatosis A condition characterized by the emergence of numerous warty growths
on the vocal cords in children and young adults. A baby
can contract juvenile laryngeal papillomatosis by being
contaminated with the human papilloma virus (HPV) during birth through the vaginal canal of a mother who has
genital warts. Each year, about 300 infants are thus born
with the virus on their vocal cords. Treatment usually
involves surgical excision. Recurrences of laryngeal papillomatosis are, unfortunately, frequent. Remission may
occur after several years.

juvenile rheumatoid arthritis See *arthritis, systemic-onset juvenile rheumatoid.*

juxta- Prefix meaning near, nearby, or close, as in juxtaspinal (near the spinal column) and juxtavesicular
(near the bladder).

juxtaarticular Near a joint. For example, a juxtaarticular fracture is a break near a joint.

juxtaposition See *apposition.*

juxtapyloric Near the pylorus, the muscular area at the
junction of the stomach and the first part of the small
intestine. For example, a juxtapyloric ulcer is located near
the pylorus.

juxtaspinal Near the spinal column. For example, juxtaspinal abscess lies adjacent to the spinal column.

juxtavesicular Near the bladder.

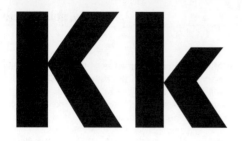

K The symbol for potassium, the major positive ion (cation) found inside cells. A proper level of potassium is essential for normal cell function. An abnormal increase in potassium (hyperkalemia) or an abnormal decrease in potassium (hypokalemia) can profoundly affect the nervous system and the heart and, if extreme, can be fatal.

kala-azar A disease of the viscera, particularly the liver, spleen, bone marrow, and lymph nodes, that is due to infection by a parasite called Leishmania. Also known as visceral leishmaniasis. *Kala-azar* is Hindi for "black fever." See also *Leishmania; leishmaniasis*.

Kaposi sarcoma A relatively rare type of skin malignancy that tends to affect elderly people and those with an abnormal immune system, as in AIDS. Kaposi sarcoma is caused by human herpesvirus 8 (HHV-8), which may be transmitted via kissing. Gay men who engage in "deep kissing" that involves much contact with saliva are at increased risk of catching HHV-8 and developing Kaposi sarcoma. Kaposi sarcoma is a highly vascular (angioblastic) tumor of the skin, characterized by soft purplish plaques and papules that form nodules, which typically start on the feet and ankles and then slowly spread across the skin of the legs, hands, and arms. In AIDS patients, these tumors can also develop internally and cause severe internal bleeding. The treatment depends on the severity of the tumor. Low dosages of radiation therapy can be effective in treating mild cases of Kaposi sarcoma. However, in more severe cases, anticancer drugs may be used to slow the spread of the tumor. The Kaposi sarcoma tumor was first described in 1872 by the dermatologist Moritz Kaposi Kohn. See also *AIDS; HIV; sarcoma*.

Kartagener syndrome A genetic syndrome that is characterized by sinusitis, bronchiectasis (widening and inflammation of the bronchi), dextrocardia (heart on the right side), and infertility. Kartagener syndrome is inherited in an autosomal recessive manner. Kartagener syndrome is usually due to mutation in the gene called DNAI1, which is in chromosome region 9p21–9p13. However, linkage studies have mapped the disease gene to 5p and 19q in some families, indicating that Kartagener syndrome is more than one genetic entity. Also known as ciliary dyskinesia syndrome.

karyotype A standard arrangement of the chromosome complement prepared for chromosome analysis. A normal female karyotype would include each of the 22 pairs of autosomes (nonsex chromosomes), arranged in numeric order, together with the two X chromosomes.

karyotyping The preparation, analysis, and interpretation of a karyotype.

karyotyping, flow See *flow karyotyping*.

Kawasaki disease A syndrome that mainly affects young children, causing fever; reddening of the eyes (conjunctivitis), lips, and mucous membranes of the mouth; ulcerative gum disease (gingivitis); swollen glands in the neck (cervical lymphadenopathy); and a rash that is raised and bright red (maculoerythematous). The rash appears in a "glove-and-sock" fashion over the skin of the hands and feet. The skin then becomes hard and swollen (edematous), and it peels off. Kawasaki disease affects the blood vessels and is now the main cause of acquired heart disease in children. It is most common in people of Asian descent, and it is both more common and more deadly in males than in females. Its cause is unknown; current theories include viral causes or an environmental toxin. Treatment usually involves intravenous immunoglobulin (IVIG). Also known as mucocutaneous lymph node syndrome.

Kb Kilobase.

KB **1** Keratodermia blennorrhagicum. **2** Ketone bodies.

Kegel exercises Exercises designed to increase muscle strength and elasticity in the female pelvis. Kegel exercises may be recommended for treatment of incompetent cervix, vaginal looseness after pregnancy and delivery, or urinary incontinence.

keloid A scar that rises quite abruptly above the rest of the skin. It is irregularly shaped, tends to enlarge progressively, and may be darker in color and harder than the surrounding skin. Keloids are a response to trauma, such as a cut to the skin. In creating a normal scar, connective tissue in the skin is repaired by the formation of collagen. This occurs in the dermis, the second layer of skin. Keloids arise when extra collagen forms. Susceptibility to keloids is genetic, and keloids are particularly common in people of African descent. If a keloid is uncomfortable or cosmetically undesirable (as in the case of a keloid scar on the face), a dermatologist may be able to reduce its prominence by using silicone pads or other methods.

keratectomy Removal of part of the cornea by surgical excision or by laser. See also *keratectomy, photorefractive*.

keratectomy, photorefractive Laser eye surgery designed to change the shape of the cornea, reducing or eliminating the need for glasses and contact lenses. The laser removes the outer layer of the cornea and then flattens it. This is intended to correct nearsightedness (myopia) and uneven curvature of the cornea that distorts vision (astigmatism). Photorefractive keratectomy is an outpatient procedure that is done in an office with numbing eye drops. It takes about 1 minute to perform and about 3 days to heal. No eye patch need be worn afterward. Abbreviated PRK. The same type of laser is used for PRK and LASIK. The major difference between the two surgeries is the way that the stroma, the middle layer of the cornea, is exposed before it is vaporized with the laser. In PRK, the top layer of the cornea, called the epithelium, is scraped away to expose the stromal layer underneath. In LASIK, a flap is cut in the stromal layer and the flap is folded back. See also *LASIK.*

keratin   A protein found in the upper layer of the skin, hair, and nails, and in animal horns.

keratitis   Inflammation of the cornea. Keratitis can occur due to abrasion trauma, infection, or underlying diseases such as Sjogren's syndrome and lupus. Keratitis can lead to blindness.

keratitis, rosacea   Inflammation of the cornea of the eye that affects about half of all people with rosacea. Symptoms include burning and grittiness of the eyes (conjunctivitis). If rosacea keratitis is not treated with medication to stop the inflammation, the damage to the cornea may impair vision. See also *rosacea.*

keratitis-ichthyosis-deafness syndrome   An inherited disorder that is characterized by keratitis (gradual destruction of the cornea of the eye, sometimes leading to blindness), ichthyosis (localized areas of disfiguring reddish thickened skin), and deafness from birth. Abbreviated KID syndrome. Another characteristic feature of KID syndrome is thin or absent scalp hair. Some patients develop cancer of the tongue, and some have subtle abnormalities of the nervous system. KID syndrome is inherited in an autosomal dominant manner and is due to mutation in the connexin-26 gene (located on chromosome 13).

kerato-   **1** Prefix referring to the cornea, as in keratitis (inflammation of the cornea) and keratoplasty (corneal transplant).   **2** Prefix referring to the nails, hair, or skin tissue, as in keratin (a protein found in the upper layer of the skin, hair, and nails, and in animal horns) and keratosis (a localized horny overgrowth of the skin).

keratoconjunctivitis   Inflammation of the eye that involves both the cornea and conjunctiva. Keratoconjunctivitis can occur due to abrasion trauma, infection, and underlying diseases such as Sjogren's syndrome and lupus.

keratoconus   A cone-shaped cornea, with the apex of the cone being forward. Keratoconus causes distorted vision. Also known as conical cornea. Treatment of keratoconus depends on the severity of the condition. Treatment options include eyeglasses, rigid contact lenses, and corneal transplantation, and combinations of these.

keratodermia blennorrhagicum   A skin disease that occurs in patients with reactive arthritis (formerly Reiter's syndrome). Abbreviated KB. Classically, the areas of the skin that are involved are the palms of the hands and the soles of the feet, although other body surfaces may also be affected. The inflammation of the skin can come and go. When the inflammation is present, it appears as patches of reddish, raised pustules that can be painful and tender. These patchy areas may group together and peel periodically. KB can be treated with topical medications, including skin softeners (emollients) and medications that clear off the peeling, dry skin (keratolytic medications). Sometimes these treatments are used along with vitamin D creams, such as calcipotriene. Emotional stress and certain medications, such as propanolol (brand name: Vasotec) and hydroxychloroquine (brand name: Plaquenil) may aggravate the condition.

keratoplasty   Corneal transplant.

keratosis   A localized horny overgrowth of the skin, such as a wart or callus. Among the common types of keratosis are actinic keratosis and senile keratosis.

keratosis, actinic   A small rough spot on the skin that can give rise to a skin cancer called squamous cell carcinoma. Actinic keratosis is due to excessive sun exposure and most frequently occurs in fair-skinned people after 40 years of age. Common locations for actinic keratosis are the face, scalp, nape of the neck, upper chest, forearms, and backs of the hands. Prevention involves minimizing sun exposure and using sunscreen. Treatments include cryosurgery (freezing), surgical removal, topical 5-fluorouracil (5-FU), and photodynamic therapy (injection into the bloodstream of a chemical that collects in the actinic keratoses to make them more sensitive to exposure to a specialized form of light). Also known as senile keratosis and solar keratosis.

keratosis follicularis   A genetic skin disease that is characterized by slowly progressive hardening of the skin (keratosis) around the hair follicles. This disorder is inherited in an autosomal dominant manner and is due to mutation in a gene called ATP2A2 on chromosome 12. Also known as Darier disease.

keratosis, seborrheic   A skin disorder that is characterized by oily skin and warts and skin lesions that appear to be "stuck on." The raised spots are usually yellow or brown. Treatment, if warranted, involves surgical or cryosurgical removal. Also known as seborrheic warts and verruca.

keratosis, senile   See *keratosis, actinic.*

keratosis, solar   See *keratosis, actinic.*

keratotic scabies   See *scabies, keratotic.*

keratotomy   A surgical cut of the cornea.

keratotomy, radial   A surgical procedure designed to flatten the cornea and thereby correct nearsightedness (myopia). It is called a radial keratotomy because the incisions resemble the spokes in a bicycle wheel.

kernicterus   A disorder that is due to severe jaundice in the newborn, with deposition of the pigment bilirubin in the brain that causes damage to the brain. Also known as bilirubin encephalopathy.

Kernig sign   A sign indicating the presence of meningitis (inflammation of the meninges covering the brain and spinal cord). The test for Kernig sign is done by having the person lie flat on the back, flex the thigh so that it is at a right angle to the trunk, and completely extend the leg at the knee joint. If the leg cannot be completely extended due to pain, this is Kernig sign.

Keshan disease   A condition caused by deficiency of the essential mineral selenium. Keshan disease is a potentially fatal form of cardiomyopathy (disease of the heart muscle). It was first observed in Keshan province in China, and it has since been found in other areas where the selenium level in the soil is low. Treatment involves selenium supplementation.

ketoacidosis   A life-threatening feature of uncontrolled diabetes that is characterized by a combination of ketosis and acidosis. Ketosis is the accumulation of substances called ketone bodies in the blood. Acidosis is increased acidity of the blood. Symptoms of ketoacidosis include slow, deep breathing with a fruity odor to the breath, confusion, frequent urination (polyuria), poor appetite, and eventually loss of consciousness. Ketoacidosis should be treated immediately and is usually done in a hospital. It may require the administration of intravenous fluids, insulin, and glucose. See also *diabetes mellitus; ketone bodies.*

ketogenic diet   A diet devised as a treatment for severe seizure disorders that do not respond to conventional medication. The ketogenic diet is almost entirely made up of fats and protein. All portions must be precisely weighed and timed. Because this diet can cause the buildup of ketone bodies in the blood, it is highly risky and should be tried only under close medical supervision. See also *ketone bodies; ketoacidosis; seizure disorders.*

ketone bodies   Acetone, acetoacetate, and B-hydroxybutyrate—three toxic, acidic chemicals that build up in the bloodstream when the body is forced to burn fat for energy instead of burning glucose. See also *ketoacidosis.*

ketonuria   A condition in which abnormally high amounts of ketone metabolites are present in the urine. Ketonuria is usually a sign of diabetes that is out of control. Ketonuria can also develop as a result of fasting, dieting, starvation, and eating disorders. See *ketoacidosis.*

KID syndrome   See *keratitis-ichthyosis-deafness syndrome.*

kidney   One of a pair of organs located in the right and left side of the abdomen. The kidneys remove waste products from the blood and produce urine. As blood flows through the kidneys, the kidneys filter waste products, chemicals, and unneeded water from the blood. Urine collects in the middle of each kidney, in an area called the renal pelvis. It then drains from the kidney through a long tube, the ureter, to the bladder, where it is stored until elimination. The kidneys also make substances that help control blood pressure and regulate the formation of red blood cells.

kidney cancer   See *cancer, kidney.*

kidney scoping   See *retrograde intrarenal surgery.*

kidney stones   Stones in the kidney or stones that originate in the kidney but have passed lower down in the urinary tract. Kidney stones are a common cause of blood in the urine and pain in the abdomen, flank, or groin. One in 20 people will have a kidney stone at some time in his or her life. The development of kidney stones is related to decreased urine volume or to increased excretion of stone-forming components, such as calcium, oxalate, urate, cystine, xanthine, and phosphate. The stones form in the urine-collecting area (pelvis) of the kidney and may range in size from tiny to "staghorn" stones the size of the renal pelvis itself. Factors that predispose people to kidney stones include reduction in fluid intake, increased exercise with dehydration, medications that cause high uric acid (hyperuricemia), and a history of gout. Pain from kidney stones is usually of sudden onset, very severe and intermittent, and not improved by changes in position, and it radiates from the back, down the flank, and into the groin. Nausea and vomiting are common. The majority of stones pass spontaneously within 48 hours. However, some stones do not. Several factors influence the ability to pass a stone, including the size of the person, prior stone passage, prostate enlargement, pregnancy, and the size of the stone. If a stone does not pass, the help of a urology specialist may be needed. Routine treatment includes relief of pain, hydration, and, if there is concurrent urinary infection, administration of antibiotics.

kidney stones, cystine See *cystine kidney stones.*

kidney transplant Replacement of a diseased, damaged, or missing kidney with a donor kidney. Patients with end-stage kidney failure are candidates for transplantation. A successful transplant frees the patient from needing dialysis and provides the kidney's other metabolic functions. The principal problems in kidney transplantation are immunologic—avoiding rejection of the transplanted kidney by the recipient's immune system. The first kidney transplant was done by the US surgeon Joseph E. Murray in 1954. It was the first successful human organ transplant. See also *transplant.*

killed polio vaccine See *polio vaccine, inactivated.*

kilobase A unit of length of DNA that is equal to 1,000 nucleotide bases. Abbreviated Kb.

kilocalorie The amount of energy required to raise the temperature of 1 liter of water 1° centigrade at sea level. In nutrition terms, the word *calorie* is commonly used instead of the more precise scientific term kilocalorie. See also *calorie.*

Kimmelstiel-Wilson disease See *diabetic nephropathy.*

kindred The extended family.

kinetic With movement, as opposed to akinetic.

kinetics 1 The rate of change in a biochemical or other reaction. 2 The study of reaction rates.

kinky hair syndrome See *Menkes syndrome.*

kinship Relationship by marriage or, specifically, a blood tie.

kissing bugs Insect carriers of the parasite Trypanosoma cruzi, which causes Chagas disease. The bugs "kiss" people, especially babies, on the lips while they are asleep, infecting them with their parasite. See also *Chagas disease.*

kissing disease Nickname for infectious mononucleosis. See also *mononucleosis.*

kit, disaster supplies See *disaster supplies.*

klebsiella A group of bacteria that normally lives in the intestinal tract, but can cause infections when the microorganism infects tissues of the body. Klebsiella are frequently the cause of infections acquired in hospitals.

Kleine-Levin syndrome A rare condition that is characterized by excessive need for sleep and food, as well as sexual disinhibition. Most patients with Kleine-Levin syndrome are adolescent males. When awake, they may be confused, irritable, and lethargic, and some have hallucinations. The cause is unknown. Most cases resolve over time without treatment. Also known as Kleine-Levin hibernation syndrome.

Klinefelter syndrome A condition in males who have XXY sex chromosomes, rather than the usual XY. Some also have additional X chromosomes, or more than one Y chromosome. XXY is one of the most common chromosomal abnormalities. It occurs in 1 in 500 male births. The signs of Klinefelter syndrome include small testes, insufficient production of testosterone, and infertility. XXY males are more likely than other males to show breast enlargement, lack of facial and body hair, and a rounded body type, and they are more likely than other males to be overweight and be taller than their fathers and brothers. Klinefelter boys tend to have learning and/or behavioral problems.

Klippel-Feil syndrome The combination of short neck, low hairline at the nape of the neck, and limited movement of the head. Klippel-Feil syndrome is due to a defect in the early development of the spinal column in the neck. Also known as Klippel-Feil sequence.

Klippel-Trenaunay-Weber syndrome A congenital malformation syndrome that is characterized by three basic features: enlargement of a single limb (asymmetric limb hypertrophy), abnormal nests of blood vessels that proliferate inappropriately and excessively (hemangiomata), and pigmented moles on the skin (nevi). Abbreviated KTW syndrome. The enlarged limb is three times more likely to be a leg than an arm, and both bone and soft tissue are enlarged. The hemangiomas range from small, innocuous capillary hemangiomas (known as strawberry marks) to huge cavernous hemangiomas. The nevi are often also dark linear streaks on the skin, due to too much pigment. There can be other abnormalities. Most persons with KTW syndrome do relatively well without treatment. Compression from an elastic stocking or sleeve can help. Skin ulcers and other skin problems can occur over the swollen limb, and they can also be treated. Treatment usually involves pain control and cosmetic applications, unless the limb reaches gigantic proportions or secondary clotting difficulties arise due to trapping and destruction of blood platelets in a huge hemangioma. In such cases amputation may become necessary. The cause of KTW syndrome is unknown.

knee A joint that permits flexibility in the middle of the lower extremity. The thigh bone (femur) meets the large shin bone (tibia) to form the main knee joint. This joint has an inner (medial) and an outer (lateral) compartment.

The kneecap (patella) joins the femur to form a third joint, called the patellofemoral joint. The patella protects the front of the knee joint. The knee joint is surrounded by a joint capsule, with ligaments strapping the inside and outside of the joint (collateral ligaments) as well as crossing within the joint (cruciate ligaments). The collateral ligaments run along the sides of the knee and limit its sideways motion. The anterior cruciate ligament (ACL) connects the tibia to the femur at the center of the knee and functions to limit the tibia's rotation and forward motion. The posterior cruciate ligament (PCL), located just behind the ACL, limits the backward motion of the tibia. All these ligaments provide stability and strength to the knee joint. A thickened cartilage pad between the two joints (meniscus) is formed by the femur and tibia. The meniscus acts as a smooth surface for the joint to move on. It serves to evenly load the surface during weight bearing, and it also aids in disbursing joint fluid for joint lubrication. The knee joint is surrounded by fluid-filled sacs called bursae, which serve as gliding surfaces to reduce friction of the tendons. Below the kneecap is a large tendon (patellar tendon) that attaches to the front of the tibia bone. Large blood vessels pass through the area behind the knee, which is called the popliteal space. The large muscles of the thigh move the knee. In the front of the thigh, the quadricep muscles extend the knee joint. In the back of the thigh, the hamstring muscles flex the knee. The knee also rotates slightly under the guidance of specific muscles of the thigh. The knee is critical to normal walking and is a weight-bearing joint. Knee pain can be caused by a number of factors, including injury, inflammation of the bursa (bursitis), strain, and problems with the sciatic nerve, which runs from the lower back to the knee. See also *bursitis; patellofemoral syndrome; sciatica.*

knee bursitis Inflammation of a fluid-filled sac (bursa) around the knee. See *bursitis.*

knee, housemaid's See *patellofemoral syndrome.*

knee jerk The reflex that is tested by tapping just below the bent knee on the patellar tendon. Normally this causes the quadriceps muscle to contract and bring the lower leg forward. It has given rise to the saying "a knee-jerk reaction." Also known as patellar reflex.

knee, secretary's See *patellofemoral syndrome.*

kneecap The patella, the small bone in the front of the knee. The patella is a little (sesamoid) bone, embedded in the tendon of insertion of the quadriceps muscle. If the patella is shattered beyond repair, it can be removed in an operation called a patellectomy and sometimes replaced with prosthetic material.

knock-knees An abnormal curve of the legs that causes the knees to touch or nearly touch while the feet are apart. The problem may arise in the bone structure, or it may develop gradually as a result of muscle abnormalities. Knock-knees can cause movement difficulties, muscle and bone strain, and pain due to overstress on the ankles. The condition can be treated via physical therapy, and in some cases it can be corrected with surgery. Also known as genu valgum.

knuckle The top of the flexed finger joint.

Koch postulates A set of criteria for judging whether a given bacterium is the cause of a given disease.

Kok disease See *hyperexplexia.*

Koplik spots Little spots inside the mouth that are highly characteristic of the early phase of measles (rubeola). The spots look like tiny grains of white sand, each surrounded by a red ring. They are often found on the inside of the cheek, opposite the first and second upper molars. See also *measles.*

Kostmann disease See *severe congenital neutropenia.*

Krabbe disease A progressive degenerative disorder of the nervous system that involves the destruction of myelin, a fatty material that surrounds and insulates nerves. Most patients have the infantile form of Krabbe disease. During the first few months of life, they seem normal, but before 6 months of age, the signs of extreme irritability, spasticity, and developmental delay become evident. Neurological deterioration leads to death (on average at 13 months of age). Other patients with Krabbe disease have a later onset of symptoms, with slower progression of the disease. The onset may be any time after 6 months and into the fifth decade of life. These patients seem not to have Krabbe disease until the symptoms of weakness and loss of vision and intellectual capacities become apparent. Krabbe disease is inherited in an autosomal recessive manner and is due to a mutation in the gene for galactosylceramidase (GALC), leading to the accumulation of galactocerebroside in tissues. Diagnosis is made by finding 5 percent or less of normal GALC activity. Prenatal diagnosis is feasible. Also known as galactocerebrosidase deficiency, GALC deficiency, and globoid cell leukodystrophy.

Krukenberg tumor A tumor of the ovary that is caused by the spread of metastatic stomach cancer.

KUB Abbreviation for kidney, ureter, and bladder.

KUB film An abdominal X-ray that shows the kidney, ureter, and bladder.

kuru A slowly progressive fatal disease of the brain that is due to an infectious agent transmitted among people in

Papua New Guinea by ritual cannibalism. Kuru is an infectious form of subacute spongiform encephalopathy and is believed to be caused by a tiny virus-like particle called a prion. It appears to be similar to bovine spongiform encephalopathy ("mad cow disease") and Creuztfeldt-Jakob disease. Also called trembling disease.

Kussmaul breathing   Air hunger, gasping. Kussmaul breathing is seen with the acidosis of diabetes mellitus that is seriously out of control. Treatment is directed toward controlling the underlying disease.

kwashiorkor   A childhood disease that is caused by protein deprivation. Early signs include apathy, drowsiness, and irritability. More advanced signs are poor growth, lack of stamina, loss of muscle mass, swelling, abnormal hair (sparse, thin, often streaky red or gray hair in dark-skinned children), and abnormal skin that darkens in irritated but not sun-exposed areas. Kwashiorkor disables the immune system, making the child susceptible to a host of infectious diseases. It is responsible for much illness and death among children worldwide. Also known as protein malnutrition and protein-calorie malnutrition (PCM).

kyphoplasty   A somewhat incorrect name for the vertebroplasty procedure. Kyphoplasty literally means "to repair the bending of the spine to curve outward from the body." Kyphosis can result when a vertebra (or several vertebrae) suffers a compression fracture from osteoporosis. Vertebroplasty is the procedure that can re-establish the height of a compressed vertebra. Sometimes, but not always, vertebroplasty can correct some of the kyphosis. See also *vertebroplasty*.

kyphoscoliosis   A combination of outward curvature (kyphosis) and lateral curvature (scoliosis) of the spine. Kyphoscoliosis can be due to musculoskeletal disease or to unknown causes. Treatment includes physical therapy and wearing a back brace, and in some cases surgery. Surgery for kyphoscoliosis may involve inserting a metal rod in the spine and restructuring some bones, and it is usually followed by wearing a back cast and then a back brace for some time.

kyphoscoliosis, idiopathic   Kyphoscoliosis that occurs during development, without a known cause.

kyphosis   Outward curvature of the spine, causing a humped back. Treatment includes physical therapy and wearing a back brace, and in some cases surgery. Surgery for kyphosis may involve inserting a metal rod in the spine and restructuring some bones, and it is usually followed by wearing a back cast and then a back brace for some time.

kyphosis, fixed   Kyphosis caused by collapse of the vertebrae, usually due to musculoskeletal disease. See also *kyphosis*.

kyphosis, juvenile   See *Scheuermann disease*.

kyphosis, mobile   Kyphosis caused by compensating for muscle weakness or structural abnormality in another area of the body. See also *kyphosis*.

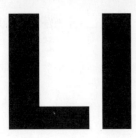

L1 through L5 The five lumbar vertebrae, which are situated between the thoracic vertebrae and the sacral vertebrae in the spinal column.

La Leche League An organization that helps and supports breastfeeding mothers with advice, ideas, and both legal and medical advocacy. Abbreviated LLL.

lab result The result of a test done in a laboratory.

lab test A test that is done in the laboratory where the appropriate equipment, supplies, and certified expertise are available.

labia Lips, the fleshy folds that surround the opening of the mouth (oral labia) or the vagina (the labia majora and labia minora).

labia majora The larger (major) outside pair of labia (lips) of the vulva (the female external genitalia). See also *labia, vaginal.*

labia minora The smaller (minor) inside pair of labia (lips) of the vulva (the female external genitalia). See also *labia, vaginal.*

labia, oral The lips around the mouth. See also *lip.*

labia, vaginal The two pairs of labia (lips)—the labia majora and labia minor—at the entrance to the vagina. Together the vaginal labia form part of the vulva, the female external genitalia.

labial Pertaining to a lip.

labial sound A sound requiring the participation of one or both lips. Also known simply as labial. All labials are consonants. Bilabial sounds, such as "p," involve both lips, whereas labiodental sounds, such as "v," involve the upper teeth and lower lip.

labile Unstable. For example, labile blood pressure is blood pressure that abnormally increases and decreases frequently.

labile diabetes See *diabetes, labile.*

labium The singular form of labia.

labor Childbirth, the process of delivering a baby and placenta from the uterus to the vagina to the outside world. There are two stages of labor. During the first stage of labor (which is called dilation), the cervix dilates fully to a diameter of about 10 cm (2 inches). The first stage of labor is divided into two phases: the latent phase and the active phase. In the latent phase, contractions become progressively more coordinated and the cervix dilates to 4 cm (approximately 1.5 inches). The latent phase averages about 8 hours for a nullipara (a woman having her first baby) and 5 hours for a multipara (a woman having a subsequent baby). The latent phase is considered distinctly abnormal if it lasts more than 20 hours in a nullipara or more than 12 hours in a multipara. In the active phase, the cervix becomes fully dilated and the presenting part of the baby descends into the midpelvis. The active phase averages about 5 hours for a nullipara and 2 hours for a multipara. In the second stage (which is called expulsion), the baby moves out through the cervix and vagina to be born. Expulsion generally lasts 2 hours for a nullipara and 1 hour for a multipara. It may last an additional hour if the woman receives an epidural. In a vaginal delivery, the woman must supplement her uterine contractions by bearing down. Also known as parturition and childbirth.

laboratory A place for doing tests and research procedures, and for preparing chemicals and some medications. Also known as lab.

labyrinth The maze of canals in the inner ear. The labyrinth is the portion of the ear that is responsible for sensing balance.

labyrinthitis Inflammation of the labyrinth of the ear, which can be accompanied by vertigo. Labyrinthitis has many potential causes including virus infection, Ménière's disease, and autoimmune disease.

laceration See *cut.*

lacrimal Pertaining to tears. For example, the lacrimal gland is a gland that secretes tears.

lacrimal gland A small almond-shaped structure that produces tears and is located just above the upper, outer corner of the eye.

lacrimation Shedding tears, or shedding more tears than is normal (for example, as a result of eye injury or irritation).

lactase The enzyme that breaks down the milk sugar lactose. Lactase is essential to digest lactose. Without enough lactase, a person is lactose intolerant.

lactase deficiency See *deficiency, lactase.*

lactation   The process of milk production. Human milk is secreted by the mammary glands, which are located within the fatty tissue of the breast. The hormone oxytocin is produced in response to the birth of a new baby, and it both stimulates uterine contractions and begins the lactation process. For the first few hours of nursing, a special fluid called colostrum is delivered; colostrum is especially high in nutrients, fats, and antibodies, to protect the newborn from infection. Thereafter, the amount of milk produced is controlled primarily by the hormone prolactin, which is produced in response to the length of time the infant nurses at the breast. See also *breastfeeding.*

lactic acid   A simple sugar that is the byproduct of glucose metabolism. When lactic acid accumulates rapidly in the muscle cells during or just after exercise, cramping can result.

Lactobacillus   A bacterium normally found in the mouth, intestinal tract, and vagina. Lactobacillus can also live in fermenting products, such as yogurt. Humans appear to have a symbiotic relationship with this bacteria: Lactobacillus has been with us so long that some types have become an important part of food digestion, although Lactobacillus can also contribute to cavities in the teeth if allowed to remain too long within the mouth.

Lactobacillus acidophilus   See *acidophilus.*

lactose intolerance   The inability to digest lactose, a component of milk and some other dairy products. The basis for lactose intolerance is the lack of an enzyme called lactase in the small intestine. The most common symptoms of lactose intolerance are diarrhea, bloating, and gas. The diagnosis may be made via a trial of a lactose-free diet or by special testing. Treatment involves avoidance of products that contain lactose or use of lactase enzyme supplements before eating. See also *deficiency, lactase.*

lacuna   An abnormal small pit, cavity, defect, or gap. For example, a lacunar infarct in the brain is an area where a stroke has left a tiny pit in the brain.

lamella   A thin leaf, plate, disk, or wafer, such as in bone tissue.

lamina   Plates or layers. For example, the lamina arcus vertebrae are plates of bone within each vertebral body.

laminaria   A thin piece of sterile seaweed that can be used to dilate the cervix.

lancet   A small, pointed knife that is used to prick a finger for a blood test.

Lancet, The   A well-known medical journal published in England. Founded in 1823, *The Lancet* is the longest-running medical journal in the world.

Landau-Kleffner syndrome   A seizure disorder with onset in childhood, in which the patient loses skills, such as speech, and develops behaviors characteristic of autism. See also *autism; epilepsy; seizure; seizure disorder.*

Landing disease   See *GM1-gangliosidosis.*

Landry ascending paralysis   A particularly virulent form of Guillain-Barre syndrome. Landry ascending paralysis often begins with a flu-like illness that brings on general physical weakness but is then characterized by rapidly progressing paralysis that starts in the legs and arms and may move on (ascend) to affect the breathing muscles and face. As with less severe forms of Guillain-Barre, the exact cause is not yet known but is presumed to be viral and/or autoimmune. Hospitalization is usually required, and treatment involves plasmapheresis and administration of intravenous immunoglobulin (IVIG). See also *demyelination; Guillain-Barre syndrome.*

Langerhans cell histiocytosis   The preferred name for what was once called histiocytosis X. This disease includes eosinophilic granuloma, Letterer Siwe disease, and Hand-Schuller-Christian disease.

Langerhans, islet of   See *islet of Langerhans.*

lanugo   Downy hair on the body of a fetus or newborn baby. Lanugo is the first hair to be produced by the fetal hair follicles, and it usually appears on the fetus at about 5 months of gestation. Lanugo is very fine, soft, and usually unpigmented. Although lanugo is normally shed before birth, around 7 or 8 months of gestation, it is sometimes present at birth. This is not a cause for concern: Lanugo disappears of its own accord within a few days or weeks.

laparoscopy   A type of surgery in which small incisions are made in the abdominal wall through which a laparoscope and other instruments can be placed to permit structures within the abdomen and pelvis to be seen. A variety of probes or other instruments can also be pushed through these small incisions in the skin. In this way, a number of surgical procedures can be performed without the need for a large surgical incision.

laparotomy   An operation to open the abdomen. For example, laparotomy is used to remove cancer of the intestines or repair bowel blockage.

large cell carcinoma   A group of lung cancers in which the cells are large and look abnormal.

large cell lymphoma See *lymphoma, large cell.*

large intestine See *intestine, large.*

laryngeal Having to do with the larynx (voice box).

laryngeal nerve palsy See *laryngeal palsy.*

laryngeal nerve, recurrent One of the branches of the vagus nerve, a long and important nerve that originates in the brain stem. After the recurrent laryngeal nerve leaves the vagus nerve, it goes down into the chest and then loops back up, to supply nerves to the larynx (the voice box). It is said to be recurrent because it returns in its course to the larynx. See also *laryngeal palsy.*

laryngeal palsy Paralysis of the larynx (voice box) that is caused by damage to the recurrent laryngeal nerve, which supplies the larynx (voice box), or its parent nerve, the vagus nerve, which originates in the brain stem and runs down to the colon. In laryngeal palsy, the larynx is paralyzed on the side where the recurrent laryngeal nerve has been damaged, unless the problem originated with damage to the vagus nerve itself. Damage to the recurrent laryngeal nerve can be the result of diseases inside the chest, such as a tumor, an aneurysm of the arch of the aorta, or an aneurysm of the left atrium of the heart.

laryngeal papilloma A warty growth in the larynx, usually on the vocal cords. Persistent hoarseness is a common symptom.

laryngeal papillomatosis The presence of numerous warty growths on the vocal cords. Laryngeal papillomatosis is most common in young children. Recurrences of laryngeal papillomatosis are, unfortunately, frequent. Remission may occur after several years.

laryngeal papillomatosis, juvenile Papillomatosis that occurs in infancy or childhood. Juvenile laryngeal papillomatosis can be caused by human papilloma virus (HPV), which is contracted at birth via the vaginal canal of a mother with genital warts.

laryngectomee A person who has had his or her larynx (voice box) removed. See also *laryngectomy.*

laryngectomy Surgery to remove part or all of the larynx. The surgeon performs a tracheostomy, creating an opening in the front of the neck (stoma). Air enters and leaves the trachea and lungs through the stoma. A tracheostomy tube keeps the new airway open.

laryngectomy, partial A laryngectomy that preserves the voice. The surgeon removes only part of the larynx (voice box)—just one vocal cord, just part of a vocal cord, or just the epiglottis—and the opening in the front

of the neck (stoma) is temporary. After a brief recovery period, the tracheostomy tube is removed, and the stoma closes up. The patient can then breathe and talk in the usual way. In some cases, however, the voice may be hoarse or weak.

laryngectomy, total A laryngectomy in which the whole larynx (voice box) is removed, and the opening in the front of the neck (stoma) is permanent. The patient breathes through the stoma and must learn to talk in a new way.

laryngitis, reflux Inflammation of the larynx (voice box) caused by stomach acid backing up into the esophagus. Reflux laryngitis is associated with chronic hoarseness and symptoms of esophageal irritation such as heartburn, chest pain, asthma, or the feeling of a foreign body in the throat (the globus phenomenon). This can lead to chronic throat clearing, difficulty swallowing, cough, spasms of the vocal cords, and growths on the vocal cords (granulomas). Reflux also increases the risk of cancer of the esophagus and larynx. See also *reflux.*

laryngomalacia An abnormally soft, floppy larynx (voice box).

laryngoscope A flexible, lighted tube that is used to examine the inside of the larynx (voice box).

laryngoscopy Examination of the larynx (voice box), either with a mirror (indirect laryngoscopy) or with a laryngoscope (direct laryngoscopy).

larynx A tube-shaped organ in the neck that contains the vocal cords. The larynx is about 5 cm (2 in.) long. It is part of the respiratory system and is located between the pharynx and the trachea. Humans use the larynx to breathe, talk, and swallow. Its outer wall of cartilage forms the area of the front of the neck referred to as the Adam's apple. The vocal cords, two bands of muscle, form a V inside the larynx. Each time a person inhales, air goes into the nose or mouth, then through the larynx, down the trachea, and into the lungs. When a person exhales, the air goes the other way. The vocal cords are relaxed during breathing, and air moves through the space between them without making any sound. The vocal cords tighten up and move closer together for speech. Air from the lungs is forced between them and makes them vibrate, producing the sound of a voice. The openings of the esophagus and the larynx are very close together in the throat. When a person swallows, a flap called the epiglottis moves down over the larynx to keep food out of the windpipe. Also known as voice box.

laser A powerful beam of light that is used in some types of surgery to cut or destroy tissue.

laser surgery, Yag   The use of a laser to punch a hole in the iris, in order to relieve increased pressure within the eye. Yag laser surgery is an outpatient procedure that may be used, for example, to treat acute angle-closure glaucoma.

laser-assisted in situ keratomileusis   See *LASIK.*

LASIK   Laser-assisted in situ keratomileusis, a kind of laser eye surgery that is designed to change the shape of the cornea to eliminate or reduce the need for glasses and contact lenses in cases of severe nearsightedness (myopia). LASIK is also coming into use to treat farsightedness (hyperopia) and astigmatism. LASIK is an outpatient procedure that is done with numbing eye drops. It takes about 1 minute to do and only a few days to heal. No eye patch need be worn after LASIK. Hormonal changes in pregnancy affect the shape and density of the cornea and can complicate the healing process and the success of LASIK. Therefore, women who plan to become pregnant within 6 months of LASIK should not have the procedure done. LASIK is similar to photorefractive keratectomy, the major difference being the way that the middle layer of the cornea is exposed before it is vaporized with the laser. In PRK, the top layer of the cornea, called the epithelium, is scraped away to expose the middle layer underneath. In LASIK, a flap is cut in the middle layer and the flap is folded back.

Lasix   See *furosemide.*

Lassa fever   See *fever, Lassa.*

lateral   **1** The side of the body or body part that is farthest from the middle or center (median) of the body. Typically, lateral refers to the outer side of the body part, but it is also used to refer to the side of a body part. For example, in references to the knee, lateral means the side of the knee farthest from the opposite knee. The opposite of lateral is medial. See also Appendix B, "Anatomic Orientation Terms."   **2** In radiology, a slang term for a lateral X-ray film.

lateral collateral ligament of the knee   The ligament that straps the outside of the knee joint. It helps provide stability and strength to the knee. See also *knee.*

lateral meniscus of the knee   A thickened crescent-shaped cartilage pad in the outer portion of the joint formed by the femur (thigh bone) and the tibia (shin bone). The lateral meniscus acts as a smooth surface for the joint to move on. The lateral meniscus is toward the outer side of the knee joint. It serves to evenly load the surface during weight-bearing, and also aids in disbursing joint fluid for joint lubrication. See also *knee.*

lateral ventricle   A communicating cavity, part of a system of four communicating cavities within the brain that are continuous with the central canal of the spinal cord. The two lateral ventricles are located in the cerebral hemispheres, one in each hemisphere. Each consists of a triangular central body and four horns. The third and fourth ventricles are located in the center of the brain. The lateral ventricles communicate with the third ventricle through an opening called the interventricular foramen. Both lateral ventricles are filled with cerebrospinal fluid.

lateral X-ray   An X-ray taken from the side of the patient.

laughing gas   See *nitrous oxide.*

lavage   Washing out. Gastric lavage, for example, is the washing out of the stomach to remove drugs or poisons.

law, Hardy-Weinberg   See *Hardy-Weinberg law.*

laxative   Something that loosens the bowels. Laxatives are used to combat constipation. They are sometimes overused, producing diarrhea. Laxatives include milk of magnesia and many others.

lb.   Abbreviation for pound (for the Latin libra), a measure of weight.

LCHAD deficiency   See *deficiency, LCHAD.*

LDL   Low-density lipoprotein.

LDL cholesterol   "Bad" low-density lipoprotein cholesterol. Elevated LDL levels are associated with an increased risk of heart disease. Lipoproteins, which are combinations of fats (lipids) and proteins, are the form in which lipids are transported in the blood. Low-density lipoproteins transport cholesterol from the liver to the tissues of the body.

L-dopa   See *levodopa.*

lead poisoning   An acute or chronic poisoning caused by the absorption of lead or any of its salts into the body. Lead poisoning is an environmental hazard that is capable of causing mental retardation, behavioral disturbance, and brain damage. Lead poisoning is formally defined in the US as at least 10 micrograms of lead per deciliter of blood. (The average level of lead, for people ages 1 to 70, is 2.3 micrograms.) Lead poisoning is more common in children than in adults because young children often put their hands and other objects in their mouths, and these objects can have lead dust on them. Furthermore, lead poisoning is more dangerous in children than in adults because children absorb more lead and the developing brain and nervous system are more sensitive to the damaging effects of lead. Lead was used in household paint until 1978, and it was also found in leaded gasoline, some types of batteries, water pipes, and pottery glazes. Lead paint and pipes are still found in many older homes, and lead is sometimes also found in water, food, household dust, and soil. Lead can be a workplace hazard for people in some occupations. A diet that is high in iron and calcium can help protect people against absorbing lead. Treatment involves chelation therapy, whereby blood is removed and metals are filtered out through a machine, then reinfused into the patient. Treatment cannot repair damage to the brain done by lead poisoning, but it may prevent further damage. Also known as plumbism.

left heart   See *heart, left.*

left heart hypoplasia syndrome   See *hypoplastic left heart syndrome.*

left ventricle   See *ventricle, left.*

leg   In popular usage, the part of the body from the top of the thigh down to the foot, and in medical terminology, the portion of the lower extremity that runs from the knee to the ankle. The leg (in the medical sense) has two bones—the tibia (shinbone) and the fibula—both of which are known as long bones. The larger of the two is the tibia. The fibula runs alongside the tibia.

leg, ankle, and foot bones   See *bones of the leg, ankle, and foot.*

leg, restless   See *restless leg syndrome.*

leg, upper   More properly called the thigh, the upper leg is the area between the knee and the hip. It has only one bone, the femur, which spans the distance from the hip to the knee.

Legg-Calvé-Perthes disease   A hip disorder in children that is due to interruption of the blood supply to the head of the femur (the ball in the ball-and-socket hip joint), causing it to deteriorate. This disease is most common between ages 6 and 9, and it tends to affect boys but is more severe in girls. Legg-Calvé-Perthes disease sometimes runs in families. The symptoms include hip and thigh pain, stiff hip, a limp, and diminution in size of the thigh. Over a period of 18 to 24 months, the blood supply usually reestablishes itself. During this period, the bone is soft and liable to fracture under pressure, causing collapse of the head of the femur. Treatment may include casting, bracing, surgery, and physical therapy. Also known as Legg disease, Legg-Perthes disease, Perthes disease, and avascular necrosis of the femoral head.

Legg-Perthes disease   See *Legg-Calvé-Perthes disease.*

Legionella   The bacterium that causes Legionnaires' disease.

Legionnaires' disease   A disease that is caused by bacteria found in plumbing, shower heads, and water-storage tanks. The disease was first identified at the 1976 American Legion convention, and subsequent outbreaks have occurred. The bacterium that causes it, now known as Legionella, thrives in the mist of condensers, air conditioners, and evaporative cooling towers, and it can infest an entire building or airplane. Travelers are especially vulnerable in the closed space in a plane. The symptoms of Legionnaires' disease are much like those of pneumonia, but they can be overwhelming and sometimes fatal. Also known as Legionella pneumonia.

leiomyoma   See *fibroid.*

leiomyosarcoma   A malignant tumor that originates in smooth muscle, the major structural component of most hollow internal organs and the walls of blood vessels. Leiomyosarcoma can occur almost anywhere in the body but is most frequently found in the uterus and gastrointestinal tract. Complete surgical excision, if possible, is the treatment of choice.

Leishmania   A group of parasites that cause several human diseases. See also *leishmaniasis.*

leishmaniasis   A parasitic disease that is spread by the bite of sand flies infected with the protozoa Leishmania. There are several forms of leishmaniasis, the most common being cutaneous and visceral leishmaniasis (known as kala-azar). The cutaneous form of the disease causes skin sores and is usually named for a geographic place (for example, Jericho boil, Baghdad button, Delhi sore). Kala-azar affects the internal organs of the body and can be fatal. See also *kala-azar.*

Lemierre's disease   A potentially lethal type of sore throat caused by the bacterium Fusobacterium necrophorum, a common inhabitant of the mouth. This disease vanished with the advent of antibiotics and then returned around the year 2000. The disease usually develops after a strep throat has created an abscess near the tonsils. Deep in the abscess, microbes that do not require oxygen (anaerobic bacteria), like Fusobacterium necrophorum, can flourish. The bacteria penetrate from the abscess into the neighboring jugular vein in the neck to cause an infected clot to form and are seeded by the bloodstream throughout the body. The keys to survival are prompt recognition of the disease, immediate use of antibiotics (to which the bacterium is responsive), and drainage of abscesses.

Lennox syndrome   See *Lennox-Gastaut syndrome.*

Lennox-Gastaut syndrome A severe form of epilepsy that usually begins in early childhood. It is characterized by frequent seizures of multiple types, mental impairment, and a slow spike-and-wave pattern seen on an EEG. The seizures are notoriously hard to treat and may lead to falls and injuries. These seizures can be reduced in frequency by treatment with lamotrigoneor with other medication. In some cases surgery may be considered.

lens The transparent structure inside the eye that focuses light rays onto the retina.

lens, intraocular See *intraocular lens.*

lens, objective In a microscope, the lens nearest to the object being examined. Most light microscopes now have a turret that bears a selection of objective lenses.

lens, ocular In a microscope, the lens closest to the eye. Also known as eyepiece. Most light microscopes are binocular, with one ocular lens for each eye.

lentigo maligna melanoma See *melanoma, lentigo maligna.*

leprosy An infectious disease of the skin, nervous system, and mucous membranes that is caused by the bacteria Mycobacterium leprae. Leprosy is transmitted via person-to-person contact. For thousands of years leprosy was one of the world's most feared communicable diseases because the nerve and skin damage often led to terrible disfigurement and disability. Today leprosy can be cured, particularly if treatment is begun early. The treatment of choice is multidrug therapy (MDT) using diaphenylsulfone (brand name: Dapsone), rifampicin (brand name: Rifadin), and clofazimine (brand name: Lamprene). Surgery can be performed to reconstruct damaged faces and limbs. Also known as Hansen's disease.

leptin A hormone that is involved in the regulation of body fat. Leptin was originally thought to signal the body to lose weight, but it may instead be a signal to the brain that there is fat on the body. A few grossly obese children have been determined to have an inability to lose weight due to a genetic inability to produce leptin. Injections of leptin have had dramatic weight loss effects. It appears that if one cannot make leptin, the brain thinks there is no fat and spurs the person on to eat more and more, in a futile effort to get the leptin signal that fat is present.

lesbian A female homosexual.

lesbianism Female homosexuality. Also known as Sapphism.

lesion An area of abnormal tissue change. Lesions vary in severity from harmless to serious.

let-down reflex An involuntary reflex during breast-feeding that causes the milk to flow freely.

lethal Deadly.

lethal gene, zygotic See *gene, zygotic lethal.*

lethargy Abnormal drowsiness, stupor.

Letterer-Siwe disease A severe disease in which histiocytes start to multiply and attack the tissues or organs of the patient, starting in infancy with a scaly, sometimes itchy rash on the scalp, ears, abdomen, and creases of the neck and face. Raw skin may provide a portal of entry for germs, leading to sepsis (bloodstream infection). Patients with Letterer-Siwe disease often have draining ears, swollen glands, enlargement of the liver and spleen, liver disease, anemia, and neutropenia (low white blood cell count). Loss of appetite, irritability, failure to thrive, and respiratory symptoms may occur. Because of their appearance, children with Letterer-Siwe disease may be misdiagnosed as being abused. Letterer-Siwe disease is the most severe form of Langerhans cell histiocytosis.

leucemia See *leukemia.*

leukemia Cancer of the blood cells. Strictly speaking, leukemia should refer only to cancer of the white blood cells (leukocytes), but in practice it can apply to malignancy of any cellular element in the blood or bone marrow, as in red cell leukemia (erythroleukemia). Treatment may involve chemotherapy, radiation therapy, biological therapy, and/or bone marrow transplantation. Also spelled leucemia. See also *accelerated phase of leukemia; leukemia, blastic phase of; leukemia, chronic phase of; leukemia, hairy cell; leukemia, lymphocytic; leukemia, myeloid; leukemia, refractory; myelodysplastic syndrome.*

leukemia, accelerated phase of See *accelerated phase of leukemia.*

leukemia, acute lymphoblastic A form of leukemia that has a sudden onset and is characterized by the presence in the blood and bone marrow of large numbers of unusually immature white blood cells that are destined to become lymphocytes (lymphoblasts). Lymphoblasts are rarely seen in the blood under normal circumstances. Abbreviated ALL. Treatment for ALL may include chemotherapy, radiation, biological therapy, and bone marrow transplantation. There is a high cure rate for ALL today, especially among children. Also known as acute lymphocytic leukemia.

leukemia, acute myeloid A quickly progressive malignancy in which there are too many immature blood-forming cells, destined to give rise to the granulocytes or monocytes in the blood and bone marrow. Abbreviated AML. AML can occur in children and adults. The early signs of AML may be similar to those of the flu or other common diseases, including fever, weakness and fatigue, loss of weight and appetite, and aches and pains in the bones or joints. Other signs may include tiny red spots in the skin, easy bruising and bleeding, frequent minor infections, and poor healing of minor cuts. In AML, the red blood cell levels may be low, causing anemia; platelet levels may be low, causing bleeding and bruising; and the white blood cell levels may be low, leading to infections. The primary treatment for AML is chemotherapy. Radiation therapy is less common, and bone marrow transplantation is coming into increasing use. The treatment of the subtype of AML called acute promyelocytic leukemia (APL) differs from that for other forms of AML; it uses all-trans-retinoic acid (ATRA), which induces a complete response in 70 percent of cases and extends survival. APL patients are then given a course of consolidation chemotherapy. Also known as acute myelogenous leukemia and acute nonlymphocytic leukemia (ANLL).

leukemia, blastic phase of A stage in chronic myeloid leukemia in which 30 percent or more of the cells in the bone marrow or blood are the malignant blast cells. See also *leukemia, chronic myeloid.*

leukemia, chronic lymphocytic The most common form of leukemia in adults, in which lymphocytes look fairly normal but are not fully mature and do not function correctly against infection. The malignant cells are found in blood and bone marrow, collect in and enlarge the lymph nodes, and may crowd out other blood cells in the bone marrow, resulting in a shortage of red cells (producing anemia) and platelets (producing bleeding and bruising). Abbreviated CLL. CLL is most common in people 60 years of age or older, and it progresses slowly. In the first stages of CLL, there are often no symptoms. As time goes on, more and more lymphocytes are made and symptoms begin to appear. Treatment may include chemotherapy, radiation, leukapheresis (a procedure to remove the extra lymphocytes), and bone marrow transplantation.

leukemia, chronic myelogenous See *leukemia, chronic myeloid.*

leukemia, chronic myeloid A malignant disease involving the white blood cells belonging to the myeloid line that is due to a chromosome rearrangement called the Philadelphia (or Ph) chromosome translocation. Abbreviated CML. CML has several phases that succeed one another. In the first phase, the chronic phase, there are few blast cells in blood and bone marrow and there may be no symptoms. This phase may last from several months to several years. Early symptoms include fatigue and night sweats. In the next phase, the accelerated

phase, there are more blast cells in blood and bone marrow and fewer normal cells. In the final phase, the blastic phase (or blast crisis), more than 30 percent of the cells in the blood or bone marrow are blast cells. Treatment may involve chemotherapy, radiation therapy, and bone marrow transplantation. Also called chronic myelocytic leukemia and chronic granulocytic leukemia.

leukemia, chronic phase of A stage in chronic myeloid leukemia in which there are few blast cells in the blood or bone marrow and few, if any, symptoms. See also *leukemia, chronic myeloid.*

leukemia, granulocytic See *leukemia, myeloid.*

leukemia, hairy cell A type of chronic leukemia in which the abnormal white blood cells appear to be covered with tiny hairs. The hairy cells are malignant B lymphocytes. Early symptoms of hairy cell leukemia include fatigue, flu-like symptoms, and sometimes an enlarged spleen. There may be too few normal blood cells of all types because of an excess of leukemic cells in the bone marrow. The deficit of different types of normal blood cells can lead to anemia, easy bleeding, and a tendency to infection. Treatment may include chemotherapy, biological therapy, and surgery (to remove the enlarged spleen). In some cases, bone marrow transplantation is done.

leukemia, lymphocytic Cancer of blood cells that are destined to become lymphocytes. The two major types of lymphocytic leukemia are acute lymphoblastic leukemia (ALL) and chronic lymphocytic leukemia (CML). Also known as lymphoid leukemia.

leukemia, myelogenous See *leukemia, myeloid.*

leukemia, myeloid Cancer of the blood cells of the myeloid line. The two major types of myeloid leukemia are acute myeloid leukemia (AML) and chronic myeloid leukemia (CML). Also known as myelogenous leukemia and nonlymphocytic leukemia.

leukemia, nonlymphocytic See *leukemia, myeloid.*

leukemia, refractory Leukemia in which the high level of white blood cells does not decrease in response to treatment.

leukemia, smoldering See *myelodysplastic syndrome.*

leukemoid reaction A benign condition in which the high number of white blood cells found on a blood test resembles the numbers seen in leukemia. For example, infectious mononucleosis can produce a leukemoid reaction.

leuko- Prefix meaning white, as in leukocyte (white blood cell).

leukocyte   A blood cell that helps the body fight infections and other diseases. Also known as white blood cell (WBC). See also *blood cell*.

leukocyte count   A white blood cell (WBC) count. See also *leukocyte*.

leukocyte, granular   See *granulocyte*.

leukocyte, polymorphonuclear   A type of white blood cell that has a nucleus that is so deeply lobated (divided) that the cell appears to have multiple nuclei. Informally called a poly. See also *blood cell; leukocyte*.

leukocytosis   A condition in which the number of white blood cells is higher than normal.

leukodystrophy   A disorder of the white matter of the brain. The white matter mainly consists of nerve fibers rather than nerve cells themselves, and it is concerned with conduction of nerve impulses.

leukodystrophy, globoid-cell   See *Krabbe disease*.

leukopenia   A shortage of white blood cells.

leukoplakia   A white spot or patch on the mucous membranes in the mouth (for instance, inside the cheeks, on the gums, on the tongue) that may become cancerous.

levo-   Prefix meaning on the left side, as in levorotation (turning or twisting to the left). The opposition of levo- is dextro-.

levocardia   Reversal of all the abdominal and thoracic organs (situs inversus) except the heart, which is still in its usual location on the left. Levocardia virtually always accompanies congenital heart disease.

levodopa   A drug (brand name: Dopar, Larodopa) that is used to treat Parkinson's disease, Parkinsonian symptoms in other disorders, restless legs syndrome, and herpes zoster. Levodopa converts to the neurotransmitter dopamine in the brain.

levothyroxine sodium   A synthetic thyroid hormone (brand names: Eltroxin, Levothroid, Levoxine, Levoxyl, Synthroid) that is used as a thyroid hormone replacement drug to treat an underactive thyroid gland (hypothyroidism). Because not all brands of levothyroxine sodium are equivalent, it is important not to switch between brand names or generic formulations.

LH   Luteinizing hormone.

LHRH   Luteinizing hormone-releasing hormone.

LHRH agonist   A compound that is similar to luteinizing hormone-releasing hormone (LHRH) in structure and can act like LHRH.

libido   1 Sexual drive.   2 In psychoanalysis, the psychic energy from all instinctive biological drives.

library   In genetics, an unordered collection of cloned DNA from a particular organism (for example, an E. coli library, a human DNA library). The relationships between these clones can be established with physical mapping. See also *genomic library*.

library, genomic   See *genomic library*.

lice, head   See *head lice*.

licensed practical nurse   See *nurse, licensed practical*.

lichen planus   A common skin disease that features small, itchy pink or purple spots on the arms or legs. The abnormal areas on the skin in lichen planus are typically polygonal, flat (hence the term planus), and itchy. Lichen planus occurs characteristically on the wrists, shins, lower back, and genitalia. Lichen planus on the scalp may lead to hair loss. The causes of lichen planus are unknown. However, it can be triggered by the use of certain drugs, such as thiazide diuretics, phenothiazines, and antimalarials. Treatment involves use of topical corticosteroids. In most cases, the disease spontaneously regresses 6 months to 2 years after onset.

ligament   A tough band of connective tissue that connects various structures, such as two bones.

ligament, anterior cruciate   See *anterior cruciate ligament*.

ligament, lateral collateral knee   See *lateral collateral ligament of the knee*.

ligament, medial collateral knee   See *medial collateral ligament of the knee*.

ligament, posterior cruciate   See *posterior cruciate ligament*.

ligaments, knee   The four strong, elastic bands of tissue that connect bone to bone in the knee. They provide strength and stability to the joint. These four ligaments connect the femur (the bone in the thigh) with the tibia (the larger bone in the lower leg); the medial collateral ligament (MCL), which provides stability to the inner (medial) aspect of the knee; the lateral collateral ligament (LCL), which provides stability to the outer (lateral) aspect of the knee; the anterior cruciate ligament (ACL), in the center of the knee, which limits rotation and the forward movement of the tibia; the posterior cruciate ligament (PCL), in the center of the knee, which limits backward movement of the tibia. Other ligaments are part of the knee capsule, which is a protective, fiber-like structure that wraps around the knee joint.

ligate   To tie, as in to ligate (tie off) an artery.

ligature   Material used to tie something in surgery. Ligatures are used to tie off blood vessels, and they may be made of silk, gut, wire, or other materials.

lightening   See *engagement.*

lightheadedness   A feeling that one is about to faint. Lightheadedness is medically distinct from dizziness, unsteadiness, and vertigo. See also *dizziness; unsteadiness; vertigo.*

lights, flashing   A sensation that is created when the clear, jelly-like substance that fills the middle of the eye (vitreous humor) shrinks and tugs on the retina. These flashes of light can appear off and on for several weeks or months. As a person ages, flashes are likely to occur increasingly often. Flashes usually do not reflect a serious problem. However, if flashing lights suddenly appear or increase, an ophthalmologist should be consulted immediately, to see whether the retina has been torn. Flashes of light that appear as jagged lines or "heat waves" in both eyes, often lasting 10 to 20 minutes, are frequently caused by migraine, a spasm of blood vessels in the brain.

limb   An arm or a leg.

lingual   Having to do with the tongue.

linkage   The tendency for genes to be inherited together as a package because of their location near one another on the same chromosome.

lip   One of the two fleshy folds that surround the opening of the mouth. The upper lip is separated from the nose by the philtrum, the area that lies between the base of the nose and the pigmented edge (called the vermillion border or the carmine margin) of the upper lip. The upper and lower lips meet at the corners (angles) of the mouth, which are called the oral commissures. The oral commissure normally lies in a vertical line below the pupil. Small blind pits are sometimes seen at the corners of the mouth; they are known as angular lip pits, and are considered normal minor variants. The lips may be abnormally thin or thick. For example, children with fetal alcohol syndrome typically have a thin upper lip and flat philtrum. If the upper lip is overgrown, the corners of the mouth appear to be downturned.

lip, cleft   See *cleft lip.*

lipectomy, suction-assisted   See *liposuction.*

lipid   A fat. Lipids have gotten a bad name, but they are vital parts of cells and, with carbohydrates and proteins, are the main constituents of cells. Lipids are easily stored in the body and serve as fuel. Among the well-known lipids are cholesterol, triglycerides, fatty acids, and steroids (such as cortisone). Lipoproteins, glycolipids, and phospholipids are all compound lipids (lipids in combination with other types of chemicals).

lipid profile   A pattern of lipids in the blood. A lipid profile usually includes the levels of total cholesterol, high-density lipoprotein (HDL) cholesterol, triglycerides, and the calculated low-density lipoprotein (LDL) cholesterol.

lipid storage disease   One in a series of disorders that are due to inborn errors in lipid metabolism. Lipid storage diseases result in the abnormal accumulation of lipids in the wrong places. Examples include Gaucher disease, Fabry disease, Niemann-Pick disease, and metachromatic leukodystrophy.

lipodystrophy, cephalothoracic   See *cephalothoracic lipodystrophy.*

lipodystrophy syndrome   A disturbance of lipid (fat) metabolism that involves the partial or total absence of fat, and often abnormal deposition and distribution of fat in the body. There are a number of different lipodystrophy syndromes. Some of them are present at birth (congenital), and others are acquired later. Some are genetic (inherited), and others are not. One lipodystrophy syndrome is associated with the protease inhibitor drugs used to treat AIDS, but how protease inhibitors induce lipodystrophy syndrome is unknown. In lipodystrophy syndrome, the face, arms, and legs become thin due to loss of subcutaneous fat, and the skin becomes dry, the lips crack, and weight drops. See also *cephalothoracic lipodystrophy; protease inhibitor.*

lipoma   A benign fatty tumor. Lipomas are common in the skin and are found anywhere on the body. They generally are not treated unless for cosmetic reasons.

lipomatosis, familial benign cervical   See *cephalothoracic lipodystrophy.*

lipoprotein   A molecule that is a combination of lipid and protein. Lipids do not travel in the blood by themselves, but they are carried through the bloodstream as lipoproteins.

liposarcoma   A type of malignant tumor that arises from fat cells in deep soft tissue, such as inside the thigh. Most frequently seen in older adults (age 40 and above), liposarcomas are the most common of all soft-tissue sarcomas. See also *sarcoma.*

liposuction   The surgical suctioning of fat deposits from specific parts of the body, the most common being the abdomen, buttocks, hips, thighs and knees, chin, upper arms, back, and calves. A hollow instrument called a cannula is inserted under the skin to break up the fat. A high-pressure vacuum is then applied to the cannula to suck out the fat. Liposuction is one of the most common cosmetic operations in the US. See also *liposuction, tumescent; liposuction, ultrasonic-assisted.*

liposuction, tumescent A form of liposuction in which several quarts of a solution are pumped below the skin in the area from which fat is to be suctioned. The saline (salt water) solution used includes the local anesthetic lidocaine to numb the area and the vessel-constrictor epinephrine (adrenaline) to help minimize bleeding. The fat is suctioned out through small suction tubes called microcannulas. Although tumescent liposuction is one of the most-used forms of liposuction, it can be fatal. It has been suggested that death occurs because of the toxicity of lidocaine or because of drug interactions related to lidocaine. See also *liposuction.*

liposuction, ultrasonic-assisted A form of liposuction in which the cannula is energized with ultrasonic energy, causing the fat to melt away on contact. This technique has an advantage in areas of scar tissue, such as the male breast, the back, and areas where liposuction has been performed before. Its disadvantages include the need for longer incisions in the skin, a potential for skin or internal burns, greater cost, and a longer time needed to complete the procedure. See also *liposuction.*

Listeria A group of parasitic bacteria that can infect both animals and humans. See also *Listeriosis.*

Listeriosis A disease that is caused by eating food contaminated with the bacterium Listeria monocytogenes. Listeriosis is an important public health problem in North America. The disease affects primarily pregnant women, newborns, and anyone who is immunocompromised. Symptoms include fever, muscle aches, nausea, and diarrhea. If infection spreads to the nervous system, symptoms such as headache, stiff neck, confusion, loss of balance, or convulsions can occur. Infection during pregnancy may appear mild but can lead to stillbirth, premature delivery, and infection of the newborn. Persons who are at risk of contracting Listeriosis can prevent the infection by avoiding certain high-risk foods and by handling food properly. Raw food from animal sources (such as beef, pork, or poultry) should be thoroughly cooked and uncooked meats should be kept separate from vegetables, cooked foods, and ready-to-eat foods. Raw vegetables should be washed thoroughly before being eaten, and raw (unpasteurized) milk or foods made from raw milk should be avoided.

liter A metric measure of capacity that is equal to the volume of 1 kilogram of water at 4° centigrade and at standard atmospheric pressure of 760 millimeters of mercury. There are 1,000 cubic centimeters, or 1 cubic decimeter, in 1 liter. A liter is a little more than 1 quart (1.057 US liquid quarts). Abbreviated L or l.

litho- Prefix meaning stone, as in lithotomy (an operation to remove a stone), or lithotripsy (a procedure to crush a stone).

lithotomy Surgical removal of a stone.

lithotripsy A procedure to break a stone into small particles that can be passed in the urine. Lithotripsy generally works well with kidney stones that are smaller than one and a half centimeters (approximately ⅝ inch) in diameter.

lithotripsy, extracorporeal shock wave A technique for shattering a kidney stone or gallstone with a shock wave that is produced outside the body. The stone breaks up after 800 to 2,000 shocks. Anesthesia may be necessary to control the pain, depending on the size and density of the stone and on the energy of the shock wave needed to break it up. The urologist may opt to place a catheter (stent) in the ureter from below to facilitate passage of the shattered fragments. Abbreviated ESWL.

lithotripsy, percutaneous nephro- A technique for removing large and/or dense stones and staghorn stones. Abbreviated PNL. In PNL, there is no incision; rather, an access port is created by puncturing the kidney through the skin, and the port is then enlarged to about one centimeter (approximately ⅜ inch) in diameter. The procedure is done under anesthesia, using real-time live X-ray control (fluoroscopy). Because X-rays are involved, an interventional radiologist may perform this part of the procedure. An endourologist then inserts instruments into the kidney via the port, to break up the stone and remove most of the debris from the stone.

lithotriptor A machine that is used to shatter kidney stones and gallstones by physical or other means, such as with shock waves. A lithotriptor is operated by a urologist or under the supervision of a urologist.

lithium A naturally occurring salt that, in purified form, is used to treat certain psychiatric disorders, especially bipolar disease The therapeutic level of lithium—the amount needed to treat bipolar disorders—is perilously close to the level that can cause toxicity. Symptoms of lithium toxicity include diarrhea, vomiting, blurred vision, loss of coordination, and loss of motor control. Treatment of lithium toxicity involves immediately reducing or discontinuing lithium use under medical supervision.

live polio vaccine See *polio vaccine, oral.*

livedo reticularis A mottled purplish discoloration of the skin. Livedo reticularis can be a normal condition that is simply more obvious when a person is exposed to the cold. It can also be an indicator of impaired circulation. Livedo reticularis has been reported in association with autoimmune diseases, such as systemic lupus erythematosus; abnormal antibodies referred to as phospholipid antibodies; and a syndrome featuring phospholipid antibodies with multiple brain strokes.

liver   The largest solid organ in the body, situated in the upper part of the abdomen on the right side. The liver has a multitude of important and complex functions, including to manufacture proteins, including albumin (to help maintain the volume of blood) and blood clotting factors; to synthesize, store, and process fats, including fatty acids (used for energy) and cholesterol; to metabolize and store carbohydrates (used as the source for the sugar in blood); to form and secrete bile that contains bile acids to aid in the intestinal absorption of fats and the fat-soluble vitamins A, D, E, and K; to eliminate, by metabolizing or secreting, the potentially harmful biochemical products produced by the body, such as bilirubin, from the breakdown of old red blood cells and ammonia from the breakdown of proteins; and to detoxify, by metabolizing and/or secreting, drugs, alcohol, and environmental toxins.

liver of pregnancy, acute fatty   See *acute fatty liver of pregnancy.*

liver transplantation   Surgery to remove a diseased liver and replace it with a healthy liver (or part of one) from a donor. The most common reason for liver transplantation in children is biliary atresia (a disease in which the ducts that carry bile out of the liver are missing or damaged). The most common reason for liver transplantation in adults is cirrhosis (a disease in which healthy liver cells are killed and replaced with scar tissue). There is no effective treatment for end-stage liver disease other than transplantation. The life of someone with kidney failure can be extended via dialysis, and someone with a failing heart can sometimes be sustained with an implantable pump, but there are no machines that can take over the liver's functions. Until such machines can be devised or until an animal liver can replace a human one or until new livers can be grown from stem cells, there is total dependence on liver transplantation. Transplanted livers may come from cadavers or living donors.

livid   Black-and-blue, as from bruising.

living will   An advance medical directive that specifies what types of medical treatment are desired. A living will can be very specific or very general. The most common statement in a living will requests that if the patient suffers an incurable, irreversible illness, disease, or condition, and the attending physician determines that the condition is terminal, life-sustaining measures that would serve only to prolong dying be withheld or discontinued. More specific living wills may include information regarding an individual's desire for services such as pain relief, antibiotics, hydration, feeding, and the use of ventilators, blood products, or cardiopulmonary resuscitation.

LLL   **1** Left lower lobe, the bottom-left lobe of the lung. **2** La Leche League.   **3** The Lawrence Livermore National Laboratory, a federal research facility that focuses on health and biomedicine, science and math education, the environment, energy, and national security.

LLQ   Left lower quadrant (quarter). For example, the LLQ of the abdomen contains the descending portion of the colon.

lobar   Having to do with a lobe. For example, lobar pneumonia is pneumonia in a single lobe of a lung.

lobe   **1** A subdivision of an organ that is divided by fissures, connective tissue, or other natural boundaries. **2** A rounded projecting portion, such as the lobe of the ear.

lobectomy   An operation to remove an entire lobe of the lung.

lobular carcinoma of the breast, infiltrating   See *breast, infiltrating lobular carcinoma of the.*

lobule   A little lobe.

local therapy   In the context of cancer, treatment that affects cells in the tumor and the area close to it. Also known as local treatment.

local treatment   See *local therapy.*

lochia   The fluid that weeps from the vagina for a week or so after childbirth. At first the lochia is primarily blood, followed by a more mucousy fluid that contains dried blood, and finally a clear-to-yellow discharge.

loci   Plural of locus.

lockjaw   See *tetanus.*

locomotion   **1** Movement from one place to another. **2** The ability to get from one place to the next. See also *locomotive system.*

locomotive system   The bones, the joints, and the muscles that contract and relax to move the joints and bones.

locus   In genetics, the place a gene occupies on a chromosome. The plural is loci.

loin   The portion of the lower back from just below the ribs to the pelvis.

long arm of a chromosome   See *chromosome.*

long QT syndrome   A genetic condition that predisposes individuals to irregular heartbeats, fainting spells, and sudden death. The irregular heartbeats are typically brought on by stress or vigorous activity. Abbreviated LQTS. LQTS is often symptomless and undiagnosed, but it is well known as a cause of sudden cardiac death in young, apparently healthy people, most notably competitive athletes. QT refers to an interval seen in an electrocardiogram (EKG) test of heart function. There are multiple genetic forms of LQTS. Romano-Ward syndrome is an autosomal dominant form of LQTS. The Jervell and Lange-Nielsen syndrome is an autosomal recessive form of LQTS and is characterized by congenital profound bilateral sensorineural hearing loss and long QT interval.

long-chain-3-hydroxyacyl-CoA dehydrogenease deficiency   See *deficiency, LCHAD.*

longevity   Lifespan. Increased longevity means a longer life.

longitudinal   Along the length of something; running lengthwise or, by extension, over the course of time.

longitudinal section   A section that is cut along the long axis of a structure. Longitudinal section is the opposite of cross-section.

longitudinal study   A study done over the passage of time. For example, a longitudinal study of children with Down syndrome might involve the study of 100 children with this condition from birth to 10 years of age. Longitudinal study is the opposite of cross-sectional (synchronic) study. Also known as diachronic study.

lordosis   Inward curvature of the spine. The spine is not supposed to be absolutely straight, so some degree of curvature is normal. When the curve exceeds the usual range, it may be due to musculoskeletal disease or simply to poor posture. Treatment usually involves physical therapy, although in severe cases surgery, casting, and/or bracing may be required. Also known as swayback.

Lou Gehrig's disease   See *amyotrophic lateral sclerosis.*

louse-borne typhus   See *typhus, epidemic.*

low blood pressure   See *hypotension.*

low placenta   See *placenta previa.*

lower GI series   A series of diagnostic X-rays of the colon and rectum, taken after the patient is given a barium enema. See also *barium enema.*

lower segment cesarean section   See *caesarean section, lower segment.*

low-set ear   See *ear, low-set.*

LP   Lumbar puncture.

LQTS   Long QT syndrome.

LSCS   Lower segment cesarean section.

lubricant   An oily or slippery substance. A vaginal lubricant may be helpful for women who feel pain during intercourse because of vaginal dryness.

lues   See *syphilis.*

LUL   Left upper lobe, the top-left lobe of the lung.

lumbar   Referring to the five lumbar vertebrae, the disks below them, and the corresponding area of the low back. The lumbar vertebrae and their disks are situated below the thoracic vertebrae and above the sacral vertebrae in the spinal column and are surrounded by soft tissues, including ligaments and large muscles.

lumbar puncture   A procedure in which cerebrospinal fluid is removed from the spinal canal for diagnostic testing or treatment. Abbreviated LP. The patient usually lies sideways for the procedure, although LPs in infants are often done upright. After local anesthesia is injected into the small of the back (the lumbar area), a needle is inserted between two vertebrae and into the spinal canal. The needle is usually placed between the third and fourth lumbar vertebrae. Spinal fluid pressure can then be measured, and cerebrospinal fluid can be removed for testing. LP is particularly helpful in the diagnosis of inflammatory diseases of the central nervous system (CNS), especially meningitis and other infections. It can also provide clues to the diagnosis of stroke, spinal cord tumor, and cancer in the CNS. An LP can also be done for therapeutic purposes, as a way of administering antibiotics, cancer drugs, or anesthetic agents into the spinal canal. Spinal fluid is sometimes removed via LP to decrease spinal fluid pressure in patients with conditions such as normal-pressure hydrocephalus or benign intracranial hypertension. Normal values for spinal fluid examination are as follows: 15–45 mg/dl protein, 50–75 mg/dl glucose, cell count of 0–5 mononuclear cells, and an initial pressure of 70–180 mm. These normal values can be altered by injury or disease of the brain, spinal cord, or adjacent tissues. Risks related to LP include headache, brain herniation, bleeding, and infection. These complications are uncommon, with the exception of headache, which can appear up to a day after LP. Headaches are less likely to occur if the patient remains lying flat for 1 to 3 hours after the procedure. The benefits of LP depend on the exact situation, but an LP can provide lifesaving information. Also known as spinal tap, spinal puncture, thecal puncture, and rachiocentesis.

lumbar vertebrae   The five vertebrae situated between the thoracic vertebrae and the sacral vertebrae in the spinal column. The lumbar vertebrae are represented by the symbols L1 through L5.

lumpectomy   The surgical removal of a small tumor, which may be benign or cancerous. In common use, lumpectomy refers especially to removal of a lump from the breast. Lumpectomy, often with chemotherapy or radiation therapy, can be an alternative to mastectomy in cases of nonmetastatic breast cancer.

lung   One of a pair of three-lobed breathing organs located within the right and left sides of the chest. The lungs remove carbon dioxide from the blood and bring oxygen into the blood. Air comes into the lungs via the trachea, traveling evenly into the left and right lungs by means of the left and right bronchi. Each bronchus branches off into several smaller bronchioles, which end in many alveolar sacs. In the tiny alveoli within these sacs, oxygen is traded for carbon dioxide in blood delivered back to the heart by the pulmonary veins. Lung function is controlled by several muscles, including the diaphragm muscle beneath the lungs and the intercostal muscles that surround the lungs.

lung, collapsed   See *atelectasis.*

lung transplant   Surgery to replace a diseased or damaged lung with a healthy lung from an organ donor. Lung transplant is sometimes done in tandem with heart transplant. See also *transplant.*

lupus   A chronic inflammatory disease that is caused by an autoimmune condition. Patients with lupus have in their blood unusual antibodies that are targeted against their own body tissues. Lupus can cause disease of the skin, heart, lungs, kidneys, joints, and nervous system. The first symptom is a red (or dark), scaly rash on the nose and cheeks, often called a butterfly rash because of its distinctive shape. As inflammation continues, scar tissue may form, including keloid scarring in patients prone to keloid formation. The cause of lupus is unknown, although heredity, viruses, ultraviolet light, and drugs may all play a role. Lupus is more common in women than in men, and although it occurs in all ethnic groups, it is most common in people of African descent. Diagnosis is made through observation of symptoms, and through testing of the blood for signs of autoimmune activity. Early treatment is essential because if lupus spreads beyond the skin, it can be painful, disabling, and fatal. A rheumatologist can provide treatment for lupus, and this treatment has two objectives: treating the difficult symptoms of the disease and treating the underlying autoimmune activity. It may include use of steroids and other anti-inflammatory agents, antidepressants and/or mood stabilizers, intravenous immunoglobulin, and, in cases in which lupus involves the internal organs, chemotherapy. See also *lupus, discoid; lupus erythematosis, systemic.*

lupus, discoid   A chronic inflammatory condition that is limited to the skin and is caused by an autoimmune disease. Up to 10 percent of persons with discoid lupus eventually develop systemic lupus erythematosus (SLE). Discoid lupus can be caused by infection with the bacterium that causes tuberculosis, and in some cases it is a reaction to tuberculosis skin testing. Heredity, viruses, ultraviolet light, and drugs may also be involved. Skin symptoms associated with discoid lupus include a malar ("butterfly") rash over the cheeks of the face; a discoid skin rash, characterized by patchy redness that can cause scarring; and photosensitivity, or skin rash in reaction to exposure to sunlight. Diagnosis of discoid lupus may be made via medical history and antinuclear antibody (ANA) testing. Treatment is directed toward decreasing inflammation and/or the level of autoimmune activity. Treatment methods include avoidance of sun exposure and use of antimalarial medications (hydroxychloroquine and others), local cortisone injections, Dapsone, and immune-suppression medications. Also known as lupus verrucosus and lupus vulgaris. See also *lupus; lupus erythematosis, systemic.*

lupus erythematosis, systemic   A form of lupus that has a tendency to involve the internal organs. Abbreviated SLE. Eleven criteria have been established for the diagnosis of SLE, including the presence of a malar ("butterfly") rash and/or other discoid skin rash; skin rash in reaction to sunlight exposure; ulceration of the mucus lining of the mouth, nose, or throat; two or more swollen, tender joints of the extremities (arthritis); inflammation of the lining tissue around the heart or lungs (pericarditis/pleuritis), usually associated with chest pain with breathing; abnormal amounts of protein or cellular elements in the urine, caused by kidney abnormalities; brain irritation manifested by seizures, severe mood swings, and/or psychosis; low counts of white or red blood cells, or platelets; abnormal results on immune-system tests, including anti-DNA or anti-Sm (Smith) antibodies, falsely positive blood test for syphilis, anticardiolipin antibodies, lupus anticoagulant, or a positive lupus erythematosis prep test; and positive results for antinuclear antibodies (ANAs) on a blood test. SLE is also often characterized by fatigue. Psychiatric symptoms closely resemble those of a bipolar disorder, which sometimes leads to misdiagnosis. SLE is eight times more common in women than in men. The causes of SLE are unknown, but heredity, infectious disease, ultraviolet light, and drugs may all play a role. Treatment is directed toward decreasing inflammation and moderating the level of autoimmune activity, and it can range from administration of anti-inflammatory medication to use of chemotherapy. Persons with SLE can help prevent flare-ups of their disease by avoiding sun exposure and by not abruptly discontinuing medications. Medication can help treat specific symptoms as well, including reducing skin rash, irritation, and scarring; reducing joint inflammation; and treating psychiatric symptoms. See also *lupus.*

LUQ   Left upper quadrant (quarter). For example, the LUQ of the abdomen contains the spleen.

Luschka, foramina of   See *foramina of Luschka.*

luteinizing hormone   A hormone that is released by the pituitary gland in response to luteinizing hormone-releasing hormone. Abbreviated LH. In females, LH controls the length and sequence of the female menstrual cycle, including ovulation, preparation of the uterus for implantation of a fertilized egg, and ovarian production of both estrogen and progesterone. In males, LH stimulates the testes to produce androgen. Also known as interstitial-cell-stimulating hormone (ICSH).

luteinizing hormone-releasing hormone   A hormone that controls the production of luteinizing hormone in men and women. Abbreviated LHRH. See also *luteinizing hormone.*

luxation   Complete dislocation of a joint. A partial dislocation is a subluxation.

Lyme disease   An inflammatory disease that is caused by the bacterium Borrelia burgdorferi, which is transmitted to humans by the deer tick. The first sign of Lyme disease is a red, circular, expanding rash, usually radiating from the tick bite, followed by flu-like symptoms and joint pains. After the B. burgdorferi has entered the bloodstream, it can infect and inflame many different types of tissues, eventually causing many diverse symptoms. Lyme disease is medically divided into three phases: early localized disease with skin inflammation; early disseminated disease with heart and nervous system involvement, including palsies and meningitis; and late disease, featuring motor and sensory nerve damage and brain inflammation and arthritis. Within hours to weeks of the tick bite, an expanding ring of unraised redness develops, with an outer ring of brighter redness and a central area of clearing, giving it the appearance of a bull's-eye. The redness of the skin is often accompanied by generalized fatigue, muscle and joint stiffness, swollen glands, and headache. Early treatment with antibiotics is the best strategy for preventing major problems due to Lyme disease. Further prevention of Lyme disease involves avoiding areas where ticks are common, wearing protective clothing and lotion, and immediately removing any ticks from the body. A vaccine for Lyme disease is available. Other treatment may include use of pain-relieving medications,

arthrocentesis to remove fluid from swollen joints, and injection of cortisone to reduce inflammation and improve function. Interestingly, Lyme disease only became apparent in 1975, when mothers of a group of children who lived near each other in Lyme, Connecticut, made researchers aware that their children were all diagnosed with rheumatoid arthritis. This unusual grouping of illness that appeared to be rheumatoid eventually led researchers to the identification of the bacterial cause of Lyme disease in 1982. The number of cases of the disease in an area depends on the number of ticks in an area and how often the ticks are infected with B. burgdorferi.

lymph   The almost colorless fluid that travels through the lymphatic system, carrying cells that help fight infection and disease.

lymph gland   See *lymph node.*

lymph node   One of many small, bean-shaped organs located throughout the lymphatic system. The lymph nodes store special cells that can trap cancer cells or bacteria that are traveling through the body through the lymph. Also known as lymph gland.

lymph node, sentinel   The first lymph node to receive lymphatic drainage from a tumor. The sentinel node for a given tumor is found by injecting a tracer substance around the tumor. This substance then travels through the lymphatic system to the sentinel node. The tracer substance may be a blue dye that can be tracked visually or a radioactive colloid that can be followed radiologically. Biopsy of the sentinel lymph node can reveal whether cancer has spread through the lymphatic system. If the sentinel node contains tumor cells, removal of more nodes in the area may be warranted. Sentinel lymph node biopsy has become a standard technique for determining the nodal stage of disease in some patients with malignant melanoma.

lymphadenitis, EBV-positive   Disease of the lymph nodes that is caused by infection with the Epstein-Barr virus (EBV) and that resembles mononucleosis. EBV-positive lymphadenitis appears in about 1 percent of all transplant patients. Treatment involves reducing the dose of immunosuppressive drugs, if any, and using antiviral medication, biological therapy, or interferon. In transplant patients, lymphadenitis may be mistaken for rejection of the new organ. See also *Epstein-Barr virus; lymphoproliferative disorders; mononucleosis.*

lymphadenitis, regional   See *cat scratch fever.*

lymphadenopathy   Abnormally enlarged lymph nodes. Commonly called swollen glands.

lymphadenopathy virus See *HIV.*

lymphadenopathy-associated virus See *HIV.*

lymphangiogram An X-ray of the lymphatic system for which a dye is injected to outline the lymphatic vessels and organs.

lymphangioma A structure that consists of a collection of blood vessels and lymph vessels that are overgrown and clumped together. Depending on its nature, a lymphangioma may grow slowly or quickly. Lymphangiomas can cause problems because of their location. For example, a lymphangioma around the larynx might cause a breathing problem.

lymphatic Pertaining to a small, thin channel that is similar to a blood vessel and that collects and carries tissue fluid (lymph) from the body. This fluid ultimately drains back into the bloodstream.

lymphatic system The tissues and organs, including the bone marrow, spleen, thymus, and lymph nodes, that produce and store cells that fight infection and disease. The channels that carry lymph are also part of this system.

lymphedema A condition in which excess fluid collects in tissue and causes swelling. Lymphedema may occur in the arm or leg after lymph vessels or lymph nodes in the underarm or groin are removed. It usually causes painless swelling. It can be treated by elevating the lower extremity, avoiding salt, and using diuretic medication.

lymphocyte A small white blood cell that plays a large role in defending the body against disease. Lymphocytes are integrally involved in many immune responses. There are two main types of lymphocytes: B cells and T cells. Lymphocytes are often present at sites of chronic inflammation.

lymphocytic Referring to lymphocytes, a type of white blood cell. For example, lymphocytic inflammation in the skin is skin that is infiltrated with lymphocytes.

lymphocytopenia Having an abnormally low number of lymphocytes. There are many causes of lymphocytopenia, ranging from medication toxicity to a variety of diseases.

lymphocytosis Having too many lymphocytes. Lymphocytosis may be a marker that infection or disease is present.

lymphoid Referring to lymphocytes, a type of white blood cell, or to tissue in which lymphocytes develop. Lymphoid tissue is full of lymphocytes, such as a lymph node.

lymphoid tissue The part of the body's immune system that helps protect it from bacteria.

lymphoma A tumor of the lymphoid tissue. The major types of lymphoma are Hodgkin's disease and non-Hodgkin's lymphoma (NHL). NHL can in turn be divided into low-grade, intermediate-grade, high-grade, and miscellaneous lymphomas. The course of NHL varies greatly, from indolent to rapidly fatal. Treatment options include chemo and radiation therapy.

lymphoma, AIDS-related A condition that occurs in people with AIDS, in which lymphoid tumors are present, presumably due to immune-system impairment. Treatment is like that of other lymphomas but must take into account the fact that the natural immunity is impaired.

lymphoma, Hodgkin's See *Hodgkin's disease.*

lymphoma, large cell Cancer of the lymphatic tissue that is characterized by unusually large cells.

lymphoma, lymphoblastic A rapidly moving, aggressive form of lymphoma that is most often seen in children or young adults. Treatment may include chemotherapy, radiation, surgery, medication, and bone marrow transplant. Precautionary treatment of the central nervous system (CNS) is usually included because of lymphoblastic lymphoma's ability to spread rapidly to the CNS.

lymphoma, non-Hodgkin's A form of lymphoma in which malignant tumors arise in the lymphatic system. Abbreviated NHL. Several subtypes of cancer are classified as NHL, all of which originate in and spread via the lymphatic system. Symptoms of NHL depend on the location of the tumor, but can include swollen, but not painful, lymph nodes; gastric distress; skin problems; night sweats; unexplained weight loss; itching; and fever. Diagnosis is made via biopsy of a swollen lymph node, although an X-ray, a sonogram, a CAT scan, or an MRI may also be helpful. Treatment may include chemotherapy, radiation, bone marrow transplantation, stem-cell rescue, use of medication, and recently, use of monoclonal antibodies, depending on the age of the patient and the type of tumor. Follow-up examinations are important after lymphoma treatment. Most relapses occur in the first 2 years after therapy.

lymphoproliferative disorders Malignant diseases of the lymphoid cells and of cells from the reticuloendothelial system. Lymphoproliferative disorders occur most often in people with compromised immune systems, such as patients with AIDS and recent transplant patients; they are often associated with Epstein-Barr virus infection. Treatment includes use of antiviral drugs, interferon, and biological therapy, as well as reduction in the dose of immunosuppressive drugs used, if any. In transplant patients, lymphoproliferative disorders may be mistaken for rejection of the new organ. See also *Epstein-Barr virus; lymphadenitis, EBV positive.*

lymphoreticulosis, benign   See *cat scratch fever.*

-lysis   Suffix indicating destruction, as in hemolysis (the destruction of red blood cells with the release of hemoglobin).

-lytic   Suffix having to do with lysis, as in hemolytic anemia (anemia due to the destruction of red blood cells).

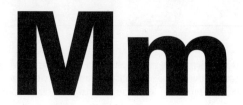

Mm

a normal variant or be a sign of pressure within the growing head during childhood, such as from hydrocephalus.

macrocytic Literally, referring to any abnormally large cell; in practice, referring to an abnormally large red blood cell. For example, macrocytic anemia is characterized by abnormally large red blood cells. The opposite of macrocytic is microcytic.

macrogenitosomia A condition in which the external sex organs are prematurely or abnormally enlarged. In males, macrogenitosomia is caused by an excess of the hormone androgen during fetal development. In females, the clitoris may be enlarged enough to resemble a small penis. Macrogenitosomia is associated with hormonal disorders that may also create changes in the internal sex organs.

M protein An antibody or part of an antibody that is found in unusually large amounts in the blood or urine of patients with multiple myeloma, a form of cancer that arises in plasma cells.

MAC 1 Mycobacterium avium complex. 2 Membrane attack complex.

Macewen operation A surgical operation to repair inguinal hernia that was designed by Scottish surgeon Sir William Macewen.

machine, heart-lung See *heart-lung machine*.

macro- Prefix meaning large or long, as in macrobiota (living organisms of a region that are large enough to be seen with the naked eye), macrocephaly (an abnormally large head), and macrosomia (an overly large body). The opposite of macro- is micro-.

macroangiopathy A disease of the blood vessels in which fat and blood clots build up in the large blood vessels, stick to the vessel walls, and block the flow of blood. Types of macroangiopathy include coronary artery disease (macroangiopathy in the heart), cerebrovascular disease (macroangiopathy in the brain), and peripheral vascular disease (macroangiopathy that affects, for example, vessels in the legs).

macrobiota The living organisms of a region that are large enough to be seen with the naked eye.

macrobiotic Referring to the macrobiota, a region's living organisms that are large enough to be seen with the naked eye.

macrobiotic diet A diet that incorporates Ayurvedic principles of food combining, is based mainly on brown rice and vegetables, and claims to lengthen life. The macrobiotic diet is strictly not recommended for pregnant women or children and may not provide sufficient protein and nutrients for others.

macrocephaly An abnormally large head. The opposite of macrocephaly is microcephaly. Macrocephaly can be

macroglossia An abnormally large tongue. Macroglossia is sometimes said to be associated with Down syndrome, but in that disorder the tongue is actually large only in relationship to a smaller-than-normal mouth cavity.

macrognathia An abnormally large jaw. Macrognathia can be associated with pituitary gigantism, tumors, and other disorders. Macrognathia can often be corrected with surgery. Also known as prognathic mandible.

macrolide antibiotic One of a family of antibiotics produced by anaerobic bacteria. The macrolide antibiotics include erythromycin and troleandomycin. See also *erythromycin*.

macroorchidism Abnormally large testes. To determine if the testes are too large, a device called an orchidometer is used that permits a testis to be compared to a series of plastic ovals (like miniature American footballs) of differing sizes. Macroorchidism is a diagnostic feature, for example, of the fragile X syndrome, the most common inherited form of mental retardation. The opposite of macroorchidism is microorchidism.

macrophage A type of white blood cell that ingests foreign material. Macrophages are key players in the immune response to foreign invaders of the body, such as infectious microorganisms. They are normally found in the liver, spleen, and connective tissues of the body.

macroscopic Large enough to be seen with the naked eye, as opposed to microscopic. For example, a macroscopic tumor is big enough to see without a microscope.

macrosomia An overly large body. A child with macrosomia has significant overgrowth, which can represent a hormone imbalance.

macula 1 A small spot. For example, a macula on the skin is a small flat spot. See also *macula lutea*.

macula lutea A small area in the retina that provides the keenest vision. It is the light-sensitive layer of tissue at the back of the eye. Also known as simply macula.

macular 1 Referring to a macule, a circumscribed change in the color of the skin that is neither elevated nor depressed. 2 Referring to the macula lutea of the retina.

macular degeneration Deterioration of the macula lutea, a common progressive disorder that causes partial or total loss of macular vision, causing difficulty in doing tasks that require fine frontal vision (such as reading and driving a car). Although some forms of macular degeneration affect young people, most macular degeneration occurs in people over 60 years of age and is termed age-related macular degeneration (AMD). There are two types of AMD: the dry type and the far more frequent wet type. Neither type causes pain. An early symptom of wet AMD is that straight lines appear wavy. This happens because the newly formed blood vessels leak fluid under the macula. The fluid raises the macula from its normal place at the back of the eye and distorts vision. Another sign that a person may have wet AMD is rapid loss of central vision. In dry AMD, loss of central vision occurs slowly. In both dry and wet AMD, the person may also notice blind spots. A person who has any of these changes in vision should consult an ophthalmologist without delay. See also *macular vision.*

macular hole A hole in the macula, the area of the retina that is responsible for fine central vision. Macular holes occur mainly in women. In time, central vision tends to worsen. A surgical procedure called vitrectomy (removal of the vitreous humor) may be considered. See also *macular vision.*

macular vision The type of fine, sharp, straight-ahead vision that enables people to read, drive, and perform other activities. As light is focused onto the macula, millions of cells change the light into nerve signals that tell the brain what is being seen. This is called macular, or central, vision.

macule A circumscribed change in the color of skin that is neither raised nor depressed. Macules are completely flat and can only be appreciated by visual inspection and not by touch. Physicians refer to flat skin spots on the skin as macules, as opposed to papules.

Magendie, foramen of See *foramen of Magendie.*

Magnesia Magnesium oxide, a chemical that is named after a town in present-day Turkey where an ore containing magnesium carbonate was mined. Magnesium carbonate can be chemically converted into magnesium hydroxide, which is the main component of the laxative Milk of Magnesia.

magnesium A mineral that is involved in many processes in the body, including nerve signaling, the building of healthy bones, and normal muscle contraction. All unprocessed foods contain magnesium. High concentrations of magnesium are found in nuts, unmilled grains, and legumes, such as peas and beans. According to the National Academy of Sciences, the recommended dietary allowance of magnesium is 420 mg per day for men and 320 mg per day for women. The upper limit for magnesium as a supplement is 350 mg daily, in addition to magnesium from food and water. See also *deficiency, magnesium; magnesium excess.*

magnesium deficiency See *deficiency, magnesium.*

magnesium excess Too much magnesium in the body. Persons with impaired kidney function should be especially careful about their magnesium intake because they can accumulate dangerous levels of magnesium. See also *magnesium.*

magnetic resonance imaging A procedure that uses a magnet linked to a computer to create pictures of areas inside the body. Abbreviated MRI. The patient slides into a tube-like chamber, which may be open or closed. The procedure takes less than an hour. There is no pain involved with an MRI, but there can be a great deal of clattering noise as the magnet moves around the walls of the tube, and many patients in closed MRI machines feel claustrophobic. In some cases sedation may be used, or the patient may listen to music through headphones to drown out the noise and reduce the mental discomfort.

Maimonides' Daily Prayer of a Physician See *Daily Prayer of a Physician.*

maintenance therapy Treatment designed to help the original primary treatment to succeed. Maintenance therapy may be given to patients who have cancer that is in remission to prevent a relapse.

major In general, something that is more than something else. For example, the teres major muscle is larger than the teres minor muscle. In anatomy, where there is a major, a minor cannot be far behind.

major depression See *depression, major.*

major histocompatability complex A cluster of genes on chromosome 6 that are concerned with antigen production and are critical to transplantation. Abbreviated MHC. The MHC includes the human leukocyte antigen (HLA) genes.

malabsorption Poor intestinal absorption of nutrients. Malabsorption can occur from diseases that injure the bowels, such as Crohn's disease, Whipple's disease, celiac disease, and many others.

malacia Softening. For example, osteomalacia is softening of bone, usually due to deficiency of calcium and vitamin D.

malady A disease or an illness, from the French *maladie,* meaning "illness."

malaise A vague feeling of discomfort, one that cannot be pinned down but is often sensed as "just not right."

malar Referring to the cheek. For example, a malar rash is a rash that appears over the cheeks.

malar bone The zygoma. See also *zygoma.*

malar rash Rash over the cheeks. See also *butterfly rash.*

malaria An infectious disease that affects many millions of people and is caused by protozoan parasites from the Plasmodium family. These parasites can be transmitted by the sting of the Anopheles mosquito or by a contaminated needle or transfusion. The symptoms of malaria include cycles of chills, fever, sweats, muscle aches, and headache that recur every few days. Other symptoms include vomiting, diarrhea, coughing, and yellowing of the skin and eyes (jaundice). Treatment includes use of oral or intravenous medication, particularly chloroquine, mefloquine (brand name: Larium), or atovaquone/proguanil (brand name: Malarone). Persons carrying the sickle cell gene have some protection against malaria. Persons with a gene for hemoglobin C (another abnormal hemoglobin like sickle hemoglobin), thalassemia trait, or deficiency of the enzyme glucose-6-phosphate dehydrogenase (G6PD) are thought also to have partial protection against malaria. Among the many names for malaria are ague, jungle fever, marsh or swamp fever, and paludism. See also *malaria, falciparum.*

malaria, falciparum The most dangerous type of malaria, which is caused by the parasite Plasmodium falciparum. Falciparum malaria is associated with high levels of parasites in the blood. Red blood cells that are infected with the parasite tend to sludge and form microinfarctions (tiny areas of dead tissue due to lack of oxygen) in capillaries in the brain, liver, adrenal gland, intestinal tract, kidneys, lungs, and other organs. Patients should be treated in a hospital setting, using intravenous medications.

male **1** Of the sex that produces sperm cells rather than eggs. **2** Having the physical appearance, by chromosome constitution or by gender identification, of the sex that produces sperm cells rather than eggs.

male breast cancer See *breast cancer, male.*

male chromosome complement The whole set of chromosomes for a human male. The large majority of males have a 46,XY chromosome complement: 46 chromosomes, including 1 X and 1 Y chromosome. A minority of males have other chromosome constitutions, such as 47,XXY (47 chromosomes, including 2 X chromosomes and 1 Y chromosome) or 47,XYY (47 chromosomes, including 1 X and 2 Y chromosomes).

male external genitalia The external genital structures of the male, comprising the penis, the male urethra, and the scrotum.

male gonad A testis, one of a pair of organs located behind the penis in a pouch of skin called the scrotum. The testes produce and store sperm and are also the body's main source of male hormones. These hormones control the development of the reproductive organs and other male characteristics, such as body and facial hair, low voice, and wide shoulders.

male internal genitalia The internal genital structures of the male that are concerned with reproduction, including the testis, epididymis, ductus deferens, seminal vesicle, ejaculatory duct, bulbourethral gland, and prostate.

male organs of reproduction The sum total of all the genital organs—internal and external—of the male that are concerned with reproduction. See also *male external genitalia; male internal genitalia.*

male pelvis The lower part of the abdomen that is located between the hip bones in a male. The male pelvis is more robust, narrower, and taller than the female pelvis. The angle of the male pubic arch and the sacrum are narrower as well.

malformation An abnormality in which the development of a structure is arrested, delayed, or misdirected early in embryonic life and the effect is permanent. See also *congenital malformation.*

malformation, arteriovenous A malformation of blood vessels in the brain, brainstem, or spinal cord that is characterized by a complex tangled web of abnormal arteries and veins connected by one or more fistulas (abnormal communications). Abbreviated AVM. An AVM has no capillary bed. The fistulas in the AVM permit high-speed, high-flow shunting of blood from the arterial to the venous side of the circulation. This creates low pressure in the arterial vessels feeding the AVM and neighboring areas of the brain that they normally supply with blood. If an AVM causes problems, it is usually before the person who has it reaches age 40. The most common symptoms include hemorrhaging (bleeding), seizures, headaches, and neurological problems such as paralysis or loss of speech, memory, or vision. Treatment for AVM may involve surgery or closing off the vessels of the AVM by nonsurgical means, using a catheter to deliver agents to block the blood vessels. These agents include permanent balloons, thrombosing (clogging) coils, sclerosing (hardening) drugs, and fast-acting embolization glue (embolization is often used before surgery). Most people with AVMs never experience problems due to them. However, AVMs that hemorrhage can lead to serious neurological problems and sometimes death.

malignancy   A tumor that is malignant (cancerous), that can invade and destroy nearby tissue, and that may spread (metastasize) to other parts of the body.

malignant   **1** Tending to be severe and become progressively worse, as in malignant hypertension.   **2** In regard to a tumor, having the properties of a malignancy. See also *malignancy*.

malignant giant cell tumor   A type of bone tumor that is characterized by massive destruction of bone near the end (epiphysis) of a long bone and causes pain and restricts movement. The most common site of malignant giant cell tumor is the knee. Diagnosis is made by examining a sample of the affected area. Treatment involves excising the affected area, usually followed by chemotherapy or radiation.

malignant melanoma   See *melanoma*.

malleability, brain   See *brain plasticity*.

malleolus   The rounded bony prominence on either side of the ankle joint.

malleus   A tiny bone in the inner ear that is shaped like a minute mallet.

malrotated ear   See *ear, slanted*.

malrotation of the intestine   Failure of the intestine to rotate normally during the development of the embryo. One of the dangers of malrotation of the intestine is that the intestine may be obstructed by abnormal bands or twist on its own blood supply, a condition called volvulus. Malrotation of the intestine is usually not apparent until the intestine becomes obstructed or twisted, generally in infants or in early childhood. Symptoms at that time may include vomiting up bile (greenish-yellow digestive fluid), abdominal pain, drawing up the legs, distention (swelling) of the abdomen, and bloody stools. This situation is considered an emergency and calls for immediate surgery to salvage the intestine and save the child.

mammary gland   One of the two half-moon–shaped glands on either side of the adult female chest, which with fatty tissue and the nipple make up the breast. Within each mammary gland is a network of sacs that produce milk during lactation and send the milk to the nipple via a system of ducts. Undeveloped mammary glands are present in female children and in males. See also *breast; lactation*.

mammogram   An X-ray of the breast that is taken with a device that compresses and flattens the breast. A mammogram can help a health professional decide whether a lump in the breast is a gland, a harmless cyst, or a tumor. A mammogram can cause pressure, discomfort, and some soreness that lasts for a little while after the procedure. If the mammogram result raises suspicions about cancer, a biopsy is usually the next step. The American Cancer Society and the American College of Surgeons currently recommend that a woman obtain her first, baseline, mammogram between the ages of 35 and 40. Between the ages of 40 and 50, a mammogram should be done every other year. After the age of 50, a mammogram should be repeated yearly. Women who are at high risk for developing breast cancer may need to obtain mammograms earlier than these recommendations and at more frequent intervals.

managed care   Any system that manages health care delivery to control costs. Typically, managed care systems rely on a primary care physician who acts as a gatekeeper for other services, such as specialized medical care, surgery, and physical therapy.

mandible   The bone of the lower jaw. The joint where the mandible meets the upper jaw at the temporal bone is called the temporomandibular joint.

maneuver, Heimlich   See *Heimlich maneuver*.

maneuver, Valsalva   See *Valsalva maneuver*.

mania   An abnormally elevated mood state that is characterized by such symptoms as inappropriate elation, increased irritability, severe insomnia, grandiose notions, increased speed and/or volume of speech, disconnected and racing thoughts, increased sexual desire, markedly increased energy and activity level, poor judgment, and inappropriate social behavior. A mild form of mania that does not require hospitalization is called hypomania. Mania that also features symptoms of depression ("agitated depression") is called mixed mania. See also *bipolar disorder*.

manic   In a state of mania.

manic depression   See *bipolar disorder*.

manic-depressive disease   See *bipolar disorder*.

MAO Monoamine oxydase, an enzyme that is active in the nervous system. All the effects of MAO are not known, but it is known that MAO acts against the neurotransmitter epinephrine.

MAO inhibitor One of a family of medications (brand names: Aurorex, Nardil, Parnate) that act to limit the activity of monoamine oxydase (MAO) in the nervous system. MAOIs are prescribed to treat depression, anxiety, migraine, and selected other conditions in patients who are not responsive to other medications. They interact with many over-the-counter medications and some foods, so patients taking MAOIs must be educated about what to avoid and must follow a restricted diet.

MAOI Monoamine oxidase (MAO) inhibitor.

map-dot-fingerprint type corneal dystrophy See *Cogan corneal dystrophy.*

maple syrup urine disease A hereditary disease that is due to deficiency of an enzyme involved in amino acid metabolism, characterized by urine that smells like maple syrup. In maple syrup urine disease, the three branched-chain amino acids (leucine, isoleucine, and valine) cannot be metabolized (processed), and they build up in the blood, causing problems with brain function and leading to mental retardation, physical disability, and death, if not treated. Treatment involves use of a special diet and monitoring of protein intake.

mapping See *gene mapping.*

mapping, gene See *gene mapping.*

marasmus See *cachexia.*

Marfan syndrome An inherited disorder of connective tissue that is characterized by abnormalities of the eyes, skeleton, and cardiovascular system. Nearsightedness (myopia) is the most common eye feature in Marfan syndrome. Displacement of the lens from the center of the pupil occurs in more than half of patients. Patients with Marfan syndrome have an increased risk for retinal detachment, glaucoma, and early cataracts. The skeleton shows bone overgrowth and lax joints. The arms and legs are unusually long, as are the fingers and toes. Due to overgrowth of the ribs, the sternum may be pushed in (pectus excavatum) or out (pectus carinatum). Scoliosis is common. Cardiovascular manifestations in Marfan syndrome include enlargement of the aorta at the level of the aortic valve, aortic aneurysm, prolapse of the mitral and triscuspid valves, and enlargement of the pulmonary artery. The major causes of disease and death in the syndrome are related to the heart and blood vessels. Marfan syndrome is inherited in an autosomal dominant manner and is caused by mutation in the FBN1 gene that encodes fibrillin 1. About 75 percent of people with Marfan syndrome have an affected parent, and 25 percent have a new gene mutation. A parent with the mutation has a 50 percent chance of transmitting it to each child. Pregnancy can be dangerous for women with Marfan syndrome because the aorta can widen. Prevention of complications is key and includes exercise, blood pressure control, monitoring of the eyes, heart, and lungs, and physical therapy. Given good medical management, the life expectancy in Marfan syndrome now approximates that for the general population. Care may be provided by a team that includes a medical geneticist, an ophthalmologist, an orthopedist, a cardiologist, and a cardiothoracic surgeon.

marijuana A common street and recreational drug that comes from the marijuana plant: the hemp plant *cannabis sativa.* The pharmacologically active ingredient in marijuana is tetra-hydro-cannabinol (THC). Marijuana is used to heighten perception, affect mood, and relax. Many people think marijuana is harmless, but it is not. Signs of marijuana use include red eyes, lethargy, and uncoordinated body movements. The long-term effects may include decrease in motivation and harmful effects on the brain, heart, lungs, and reproductive system. People who smoke marijuana are also at increased risk of developing cancer of the head and neck.

mark, strawberry See *hemangioma, capillary.*

marker **1** See *gene marker.* **2** A blood marker or a tumor marker. See also *blood marker; tumor marker.*

marker, blood See *blood marker.*

marker chromosome See *chromosome, marker.*

marker, gene See *gene marker.*

marker, tumor See *tumor marker.*

Maroteaux-Lamy syndrome A form of mucopolysaccharidosis with onset before age 3 that is characterized by an inability to metabolize dermatin sulfate. This leads to abnormal accumulation of dermatin sulfate, mostly in the peripheral tissues. The result is mild to severe changes in muscle, bone, skin, and other tissues, particularly the heart. Diagnosis is made through examination of leukocytes and cultured skin fibroblasts, or 24-hour urine collection to search for high levels of dermatin sulfate. There is no current treatment for Maroteaux-Lamy syndrome, but individual symptoms and problems may respond to physical therapy, medication, or surgery. Due to the heart damage caused by the syndrome, death usually occurs before the patient is age 40. Also known as mucopolysaccharidosis type VI. See also *mucopolysaccharidosis.*

marriage, cousin See *consanguinity.*

marrow See *bone marrow.*

marsh fever See *malaria.*

Martin-Bell syndrome See *fragile X syndrome.*

MASA syndrome A syndrome named for its characteristics: mental retardation, aphasia, shuffling gait, and adducted thumbs. Features of the syndrome include mental retardation and aphasia (lack of speech); adducted (clasped) thumbs, absent extensor pollicis longus and/or brevis muscles to the thumb, shuffling gait, and leg spasticity; small body size; and lumbar lordosis (swayback). MASA is inherited as an X-linked trait, and so it affects mainly boys. Also known as clasped thumbs and mental retardation, congenital clasped thumbs with mental retardation, adducted thumbs with mental retardation, and Gareis-Mason syndrome. See also *adducted thumbs.*

mask of pregnancy See *melasma.*

masklike face See *face, masklike.*

masochism The derivation of pleasure from one's own pain. Masochism is considered a sexual disorder (paraphilia). Named after the 19th-century Austrian writer Leopold von Sacher-Masoch.

MASS syndrome Mitral valve, aorta, skeleton, and skin syndrome, a heritable disorder of connective tissue that is characterized by involvement of all those structures. MASS syndrome is due to a mutation in the fibrillin 1 gene FBN1, the same gene that is mutated in Marfan syndrome.

massage The therapeutic practice of manipulating the muscles and limbs to ease tension and reduce pain. Massage can be a part of physical therapy or practiced on its own. It can be effective for reducing the symptoms of disorders of or pain in the muscles and nervous system, and it is often used to reduce stress.

massage therapist A person who practices therapeutic massage. In many US states, massage therapists can be licensed after completing a specified training program. Licensed therapists may practice independently or in medical settings.

masseter The muscle that raises the lower jaw.

mast cell A connective tissue cell whose normal function is unknown but that is frequently injured during allergic reactions. When a mast cell is injured, it releases strong chemicals, including histamine, into the tissues and blood. These chemicals are very irritating and cause itching, swelling, and fluid leaking from cells. They can also cause muscle spasm, leading to lung and throat tightening (as is found in asthma) and loss of voice.

mastalgia Pain in the breast or mammary gland, whether serious or not. Mastalgia has many causes including injury, infection, and plugged milk ducts.

mastectomy A general term for removal of the breast, usually to remove cancerous tissue. The operation can be done in a hospital or in an outpatient clinic, depending on how extensive it needs to be. The procedure itself takes from 2 to 3 hours, and full recovery takes 3 to 5 weeks. Drainage shunts are left in the surgical incision for a few days after the operation; they are removed in 3 to 5 days if the area is healing normally. After a mastectomy, reconstructive surgery may be performed to restore a more normal appearance. Many patients choose to avoid reconstructive surgery and instead wear special undergarments. In cases of nonmetastatic breast cancer, a lumpectomy, radiation, chemotherapy, or a combination of these treatments may prove a viable alternative to mastectomy. If a lumpectomy is chosen, the surgeon may remove some lymph node tissue from under the arms to make sure cancer has not spread.

mastectomy, double Removal of both breasts.

mastectomy, Halsted A radical mastectomy. See *mastectomy, radical.*

mastectomy, modified radical Removal of the breast tissue and the axillary lymph nodes, which are under the arms.

mastectomy, partial Surgical removal of only enough breast tissue to be sure that the margins of the tissue removed are free of cancer. Also known as segmental mastectomy.

mastectomy, preventive Removal of one or both breasts without the current presence of cancer. This surgery is sometimes chosen as a preventive measure by women who have a strong family history of breast cancer.

mastectomy, prophylactic See *mastectomy, preventive.*

mastectomy, radical Removal of all breast tissue, from just under the collarbone to the abdomen, including the chest wall muscles and the axillary lymph nodes in the armpit. In a trial begun in 1971, the efficacy of radical mastectomy was compared with that of total mastectomy. This historic trial spelled the end of radical mastectomy and started the trend toward less extensive surgery, which has culminated in the lumpectomy, leading to a vast improvement in the quality of life for women with breast cancer. Also known as Halstead mastectomy.

mastectomy, segmental A partial mastectomy. See *mastectomy, partial.*

mastectomy, simple Removal of one or both breasts, but not the lymph nodes. Also known as a total mastectomy.

mastectomy, subcutaneous Removal of breast tissue, using a minimal incision. This type of mastectomy may be used to remove small areas of suspicious or cancerous tissue, but it can also be a cosmetic surgery procedure. For example, subcutaneous mastectomy can reduce the volume of enlarged male breasts or be part of a female-to-male sex-change procedure.

mastectomy, total A simple mastectomy. See *mastectomy, simple.*

masticate To chew.

mastitis Inflammation of one or more mammary glands within the breast, usually in a lactating woman. Mastitis can be felt as a hard, sore spot within the breast. Mastitis can be caused by an infection in the breast or by a plugged milk duct. Treatment includes resting and applying warm compresses to the affected area, for those who are lactating, nursing or expressing milk frequently. If a woman has recurring mastitis during nursing, she should contact a lactation expert through an obstetrician, a midwife, or the La Leche League.

mastoid The rounded protrusion of bone just behind the ear. The mastoid was once thought to look like a breast (hence its name).

mastoiditis Inflammation of the mastoid, which often occurs secondarily to ear infection.

maternal mortality ratio The number of registered maternal deaths per 100,000 registered live births. The maternal mortality ratio in the US in 2001 was 2.0, or 2 mothers dying per 100,000 live births.

maternal serum alpha-fetoprotein The presence of alpha-fetoprotein (AFP), a plasma protein that is normally produced by the fetus, in the mother's blood. Abbreviated MSAFP. MSAFP serves as the basis for some valuable tests. AFP is manufactured principally in the fetus's liver but is also found in the fetal gastrointestinal tract and in the yolk sac, a structure that is temporarily present during embryonic development. The level of AFP is typically high in the fetus's blood, goes down in the baby's blood after birth, and by 1 year of age is virtually undetectable. During pregnancy, AFP crosses the placenta from the fetal circulation and appears in the mother's blood. The MSAFP can be screened to detect a number of disorders, including open neural tube defects, such as anencephaly and spina bifida, in which case MSAFP tends to be high; Down syndrome, in which case MSAFP tends to be low; and other chromosome abnormalities.

matter, gray See *gray matter.*

matter, white See *white matter.*

maxilla The major bone of the upper jaw.

MCAT Medical College Admissions Test.

McBurney point The most tender area of the abdomen of patients in the early stage of appendicitis.

McCune-Albright syndrome See *polyostotic fibrous dysplasia.*

MD Abbreviation for the Latin *Medicinae Doctor,* "doctor of medicine."

measles An acute and highly contagious viral disease characterized by fever, runny nose, cough, red eyes, and a spreading skin rash. Measles is a potentially disastrous disease that can be complicated by ear infections, pneumonia, encephalitis (which can cause convulsions, mental retardation, and even death), the sudden onset of low blood platelet levels with severe bleeding (acute thrombocytopenic purpura), or a chronic brain disease that occurs months to years after an attack of measles (subacute sclerosing panencephalitis). During pregnancy, exposure to the measles virus may trigger miscarriage or premature delivery. Treatment includes rest and use of calamine lotion or other anti-itching preparations to soothe the skin, nonaspirin pain relievers for fever, and in some cases antibiotics. Measles can often be prevented through vaccination. Also known as rubeola, hard measles, seven-day measles, eight-day measles, nine-day measles, ten-day measles, and morbilli. See also *measles encephalitis; measles immunization; measles syndrome, atypical; MMR.*

measles encephalitis Inflammation of the brain due to infection with the measles virus. Measles encephalitis occurs in approximately 1 in 1,000 cases of measles, starting up to 3 weeks after onset of the rash and causing high fever, convulsions, and coma. It usually runs a blessedly short course, with full recovery within a week, but it may eventuate in central nervous system impairment or death.

measles immunization A vaccine for measles only. Single-virus vaccines may be safer than multivirus vaccines for children with known or suspected brain disorders or compromised immune systems, and they are generally given after 1 year of age. For other children, the measles vaccine is usually administered as a multivirus vaccine (MMR), along with vaccines for mumps and rubella. See also *MMR.*

measles, mumps, rubella vaccine See *MMR.*

measles syndrome, atypical An altered type of measles that begins suddenly, with high fever, headache, cough, and abdominal pain. The rash may appear 1 or 2 days later, often beginning on the limbs. Abbreviated AMS. With AMS, swelling (edema) of the hands and feet may occur, and pneumonia is common, sometimes persisting for 3 months or more. AMS occurs in people who were incompletely immunized against measles. It often occurs in people who were given the old killed-virus measles vaccine, which does not provide complete immunity and is no longer available, or attenuated (weakened) live measles vaccine that was inactivated due to improper storage. AMS can be confused with other illnesses, including Rocky Mountain spotted fever, meningococcal infection, various types of pneumonia, appendicitis, and juvenile rheumatoid arthritis.

measly tapeworm See *Taenia solium.*

meatus An opening or a passageway. For example, the meatus of the ear is the opening to the ear canal.

meatus, female urethral The meatus (opening) of the female urethra, the transport tube that leads from the bladder to discharge urine outside the body. The female urethral meatus is above the vaginal opening.

Meckel's diverticulum See *diverticulum, Meckel's.*

meconium Dark, sticky material that is normally present in the intestine at birth and passed in the feces after birth, after trypsin and other enzymes from the pancreas have acted on it. The passage of meconium before birth can be a sign of fetal distress.

meconium ileus Obstruction of the intestine (ileus) due to overly thick meconium. Meconium ileus results from a deficiency of trypsin and other digestive enzymes from the pancreas, as in cystic fibrosis.

MEDEVAC See *MEDVAC.*

medial The side of the body or the side of a body part that is nearest to the middle or center (median) of the body. For example, when referring to the knee, medial would mean the side of the knee that is closest to the other knee. The opposite of medial is lateral. See also Appendix B, "Anatomic Orientation Terms."

medial collateral ligament of the knee The ligament that straps the inner side of the knee joint, providing stability and strength. See also *knee.*

medial meniscus of the knee A thickened, crescent-shaped cartilage pad in the inner portion of the joint formed by the femur (the thigh bone) and the tibia (the shin bone). The medial meniscus is in the inner side,

whereas the lateral meniscus is in the outer side of this knee joint. The meniscus acts as a smooth surface for the joint to move on, serves to evenly load the surface during weight-bearing, and aids in disbursing joint fluid for joint lubrication. See also *knee.*

median The middle, as in the median strip in a highway. For example, the median nerve is the nerve the runs through the middle of the wrist.

mediastinoscopy A procedure in which the physician inserts a tube into the chest to view the organs in the mediastinum. The tube is inserted through an incision above the breastbone. Also known as mediastinotomy.

mediastinotomy See *mediastinoscopy.*

mediastinum The area between the lungs. The organs in the mediastinum include the heart and its large veins and arteries, the trachea, the esophagus, the bronchi, and lymph nodes.

Medicaid A number of US programs of public assistance for persons whose income is insufficient to pay for health care, regardless of age. Medicaid is administered on a state level, with the federal government providing matching funds to state Medicaid programs. Services and options can vary from state to state. Disabled persons who receive Social Security income (SSI), among others, are automatically eligible for Medicaid. To apply for Medicaid, one should contact the local Social Security, public health, or disability services office.

Medical College Admissions Test A test that is required of all applicants to medical school in the US and Canada, which assesses applicants' science knowledge, reasoning, and communication and writing skills. It is given under the aegis of the Association of American Medical Colleges. Abbreviated MCAT.

medical directive, advance See *advance directive.*

Medical Literature Analysis and Retrieval System See *MEDLARS.*

medical symbol See *Aesculapius.*

Medicare The US government's national health insurance program for people aged 65 and older who have worked for at least 10 years in Medicare-covered employment, and who are citizens or permanent residents of the US. Medicare Part A covers inpatient hospital stays, and Medicare Part B covers physician and outpatient services. Currently, Medicare does not cover the cost of prescription drugs.

medication **1** A drug that is used to medicate, a medicine, or a medicament or medical substance. Although the terms medication and drug are sometimes used interchangeably, the term medication is not used to speak of a recreational substance. **2** The administration of a drug or medicine.

medicine, occupational See *occupational medicine.*

medicine, transfusion See *transfusion medicine.*

MedicineNet.com A premier online health and medical information website. MedicineNet.com provides easy-to-read, in-depth, authoritative medical information for consumers. Since 1996, MedicineNet.com has become nationally-recognized for providing quality information that is produced by a network of board-certified physicians from across the US.

Medigap An insurance policy in the US that supplements Medicare benefits, presumably filling the gaps in health care coverage. Many Medigap policies are mainly intended to cover the cost of prescription drugs. Some actually duplicate Medicare coverage, however, and may be unnecessary.

meditation A typically self-directed practice for relaxing the body and calming the mind. Most meditative techniques have come to the West from Eastern religious practices, particularly India, China, and Japan, but can be found in many cultures of the world. Until recently, the primary purpose of meditation has been religious, although its health benefits have long been recognized. During the past several decades, meditation has been further explored as a way of reducing stress on both the mind and body.

Mediterranean anemia See *thalassemia major.*

Mediterranean fever See *familial Mediterranean fever.*

MEDLARS Medical Literature Analysis and Retrieval System, a computer system of the US National Library of Medicine (NLM) that allows rapid access to NLM's store of biomedical information. Today, through the Internet and World Wide Web, MEDLARS search services are available around the world without charge. See also *MEDLINE.*

MEDLINE The best-known bibliographic database of the US National Library of Medicine (NLM), which lets anyone with computer access query the NLM's store of journal references on specific topics. MEDLINE currently contains 11 million references, going back to the mid-1960s. The MEDLINE database covers the fields of medicine, nursing, dentistry, veterinary medicine, the health care system, and the preclinical sciences. Through the

World Wide Web, some 350,000 MEDLINE searches are performed each day by health professionals, scientists, librarians, and the general public. A new Web service, called MEDLINEplus, links users to sources of consumer health information. MEDLINE and MEDLINEplus are part of the MEDLARS system. See also *MEDLARS.*

medulla The innermost part. For example, the adrenal medulla is the innermost part of the adrenal gland, the renal medulla is the inner part of the kidney, and the spinal medulla is the part of the spinal cord that is lodged deep within the vertebral canal.

medulla, adrenal The innermost portion of the adrenal gland, which makes epinephrine (adrenaline) and norepinephrine (noradrenaline). Epinephrine is secreted in response to low blood levels of glucose as well as exercise and stress; it causes the breakdown of the storage product glycogen to the sugar glucose in the liver, facilitates the release of fatty acids from adipose (fat) tissue, causes dilation (widening) of the small arteries within muscle, and increases the output of the heart. Norepinephrine acts to narrow blood vessels and raise blood pressure.

medulla oblongata The base of the brain, which is formed by the enlarged top of the spinal cord. The medulla oblongata directly controls breathing, blood flow, and other essential functions.

medulloblastoma A type of brain tumor that tends to occur in children, arise in the cerebellum (in the lower part of the brain), and spread along the spine. Medulloblastoma is the most common type of primary brain tumor in childhood. Medulloblastomas occasionally metastasize outside the central nervous system, usually to bone. Surgery and radiotherapy have been the mainstays of treatment, and chemotherapy is now sometimes used as well. Currently, up to half of the children with medulloblastomas are free of the disease 10 years after the diagnosis.

MEDVAC Acronym for medical evacuation. MEDVAC typically refers to a team that has the skills necessary for proper medical evacuation in emergency situations. Also known as MEDEVAC.

mega- Prefix meaning abnormally large, as in megalocephaly (an overly large head) and megacardia (an enlarged heart).

megacolon An abnormally enlarged colon. Megacolon is a serious problem of the newborn. It can be caused by abnormal innervation of the colon and frquently requires surgery.

megakaryocyte　A giant cell in the bone marrow that is the ancestor of blood platelets, which are essential to normal blood clotting.

megavitamin therapy　The use of massive doses of vitamins to treat disease. Because overuse of vitamins can cause disease, most physicians consider megavitamin therapy controversial. See also Appendix C, "Vitamins"; *orthomolecular medicine; vitamin therapy.*

Meibomian cyst　See *cyst, Meibomian.*

Meibomian glands　See *glands, Meibomian.*

meibomianitis　Inflammation of the little glands in the tarsus of the eyelids. Chronic inflammation of these glands leads to cysts of the Meibomian glands, called chalazions. Also known as meibomitis.

meibomitis　See *meibomianitis.*

meiosis　The process chromosomes undertake during germ-cell formation to halve the chromosome number from 46 to 23. In meiosis, the 46 chromosomes in the cell divide to make two new cells with 23 chromosomes each. Before meiosis is complete, however, chromosomes pair with their corresponding chromosomes and exchange bits of genetic material. In women, X chromosomes pair; in men, the X and Y chromosomes pair. After the exchange, the chromosomes separate, and meiosis continues.

meiotic　Pertaining to meiosis.

meiotic nondisjunction　Failure of two members of a chromosome pair to separate from one another during meiosis, causing both chromosomes to go to a single daughter cell. Meiotic nondisjunction is responsible for the extra chromosome 21 in trisomy 21 (Down syndrome) and for extra and missing chromosomes that cause other birth defects and many miscarriages.

melan-　Prefix meaning dark or black, as in melancholia (a dark and gloomy mood) and melanin (a dark pigment).

melancholia　An old term for depression.

melanin　The pigment that gives human skin, hair, and eyes their color. Dark-skinned people have more melanin in their skin than light-skinned people have. Melanin is produced by cells called melanocytes. It provides some protection again skin damage from the sun, and the melanocytes increase their production of melanin in response to sun exposure. Freckles, which occur in people of all races, are small, concentrated areas of increased melanin production.

melanocyte　A cell in the skin that produces and contains the pigment melanin.

melanoma　The most dangerous form of skin cancer, a malignancy of melanocytes, the cells that produce pigment in the skin. Melanoma is most common in people with fair skin, but it can occur in people with all skin colors. Most melanomas present as dark, mole-like spots that spread and, unlike moles, have irregular borders. The tendency toward melanoma may be inherited, and the risk increases with overexposure to the sun and sunburn. Fair-skinned people and people with a family history of melanoma should always use a high-SPF sunscreen when outdoors. Anyone who has concern about an unusual mole-like spot should see a physician. Detected early, melanoma is almost always treatable. Undetected, melanoma can spread rapidly and be fatal. Malignant melanoma is classified into four clinical types: acral-lentiginous melanoma, lentigo maligna melanoma, nodular melanoma, and superficial spreading melanoma.

melanoma, acral-lentiginous　One of the four clinical types of malignant melanoma, which is uncommon in white people but the most common type in nonwhite people. Acral-lentiginous melanoma starts as an irregular enlarging black flat spot (macule), most often on the palm of the hand and the sole of the foot, less often on a mucosal surface, such as the vulva or vagina.

melanoma, amelanotic　A colorless melanoma that is detectable only on close examination of the skin.

melanoma, choroidal　See *melanoma, ocular.*

melanoma, juvenile　A benign raised pink or red scaly area that appears on a child's skin, usually on the cheek, before puberty. Also known as benign compound nevus or a spindle and epithelioid cell nevus.

melanoma, lentigo maligna　One of the four clinical types of malignant melanoma and the slowest growing type. Lentigo maligna melanoma typically begins as a patch of mottled pigmentation that is dark brown, tan, or black on sun-exposed skin, such as on the face.

melanoma, nodular　One of the four clinical types of malignant melanoma, which typically presents as a raised, distinct, bluish-black tumor that may be encircled by particularly pale skin, most often in middle-aged or older adults.

melanoma, ocular　A malignant melanoma that arises from a structure within the eye. The most common sites for ocular melanoma are the choroid, the ciliary body, and the iris. The tumor may metastasize (spread), most often to the liver. Ocular melanoma tends to occur after age 40.

melanoma, superficial spreading　One of the four clinical types of malignant melanoma, the most common type in white people, which typically presents as a raised, irregular, colored area that starts in a mole-like shape and spreads across the skin.

MELAS syndrome Mitochondrial encephalopathy, lactic acidosis, and stroke-like episodes syndrome, a rare form of dementia caused by mutations in the genetic material (DNA) in the mitochondria. Most DNA is in the chromosomes in the cell nucleus, but another important cell structure that carries DNA is the mitochondrion. Much of the DNA in the mitochondrion is used to manufacture proteins that help to produce energy. As a result of the disturbed function of their cells' mitochondria, patients with MELAS syndrome develop brain dysfunction (encephalopathy), with seizures and headaches, as well as muscle disease, with a buildup of lactic acid in the blood (lactic acidosis), temporary local paralysis (stroke-like episodes), and abnormal thinking (dementia). MELAS syndrome is diagnosed via muscle biopsy that shows characteristic ragged red fibers. Brain biopsy shows stroke-like changes. MELAS syndrome can affect people at different times of life, but most patients show symptoms before age 20. Patients are treated according to which areas of the body are affected at a particular time. There is no known cure for MELAS, which is progressive and fatal.

melasma Pigmentation of the cheeks of the face (malar area) that occurs in half of women during pregnancy. Melasma darkens due to sun exposure. Also known as the mask of pregnancy.

melatonin A hormone that is produced by the pineal gland and is intimately involved in regulating the sleeping and waking cycles, among other processes. Some people who have chronic insomnia use melatonin supplements. However, melatonin is not recommended for all patients with sleep problems, so one should consult a physician before taking it.

melena Stool or vomit that is stained black by blood pigment or dark blood products.

melorheostosis A rare bone condition that usually begins in childhood and is characterized by thickening of the bones (sclerosis) of a limb. Pain is frequent in the involved limb, and the affected bone can have the appearance of dripping candle wax on an X-ray.

membrane A very thin layer of tissue that covers a surface.

membrane attack complex An abnormal activation of the complement (protein) portion of the blood that forms a cascade reaction and brings blood proteins together, binds them to the cell wall, and then inserts them through the cell membrane. Abbreviated MAC. MAC allows water, ions, and other small molecules to move freely into and out of a cell, and it quickly results in cell death.

membranous gingivitis, acute See *acute membranous gingivitis.*

memory The ability to recover information about past events or knowledge, and/or the process of doing so. Memory is often divided into short-term (also known as working, or recent, memory) and long-term memory: Short-term memory recovers memories of recent events, and long-term memory is concerned with the more distant past. Some medical disorders, such as Alzheimer's disease, damage the cognitive systems that control memory. Usually, long-term memory is retained and short-term memory is lost; conversely, memories may become jumbled, leading to mistakes in recognizing people or places that should be familiar. See also *memory, anterograde; memory, long-term; memory, short-term.*

memory, anterograde A condition in which the short-term memory for things following an event or brain injury is affected. The opposite of retrograde memory.

memory B cells Secondary immune-system components that have an affinity for a particular antigen. Like other B cells, memory B cells originate from lymphocytes that develop and are activated in the bone marrow. They become antigen specific when they are stimulated by interleukin-4 (IL-4).

memory, long-term The ability to permanently store, manage, and retrieve information for later use. Items of information stored as long-term memory may be available for a lifetime.

memory, recent See *memory, short-term.*

memory, retrograde Memory for things prior to an event or brain injury. The opposite of anterograde memory.

memory, short-term The ability to temporarily store and manage information that is required to carry out complex cognitive tasks such as learning, reasoning, and comprehension. Short-term memory is involved in the selection, initiation, and termination of information-processing functions, such as encoding, storing, and retrieving data. One test of short-term memory is memory span: the number of items, usually words or numbers, that a person can retain and recall. Also known as recent, or working, memory. See also *memory; memory span.*

memory span The number of items, usually words or numbers, that a person can retain and recall. Memory span is a test of working memory (short-term memory). In a typical test of memory span, an examiner reads a list of random numbers aloud at about the rate of one number per second. At the end of a sequence, the person being tested is asked to recall the items, in order. The average memory span for normal adults is seven.

memory, working See *memory, short-term.*

menarche The time in a girl's life when menstruation first begins. During the menarche period, menstruation may be irregular and unpredictable. Mood, weight, activity level, and growth rate may fluctuate with the hormone levels as well. Also known as female puberty.

Mendel, Gregor The father of genetics, the great Moravian/Bohemian biologist who in the 19th century set forth the basic laws that constitute the foundation of classical genetics. Gregor Mendel was a monk who lived in an Augustinian monastery where teaching and research were emphasized and where he was given the freedom to pursue scientific studies in the diverse fields that interested him: mathematics, botany, physics, and meteorology. Mendel's meticulous controlled experiments with breeding peas in the monastery garden led him to conclude that the heritable units (now called genes) were not blends of parental traits, but rather were separate physical entities passed individually from one generation to the next.

Mendelian Referring to Gregor Mendel or his theories.

Mendelian inheritance The manner by which genes and traits are passed from parents to their children. The modes of Mendelian inheritance are autosomal dominant, autosomal recessive, X-linked dominant, and X-linked recessive. Also known as classical or simple genetics.

Ménière's disease A condition that is characterized by recurrent vertigo accompanied by ringing in the ears (tinnitus) and deafness. Symptoms include vertigo, dizziness, nausea, vomiting, loss of hearing in the affected ear, and abnormal eye movements. Ménière's disease is due to dysfunction of the semicircular canals (endolymphatic sac) in the inner ear. Treatment usually includes use of medications, such as anticholinergic drugs or antihistamines, to relieve the vertigo. Diuretics may also be used to lower the pressure in the endolymphatic sac. Also known as recurrent aural vertigo. See also *vertigo*.

meningeal Pertaining to the meninges.

meningeal carcinoma See *meningitis, neoplastic*.

meningeal metastases See *meningitis, neoplastic*.

meninges The three membranes that cover the brain and spinal cord (singular: meninx). The outside meninx is called the dura mater, and is the most resilient of the three meninges. The center layer is the pia mater, and the thin innermost layer is the arachnoid. Inflammation of the meninges (meningitis) can occur due to bacterial infection. See also *meningitis*.

meningioma A common type of slow-growing, usually benign brain tumor that arises from the dura, one of the meninges, the membranes covering the brain and spinal

cord. A meningioma may occur wherever there is dura (the outermost of the three meninges), but the most common sites are over the cerebral hemispheres of the brain. Meningiomas are the only brain tumors that are more common in women than in men. They tend to occur in people between ages 40 and 60 but can occur at any age. A person may have several meningiomas. Very rarely do meningiomas become malignant. The symptoms depend on the location of the tumor. Treatment ranges from observation to neurosurgical resection.

meningitis Inflammation of the meninges, the three membranes that envelop the brain and the spinal cord. Meningitis can be caused by infection by bacteria, viruses, and protozoa. Other causes include cancer (metastasis to the meninges), inflammatory diseases, and drugs. In some cases the cause of meningitis cannot be determined. The treatment depends on the cause of the meningitis.

meningitis, aseptic See *meningitis, viral*.

meningitis, bacterial Inflammation of the meninges due to a bacterial infection. Haemophilus influenzae type B (HIB) was the leading cause of bacterial meningitis before the 1990s, but new vaccines given to children as part of their routine immunizations have reduced the occurrence of invasive disease due to H. influenzae. Streptococcus pneumoniae and Neisseria meningitidis are now the leading causes of bacterial meningitis. High fever, headache, and stiff neck are common symptoms of bacterial meningitis in anyone over the age of 2 years. In newborns and small infants, the classic symptoms of fever, headache, and neck stiffness may be absent and the infant may only appear to be inactive, irritable, vomiting, or feeding poorly. A sample of spinal fluid obtained via lumbar puncture can be examined to confirm the diagnosis and fully identify the bacteria involved and their antibiotic sensitivity. Treatment is started as early as possible, in the hospital. Appropriate antibiotic treatment has reduced the risk of death from most common types of bacterial meningitis to below 15 percent, although the risk is higher among the elderly.

meningitis, benign recurrent aseptic See *meningitis, Mollaret*.

meningitis, cryptococcal Inflammation of the meninges due to infection with the fungal organism Cryptococcus neoformans, which is found mainly in dirt and bird droppings. Most people have been exposed to this organism at some time, but normally it causes no problems. Often associated with AIDS, cryptococcal meningitis is considered an opportunistic infection: a disease that emerges most often when the immune system is compromised in some way. Diagnosis is made via observation of symptoms, lumbar puncture, and cryptococcal titre. Treatment takes place in the hospital and usually consists of intravenous doses of the antibiotic amphotericin B. After the infection is under control, patients usually remain on a maintenance dose of fluconazole (brand name: Diflucan) to prevent reinfection.

meningitis, infectious Inflammation of the meninges due to bacterial, viral, or protozoan infection. Most of the agents known to cause meningitis are infectious, but very few people exposed to them develop meningitis. Those at greatest risk for infectious meningitis include people with AIDS, infants, transplant patients, and others whose immune systems may be compromised. For this reason, infectious meningitis patients are almost always isolated until the risk of spreading the illness to others has passed.

meningitis, Kernig sign of See *Kernig sign.*

meningitis, meningococcal Inflammation of the meninges due to infection with the bacterium Neisseria meningitidis. Meningococcal meningitis typically starts like the flu, with the sudden onset of an intense headache, fever, sore throat, nausea, vomiting, and malaise. But, unlike with the flu, a stiff neck and intolerance of lights are frequent symptoms of meningococcal meningitis. Within hours of the first symptoms, the disease can progress to delirium, coma, or convulsions and invade the bloodstream, setting off a bodywide infection that attacks organs and can cause circulatory collapse, a hemorrhagic rash, and gangrene. Meningococcal meningitis is a medical emergency. Diagnosis is made through examination of the fluid obtained via a spinal tap. Treatment includes use of appropriate antibiotics, usually in the hospital. The disease is highly contagious; it can be spread by a cough or sneeze, a kiss, or even a drink from a contaminated cup. Meningococcal meningitis has a high fatality rate: up to 15 percent with treatment and as high as 50 percent without treatment. A disproportionate number of victims are children or young adults, with the greatest number being college freshmen who live in dormitories. A federal health advisory panel in the US recommends that college freshmen be informed about the disease and about the availability of the vaccine, which is effective against most of the strains that infect college students.

meningitis, Mollaret Inflammation of the meninges due to unknown causes, distinguished from viral meningitis by its recurrent character with symptom-free intervals between episodes. Symptoms of Mollaret meningitis, which last from 1 to 7 days, include headache, neck ache, fever, and neck stiffness. With this type of meningitis, there is usually rapid onset of symptoms and resolution without residual damage to the nervous system. Symptom-free periods may last from weeks to years. A distinctive feature of Mollaret meningitis is the presence of peculiar cells in the spinal fluid, called Mollaret cells, that are most often visible in the first day of the attack. Other causes of meningitis are typically excluded through testing, including tests of the brain, blood, and spinal fluid. There is no specific treatment for Mollaret meningitis, but medications for pain, colchicine, and acyclovir are often used. The long-term outcome for a patient with Mollaret meningitis is excellent. Also known as benign recurrent aseptic meningitis.

meningitis, neoplastic Inflammation of the meninges due to cancer that has spread from the original (primary) tumor to the meninges. The name neoplastic meningitis is a misnomer because the condition is not inflammatory. It is more properly called meningeal carcinoma or meningeal metastases.

meningitis, viral Inflammation of the meninges that is due to a virus, such as mumps virus or coxsackievirus, that is shed in the feces, sputum (spit), and nasal discharges. Viral meningitis is contagious, and it occurs most frequently in children. It can be a complication of common childhood diseases, including chickenpox. Symptoms include fever, headache, stiff neck, nausea, vomiting, drowsiness, and confusion. Babies with viral meningitis may be irritable and difficult to awaken, and they may feed poorly. Most patients with viral meningitis recover completely. Treatment, if warranted, involves use of antiviral drugs. Viral meningitis can often be prevented by improved hygiene. Also known as aseptic meningitis.

meningocele Protrusion of the membranes of the spinal cord or brain through a defect in the vertebral column or skull. This term is more broad than the similar term menigomyelocele, which only means protrusion of the membrane of the spinal cord through the vertebral column.

meningococcal meningitis See *meningitis, meningococcal.*

meningomyelocele Protrusion of the spinal cord and the membranes covering it through a defect in the vertebral column. The defect is due to failure of the neural tube to close during fetal development. The infant has a hole in the lumbar spine through which a skin-covered sac containing the meninges and part of the spinal cord bulge. Abbreviated MM. MM may be suspected prenatally if the mother's serum alpha-fetoprotein (AFP) is elevated, and it can be confirmed via ultrasound. Delivery of an infant with MM should ideally be done by C-section, to protect the skin covering the sac and prevent infection of the spinal cord. Surgery is then done to repair the defect and, if needed, a shunt is inserted to treat hydrocephalus, which commonly accompanies MM. The baby may still have neurological deficits involving loss of nerve control over the bowel, bladder, and legs. For a family that has already produced a child with MM, the risk of having another child with MM is increased. Folic acid intake during the childbearing years lowers the risk of bearing a child with MM. Also known as myelomeningocele. See also *alpha-fetoprotein; meninges; neural tube defect; spina bifida cystica.*

meniscus, lateral knee See *lateral meniscus of the knee.*

meniscus, medial knee See *medial meniscus of the knee.*

Menkes syndrome A genetic disorder that is characterized by fragile, twisted hair and progressive deterioration of the brain. Menkes syndrome is due to an error in copper transport that results in copper deficiency. The gene responsible for the syndrome is called ATP7A, on the X chromosome in region Xq12-13. Females are carriers of Menkes syndrome, and their sons who have the gene have the disease. If the disorder is recognized early, injections of copper can prevent further brain damage. Also known as kinky hair syndrome and copper transport disease.

meno- Prefix meaning pertaining to the menses.

menometrorrhagia Excessive uterine bleeding, both at the usual time of menstrual periods and at other irregular intervals. Menometrorrhagia can be a sign of a number of different disorders, including hormone imbalance, endometriosis, benign fibroid tumors in the uterus, and cancer. Women who have abnormal menstrual bleeding should consult a physician to rule out these conditions. Anemia may also result from the excessive uterine bleeding. Treatment depends on the cause: If there does not appear to be a dangerous cause, such as cancer, then hormone supplementation or the therapeutic use of birth control pills to better control the menstrual cycle may be recommended. See also *menorrhagia; metrorrhagia.*

menopause The time for a woman, usually in middle age, when menstrual periods end. When there has been no menstruation for 12 consecutive months, and no other biological or physiological cause can be identified, the childbearing years have probably ended and menopause has begun. Natural menopause occurs when the ovaries begin decreasing their production of the sex hormones estrogen and progesterone. The timing of menopause varies. In the Western world, the average age is now 51, but menopause can occur from the 30s onward. Factors that influence the time of menopause include heredity and cigarette smoking. Smokers and former smokers reach menopause an average of 2 years before women who have never smoked. There is no relationship between the time of a woman's first period and her age at menopause, nor

is the age of menopause influenced by a woman's ethnicity, height, number of children, or use of oral contraceptives. Changes associated with menopause include night sweats, mood swings, vaginal dryness, fluctuations in sexual desire (libido), forgetfulness, trouble sleeping, and fatigue (probably due to the loss of sleep). Problems that have not been proven to be due to the menopause include headache, dizziness, palpitations of the heart, and depression. Estrogen replacement therapy (ERT) is sometimes used to treat symptoms associated with menopause. ERT reduces or stops short-term changes such as hot flashes, disturbed sleep, and vaginal dryness. ERT can also prevent osteoporosis, a consequence of lowered estrogen levels. Vaginally used ERT products help with vaginal dryness, more severe vaginal changes, and bladder effects only. The use of ERT by itself is associated with an increase in the risk of endometrial cancer (cancer of the lining of the uterus). However, by taking the hormone progestogen along with estrogen, the risk of endometrial cancer is reduced substantially. Progestogen protects the uterus by keeping the endometrium from thickening, an effect caused by estrogen. The combination therapy of estrogen plus progestogen is called hormone replacement therapy (HRT). Also known as change of life. See also *estrogen replacement therapy; hormone replacement therapy; menopause transition; menopause, induced.*

menopause, chemical Menopause that is induced by chemotherapy or by other chemicals or medications. See also *menopause; menopause, induced.*

menopause, induced Menopause that is caused by surgical removal of the ovaries, or grave damage to the ovaries by radiation, chemotherapy, or medication. Because of the abrupt cutoff of ovarian hormones, induced menopause causes the sudden onset of hot flashes and other menopause-related symptoms, such as vaginal dryness and a decline in sex drive. Induced menopause before age 40 carries with it a greater risk for heart disease and osteoporosis because more years are spent beyond the protective cover of estrogen. Estrogen replacement therapy (ERT) may be used to treat symptoms associated with induced menopause, as may hormone replacement therapy (HRT). See also *menopause; menopause chemical.*

menopause, natural Menopause that occurs when the ovaries naturally decrease their production of the sex hormones estrogen and progesterone. See also *menopause.*

menopause, radiation See *menopause, induced.*

menopause, surgical See *menopause, induced.*

menopause transition Changes in female hormone production that begin about 6 years before the natural menopause. The levels of hormones produced by the aging ovaries fluctuate, leading to irregularity in the length of menstrual periods, the time between periods, and the level of period flow, as well as to hot flashes. Other changes associated with the menopause transition include night sweats, mood swings, vaginal dryness, fluctuations in sexual desire (libido), forgetfulness, trouble sleeping, and fatigue (probably due to loss of sleep). Estrogen replacement therapy (ERT) or hormone replacement therapy (HRT) may be considered if the symptoms accompanying menopause transition are particularly severe. Also known as perimenopause. See also *menopause.*

menorrhagia Excessive uterine bleeding or menstruation at the expected intervals of menstruation but that lasts longer than usual. Menorrhagia can cause significant anemia. It may also be a sign of underlying disease, such as hormone disorder, uterine fibroids, or cancer of the uterus. See also *menometrorrhagia; metrorrhagia.*

menorrhea See *menstruation.*

menstrual cramps Cramping in the lower abdomen, usually in the first or second day of the menstrual cycle, that is caused by contractions of the uterus as it expels its unneeded contents and by the passage of clotted blood through the cervix. Ibuprofen or other pain relievers can reduce the severity of menstrual cramps, and some women report that exercise is also helpful. Severe menstrual cramps, particularly if paired with excessive bleeding or passage of large blood clots, can occasionally be a sign of endometriosis or other disorders of the female reproductive tract. Also known as dysmenorrhea.

menstrual cycle The monthly cycle of changes in the ovaries and the lining of the uterus (endometrium), starting with the preparation of an egg for fertilization. When the follicle of the prepared egg in the ovary breaks, it is released for fertilization, and ovulation occurs. Unless pregnancy occurs, the cycle ends with the shedding of part of the endometrium (menstruation). Although it is actually the end of the physical cycle, the first day of menstrual bleeding is designated as "day 1" of the menstrual cycle in medical parlance.

menstrual irregularity Abnormality in the normal menstrual cycle, which is about 4 weeks long, often follows the phases of the moon, and has a length that varies from 3 to 7 days but is usually consistent. Girls and teenagers who menstruate usually have menstrual irregularity. It is not a cause for concern unless regular menstruation has been established and is then lost. Some adult women also have irregular cycles. This can be a benign condition, but it can also be due to problems in the uterus or ovaries, including cancer. Adults with menstrual irregularity should see a physician to rule out disease or other problems. In some cases, medication, such as birth control pills, can be used to regulate a chronically irregular cycle.

menstrual spotting The presence of apparent menstrual blood during the wrong parts of the menstrual cycle. Some women have a tendency to bleed around the time of ovulation, which occurs at about the 14th day after the first day of menstrual bleeding. In other women, spotting can be a sign of internal problems, including fibroid tumors of the uterus. Although spotting is usually benign, its onset is always a reason to see a physician, who can rule out problems.

menstrual synchronization A phenomenon that occurs when two or more menstruating women live or otherwise spend a lot of time together, in which the menstrual cycles of the women gradually become synchronized. The mechanism and reason for this effect is unknown, although current research suggests that it is due to the effects of female pheromones on other women's ovulation cycles.

menstruation Bleeding that occurs each month if pregnancy does not occur. Also known as menorrhea and menses. See also *menstrual cycle.*

menstruation, anovular Menstruation that occurs without ovulation. Usually in anovular menstruation the egg that remains in the ovary simply disintegrates, but in some circumstances it is fertilized and a life-threatening ovarian pregnancy results.

menstruation, cessation of The ending of a woman's menstrual cycles. Menstruation ends naturally in middle age with the onset of menopause. It can also end suddenly as a result of induced menopause. Cessation of menstruation in nonmenopausal women may be due to pregnancy, illness, disorders of the hypothalamus or pituitary gland, medication, stress, overexercise, or malnutrition, among other causes. In particular, it can be a symptom of anorexia, signaling potentially dangerous changes in the body's hormonal system. Cessation of menstruation in women who have established a regular menstrual cycle, or in girls or teens who show other signs of anorexia, is a cause for medical concern. Also known as amenhorrhea.

menstruation, retrograde Menstruation in which blood flows from the uterus into the Fallopian tubes, and potentially into the abdomen. This condition can lead to endometriosis.

mental 1 Pertaining to the mind. 2 Pertaining to the chin.

mental child injury   See *child abuse, emotional.*

mental illness   Any disease that affects the central nervous system, causing disturbances of thought or behavior. Mental illnesses can be caused by genetic, metabolic, structural, viral, bacterial, or environmental causes. The term mental illness is also used to describe emotional disturbances caused by traumatic or distressing events or by poor adjustment to normal life stresses. Treatment depends on the root cause of the illness and may include use of medication, surgery (as in the case of brain tumors and some types of epilepsy), and various forms of therapy to help patients rebuild life skills.

mental retardation   The condition of having an IQ measured as below 70 to 75 and significant delays or lacks in at least two areas of adaptive skills. Mental retardation is present from childhood. Between 2 and 3 percent of the general population meet the criteria for mental retardation. Causes of mental retardation include fetal alcohol syndrome and fetal alcohol effect; brain damage caused by the use of prescription or illegal drugs during pregnancy; brain injury and disease; and genetic disorders, such as Down syndrome and fragile X syndrome. Most people with mental retardation are mildly affected. These individuals have an IQ over 50 and are usually able to work, care for themselves, and live independently. About 13 percent require more intensive help as adults. Treatment of mental retardation depends on the underlying cause. In some cases, such as phenylketonuria and congenital hypothyroidism, special diets or medical treatments can help. In all cases, special education starting as early in infancy as possible can help people with mental retardation maximize their abilities.

mental retardation, aphasia, shuffling gait, and adducted thumbs syndrome   See *MASA syndrome.*

mesentery   In general, a fold of tissue that attaches organs to the body wall. The word mesentery usually refers to the small bowel mesentery, which anchors the small intestines to the back of the abdominal wall. Blood vessels, nerves, and lymphatics branch through the mesentery to supply the intestine. Other mesenteries exist to support the sigmoid colon, appendix, transverse colon, and portions of the ascending and descending colon.

mesoderm   The middle of the three primary germ cell layers (the other two being the ectoderm and endoderm) that make up a very young embryo. The mesoderm differentiates (specializes) to give rise to a number of tissues and structures, including bone, muscle, connective tissue, and the middle layer of the skin. Some cells in mesodermal tissues retain the capacity to differentiate in diverse directions. For example, some cells in the bone marrow (mesoderm) can become liver (endoderm). See also *differentiation; ectoderm; embryo; endoderm.*

mesodermal   Pertaining to the mesoderm or to tissues derived from the mesoderm.

mesothelioma   A malignant tumor of the mesothelium, the thin lining of the surface of the body cavities and the organs that are contained within them. Most mesotheliomas begin as one or more nodules that progressively grow to form a solid coating of tumor surrounding the lung, abdominal organs, or heart. Mesothelioma occurs most commonly in the chest cavity and is associated with exposure to asbestos in up to 90 percent of cases. It has been shown that some inhaled asbestos fibers quickly work their way through the lung tissue and into the chest (pleural) cavity. Asbestos fibers that are swallowed can penetrate the wall of the intestine and appear in the abdominal (peritoneal) cavity. The risk of mesothelioma increases with the intensity and duration of exposure to asbestos. Family members and others living with asbestos workers may also have an increased risk of developing mesothelioma and possibly other asbestos-related diseases. This risk may be the result of exposure to asbestos dust brought home on the clothing and hair of asbestos workers. Mesothelioma is currently difficult to treat in most cases, and survival beyond 2 years is unusual.

messenger RNA   The key intermediary in gene expression, which translates the DNA's genetic code into the amino acids that make up proteins. Abbreviated mRNA.

metabolic disease   A genetic disorder of biochemistry, such as albinism, cystinuria, phenylketonuria (PKU), and some forms of gout, sun sensitivity, and thyroid disease. There are hundreds of known metabolic diseases, and there are surely many more yet to be discovered. Advances in the diagnosis and treatment of metabolic diseases have improved the outlook for many of these conditions so that early diagnosis, if possible in infancy, can be helpful. Many metabolic diseases cause infants to have symptoms such as sluggishness (lethargy), poor feeding, apnea (stopping breathing) or tachypnea (fast breathing), and recurrent vomiting. Any infant with these findings, particularly a full-term infant, should be seen immediately by a physician. Laboratory testing for metabolic disorders might include specific blood tests for known conditions or general tests that indicate metabolic problems. General indicators include hypoglycemia (low blood sugar), which is the predominant finding in a number of metabolic diseases , and jaundice (yellowing) or other evidence of liver disease, which is a sign of another important group of inborn errors of metabolism. Specific patterns of birth defects characterize yet another group of inherited metabolic disorders. The great number, complexity, and varied features of metabolic diseases would fill a large book if each were considered in any detail. Although most of these disorders are individually rare, together they represent a major source of human disease and suffering. Also known as inborn error of metabolism.

metabolic rate, basal   See *basal metabolic rate.*

metabolism   The whole range of biochemical processes that occur within a living organism. Metabolism consists of anabolism (the buildup of substances) and catabolism (the breakdown of substances). The term metabolism is commonly used to refer specifically to the breakdown of food and its transformation into energy.

metabolism, inborn error of   See *metabolic disease.*

metacarpal   One of the five cylindrical bones that extend from the wrist to the fingers.

metaphase chromosome   A chromosome in the stage of its cell life in which it is most condensed and easiest to see separately. Because metaphase chromosomes are easier to study than others, they are often chosen for karyotyping and chromosome analysis.

metastases, meningeal   See *meningitis, neoplastic.*

metastasis   **1** The spread of cancerous cells from one part of the body to another. The cells may be carried by the lymphatic system or in the blood. Cells that have metastasized are like those in the original (primary) tumor. For example, if the cancer begins in the stomach and spreads to the pancreas, the cancer cells in the pancreas are stomach cancer cells.   **2** A tumor that is spreading via metastasis. The plural of metastasis is metastases.

metastasize   The process cancer cells go through in spreading from one part of the body to another. See also *metastasis.*

metatarsal   One of the five cylindrical bones that extend from the heel to the toes.

methadone   A synthetic opiate. The most common medical use for methadone is as a legal substitute for heroin in treatment programs for drug addiction.

methemoglobin   A form of hemoglobin that is incapable of carrying oxygen. Sometimes found in the blood after certain poisonings, such as with acetanilid or potassium chlorate.

methimazole   An antithyroid medication (brand name: Tapazol) that is prescribed to treat hyperthyroidism. Also known as thiamazole.

methotrexate   An anti-inflammatory drug (brand names: Rheumatrex, Trexall) that is used to treat rheumatoid arthritis, severe psoriasis, reactive arthritis, and severe asthma. In high doses it is also used as a part of cancer chemotherapy programs. Methotrexate is an effective but potentially dangerous medication. People taking methotrexate must have their lung, liver, and kidney function monitored regularly, and they need blood testing to be done frequently as well. Methotrexate interacts dangerously, and potentially fatally, with many other medications, including prescription and over-the-counter nonsteroidal anti-inflammatory drugs, even aspirin and ibuprofen. Folic acid supplements are sometimes used to counteract side effects of methotrexate. Methotrexate should be taken on an empty stomach.

metrorrhagia   Uterine bleeding at irregular intervals, particularly between periods. Metrorrhagia can cause significant anemia. It may also be a sign of underlying disease, such as hormone disorder, uterine fibroids, or cancer of the uterus. See also *menometrorrhagia; menorrhagia.*

MHC   Major histocompatability complex.

MI   Myocardial infarction. See *heart attack.*

micro-   Prefix meaning small, as in microcephaly (small head) and microsomia (small body). The opposite of micro- is macro-.

microangiopathy   A disease of the capillaries (very small blood vessels), in which the capillary walls become so thick and weak that they bleed, leak protein, and slow the flow of blood. For example, diabetics may develop microangiopathy in many areas, including the eye.

microbe   A minute organism. Microbes include bacteria, fungi, and protozoan parasites, and they are best seen with a microscope.

microcephaly   An abnormally small head due to failure of brain growth. Microcephaly is an ominous sign because it is almost always associated with developmental delay and mental retardation. The reason the head is abnormally small is that the brain does not grow enough to cause the skull to enlarge. Many factors can impair the growth of the brain, including intrauterine infections (such as rubella, cytomegalovirus, and toxoplasmosis), intrauterine chemical exposure (such as in fetal alcohol syndrome), excessive radiation exposure (as in an atomic bomb explosion), chromosome abnormalities (such as trisomy 13 and trisomy 18), and genetic syndromes (such as Fanconi syndrome and Williams syndrome). The opposite of microcephaly is macrocephaly.

microcystic corneal dystrophy   See *Cogan corneal dystrophy.*

microcytic   Literally, referring to any abnormally small cell; in practice, referring to an abnormally small red blood cell. For example, microcytic anemia is characterized by small red blood cells. The opposite of microcytic is macrocytic.

microdeletion Loss of a tiny piece—a piece that may be too small to be seen readily through a microscope—from a chromosome. Microdeletions can be detected via high-resolution chromosome banding, molecular chromosome analysis (with FISH), or DNA analysis. Disorders caused by microdeletions include Angelman, DiGeorge, Prader-Willi, and Williams syndromes.

microhematuria See *blood in the urine.*

microorchidism Abnormally small testes. To determine if the testes are too small, a device called an orchidometer is used that permits a testis to be compared to a series of plastic ovals (like miniature American footballs) of differing sizes. Microorchidism is a diagnostic feature, for example, of Prader-Willi syndrome and certain other multiple malformation syndromes. Microorchidism may also result from shrinkage (atrophy) of the testis due to damage, as from mumps. The opposite of microorchidism is macroorchidism. See also *micropenis.*

micropenis An abnormally small penis. In medical practice, the dimension of the penis that is measured is the length. The measurement is taken along the upper surface of the shaft of the penis to the tip, using a measuring tape or, preferably, a ruler. The ruler is pressed firmly into the soft tissue over the pubic bone (the symphysis pubis) because in obese boys and men, a seemingly small penis may be partly engulfed by the fat pad at its base and actually be normal in length. Normal standards are available for penis length. True micropenis may reflect failure of normal hormonal stimulation or failure of normal development (a birth defect). See also *microorchidism.*

microphallus See *micropenis.*

microphthalmia An abnormally small eye. Microphthalmia is a congenital malformation of the globe, a birth defect of the eye. A related term, anophthalmia, indicates that there is no eye at all. Also known as microphthalmos.

microscope An optical instrument that augments the power of the eye to see small objects. Most optical microscopes today are compound microscopes.

microscope, compound A microscope that consists of two microscopes in series, the first serving as the ocular lens (close to the eye), and the second serving as the objective lens (close to the object to be viewed).

microscope, electron A microscope in which an electron beam replaces light to form the image. Electron microscopy (EM) has both pluses (greater magnification and resolution than optical microscopes) and minuses (you are not really "seeing" objects, but rather their electron densities, so artifacts may abound).

microscope, fluorescent A microscope that is equipped to examine material that fluoresces under ultraviolet (UV) light.

microscope, simple A microscope that has a single converging lens.

microscopic Too small to be seen without the aid of a microscope, as opposed to macroscopic. For example, a microscopic tumor is too small to be seen without a microscpe.

microscopic anatomy See *anatomy, microscopic.*

microsomia A body that is too small. A child with microsomia has significant undergrowth.

micturate To urinate.

micturition Urination; the act of urinating.

micturition syncope The temporary loss of consciousness upon urinating. See also *syncope; vasovagal reaction.*

middle ear See *ear, middle.*

middle ear infection See *otitis media.*

midwife A trained person who assists women during childbirth. Many midwives also provide prenatal care for pregnant women, birth education for women and their partners, and care for mothers and newborn babies after the birth. Depending on local law, midwives may deliver babies in the mother's home, in a birthing center or clinic, or in a hospital. Most midwives specialize in normal, uncomplicated deliveries, referring women with health problems that could require hospitalization during birth to a hospital-based obstetrician. Others work with physicians as part of a team. Legal qualifications required to practice midwifery differ among the US states and various countries.

midwife assistant A person who assists a midwife with prenatal care, childbirth education, delivery, and postnatal care. Also known as doula and labor assistant.

midwife, certified A midwife who has been certified by his or her state or national agency for credentialing midwives.

midwife, certified nurse A person with an associate's, bachelor's, or master's degree in nursing who has also completed specialized training in midwifery. Abbreviated CNM. In the US, CNMs must earn certification from the American College of Nurse Midwives.

midwife, certified professional A midwife who has completed a degree in midwifery at a credentialed educational institution. Abbreviated CPM.

migraine Usually, periodic attacks of headaches on one or both sides of the head that may be accompanied by nausea, vomiting, increased sensitivity of the eyes to light (photophobia), increased sensitivity to sound (phonophobia), dizziness, blurred vision, cognitive disturbances, and other symptoms. Some migraines do not include headache, and migraines may or may not be preceded by auras.

migraine, abdominal An attack of abdominal pain that may be preceded by a migraine aura and accompanied by nausea, vomiting, and cognitive disturbance.

migraine aura A sensory phenomenon that may occur before a migraine. Visual auras may include flashing lights, geometric patterns, or distorted vision. Some people may have aural auras that involve hearing sounds (usually buzzing) that are not actually present, olfactory auras that involve smelling odors that are not actually present, or tactile auras that appear as premonitory physical sensations. Auras are caused by unusual activity in the brain. The auras experienced by migraine sufferers are similar to those associated with epilepsy.

migraine, classic A migraine with an aura. Such migraines account for no more than 20 percent of migraines. See also *migraine*.

migraine, common A migraine without an aura. This is the most frequent type of migraine, accounting for about 80 to 85 percent of migraines. See also *migraine*.

migraine headache The most common type of vascular headache, thought to be caused by abnormal sensitivity of arteries in the brain to various triggers that result in arterial spasms. Other arteries in the brain and scalp then open, and throbbing pain is perceived in the head. The tendency to migraine is inherited and appears to involve serotonin. This brain chemical (neurotransmitter) is involved in the transmission of nerve impulses that trigger the release of substances in the blood vessels. These nerve impulses cause the flashing lights and other sensory phenomena, known as auras, that may accompany migraines. Not all severe headaches are migraines and not all migraines are severe. Factors known to make migraines worse in some patients include stress, food sensitivities, menstruation, and the onset of menopause. Most patients feel better if they lie down and avoid bright lights. Preventive measures can include taking preventive medication (usually an antispasmodic) and avoiding any known migraine triggers. Medication that can ease the pain of a current migraine is also available. See also *headache; headache, vascular*.

migraine, ocular A migraine involving the eyes, with or without headache. An ocular migraine usually affects only one eye at a time. Image distortion generally begins in the center of the image and then moves to one side. Images "gray out" or look wavy, and sight may be lost temporarily. See also *migraine, ophthalmic*.

migraine, ophthalmic A migraine involving the eyes but without headache. Flashes of light may appear as jagged lines or "heat waves" in one or both eyes. Ophthalmic migraines often last 10 to 20 minutes.

migrainous neuralgia See *cluster headache*.

miliary aneurysm A tiny aneurysm. Miliary aneurysms tend to affect minute arteries in the brain or in the retina of the eye. They can bleed and lead to impaired function of the brain or eye.

miliary tuberculosis The presence of numerous sites of tuberculosis infection, each of which is minute, due to dissemination of infected material through the bloodstream in a process somewhat like the metastasis of a malignancy.

milk teeth See *primary teeth*.

mineralocorticoid A group of hormones that regulate the balance of water and electrolytes (ions such as sodium and potassium) in the body. The mineralocorticoid hormones act on the tubules of the kidney. The most important mineralocorticoid hormone is aldosterone.

minor In general, something that is less than something else. For example, the teres minor muscle is smaller than the teres major muscle.

minor salivary gland A small gland that produces saliva. The mouth and palate contain numerous minor salivary glands.

minoxidil A medication (brand names: Loniten, Rogaine) that was originally developed to treat high blood pressure as an oral medication and is now also prescribed in lotion form to promote hair growth. Side effects of the oral form can include increased heart rate, edema, and nausea. Side effects of the lotion are itching or irritation of the scalp.

miosis Contraction of the pupil. The opposite of miosis is mydriasis.

miscarriage Inadvertent loss of a pregnancy before the fetus is viable. A considerable proportion of pregnancies end in miscarriage. Also known as spontaneous abortion.

miscarriages, multiple More than one miscarriage for a woman. In multiple miscarriages, there is about a

5 percent chance that one member of the couple is carrying a chromosome translocation that is responsible for the miscarriages. Other causes of multiple miscarriage include Rh incompatibility, exposure to toxic substances that harmed the embryo, and physical problems in the mother that make it difficult for her to carry a fetus to term, such as antiphospholipid syndrome.

missense mutation   A genetic change that results in the substitution of one amino acid in protein for another. A missense mutation is responsible for sickle hemoglobin, the molecular basis of sickle cell trait and sickle cell anemia.

mite-borne typhus   See *typhus, scrub.*

mitochondria   Structures located in the cell's cytoplasm outside the nucleus. Mitochondria are responsible for energy production. Each consists of two sets of membranes: a smooth, continuous outer coat and an inner membrane arranged in tubules or in folds that form plate-like double membranes (cristae). The mitochrondria are the principal energy source of the cell. They not only convert nutrients into energy but also perform many other specialized tasks. Each mitochondrion has a chromosome that is made of DNA but is otherwise quite different from the better-known chromosomes in the nucleus. The mitochondrial chromosome is much smaller than other chromosomes. It is round, whereas the chromosomes in the nucleus are shaped like rods. There are many copies of the mitochondrial chromosome in every cell, whereas there is normally only one set of chromosomes in the nucleus. All mitochondrial chromosomes are inherited from the mother.

mitochondrial   Referring to mitochondria.

mitochondrial disease   A mutation in the mitochondrial chromosome that is responsible for a disease. Known mitochondrial diseases include the eye disease Leber hereditary optic atrophy; myoclonus epilepsy with ragged red fibers (MERRF); and mitochondrial encephalopathy, lactic acidosis, and stroke-like episodes syndrome (MELAS syndrome).

mitochondrial DNA   The DNA of the mitochondria. Abbreviated mtDNA. There are 2 to 10 copies of the mtDNA genome in each mitochondrion. The mtDNA molecule is double-stranded and circular. It is very small compared to the chromosomes in the nucleus, and so it contains only a limited number of genes. It is specialized in the information it carries, and it encodes a number of the subunits in the mitochondrial respiratory-chain complex that the cell needs in order to respire. It also contains genes for some ribosomal RNAs and transfer RNAs. Mutations in mtDNA can cause disease. These mutations often impair the function of oxidative-phosphorylation

enzymes in the respiratory chain. This is especially manifest in tissues with a high energy expenditure, such as those of the brain and muscle. All mtDNA comes from the oocyte at fertilization. Therefore, inherited mtDNA mutations are transmitted from the mother to both male and female offspring. The higher the level of mutant mtDNA in the mother's blood, the higher the frequency of clinically affected offspring and the more severely the children tend to be affected. Each cell in the body contains different mtDNA populations. Due to the presence of multiple mitochondria in cells, each cell contains several mtDNA copies. This produces tissue variation, so a mutation in mtDNA versus normal mtDNA can vary widely among tissues in an individual. Accordingly, the percentage of mutant mtDNA must be above a certain threshold to produce clinical disease. The threshold varies from tissue to tissue because the percentage of mutant mDNAs needed to cause cell dysfunction varies according to the oxidative requirements of the tissue.

Mitochondrial encephalopathy, lactic acidosis, and stroke-like episodes   See *MELAS syndrome.*

mitochondrial encephalopathy, MELAS   See *MELAS syndrome.*

mitochondrial genome   See *genome, mitochondrial.*

mitochondrial inheritance   See *inheritance, mitochondrial.*

mitochondrial myopathy   A form of muscle disease that leads to progressive muscle weakness. More than 25 types of enzyme abnormalities have been defined that fall into this category. They result in a disease of cell metabolism and are defined via a biopsy of muscle tissue that shows ragged red fibers under microscopic examination.

mitochondrion   Singular of mitochondria.

mitosis   The ordinary division of a body cell (a somatic cell) to form two daughter cells, each with the same chromosome complement as the parent cell.

mitotic   Pertaining to mitosis.

mitotic nondisjunction   The failure in mitosis for the two members of a chromosome pair to separate (to disjoin) normally so that both chromosomes go to one daughter cell while none go to the other daughter cell. See also *mitosis.*

mitral insufficiency   Malfunction of the mitral valve, which permits the backflow of blood (regurgitation) from the left ventricle into the left atrium. Most mitral insufficiency is mild and requires no treatment. When severe, however, treatment with medications and sometimes surgery is necessary.

mitral prolapse See *mitral valve prolapse.*

mitral regurgitation Backflow of blood from the left ventricle to the left atrium due to mitral valve insufficiency.

mitral valve A valve in the heart that is situated between the left atrium and the left ventricle. The mitral valve permits blood to flow from the left atrium into the left ventricle, but not in the reverse direction. The mitral valve has two flaps (cusps). It is so named because it looks like a bishop's miter (headdress). Also known as bicuspid valve.

mitral valve, aorta, skeleton, and skin syndrome See *MASS syndrome.*

mitral valve prolapse Drooping down or abnormal bulging of the mitral valve's cusps during the contraction of the heart.

mittelschmerz Pain due to ovulation that usually occurs at the midpoint between the menstrual periods. From the German *mittel,* meaning "middle," and *schmerz,* meaning "pain."

mixed connective tissue disease A mixture of three diseases of connective tissue (the framework for the cells of the body): systemic lupus erythematosus, scleroderma, and polymyositis. Patients with mixed connective tissue disease typically have features of each of these three component diseases. They also typically have very high blood levels of antinuclear antibodies (ANAs) and antibodies to ribonucleoprotein (anti-RNP). The symptoms often eventually become dominated by features of one of the three component illnesses, most commonly scleroderma. The treatment for mixed connective tissue disease depends on which features are causing symptoms. Treatment is often directed at suppressing the inflammation in the tissues by using anti-inflammatory and immunosuppressive medications. These medications include nonsteroidal anti-inflammatory drugs, cortisone drugs/steroids (such as prednisone), and cytotoxic drugs (such as methotrexate, azathioprine, and cyclophosphamide). Organ damage, such as to the kidneys, can require additional specific treatment.

mixed mania A state of mind that is characterized by symptoms of both mania and depression and is seen in bipolar disorders. Mixed mania is more common in bipolar children and women than in men. A person experiencing mixed mania may feel agitated, angry, irritable, and depressed all at once. Because it combines a high activity level with depression, mixed mania poses a particular danger of suicide or self-injury. Treatment involves use of mood-stabilizing medication, sometimes accompanied by antidepressant or neuroleptic medication. Also known as

agitated depression. See also *bipolar disorder; depression; mania.*

MMR Measles, mumps, rubella vaccine, a combination vaccine.

MND Motor neuron disease.

modifiers, biological response See *biological response modifiers.*

Mohs surgery A type of surgery that is used for the treatment of skin cancer, especially basal cell or squamous cell carcinoma of the skin. Mohs surgery is designed to remove all the cancerous tissue while removing as little of the healthy tissue as possible. This type of surgery is especially helpful when the physician is not sure of the shape and depth of a tumor. In addition, this method is used to remove large tumors, tumors in hard-to-treat places, and cancers that have recurred. Mohs surgery is microscopically controlled. The area of skin is removed under local anesthetic and is then carefully oriented and serially examined under a microscope to ensure that all of the tumor has been removed. If the tumor has not all been removed, the procedure is repeated until the entire tumor is removed.

molar 1 One of the large teeth at the back of the mouth. The molars are well adapted to grinding. 2 Relating to or associated with a mass within the uterus that is formed by degeneration of partly developed products of conception.

molar pregnancy See *hydatidiform mole.*

mold One of a large group of fungi that can proliferate on food or in moist areas. Household mold is a common trigger for allergies.

mole 1 A pigmented spot on the skin. A type of nevus. 2 A mass within the uterus that is formed by partly developed products of conception.

mole, hydatidiform See *hydatidiform mole.*

molecule The smallest unit of a substance that can exist alone and retain the character of that substance.

molecules, recombinant DNA A combination of DNA molecules of different origin that are joined by using recombinant DNA technology.

Mollaret meningitis See *meningitis, Mollaret.*

mongolism See *Down syndrome.*

monilia A yeast-like fungus that is now known as Candida. See also *Candida albicans; candidiasis.*

monitor, Holter See *Holter monitor.*

mono **1** Abbreviation for infectious mononucleosis. See *mononucleosis.* **2** Prefix meaning one or single, as in monochromatic (one color) and monoclonal (derived from a single cell).

monoamine oxydase See *MAO.*

monoarticular Involving just one joint, as opposed to polyarticular.

monochromat A person with one of the many forms of colorblindness. See also *colorblindness.*

monochromatism **1** Total inability to perceive color due to the lack of or damage to the cones of the eye that perceive color, or the inability of the nerves to translate information received from the cones. A person with true monochromatism perceives only black, white, and shades of gray. Complete monochromatism is usually an inherited condition. **2** One of the many types of colorblindness that affects perception of certain colors only. See also *colorblindness.*

monoclonal Derived from a single cell and cells identical to that cell.

monoclonal antibody An antibody produced by a single clone of cells. A monoclonal antibody is therefore a single pure type of antibody. Monoclonal antibodies can be made in large quantities in the laboratory and are a cornerstone of immunology. Monoclonal antibodies are increasingly coming into use as therapeutic agents.

monocyte A white blood cell that has a single nucleus and can take in (ingest) foreign material.

mononeuritis Inflammation of a single nerve. The many causes of mononeuritis include diabetes mellitus, carpal tunnel syndrome, rheumatoid arthritis, and Lyme disease. The treatment for mononeuritis depends on the underlying cause. See also *mononeuritis multiplex.*

mononeuritis multiplex Inflammation of two or more nerves, typically in unrelated parts of the body. Mononeuritis multiplex causes a loss of function in the muscle tissue that is innervated by the affected nerves. For example, sudden loss of the ability to lift the foot normally while walking (foot drop) can be caused by mononeuritis multiplex, when it is accompanied by loss of nerve function elsewhere in the body. There are many causes of mononeuritis multiplex, including diabetes mellitus; infections, such as AIDS, Lyme disease, and leprosy; sarcoidosis; and connective tissue diseases, such as rheumatoid

arthritis, systemic lupus erythematosus, vasculitis, Churg-Strauss syndrome, cryoglobulinemia, and Sjogren syndrome. The treatment for mononeuritis multiplex depends on the underlying cause.

mononucleosis Chronic infection with the Epstein-Barr virus (EBV, human herpesvirus 4 [HHV-4]) in which there is an increase of white blood cells that have a single nucleus (monocytes). The infection can be spread by saliva. Its incubation period is 4 to 8 weeks. Symptoms include fever, fatigue, sore throat, and swollen lymph glands. Mononucleosis can cause liver inflammation (hepatitis) and spleen enlargement; a person with mononucleosis should avoid vigorous contact sports to prevent spleen rupture. It is less severe in young children than in others. Most people exposed to EBV do not develop mononucleosis; most adults carry an antibody against EBV in their blood, which means they have been infected with EBV at some time. Treatment includes rest, pain medication, and in some cases antiviral medication. Also known as mono and the kissing disease. See also *Epstein-Barr virus.*

monosomy Missing one chromosome from a pair. For example, if a female has one X chromosome (X monosomy) rather than two, she has Turner syndrome.

monostotic fibrous dysplasia Excessive growth in a single bone of hard-fibrous tissue that replaces the normal bone tissue. Symptoms of monostotic fibrous dysplasia may include pain and fracture of the bone. Most cases are diagnosed in adolescence or young adulthood and remain unchanged throughout life. The outlook is usually very good. Monostotic fibrous dysplasia appears to be a different disorder from polyostotic fibrous dysplasia.

monozygous twins Identical twins. They are called monozygous because they originate from a single fertilized egg (zygote).

morbidity Illness, disease.

morbilli See *measles.*

morgue A place where dead bodies are kept before autopsy, funeral, or burial.

morning sickness The common phenomenon of nausea between the 6th and 12th weeks of pregnancy. Symptoms include nausea and vomiting. Morning sickness is believed to be caused by hormonal changes and metabolic changes that involve carbohydrate digestion. Suggested treatment includes eating crackers or other high-carbohydrate foods first thing in the morning (even before getting out of bed); eating small, frequent meals; drinking extra fluids between meals; and avoiding fatty foods. If morning sickness is extreme enough to lead to weight loss during pregnancy, the condition is termed hyperemesis gravidarum, and it requires immediate medical treatment. See also *hyperemesis gravidarum*.

morning-after pill See *contraceptive, emergency*.

morphine A powerful narcotic agent that has strong analgesic (pain relief) action and other significant effects on the central nervous system. It is dangerously addicting. Morphine is a naturally occurring member of a large chemical class of compounds called alkaloids. The name, which derives from Morpheus (the mythologic god of dreams) was coined in 1805 by German apothecary Adolf Serturner to designate the main alkaloid in opium. Opium comes from the poppy plant.

morphology 1 Literally, the study of form (structure). 2 A form itself.

Morquio syndrome A form of mucopolysaccharidosis that is characterized by an inability to break down keratin sulfate, which leads to abnormal accumulation of keratin sulfate in muscle and skeletal tissues. This in turn can lead to abnormalities of the skeleton, muscles, skin, teeth, and muscular organs. Diagnosis is made by examining leukocytes and cultured skin fibroblasts or by checking urine for high levels of keratin sulfate. There is currently no treatment for Morquio syndrome, but physical therapy, medication, and sometimes surgery can reduce discomfort and enhance the patient's ability to move. Morquio syndrome is inherited in an autosomal recessive manner. Also known as mucopolysaccharidosis type IV (MPS4). See also *mucopolysaccharidosis*.

mortality 1 The condition of being mortal, of eventually having to die. The opposite of mortality is immortality. 2 The rate of death.

mortality rate, fetal See *fetal mortality rate*.

mortality rate, infant See *infant mortality rate*.

mortality rate, maternal See *maternal mortality rate*.

mortality rate, neonatal See *neonatal mortality rate*.

mosaic A person or a tissue that contains two or more types of genetically different cells. All females are mosaics because of X-chromosome inactivation (lyonization). Mosaic patterns can affect the way genetic disorders are expressed. For example, about 5 percent of people with Down syndrome have a mosaic variant in which only some cells have an extra chromosome 21. Compared to others with Down syndrome, these individuals have fewer clinical symptoms, are more likely to have a normal IQ, and are less likely to have heart and other problems that can be associated with Down syndrome.

mother 1 The female parent. 2 To produce offspring as a female, to attribute the maternity of. 3 A cell or another structure from which similar cells or structures are formed. Such a cell might be referred to as the mother cell. 4 To provide maternal protection, guidance, and nurturing to a child or children.

motility study, antro-duodenal A study for detecting and recording the contractions of the muscles of the stomach and the first part of the small intestine (the duodenum). An antro-duodenal motility study is performed to diagnose problems in the way the muscles of the stomach and small intestine are working. To conduct the study, a tube is passed through the nose, throat, esophagus, and stomach until the tip of the tube lies in the small intestine. The tube senses when the muscles of the stomach and small intestine contract and squeeze the tube tightly. The contractions are recorded for analysis by a computer.

motion, range of See *range of motion*.

motion sickness A disorder of the sense of balance and equilibrium and, hence, the sense of spatial orientation that is caused by repeated motion such as from the swell of the sea, the movement of a car, or the motion of a plane in turbulent air. Motion sickness is due to irritation of a portion of the inner ear called the labyrinth. The symptoms of motion sickness include nausea, vomiting, and vertigo. Other common signs of motion sickness are sweating and a general feeling of discomfort and not feeling well (malaise). Symptoms usually stop when the motion that causes it ceases. However, some people suffer symptoms for even a few days after the trip is over.

motor Something that produces or refers to motion. For example, a motor neuron is a nerve cell that conveys an impulse to a muscle for contraction, which then moves a joint.

motor neuron disease A group of related diseases of the nervous system that are characterized by steadily progressive deterioration of the motor neurons in the brain, brainstem, and spinal cord. Abbreviated MND. Motor neurons are the nerve cells along which the brain sends instructions, in the form of electrical impulses, to the muscles. The degeneration of motor neurons leads to weakness and wasting of muscles. MND usually first affects the arms or legs. Then shoulders and other muscles may be affected. Weakness and wasting in the muscles of the face and throat may cause problems with speech, chewing, and swallowing. MND does not affect touch, taste, sight, smell, or hearing, nor does it directly affect bladder, bowel, or sexual function. In the vast majority of cases, the intellect remains unchanged. Subtypes of MND are distinguished by the major site of degeneration of the motor neurons—for example, amyotrophic lateral sclerosis (Lou Gehrig's disease), progressive spinal muscular atrophy, progressive bulbar palsy, and primary lateral sclerosis.

mountain sickness   See *altitude sickness.*

mouth, trench   See *acute membranous gingivitis.*

movement, fetal   See *fetal movement.*

MPH   Master of public health, a degree designating successful training in analyzing past, present, and future public health issues.

MPS   **1** Mucopolysaccharidosis.   **2** Myofascial pain syndrome.

MPS1   Mucopolysaccharidosis type I. See *Hurler syndrome.*

MPS2   Mucopolysaccharidosis type II. See *Hunter syndrome.*

MPS3   Mucopolysaccharidosis type III. See *Sanfilippo syndrome.*

MPS4   Mucopolysaccharidosis type IV. See *Morquios syndrome.*

MRC   **1** Medical Research Council.   **2** Medical Reserve Corps.

MRI   Magnetic resonance imaging.

mRNA   Messenger RNA.

MS   Multiple sclerosis.

MSAFP   Maternal serum alpha-fetoprotein.

MSUD   Maple syrup urine disease.

mtDNA   Mitochondrial DNA.

mucocutaneous lymph node syndrome   See *Kawasaki disease.*

mucolipidosis   One of a group of storage diseases in which both lipids and substances called mucopolysaccharides accumulate in the tissues of the body. Four different mucolipidoses have been identified, numbered I through IV. All four are lysosomal disorders—that is, the lysomes are organelles within the cell that contain enzymes that can digest (lyse) substances—and all are inherited in an autosomal recessive manner.

mucolipidosis I   A type of mucolipidosis that is characterized by deficiency of the enzyme neuraminidase (sialidase). There are two forms of the disease. One form is characterized by cherry red spots in the eyes, gradual loss of vision, progressive debilitating myoclonus (muscle spasms), and normal intelligence. The other form of the disease, in addition to featuring the symptoms of the first form, causes a coarse face, bony abnormalities, and sometimes early death. Also known as sialidosis.

mucolipidosis II   See *I-cell disease.*

mucolipidosis III   A type of mucolipidosis that is characterized by deficiency of the enzyme N-acetylglucosamine-1-phosphotransferase and features of Hurler syndrome, but with much slower progression. Also known as pseudo-Hurler polydystrophy.

mucolipidosis IV   A type of mucolipidosis that is due to mutation in the gene that encoded mucolipin-1. Most patients with mucolipidosis IV have developmental delay, mental retardation, clouding of the cornea of the eye, and severe visual impairment.

mucopolysaccharidosis   One of several inherited metabolic disorders that affect carbohydrate use by the body. Abbreviated MPS. Substances derived from carbohydrates that are called mucopolysacchardes, or glycosaminoglycans (GAGs), accumulate in body tissues because the body lacks the specific enzymes needed to metabolize or digest them. This accumulation damages and distorts tissues, stunts growth, limits muscle and joint movement, and may cause mental retardation. MPS is believed to occur in about 1 in every 25,000 births. It usually becomes obvious in early childhood and leads to death before middle age. There are currently no treatments available for any form of MPS, although enzyme replacement therapies are being researched and bone-marrow transplants have been tried on patients with MPS type I (Hurler syndrome) with some limited success. See also *Hunter syndrome; Hurler syndrome; Maroteaux-Lamy syndrome; Morquio syndrome; Sanfilippo syndrome.*

mucopolysaccharidosis type I   Also known as Hurler syndrome, Scheie syndrome, and Hurler-Scheie syndrome. See also *Hurler syndrome.*

mucopolysaccharidosis type II   See *Hunter syndrome.*

mucopolysaccharidosis type III   See *Sanfilippo syndrome.*

mucopolysaccharidosis type IV   See *Morquio syndrome.*

mucopolysaccharidosis type VI See *Maroteaux-Lamy syndrome.*

mucosa Having to do with a mucous membrane. For example, the oral mucosa is the mucous membrane that lines the mouth and throat.

mucositis Inflammation of the mucous membranes lining the digestive tract from the mouth to the anus. Mucositis is a common side effect of chemotherapy and of radiotherapy that involves any part of the digestive tract. Mucositis affects the rapidly dividing mucosal cells that line the mouth, throat, stomach, and intestines, which normally have a short lifespan. If a therapy destroys these cells, they may not be replaced right away, in which case mucositis results. A person with mucositis may have raw sores (ulcers) in the mouth and throat and feel like he or she has a a sunburn in the throat.

mucous Pertaining to mucus, a thick fluid produced by the lining of some tissues of the body.

mucoviscidosis See *cystic fibrosis.*

mucus A thick fluid that is produced by the lining of some organs of the body.

multifactorial In medicine, referring to multiple factors in heredity or disease. For example, traits and conditions that are caused by more than one gene occurring together are multifactorial, and diseases that are caused by more than one factor interacting (for example, heredity and diet in diabetes) are multifactorial.

multifactorial inheritance A hereditary pattern seen when more than one genetic factor is involved in the causation of a condition. Many common traits and many common diseases are inherited in a multifactorial manner.

multi-infarct dementia Dementia that is brought on by a series of strokes.

multipara A woman who has had two or more pregnancies resulting in potentially viable offspring. The term para refers to births. A para III has had three such pregnancies; a para VI or more is also known as a grand multipara.

multiparous 1 Having two or more offspring at one birth. 2 Related to a multipara. See also *uniparous.*

multiple enchondromatosis A condition characterized by benign masses of cartilage, called enchondromas, growing within bones. The enchondromas tend to be in the bones of the hands and feet and the long bones of the arms and legs. They can cause pain, deform and shorten a limb, and predispose a person to fractures. This disorder is caused in at least some, if not all, cases by mutation in the gene for the parathyroid hormone receptor (PTHR1). Surgery can help to correct limb-length inequality if it occurs. Also known as Ollier's disease.

multiple myeloma A bone marrow cancer that involves a type of white blood cell called a plasma (or myeloma) cell. The tumor cells in myeloma can form a single collection (plasmacytoma) or many tumors (multiple myeloma). Plasma cells are normally part of the immune system; they make antibodies. Because myeloma patients have an excess of identical plasma cells, they have too much of one type of antibody. As myeloma cells increase in number, they damage and weaken the bones, causing pain and often fractures. When bones are damaged, too much calcium is released into the blood, leading to loss of appetite, nausea, thirst, fatigue, muscle weakness, restlessness, and confusion. Myeloma cells prevent the bone marrow from forming normal plasma cells and other white blood cells that are important to the immune system, so patients with multiple myeloma may not be able to fight infections. Myeloma cells can also prevent the growth of new red blood cells in the marrow, causing anemia. Excess antibody proteins and calcium may prevent the kidneys from filtering and cleaning the blood properly. Also known as plasma cell myeloma and myeloma.

multiple personality disorder See *dissociative disorder.*

multiple sclerosis A disease that is characterized by loss of myelin (demyelinization). Abbreviated MS. Myelin, the coating of nerve fibers, is composed of lipids (fats) and protein. It serves as insulation and permits efficient nerve fiber conduction. In MS, demyelinization usually affects white matter in the brain, but sometimes it extends into the gray matter. When myelin is damaged, nerve fiber conduction is faulty or absent, and nerve cell death may occur. Impaired bodily functions or altered sensations associated with those demyelinated nerve fibers give rise to the symptoms of MS, which range from numbness to paralysis and blindness. People with MS experience attacks of symptoms that may last days, months, or longer. For many patients, the disease is progressive and leads to disablement, although some cases enter long, perhaps even permanent, remission. The cause of MS is unknown, although viral activity is suspected. Most patients are diagnosed between the ages of 20 and 40. Until recently, treatment had focused on preventing attacks. Steroids, interferon, and medications to treat specific symptoms (such as fatigue, depression, and vertigo) are standard, along with lifestyle changes to avoid stress and other triggers. New treatment options are under development, most of which involve immune system modulation or support. Some patients also use antiviral medications.

multiple symmetric lipomatosis See *lipomatosis, familial benign cervical.*

mumps An acute viral illness that is caused by the paramyxovirus and that usually presents with inflammation of the salivary glands, particularly the parotid glands. A child with mumps often looks like a chipmunk with a full mouth due to the swelling of the salivary glands near the ears. Mumps can also cause inflammation of other tissues, most frequently the covering and substance of the central nervous system (meningoencephalitis), the pancreas (pancreatitis), and, especially after adolescence, the ovaries (oophoritis) or the testes (orchitis). The mature testes are particularly susceptible to damage from mumps, which can lead to infertility. Mumps spreads easily through airborne particles of human saliva. Treatment involves rest and use of nonaspirin pain relievers to ease pain in swollen areas. Rarely, mumps can cause a form of meningitis, in which case hospitalization may be necessary. Mumps can be prevented via a vaccine. See also *meningitis; MMR; mumps immunization.*

mumps immunization A vaccination for mumps. Mumps immunization may be given individually, or together with the measles and rubella vaccines, in the MMR immunization. See also *MMR.*

mumps in pregnancy Mumps contracted in pregnancy, which can cause early miscarriage or birth defects. The most common birth defect associated with mumps is congenital deafness. Mumps vaccination is not recommended during or shortly before pregnancy because it is a live attenuated vaccine, so carries a risk of causing mumps infection.

Munchhausen by proxy A form of Munchhausen syndrome in which a parent feigns illness in a child. In some cases the parent is simply overanxious or poorly informed. In others, a misdirected desire for attention or psychiatric illness is the cause. In a very few cases, the parent actually causes the child's illness, as by injecting toxic substances. See also *Munchhausen syndrome.*

Munchhausen syndrome Recurrent feigning of catastrophic illnesses. Some patients with Munchhausen syndrome actually cause their own illness, as by secretly drinking or injecting substances. Munchhausen syndrome may be caused by a misdirected desire for attention, although in some cases it arises in actual psychiatric illness. It is named for the fictitious Baron Munchhausen, who told tall tales. See also *body dysmorphic disorder; hypochondria; Munchhausen by proxy.*

murine typhus See *typhus, murine.*

murmur, heart See *heart murmur.*

muscle The tissue of the body that functions primarily as a source of power. There are three types of muscle in the body: Muscle that is responsible for moving extremities and external areas of the body is called skeletal muscle, heart muscle is called cardiac muscle, and muscle in the walls of arteries and the bowel is called smooth muscle. See also *cardiac muscle; skeletal muscle; smooth muscle.*

muscle, abdominal See *abdominal muscle.*

muscle, abductor Any muscle that pushes away from the midline of the body. For example, the abductor muscles of the arms allow the arms to be raised from one's sides. Abductor muscles are opposed by adductor muscles. To keep these similar-sounding terms straight, medical students learn to speak of "A B ductors" versus "A D ductors."

muscle, adductor Any muscle that pulls inward toward the midline of the body. For example, the adductor muscles of the leg serve to pull the legs together. Adductor muscles are opposed by abductor muscles. To keep these similar-sounding terms straight, medical students learn to speak of "A B ductors" versus "A D ductors."

muscle, central core disease of See *central core disease of muscle.*

muscle, infraspinatus See *infraspinatus muscle.*

muscle, papillary A small muscle within the heart that anchors the heart valves. The anchor ropes are the chordae tendineae, thread-like bands of fibrous tissue that attach on one end to the edges of the tricuspid and mitral valves of the heart and on the other end to the papillary muscles.

muscle, piriformis A muscle that begins at the front surface of the sacrum (the V-shaped bone between the buttocks, at the base of the spine) and passes through the greater sciatic notch to attach to the top of the thighbone (femur) at its bony prominence (the greater trochanter). The gluteus maximus muscle covers the piriformis muscle in the buttocks.

muscle, subscapularis A muscle that moves the arm by turning it inward (internal rotation). The tendon of the subscapularis muscle is one of four tendons that stabilize the shoulder joint and constitute the rotator cuff.

muscle, supraspinatus A muscle that is responsible for elevating the arm and moving it away from the body. The tendon of the supraspinatus muscle is one of four tendons that stabilize the shoulder joint and constitute the rotator cuff.

muscle, teres minor   A muscle that assists in the lifting of the arm during outward turning (external rotation) of the arm. The tendon of the teres minor muscle is one of four tendons that stabilize the shoulder joint and constitute the rotator cuff.

muscular   Having to do with muscles or endowed with above-average muscle development. For example, the muscular system is all the muscles of the body, collectively.

muscular atrophy, post-polio   Muscle-wasting that occurs after the initial acute polio illness.

muscular dystrophy   One of a group of genetic diseases characterized by progressive weakness and degeneration of the skeletal or voluntary muscles that control movement. Abbreviated MD. The muscles of the heart and some other involuntary muscles are also affected in some forms of MD, and a few forms involve other organs as well. The major forms of MD include Duchenne MD, Becker MD, limb-girdle MD, facioscapulohumeral MD, congenital MD, oculopharyngeal MD, distal MD, Emery-Dreifuss MD, and myotonic dystrophy. MD can affect people of all ages. Although some forms first become apparent in infancy or childhood, others may not appear until middle age or later. Duchenne MD is the most common kind of MD that affects children. Myotonic dystrophy is the most common kind of MD in adults. There is no specific treatment for any of the forms of MD. Physical therapy to prevent contractures (a condition in which shortened muscles around joints cause abnormal and sometimes painful positioning of the joints), use of orthoses (orthopedic appliances used for support), and corrective orthopedic surgery may be needed to improve the quality of life in some cases. The prognosis with MD depends on the type of MD. Some cases may be mild and very slowly progressive, giving the patient a normal lifespan, and other cases may have more marked progression of muscle weakness, functional disability, and loss of ambulation. Life expectancy depends on the degree of progression and late respiratory deficit. In Duchenne MD, death usually occurs in the late teens to early 20s. See also *myotonic dystrophy.*

muscular dystrophy, Becker   A form of muscular dystrophy (MD) that is similar to Duchenne MD but milder. Patients with Becker MD produce a little of the key protein, dystrophin, whereas those with Duchenne make none. Progression of Becker MD is slower and symptoms tend to appear later than progression of Duchenne MD. Both Becker and Duchenne MD result from mutations in the huge gene on the X chromosome (in Xp21.2) that encodes dystrophin.

muscular dystrophy, congenital   A form of muscular dystrophy (MD) that is present at birth. Various types of congenital MD have been identified, each caused by a different genetic error. Congenital MD can affect males or females. Diagnosis is initially made via observation of general muscle weakness (hypotonia). See also *dystrophy, myotonic.*

muscular dystrophy, distal   One of two genetic muscle diseases characterized by wasting of the muscles that are most distant from the midline, such as those of the hands and feet. The first type of distal muscular dystrophy (MD) starts in infancy, does not progress after adolescence, and is not debilitating. The second type of distal MD starts after age 40, affects the muscles of the hands and feet and then the muscles closer to the trunk, but does not shorten the lifespan. Both types of distal MD are inherited in an autosomal dominant manner and affect males and females. Also known as distal myopathy and distal hereditary myopathy.

muscular dystrophy, Duchenne   The best-known form of muscular dystrophy, which is due to mutation in a gene on the X chromosome that prevents the production of dystrophin, a normal protein in muscle. Abbreviated DMD. DMD affects boys and, very rarely, girls. DMD typically appears after two years of age with weakness in the pelvis and upper limbs, resulting in clumsiness, frequent falling, an unusual gait, and general weakness. Some patients also have mild mental retardation. As DMD progresses, the patient may need a wheelchair. Most patients with DMD die in their early 20s because of muscle-based breathing and heart problems. There is no cure for DMD. Current treatment is directed toward symptoms, such as assisting with mobility, preventing scoliosis, and providing pulmonary therapy. Gene replacement with dystrophin minigenes is being investigated, but no cure appears to be around the corner.

muscular dystrophy, Emory-Dreifuss   A form of muscular dystrophy (MD) that begins in childhood or the teen years. It is a slowly progressing disorder that begins in the upper arms or upper legs. Contractures of the limbs are common, as are serious heart problems. Emory-Dreifuss MD is caused by mutation in the gene that encodes emerin in region Xq28 on the X chromosome. Although only males have the muscle problems associated with Emory-Dreifuss MD, females may have the heart problems. Therefore, female relatives of males with this disorder should have regular heart checkups.

muscular dystrophy, facioscapulohumeral   A form of muscular dystrophy that begins before age 20, with slowly progressive weakness of the muscles of the face, shoulders, and feet. The severity of the disease is variable.

Abbreviated FSMD. Although most people with FSMD retain the ability to walk, about 20 percent of affected individuals require wheelchairs. Life expectancy for FSMD is not shortened. The diagnosis can be confirmed with a DNA test. FSMD is inherited in an autosomal dominant manner. Offspring of an affected individual have a 50 percent chance of inheriting the mutant chromosome. About 10 to 30 percent of cases are due to new mutations. Prenatal testing is available.

muscular dystrophy, limb-girdle   A form of muscular dystrophy (MD) that may begin in childhood or anytime later, with slowly progressive weakness and wasting of the muscles in the hips or shoulders. Limb-girdle MD is caused by a number of genetic defects and can affect both males and females.

muscular dystrophy, myotonic   See *dystrophy, myotonic.*

muscular dystrophy, oculopharyngeal   A form of muscular dystrophy (MD) that begins in the muscles of the eyes and throat. It usually appears between the ages of 40 and 60, and it progresses slowly. Oculopharyngeal MD is inherited in an autosomal dominant manner and affects both males and females. It may actually involve more than one disease. One cause of oculopharyngeal MD is mutation in the PABP2 gene on chromosome 14, which encodes poly(A)-binding protein-2.

muscular dystrophy, tibial   A form of muscular dystrophy (MD) in which weakness is usually confined to the anterior compartment (the front part) of the lower leg and, in particular, to the tibialis anterior muscle. The weakness usually starts at age 35 to 45, or even much later. Tibial MD, which was discovered in the 1990s, is inherited in an autosomal dominant manner. It is due to mutation in the gene that encodes titin, a giant filamentous protein that is essential to muscle structure, development, and elasticity.

mutagen   Something that is capable of mutating DNA. Among the known mutagens are radiation, certain chemicals, and some viruses.

mutant   An individual with a mutant (changed) gene.

mutation   A change in a gene. Mutations can be caused by many factors, including random chance and environmental insult. See also *missense mutation; point mutation.*

mute   **1** A person who does not speak, either because of an inability to speak or an unwillingness to speak. The term is specifically applied to a person who, due to profound congenital or early deafness, is unable to use articulate

language and so is deaf-mute.   **2** The condition of not speaking. See also *apraxia of speech; autism; elective mutism; selective mutism.*   **3** In speech, a letter that is silent, or an element of speech that is formed by a position of the mouth that stops the passage of the breath, such as the letters p, b, d, k, and t.

mutism   The inability or unwillingness to speak. See also *apraxia of speech; autism; elective mutism; selective mutism.*

mutism, akinetic   A state in which a person is unable to speak (mute) or move (akinetic). Akinetic mutism is often due to damage to the frontal lobes of the brain.

myalgia   Pain in the muscles or within muscle tissue.

myalgia, epidemic   See *Bornholm disease.*

myasthenia gravis   An autoimmune neuromuscular disorder that is characterized by fatigue and exhaustion of muscles. Abbreviated MG. MG is caused by a mistaken immune response to the body's own nicotinic acetylcholine receptors, which are found in junctions between muscles and the nervous system. The body produces antibodies that attack these receptors, preventing signals from reaching the muscles. There is currently no cure for myasthenia gravis, but today only about 10 percent of patients with MG die. A number of treatments are available that help, including steroids and other immunosuppressive medications and cholinergic medications.

mycobacterium avium complex   A serious opportunistic infection that is caused by two similar bacteria, Mycobacterium avium and Mycobacterium intercellulare, which are found in the soil and in dust particles. Abbreviated MAC. In persons with suppressed immune systems, such as people with AIDS, MAC can spread through the bloodstream to infect lymph nodes, bone marrow, the liver, the spleen, spinal fluid, the lungs, and the intestinal tract. Typical symptoms of MAC include night sweats, weight loss, fever, fatigue, diarrhea, and enlarged spleen. Clarithromycin, azithromycin, ethambutal, rifampin, clofazimine, and rifabutin are some of the antibiotics that are commonly used in MAC prevention (for persons with suppressed immune systems) and treatment.

mycoplasma   A large group of bacteria, with more than 70 types identified. Mycoplasma are very simple one-celled organisms without outer membranes. They penetrate and infect individual cells. Mycoplasma hominis and Mycoplasma pneumoniae are examples of mycoplasma bacteria that occur in humans.

mycoplasma hominis   A common inhabitant of the vagina that can cause infections of the female and male genital tracts. Treatment involves use of antibiotics, including tetracycline and erythromycin.

mycoplasma pneumoniae   A mycoplasma that can infect the upper respiratory tract and the lungs. Mycoplasma pneumoniae is a major cause of respiratory infection in children of school age and young adults. It is also a common cause of pneumonia in persons with HIV. Treatment involves use of antibiotics, including tetracycline and erythromycin.

mycosis fungoides   A type of non-Hodgkin's lymphoma that first appears on the skin. Also known as cutaneous T-cell lymphoma.

mydriasis   Dilation of the pupil. The opposite of myadriasis is miosis.

myelin   The fatty substance that covers and protects nerves. Myelin is a layered tissue that surrounds the nerve fibers (axons). This sheath around the axons acts like a conduit in an electrical system, ensuring that messages sent by axons are not lost en route.

myelitis   Inflammation of the spinal cord, such as from infection or immune inflammation.

myelodysplastic syndrome   One of a group of disorders characterized by abnormal development of one or more of the cell lines that are normally found in the bone marrow. Patients can develop a variety of symptoms related to anemia, low or high white blood cell count, infections, and bleeding problems. Myelodysplastic syndrome may progress and become acute leukemia. The seven well-recognized myelodysplastic syndromes include refractory anemia, refractory anemia with ringed sideroblasts, refractory anemia with excess blasts, refractory anemia with excess blasts in transformation, chronic myelomonocytic leukemia, chronic myelomonocytic leukemia in transformation, and unclassified myelodysplastic syndrome. Also known as preleukemia or smoldering leukemia.

myeloencephalitis   See *encephalomyelitis.*

myelofibrosis   Spontaneous scarring (fibrosis) of the bone marrow. Myelofibrosis can be associated with a variety of diseases, primarily myeloproliferative (preleukemic) disorders. Also known as agnogenic myeloid metaplasia.

myelofibrosis, acute   A disorder that is characterized by acute inadequate blood cell production (pancytopenia) and marrow fibrosis but no enlargement of the spleen or liver.

myelogenous   See *myeloid.*

myelogram   An X-ray test of the spinal cord and the bones of the spine. A myelogram is used to detect impingement of the spinal cord by bone, disc, or other tissues.

myeloid   Referring to myelocytes, a type of white blood cells. Also known as myelogenous.

myeloma   See *multiple myeloma.*

myelomeningocele   See *meningomyelocele.*

myeloproliferative disorder   One of the malignant diseases of certain bone marrow cells, including those that give rise to the red blood cells, the granulocytes, and the blood platelets. The myeloproliferative disorders include myelophthisic anemia, erythroblastic leukemia, leukemoid reaction, myelofibrosis, myeloid metaplasia, polycythemia vera, and thrombocytosis.

myocardial infarction   See *heart attack.*

myocardial infarction, acute   See *acute myocardial infarction.*

myocarditis   Inflammation of the heart muscle. Inflammation of heart muscle can be caused by viruses, medications, parasites, or underlying diseases. Treatment depends on the cause.

myocardium   The heart muscle.

myoclonic twitch   A rapid, involuntary muscle contraction, particularly near the eye. Myoclonic tics resemble and may be mistaken for tics. Like tics, they tend to occur more often when the person is under stress; unlike tics, they are not preceded by any sensation and they cannot be delayed.

myoclonus   The shock-like, involunatary contraction of a muscle. See also *myoclonic twitch.*

myofascial pain syndrome   A condition that is characterized by chronic pain in the muscle tissues and is similar to fibromyalgia. Abbreviated MPS. MPS is sometimes the aftermath of injury. Pain medication, anti-inflammatory medication, and therapies aimed at relaxing the muscle tissues (such as massage, chiropractic, and some forms of acupuncture) have been reported as beneficial. See also *fibromyalgia.*

myoglobin   The pigment in muscle that carries oxygen.

myoma   A tumor of muscle. Myoma can refer specifically to a benign tumor of uterine muscle, also called a leiomyoma or a fibroid.

myomectomy   Surgery to remove a fibroid from the uterus.

myometrium   The muscular outer layer of the uterus.

myopathic   pseudo-obstruction   See *pseudo-obstruction, myopathic.*

myopathy   Any and all diseases of muscle.

myopathy, mitochondrial   See *MELAS syndrome.*

myopia   Nearsightedness, the inability to see distant objects well. Myopia can be caused by either a longer-than-normal eyeball or a condition that prevents light rays from focusing on the retina. Most forms of myopia can be managed with corrective lenses. Surgery is available to permanently correct some forms of myopia.

myositis   Inflammation of muscle tissue. There are many causes of myositis, including injury, medications, and diseases, such as dermatomyositis. Myositis may require no treatment, stopping medications, or treatment of an underlying disease, if present.

myotonic dystrophy   See *dystrophy, myotonic.*

myringotomy   A tiny surgical incision in the eardrum. A myringotomy can be used to drain any fluid behind the eardrum and to remove thickened secretions. A small plastic ear tube is often inserted into the eardrum to keep the middle ear aerated for a prolonged period of time. These ventilating tubes usually remain in place for 6 months to several years. Eventually, they move out of the eardrum (extrude) and fall into the ear canal.

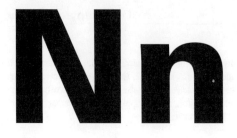

Nn

Na The chemical symbol for sodium. The symbol for sodium chloride (table salt) is NaCl. See also *sodium.*

nadir The lowest point. The nadir may refer, for example, to the lowest blood count after chemotherapy or the lowest concentration of a drug in the body.

nail **1** A piece of metal that is used to hold two or more pieces of bone together (for example, after a fracture). **2** The horny plate on the end of the finger (fingernail) or toe (toenail). Each nail has a body, lateral nail folds on its sides, a lunula (the little moon-shaped feature at the base), and a proximal skin fold at its base. See also *fingernail; nail care; toenail.*

nail care Care of the fingernails and toenails. Many nail problems are due to poor nail care. Recommendations for maintaining nail health include keeping nails clean and dry to keep bacteria and other infectious organisms from collecting under the nails, cutting nails straight across with only slight rounding at the tip, using a fine-textured file to keep nails shaped and free of snags, and avoiding nail-biting. It is a good idea to soak toenails that are thick and difficult to cut in warm salt water (1 tsp. salt to 1 pint of water) for 5 to 10 minutes, and apply a 10 percent urea cream (available at drugstores, without a prescription) before trimming. One should not "dig out" ingrown toenails, especially if they are sore; instead, a physician should provide treatment. Nail changes, swelling, and pain can signal serious problems that should be reported to a physician.

nail fungus See *onychomycosis.*

nail-patella syndrome A hereditary condition that is characterized by abnormally formed or absent nails and underdeveloped or absent kneecaps. Abbreviated NPS. Other features of NPS include iliac horns; elbow abnormalities that interfere with full range of motion (pronation and supination); and kidney disease that resembles glomerulonephritis, which can be progressive and lead to kidney failure. NPS is inherited as an autosomal dominant trait. In a pioneering autosomal linkage, the gene for NPS was found to be linked genetically to the ABO blood group locus in chromosome region 9q34. NPS is caused by mutations in a gene LMX1B (the LIM homeo box transcription factor 1, beta gene). Also known as Fong disease and Turner-Kieser syndrome.

nails, jogger's See *jogger's nails.*

nails, ringworm of the See *onychomycosis.*

nails, white spots on the See *jogger's nails.*

nanism See *dwarfism.*

narcolepsy A neurological disorder that is marked by the recurrent, sudden, uncontrollable compulsion to sleep. Narcolepsy is often associated with cataplexy (a sudden loss of muscle tone and paralysis of voluntary muscles associated with a strong emotion), sleep paralysis (immobility of the body that occurs in the transition from sleep to wakefulness), hypnagogic hallucinations (presleep dreams), and automatic behaviors (such as doing something "automatically" and not remembering afterward how one did it). The causes of narcolepsy are unknown. Narcolepsy is not a fatal disorder in itself, but it can lead to fatalities. For example, a narcoleptic may fall asleep while driving. Also known as excessive daytime sleepiness, hypnolepsy, sleeping disease, paroxysmal sleep, and Gelineau syndrome.

nares The nostrils.

nasal Having to do with the nose.

nasal decongestant A drug that shrinks the swollen membranes in the nose, making it easier to breath. Decongestants can be taken orally or as nasal drops or spray. Nasal decongestants should not be used for more than 5 days in a row without the physician's consent, and then usually only when accompanied by a nasal steroid. When nasal decongestants are used for a long time and then discontinued, symptoms often worsen (a rebound effect) because the tissues become dependent on the medication.

nasal passage A channel for airflow through the nose. The walls of the nasal passages are coated with respiratory mucous membranes, which contain innumerable tiny hair-like cells that move waves of mucus toward the throat. Dust, bacteria, and other particles inhaled from the air are trapped by the mucus in the nose, carried back, swallowed, and dropped into the gastric juices so that any potential harm they might do is nullified. The organs of smell are made up of patches of tissue called olfactory membranes. The olfactory membranes are about the size of a postage stamp and are located in a pair of clefts just under the bridge of the nose. Most air breathed in normally flows through the nose, but only a small part reaches the olfactory clefts to get a response to an odor. When a person sniffs to detect a smell, air moves faster through the nose, increasing the flow to the olfactory clefts and carrying more odor to these sensory organs.

nasal septum　The dividing wall that runs down the middle of the nose, separating the two nasal cavities, each of which ends in a nostril. The nasal septum is composed of bone, cartilage, and membranes.

nasal septum, deviated　Failure of the nasal septum to be in the center of the nose and divide the nasal passages evenly. Deviation of the nasal septum may be congenital (present at birth) or acquired (occur later). The major problem it causes is airway obstruction. A deviated septum can be corrected with surgery.

nasal septum, perforated　A condition in which the dividing wall between the two main nasal passages has been eroded away, resulting in a communication between the passages. Perforated nasal septum can be caused by a number of conditions, including repeated inhalation of cocaine and other harmful drugs. It can usually be repaired with surgery.

naso-　Prefix referring to the nose, as in nasogastric tube (a tube that is passed through the nose and to the stomach).

nasogastric　Referring to the passage from the nose to the stomach. Abbreviated NG.

nasogastric tube　A tube that is passed through the nose and down through the nasopharynx and esophagus into the stomach. Abbreviated NG tube. It is a flexible tube made of rubber or plastic, and it has bidirectional potential. It can be used to remove the contents of the stomach, including air, to decompress the stomach, or to remove small solid objects and fluid, such as poison, from the stomach. An NG tube can also be used to put substances into the stomach, and so it may be used to place nutrients directly into the stomach when a patient cannot take food or drink by mouth.

nasopharynx　The area of the upper throat that lies behind the nose. See also *oropharynx*.

National Academy of Sciences　A nonprofit, self-perpetuating society of distinguished scholars engaged in scientific and engineering research, dedicated to the furtherance of science and technology, and to their use for the general welfare. The US Congress granted the NAS a charter in 1863 with the authority that requires it to advise the federal government on scientific and technical matters.

national board exam　In medicine, the United States Medical Licensing Examination (USMLE), an exam sponsored by the Federation of State Medical Boards (FSMB) of the US and the National Board of Medical Examiners (NBME). It has replaced the examinations previously used to fulfill examination requirements for medical licensure. The national board exam provides a common

evaluation system for all applicants for medical licensure. Results of the exam are reported to medical licensing authorities in the US for use in granting licenses to practice medicine.

National Institutes of Health　An important US agency that is devoted to medical research. Abbreviated NIH. Administered by the Department of Health and Human Services (HHS), the NIH consists of 24 separate institutes and centers that represent the NIH's program activities:

- **Center for Information Technology (CIT)**　As the NIH's computing technology arm, the CIT seeks to develop, promote, and spread the use of high-tech tools in biomedical science.

- **Center for Scientific Review (CSR)**　The CSR provides staff and procedural support to the director of the NIH for running the grant approval process. It handles scientific review of most NIH grant applications, proposals, fellowships, and projects. Formerly known as the Division of Research Grants.

- **Fogarty International Center (FIC)**　The FIC serves as NIH's coordinating body for international medical research and cooperation. It supports research partnerships between US biomedical scientists and their counterparts around the world.

- **National Cancer Institute (NCI)**　The NCI's mission is to lead a national effort against cancer. The NCI conducts basic and clinical biomedical research, trains practitioners, and conducts and supports programs to prevent, detect, diagnose, treat, and control cancer. It also provides practitioners, patients, and the public with information about cancer detection and treatment.

- **National Center for Research Resources (NCRR)**　The NCRR conducts biomedical research and shares its resources and findings with others in the fields of biomedical technology, clinical research, comparative medicine, and research infrastructure.

- **National Eye Institute (NEI)**　The NEI conducts and supports research, training, and other programs related to eye diseases, visual disorders, mechanisms of visual function, preservation of sight, blindness, and the health problems and special needs of the visually impaired.

- **National Heart, Lung, and Blood Institute (NHLBI)**　The NHLBI leads a national research program that deals with diseases of the heart, blood vessels, lungs, and blood. It also supports basic clinical, population-based, and health-education research in the area of transfusion medicine.

- **National Human Genome Research Institute (NHGRI)** The NHGRI supports the role of NIH in the Human Genome Project. The NHGRI also develops and implements technology for understanding, diagnosing, and treating genetic diseases.

- **National Institute of Allergy and Infectious Diseases (NIAID)** The NIAID's specialty is research into and research training about infectious, immune-system, and allergic diseases.

- **National Institute of Arthritis and Musculoskeletal and Skin Diseases (NIAMS)** The NIAMS specializes in research into the normal structure and function of bones, muscles, and skin, as well as diseases that affect these tissues.

- **National Institute of Child Health and Human Development (NICHD)** The NICHD supports and conducts research on fertility, pregnancy, child growth and development, and medical rehabilitation for children affected by disease or disability.

- **National Institute of Dental Research (NIDR)** The NIDR leads a national research program aimed at understanding, treating, and preventing dental and craniofacial diseases.

- **National Institute of Diabetes and Digestive and Kidney Diseases (NIDDK)** The NIDDK conducts national programs in diabetes, endocrinology, and metabolic diseases; digestive diseases and nutrition; and kidney, urologic, and hematologic diseases.

- **National Institute of Environmental Health Sciences (NIEHS)** The NIEHS conducts research into interactions between environmental exposure, genetic susceptibility, and age that can cause disease or disability.

- **National Institute of General Medical Sciences (NIGMS)** The NIGMS supports basic biomedical research that is not targeted to specific diseases or disorders. Among its most significant research results has been the development of recombinant DNA technology, forming the basis for the biotechnology industry.

- **National Institute of Mental Health (NIMH)** The NIMH leads a national program of research into the causes, treatment, and prevention of mental illness. It conducts basic research on the brain and behavior, as well as clinical, epidemiological, and services research.

- **National Institute of Neurological Disorders and Stroke (NINDS)** The NINDS supports and conducts research and research training on the normal structure and function of the nervous system, and on the causes, prevention, diagnosis, and treatment of neurological disorders.

- **National Institute of Nursing Research (NINR)** The NINR supports research into clinical patient care aimed at understanding and mitigating the effects of acute and chronic illness and disability, promoting healthy behaviors, preventing the onset or worsening of disease, and improving the clinical environment.

- **National Institute on Aging (NIA)** The NIA leads a national program of research on the biomedical, social, and behavioral aspects of the aging process; the prevention of age-related diseases and disabilities; and health promotion for older Americans.

- **National Institute on Alcohol Abuse and Alcoholism (NIAAA)** The NIAAA conducts research into improving the treatment and prevention of alcoholism and alcohol-related problems.

- **National Institute on Deafness and Other Communication Disorders (NIDCD)** The NIDCD conducts and supports biomedical research and research training on normal mechanisms as well as diseases and disorders of hearing, balance, smell, taste, voice, speech, and language.

- **National Institute on Drug Abuse (NIDA)** The NIDA conducts and supports research on the causes, prevention, and treatment of drug abuse and addiction.

- **National Library of Medicine (NLM)** The world's largest medical library, the NLM collects, organizes, and makes available biomedical science information to investigators, educators, and practitioners. It also carries out programs to strengthen medical library services in the US. Its electronic databases, including MEDLINE, are used extensively throughout the world.

- **Warren Grant Magnuson Clinical Center**
As the clinical research facility of NIH, this
center provides the patient care, services, and
facilities to support human subjects research
by the NIH. Also known as the National
Institutes of Health Clinical Center (NIHCC).

natriuresis   The excretion of an excessively large
amount of sodium in the urine. Natriuresis is similar to
diuresis (the excretion of an unusually large quantity of
urine), except that in natriuresis the urine is exceptionally
salty. Natriuresis occurs with some diuretics and diseases
(as of the adrenal gland) and can lead to the salt-losing
syndrome characterized by dehydration, vomiting, low
blood pressure, and the risk of sudden death. See also
diuresis.

natriuretic   An agent or disease that promotes natriuresis. For example, a diuretic with natriuretic action
could be helpful for someone retaining water and salt. See
also *diuretic.*

natural family planning   Birth control without the use
of contraceptive medications or barrier methods. There
are several natural family planning methods. If applied
exactly, their efficiency comes close to that of barrier
methods, but not to that of birth control pills, Depo-
Provera, Norplant, or the IUD. The most common natural
family planning method is the use of basal temperature to
detect ovulation, accompanied by abstention from intercourse during and after ovulation. Because a sperm may
live in the female's reproductive tract for up to 7 days and
the egg remains fertile for about 24 hours, a woman can
get pregnant within a substantial window of time—from
7 days before ovulation to 3 days after it. Also known as
the basal temperature method, fertility awareness, periodic abstinence, and the rhythm method. See also *birth
control.*

natural killer cell   A cell that can react against and
destroy another cell without prior sensitization to it.
Abbreviated NK cell. NK cells are part of our first line of
defense against cancer cells and virus-infected cells. NK
cells are small lymphocytes that originate in the bone
marrow and develop without the influence of the thymus.
An NK cell attaches to a target cell, releases chemicals that
breach its cell wall, and causes it to lyse (break up).

natural menopause   See menopause.

naturopath   A person who practices naturopathy. A
naturopathic doctor (ND) has been trained to care for
well and ailing patients by using naturopathic methods. In
some US states, NDs must complete a program equivalent
to the training received by MDs, and they are therefore
licensed to practice medicine. In other states, the term ND
is neither defined nor regulated. See also *naturopathy.*

naturopathic   Pertaining to naturopathy.

naturopathy   A system of therapy that is based on preventive care and on the use of physical forces such as
heat, water, light, air, and massage as primary therapies
for disease. Some naturopaths use no medications, either
pharmaceutical or herbal. Some recommend herbal
remedies only. A few who are licensed to prescribe may
recommend pharmaceuticals in cases in which they feel
their use is warranted.

nausea   Stomach queasiness, the urge to vomit. Nausea
can be brought on by many causes, including systemic illnesses (such as influenza), medications, pain, and inner
ear disease.

navel   See *bellybutton.*

NCI   National Cancer Institute. See *National Institutes
of Health.*

ND   Naturopathic doctor. See *naturopath.*

nearsightedness   See *myopia.*

nebulization   The conversion of a medication into an
aerosol or a spray to deliver the medication, for example,
to the lungs.

nebulization, heated   Administration of medication
via fine spray that has been heated to increase its water
content.

nebulizer   A device for administering a medication by
spraying a fine mist. Also known as atomizer.

Necator americanus   The American hookworm, the
cause of hookworm disease in people. See also *hookworm.*

neck, stiff   See *torticollis.*

necropsy   See *autopsy.*

necrosis   The death of living cells or tissues. Necrosis
can be due, for example, to lack of blood flow (ischemia).
From the Greek nekros, meaning "dead body."

necrosis, coagulation   Tissue death that is due to clots
in the bloodstream blocking the flow of blood to the
affected area.

necrosis, gangrenous   Tissue death that is due to the
combined effects of blood-flow stoppage and bacterial
infection.

necrotic   Dead. For example, necrotic tissue is dead
tissue.

necrotizing fasciitis Severe bacterial infection of the fascia, the tissues that line and separate muscles, that causes extensive tissue death. Necrotizing fasciitis can be caused by several different types of bacteria, particularly by virulent strains of streptococcus and staphylococcus. The rapid spread and destruction of tissue occurs because of substances produced by the bacteria. Treatment involves the use of high-dose antibiotics and surgical removal of dead and infected tissue to help control the infection. Also known as flesh-eating bacteria.

needle aspiration, fine See *fine needle aspiration.*

needle biopsy See *biopsy, needle.*

needle biopsy, stereotactic See *biopsy, stereotactic needle.*

negative, false See *false negative.*

neglect, child See *child neglect.*

Neisseria A group of bacteria that includes the bacterium that causes gonorrhea.

nematode A parasitic roundworm.

neo- Prefix meaning new, as in neonate (a newborn baby) and neoplasm (an abnormal new growth, a tumor).

neonatal Pertaining to the newborn period, specifically the first 4 weeks after birth.

neonatal jaundice See *jaundice, neonatal.*

neonatal mortality rate The number of children under 28 days of age who die, divided by the number of live births that year. The neonatal mortality rate in the US was 8.4 per 1,000 live births in 1980, and it declined to 6.9 per 1,000 live births in 2000.

neonatal sepsis A bacterial infection of the blood in a neonate, an infant younger than 4 weeks of age. Babies with sepsis may be listless, overly sleepy, floppy, weak, and very pale. Neonatal sepsis is life threatening.

neonate A newborn baby, specifically a baby in the first 4 weeks after birth. After a month, a baby is no longer considered a neonate.

neonatologist A specialist who cares for newborns.

neonatology The art and science of medical care for newborns.

neoplasia Abnormal new growth of cells.

neoplasm A tumor.

neoplastic Pertaining to a tumor or the process of tumor formation.

nephrectomy Surgery to remove all or part of the kidney, for example, because of cancer.

nephrectomy, partial Removal of part of a kidney, but not the entire kidney.

nephrectomy, radical Surgery to remove the kidney, the adrenal gland, the nearby lymph nodes, and other surrounding tissue.

nephrectomy, simple Surgery to remove only the kidney that is diseased.

nephritis Inflammation of the kidney, which causes impaired kidney function. Nephritis can be due to a variety of causes, including kidney disease, autoimmune disease, and infection. Treatment depends on the cause.

nephritis, acute Sudden kidney inflammation. Diagnosis is usually made by finding protein or urine in the blood.

nephritis, infective tubulointerstitial Inflammation of the kidney that is due to infection. Symptoms include nausea, pain in the kidney area, fever, and chills. Early diagnosis is essential to save the kidneys. Treatment involves use of antibiotics or antiviral medications.

nephritis, interstitial Nephritis that is due to disorders of the connective tissue within the kidney, exposure to toxic substances, transplant rejection, urinary blockage, or other factors. Symptoms include fever, pain in the kidney area, blood or protein in the urine, and eventually kidney failure. Treatment depends on the cause.

nephritis, lipomatous A disorder in which the nephrons (the functional components of the kidneys that manage the balance of important ions in the blood stream, especially potassium and sodium, as well as its acidity) are gradually replaced with fatty tissues. This prevents proper filtration of wastes and eventually results in kidney failure. Treatment is dialysis or kidney transplantation.

nephro- Having to do with the kidney, as in nephrology (the art and science of the care of the kidneys) and nephropathy (any kidney disease).

nephrolith A kidney stone.

nephrolithiasis The process of forming a stone in the kidney or lower down in the urinary tract. Also known as urolithiasis. See also *kidney stones.*

nephrolithotripsy, percutaneous See *percutaneous nephrolithotripsy.*

nephrologist   A medical practitioner whose specialty is nephrology.

nephrology   The art and science of the care of the kidneys.

nephron   A key unit of the kidney, a tiny funnel-like structure that filters wastes as they enter and progress through the kidney.

nephropathy   Any kidney disease.

nephropathy, diabetic   See *diabetic nephropathy*.

nephrosclerosis   Hardening (sclerosis) of the kidney, usually due to hardening of the blood vessels within it (atherosclerosis).

nephrosis   Any degenerative disease of the kidney tubules, the tiny canals that make up much of the substance of the kidney. Nephrosis can be caused by kidney disease, or it may be a complication of another disorder, particularly diabetes. Diagnosis is made via urine testing for the presence of protein, blood testing for lower-than-normal levels of protein, and observation of edema. Treatment usually involves use of cortisone-like drugs. Also known as nephrotic syndrome.

nephrotic syndrome   See *nephrosis*.

nephrotomogram   A series of X-rays of the kidneys that are taken from different angles to clearly show the kidneys, without the shadows of the organs around them.

nerve   A bundle of fibers that uses electrical and chemical signals to transmit sensory and motor information from one body part to another. The fibrous portions of a nerve are covered by a sheath called myelin and/or a membrane called neurilemma. (Note that entries for specific nerves can be found under the names of the particular nerves. For example, the optic nerve is not under "nerve, optic" but rather under "optic nerve.")

nerve, afferent   See *afferent nerve*.

nerve cell   See *neuron*.

nerve compression   "Pinching" of a nerve that is due to too much pressure on it. For example, a woman's sciatic nerve may be painfully compressed by the weight and position of the fetus during the latter part of pregnancy.

nerve, efferent   See *efferent nerve*.

nerve growth factor   A naturally occurring substance that enhances the growth and survival of cholinergic nerves.

nerve, pinched   A compressed nerve, as between two vertebrae or within a joint, causing discomfort, pain, or impairment of sensation. Treatment involves physical therapy and sometimes surgery. See also *nerve compression*.

nerves, cranial   See *cranial nerves*.

nervous colon syndrome   See *irritable bowel syndrome*.

nervous system   The sum total of the tissues that use electrical and chemical means to record and distribute information within a body. The nervous system has two distinct parts: central and peripheral. The central part is made up of the brain and spinal cord; together they are the central nervous system (CNS). The peripheral part of the nervous system is said to be peripheral because it is outside the CNS. The function of the peripheral nervous system is to transmit information back and forth between the CNS and the rest of the body. The human nervous system contains approximately 10 billion nerve cells (neurons). These neurons are the basic building blocks of the nervous system. A neuron consists of the nerve cell body and various extensions, or processes, from the cell body. These extensions are the dendrites (branches off the cell that receive electrical impulses), the axon (the electrical wiring and conduit tube that conducts impulses), and specialized endings (terminal areas to transfer impulses to receivers on other nerves or muscles). See also *central nervous system; peripheral nervous system*.

nervous system, autonomic   See *autonomic nervous system*.

nervous system, central   See *central nervous system*.

nervous system, parasympathetic   See *parasympathetic nervous system*.

nervous system, peripheral   See *peripheral nervous system*.

nervous system, sympathetic   See *sympathetic nervous system*.

neural   Having to do with nerve cells (neurons).

neural tube defect   A major birth defect caused by abnormal development of the neural tube, the structure that is present during embryonic life that gives rise to the central nervous system. Abbreviated NTD. NTDs are among the most common birth defects resulting in infant death and serious disability. There are a number of different types of NTDs, including anencephaly, spina bifida, and encephalocele. In anencephaly there is absence of the cranial vault (the skull) and absence of most or all of the cerebral hemispheres of the brain. Encephalocele is a hernia of part of the brain, and the membranes covering it (meninges), through a skull defect. Spina bifida is an opening in the vertebral column encasing the spinal cord. Through this opening, the spinal cord and the meninges may herniate to create a meningomyelocele. All pregnancies are at risk for NTDs. Factors that increase the risk include a prior NTD in the family and type 1 diabetes in the mother. More than half of NTDs can be prevented if women consume supplements that contain folic acid before and during the early weeks of pregnancy in addition to getting folate in their diets. The US Public Health Service, Centers for Disease Control and Prevention (CDC), and American Academy of Pediatrics recommend that all women of childbearing age who are capable of becoming pregnant consume 400 (0.4 mg) μ of folic acid daily. Because the risk for NTDs is not totally eliminated by folic acid use, routine prenatal screening for NTDs is still advisable.

neuralgia Pain along the course of a nerve; for example, with and after shingles. See also *neuralgia, postherpetic.*

neuralgia, facial Severe pain that usually occurs in bursts along the path of the trigeminal nerve, the chief sensory nerve of the face.

neuralgia, postherpetic The most common complication of shingles, persistence of the pain associated with shingles beyond 1 month, even after the rash is gone. The pain can be severe and debilitating, and it occurs primarily in persons over age 50. There is some evidence that treating shingles with steroids and antiviral agents can reduce the duration and occurrence of postherpetic neuralgia. However, the decrease is minimal. The pain of postherpetic neuralgia can be reduced with a number of medications. Tricyclic antidepressant medications, such as amitriptyline (brand name: Elavil), as well as anti-seizure medications such as gabapentin (brand name: Neurontin) or carbamazipine (brand name: Tegretol), have been used. Capsaicin cream, a derivative of hot chili peppers, or lidocaine patches can be applied on the area after all the blisters have healed, to reduce pain. Acupuncture and electric nerve stimulation through the skin can be helpful for some patients.

neuritis Inflammation of nerves. There are many causes of neuritis, including various viruses and local irritation of a nerve by adjacent tissues.

neuroblastoma A childhood form of cancer that arises in the adrenal gland or in tissue in the nervous system that is related to the adrenal gland. Neuroblastoma is the most common solid tumor outside the brain in infants and children. It is often present at birth but may not be detected until later in infancy or childhood. The most common symptoms are the result of pressure by the tumor or bone pain from metastases. Protruding eyes and dark circles around the eyes are common and are caused by cancer that has spread to the area behind the eye. Neuroblastomas may compress the spinal cord, causing paralysis. Approximately 70 percent of all children with neuroblastoma have metastases by the time the disease is diagnosed. The prognosis for neuroblastoma is related to the age at diagnosis (the younger, the better the prognosis), clinical stage of the disease at diagnosis, and whether the child has lymph node involvement by the tumor. Screening infants for neuroblastoma is not warranted because it does not decrease the morbidity (illness) or mortality rate.

neurodermatitis Scaly patches of skin on the head, lower legs, wrists, or forearms that are caused by a localized itch that becomes intensely irritated when scratched.

neurofibromatosis A genetic disorder of the nervous system that primarily affects the development and growth of neural (nerve) cell tissues, causes tumors to grow on nerves, and may produce other abnormalities. Neurofibromatosis consists of two very different disorders: neurofibromatosis type 1 (NF1) and neurofibromatosis type 2 (NF2).

neurofibromatosis type 1 A genetic disorder that is characterized by a number of skin characteristics, including multiple café au lait (coffee with milk) spots, multiple benign tumors called neurofibromas on the skin, plexiform neurofibromas (thick and misshapen nerves due to the abnormal growth of cells and tissues that cover the nerve), and freckles in the armpit and groin. Abbreviated NF1. The café au lait spots increase in number and size with age. Ninety-seven percent of people with NF1 have 6 or more café au lait spots by age 20. The skin neurofibromas appear later, usually in the second decade of life. Patients with NF1 have an increased risk of scoliosis, optic gliomas (benign tumors on the optic nerve), epilepsy, and learning disabilities. The risk of malignant degeneration of neurofibromas is lower than 5 percent. NF1 is inherited in an autosomal dominant manner and is due to mutation of the NF1 gene (in chromosome band 17q11) that encodes a protein called neurofibromin. Half of cases are due to new mutations in the NF1 gene. Prenatal testing is available. Also known as von Recklinghausen disease.

neurofibromatosis type 2 A genetic disorder that is characterized by the growth of benign tumors of both acoustic nerves (the nerves to the ears). These tumors, called acoustic neuromas, cause tinnitus (ringing in the ears), hearing loss, and problems with balance. Abbreviated NF2. Other findings in NF2 include similar benign tumors of other nerves, meningiomas, and juvenile cataracts. NF2 is inherited in an autosomal dominant manner and is due to mutation in the NF2 gene (in chromosome band 22q12.2), which encodes the protein merlin. About half of people with NF2 have a new gene mutation. Prenatal testing is available. Also known as bilateral acoustic neurofibromatosis and central neurofibromatosis.

neurogenic　Giving rise to or arising from the nerves or the nervous system. For example, neurogenic pain is pain that originates in the nerves, as opposed to muscle pain, bone pain, etc.

neurological　Having to do with the nerves or the nervous system as, for example, a neurological exam.

neurologist　A physician who specializes in the diagnosis and treatment of disorders of the nervous system.

neurology　The medical specialty concerned with the diagnosis and treatment of disorders of the nervous system, which includes the brain, the spinal cord, and the nerves.

neuroma　A benign tumor that arises from a nerve as, for example, an acoustic glioma or optic glioma.

neuroma, acoustic　A benign tumor of the hearing and balance nerves near the inner ear. Aside from hearing and balance, these tumors can impinge on the facial nerve, causing facial paralysis, and press on nearby brain structures and be life-threatening. Acoustic neuromas may be removed by surgery or shrunk by radiosurgery. Bilateral acoustic neuromas are associated with neurofibromatosis type 2 (NF2).

neuron　A nerve cell that receives and sends electrical signals over long distances within the body. A neuron receives electrical input signals from sensory cells (called sensory neurons) and from other neurons. The neuron sends electrical output signals to muscle neurons (called motoneurons or motor neurons) and to other neurons. A neuron that simply signals another neuron is called an interneuron.

neuron-specific enolase test　A test for an enzyme that has been detected in the blood of patients with certain tumors, including neuroblastomas, small-cell lung cancers, medullary thyroid cancers, carcinoid tumors, pancreatic endocrine tumors, and melanomas. Abbreviated NSE test. Measurement of NSE levels as a tumor marker in patients with these types of tumors can provide information about the extent of the disease and the patient's prognosis and response to treatment.

neuropathic pseudo-obstruction　See *pseudo-obstruction, neuropathic.*

neuropathy　Any disease or malfunction of the nerves.

neuropathy, accessory　See *accessory neuropathy.*

neuropathy, diabetic　See *diabetic neuropathy.*

neuropathy, hypoglossal　See *hypoglossal neuropathy.*

neuropsychologist　A psychologist who has completed special training in the neurobiological causes of brain disorders and who specializes in diagnosing and treating these illnesses by using a predominantly medical (as opposed to psychoanalytical) approach.

neurosurgeon　A physician who specializes in surgery on the brain and other parts of the nervous system.

neurosyphilis　Neurological complications in the third (tertiary) and final phase of syphilis, which involve the central nervous system and can include psychosis, pain, and loss of physical control over a variety of bodily functions.

neurosyphilis, tabes　The slowly progressive degeneration of the spinal cord that occurs in the tertiary phase of syphilis, a decade or more after a person contracts the infection. Among the features of tabes neurosyphilis are sharp, lightning-like pain; wobbliness (ataxia); deterioration of the optic nerve, leading to blindness; urinary incontinence; loss of the sense of position; and degeneration of the joints. Also known as tabes dorsalis.

neurotoxic　Poisonous to nerves or nerve tissue.

neurotoxin　Any substance that is capable of causing damage to nerves or nerve tissue. For example, arsenic and lead are neurotoxins.

neutropenia　A marked decrease in the number of neutrophils (white blood cells). Neutropenia is a sign of impaired immune system response. See also *agranulocytosis; agranulocytosis, infantile genetic; granulocytopenia; severe congenital neutropenia.*

neutropenia, severe congenital　See *severe congenital neutropenia.*

neutrophil　A type of white blood cell, a granulocyte that is filled with microscopic granules, little sacs containing enzymes that digest microorganisms.

neutrophilia　Too many neutrophils in the blood. Neutrophilia may be due merely to a shift of neutrophils into the circulating blood as occurs, for example, with vigorous exercise and with cortisone medications. A true increase in neutrophil production usually reflects infection, particularly bacterial infection.

nevus A pigmented spot on the skin, such as a mole. The plural of nevus is nevi.

nevus araneus See *spider vein.*

new variant Creutzfeldt-Jakob disease A human disease that is thought to be due to the same infectious agent as bovine spongiform encephalopathy (BSE), or mad cow disease. Abbreviated nvCJD, this disease represents a new variant of Creutzfeld-Jakob disease. Both the human and bovine disorders are invariably fatal brain diseases with unusually long incubation periods and are due to an unconventional transmissible agent, a prion. Deposition of amyloid (a glassy-looking substance) in the brain causes the breakdown of brain tissue, leaving the brain with a "spongy" (spongiform) appearance. See also *Creutzfeldt-Jakob disease; prion.*

newborn screening Testing of newborns to screen for serious treatable diseases, many of which are genetic. Which newborn screening tests are done in the US are determined on a state-by-state basis. The most common newborn screening tests in the US are for hypothyroidism, phenylketonuria (PKU), galactosemia, and sickle cell disease. Testing for hypothyroidism and PKU is required in virtually all states, and testing for galactosemia and sickle cell disease is required in most states. Some states mandate tests for other conditions, including deafness, maple syrup urine disease, homocystinuria, congenital adrenal hyperplasia, tyrosinemia, cystic fibrosis, and toxoplasmosis. See also *cystic fibrosis; galactosemia; homocystinuria; hypothyroidism, congenital; maple syrup urine disease; phenylketonuria; sickle cell disease; toxoplasmosis; tyrosinemia.*

NF1 Neurofibromatosis type 1.

NF2 Neurofibromatosis type 2.

NG tube See *nasogastric tube.*

NHL Non-Hodgkin's lymphoma. See *lymphoma, non-Hodgkin's.*

niacin Nicotinic acid, one of the water-soluble B vitamins. See also Appendix C, "Vitamins."

niacin deficiency See *pellagra.*

niacin for high cholesterol Niacin given to lower cholesterol. Niacin lowers the total cholesterol, LDL cholesterol (by 10 to 20 percent), and triglyceride levels (by 20 to 50 percent), and it raises the HDL cholesterol level (by 15 to 35 percent). All patients taking niacin to lower their serum cholesterol should be closely monitored by a physician to avoid complications. A common side effect of niacin is flushing or hot flashes, which result from the widening of blood vessels. Most patients develop a tolerance to flushing, and in some patients, it can be decreased by taking the niacin during or after meals. The effectiveness of high blood pressure medicines may also be increased for people on niacin. If a patient is taking high blood pressure medication, it is important to have a blood pressure monitoring system while the patient is getting used to the new niacin regimen. Gastrointestinal symptoms, including nausea, indigestion, gas, vomiting, diarrhea, and the activation of peptic ulcers, have been seen with the use of niacin. Other major adverse effects include liver problems, gout, and high blood sugar. Niacin is usually not recommended with diabetes, because of the effect on blood sugar.

nicotinic acid See *niacin.*

nictitate To wink. For example, nictitating spasm is spasm of the eyelid with continuous winking.

nidus In medicine, any structure that resembles a nest in appearance or function. For the Latin for "nest." A nidus is a breeding place where bacteria, parasites, and other agents of a disease lodge and develop. For example, a nidus of infection is a focus of infection. A nidus is also the nucleus or origin of a nerve. The nidus avis cerebelli is a deep sulcus (groove) on each side of the inferior vermis (a wormlike structure in the brain), separating it from the adjacent lobes of the cerebral hemispheres.

Niemann-Pick disease A biochemical disorder of a fat (lipid) called sphingomyelin that is characterized by progressive enlargement of the liver and spleen (hepatosplenomegaly), enlarged lymph nodes (lymphadenopathy), anemia, and mental and physical deterioration. Niemann-Pick disease is inherited in an autosomal recessive manner. The classical form of the disease has its onset in very early infancy, and death usually occurs before age 3. The lipid accumulates in cells (called reticuloendothelial cells) in the liver, spleen, and central nervous system. The neurological features of Niemann-Pick disease include mental retardation, spasticity, seizures, jerks, eye paralysis (ophthalmoplegia), and ataxia (wobbliness). Growth is retarded. Other features are hepatosplenomegaly, jaundice, hepatic (liver) failure, and ascites (fluid in the abdomen). Eye hallmarks include a "cherry red spot" in the macula in the center of the retina and cloudy cornea. Bruising occurs easily, and coronary artery disease occurs early. The sphingomyelin accumulation is due to deficiency of the enzyme sphingomyelinase. The gene for this enzyme and hence the location of the gene for this disease is in chromosome region 11p15.4–11p15.1.

night blindness See *nyctanopia.*

night sweats   Severe hot flashes that occur at night and result in a drenching sweat. Night sweats can have many different causes, including medications, infections, and cancers.

NIH   National Institutes of Health.

Nipah virus   A virus that infects pigs and people, in whom it causes a sometimes fatal form of viral encephalitis. Symptoms include high fever and aches, coma, and sometimes death. It is not known how Nipah virus is transmitted. It may be carried from pigs to humans by mosquitoes.

nipple   The pigmented projection on the surface of the chest in the male and the breast in the female. In the mature female, ducts that conduct milk from the mammary glands to the surface of the breast exit through the nipple. The surrounding flat area of pigmentation is the areola.

nipple absence   See *athelia.*

nipple, supernumerary   An extra nipple. Supernumerary nipples are usually smaller than normal and vestigial (nonfunctional, without accompanying mammary glands). They tend to occur along a roughly curved line that extends from near the armpit, through the center of the normal breast, and down to the lower abdomen. This distribution is very similar to the location of nipples on mammals that have multiple nipples along the underbelly. Supernumerary nipples do not cause problems and do not need to be removed.

nitrogenous base   A molecule that contains nitrogen and has the chemical properties of a base. The nitrogenous bases in DNA are adenine (A), guanine (G), thymine (T), and cytosine (C). The nitrogenous bases in RNA are the same, with one exception: adenine (A), guanine (G), uracil (U), and cytosine (C).

nitrosourea   One of a group of anticancer drugs that can cross the blood–brain barrier.

nitrous oxide   A gas that can cause general anesthesia and that should be administered with other anesthetic agents. Nitrous oxide is not used alone today because the concentration of nitrous oxide needed to produce anesthesia is close to the concentration that seriously lowers the blood oxygen level, creating a hazardous hypoxic state. Nitrous oxide is used sometimes as a recreational drug for its euphoric effect. Also known as laughing gas and nitrous.

nits   Lice eggs. Nits are hard to see, and they are often confused with dandruff or hair-spray droplets. Nits firmly attach to the hair shaft with a glue-like substance. They are oval and range in color from yellow to white. Nits take about a week to hatch. All nits must be removed to prevent reinfestation with lice. They can be removed with a special comb or with the fingers. Topical preparations are available that loosen the glue that binds them to the hair, making removal easier. See also head lice.

NK cell   Natural killer cell.

NMR   Nuclear magnetic resonance, an imaging technique that does not use radiation, but instead employs large magnetic forces to produce detailed images of body tissues.

nocardiosis   Infection with Nocardia bacterium, which tends to strike the lungs, brain, and skin, particularly in people with an impaired immune system. Nocardia is in the soil and in dust particles. The inhalation of Nocardia spores usually initiates nocardiosis in the lung. The skin form of nocardiosis is contracted through soil contamination of wounds. There is no evidence for person-to-person transmission of Nocardia. The combination of the antibiotics trimethoprim and sulfamethoxazole (TMP-SMX) is used to treat nocardiosis. However, resistance to TMP-SMX is becoming more common.

nocturia   Excessive urinating at night. Nocturia can be normal and more common with aging. Nocturia can also be a sign of an underlying condition, such as diabetes or urinary infection.

nocturnal amblyopia   See *nyctanopia.*

nocturnal enuresis   See *bedwetting.*

node   A knot, a collection of tissue. For example, a lymph node is a collection of lymphoid tissue. See also *nodule.*

node, atrioventricular   See *atrioventricular node.*

node, AV   See *atrioventricular node.*

node, Heberden's   See *Heberden's node.*

node, Osler   See *Osler node.*

node, SA   See *sinoatrial node.*

node, sentinel lymph   See *lymph node, sentinel.*

node, sinoatrial   See *sinoatrial node.*

node, sinus   See *sinoatrial node.*

nodular   Bumpy.

nodular hyperplasia of the prostate   See *benign prostatic hyperplasia.*

nodular melanoma   See *melanoma, nodular.*

nodule   A small collection of tissue that is palpable (can be felt) at any level of the skin (in the epidermis, dermis, or subcutis). Nodules characteristically range in size from 1 to 2 cm in diameter.

noncompliance   Failure or refusal to comply. In medicine, the term noncompliance is commonly used in regard to a patient who does not take a prescribed medication or follow a prescribed course of treatment. A person who demonstrates noncompliance is said to be noncompliant.

nondisjunction   Failure of paired chromosomes to separate (to disjoin) during cell division, so that both chromosomes go to one daughter cell and none go to the other. Nondisjunction causes errors in chromosome number, such as trisomy 21 (Down syndrome) and monosomy X (Turner syndrome). It is also a common cause of early spontaneous abortions.

non-Hodgkin's lymphoma   See *lymphoma, non-Hodgkin's.*

nonmelanoma skin cancer   Skin cancer that does not involve melanocytes. Basal cell cancer and squamous cell cancer are nonmelanoma skin cancers.

Nonoxynol-9   A potent spermicide (sperm-killing agent) used as a contraceptive.

nonpathogenic   Incapable of causing disease. For example, nonpathogenic E. coli are E. coli bacteria that do not cause disease, but instead live naturally in the large intestine.

non-rapid eye movement sleep   See *NREM sleep.*

nonseminoma   A type of testicular cancer that arises in specialized sex cells called germ cells. Nonseminomas include embryonal carcinoma, teratoma, choriocarcinoma, and yolk sac tumor.

non-small cell lung cancer   Cancer of the lung that is not small cell carcinoma. It may be bronchogenic carcinoma, squamous cell carcinoma, adenocarcinoma, or large cell carcinoma of the lung. The distinction between small and non-small cell lung cancers is made under the microscope. Knowing which type a patient has is important for proper therapy. The treatment options for non-small cell lung cancer are generally different than those for small cell lung cancer, and surgical treatment is an option in early stages of non-small cell lung cancer.

nonsteroidal anti-inflammatory drug   See *NSAID.*

nonsyndromic   Not part of a syndrome. Hearing loss, for instance, can be syndromic or nonsyndromic.

Noonan syndrome   A congenital malformation syndrome that is characterized by mildly short stature, a congenital heart defect, a broad or webbed neck, an unusual chest shape (prominent above and caved in below), low-set nipples, a characteristic facial appearance, and, in boys, testes that do not descend normally into the scrotum (cryptorchidism). Abbreviated NS. Many types of heart defects occur in NS. The most common defect is pulmonary valve stenosis (a narrow valve between the right ventricle and pulmonary artery), and hypertrophic cardiomyopathy is the second most common. Although NS was once called Turner-like syndrome, it is a distinctive entity that affects both males and females and carries an elevated risk of developmental and language delay, learning disabilities, hearing loss, and mild mental retardation. NS is inherited in an autosomal dominant manner. It is relatively common, with an estimated incidence of 1 in 1,000–2,500 live births. A gene for NS has been mapped to chromosome 12q24.1. About half of cases of NS are due to mutations in a gene called PTPN11 that encodes the protein-tyrosine phosphatase, non-receptor type 11. This protein appears to be essential in the pathways that control developmental processes, including the formation of the pulmonary valves and in modulating cell proliferation, differentiation, and migration.

normal pressure hydrocephalus   See *hydrocephalus, normal pressure.*

normal range   Characteristic of 95 percent of values from a normal population. The remaining normal results fall outside the normal range, as do any truly abnormal results. The normal range for a particular test result, condition, symptom, or behavior may differ, based on the patient's age, size, sex, ethnicity, or culture.

Norplant   A contraceptive device that consists of six matchstick-sized rods that can be implanted in a woman's upper arm. The rods release hormones that prevent conception for 5 years. Norplant is the most effective reversible form of contraception. Common side effects include irregular menstrual periods and spotting between periods. See also *birth control; contraception.*

North Asian tick-borne rickettsiosis   See *rickettsiosis, North Asian tick-borne.*

Norwalk virus   A family of small round viruses that are an important cause of viral gastroenteritis (viral inflammation of the stomach and intestines). Only the common cold is reported more frequently than Norwalk virus as a cause of disease. Norwalk viruses are transmitted via fecal contamination of water and foods. Water is the most common source of outbreaks and may include water from municipal supplies, wells, lakes, pools, and water stored aboard cruise ships. Shellfish and salad ingredients are the foods that are most often implicated. Eating raw or insufficiently steamed clams and oysters poses a high risk for infection with Norwalk virus. Norwalk disease is a mild and brief illness that develops 1 or 2 days after contaminated food or water is consumed, and symptoms, including nausea, vomiting, diarrhea, and abdominal pain, last for 24 to 60 hours. Illness severe enough to require hospitalization is unusual.

nose   The external midline projection from the face. The purpose of the nose is to warm, clean, and humidify the air that a person breathes. In addition, it helps a person to smell and taste. The nose is divided into two passageways by a partition called the septum. Opening to these passageways are the nostrils. Bony projections, called turbinates, protrude into each breathing passage; they help to increase the surface area of the inside of the nose. There are three turbinates on each side of the nose (the inferior, middle, and superior turbinates). The sinuses are four paired air-filled chambers that empty into the nasal cavity.

nose job   See *rhinoplasty.*

nose picking   Using the finger to remove debris from within the nose. Compulsive nose picking, known medically as rhinotillexomania, is common among children.

nose, runny   The production of extra mucus by the nose. Rhinorrhea is the medical term for this common problem. The nose makes extra mucus whenever something that is in the nose, such as pollen or dust, needs to be removed. Mucus formation is also part of the histamine reaction to allergies and of the body's defenses during respiratory infections. Although many over-the-counter medications are available to treat a runny nose, it is usually best to allow the mucus to perform its function until the underlying condition is resolved.

nosebleed   Bleeding from the blood vessels of the nose. The nose is rich in blood vessels and is situated in a vulnerable position on the face. As a result, any trauma to the face can cause bleeding, which may be profuse. Nosebleeds can also occur spontaneously when the nasal membranes dry out, crust, and crack, as is common in dry climates or during winter months, when the air is dry and warm from household heaters. People have increased susceptibility to nosebleeds if they are taking medications that prevent normal blood clotting, such as warfarin (brand name: Coumadin), aspirin, or any anti-inflammatory medication. Other predisposing factors include infection,

trauma, allergic and nonallergic rhinitis, hypertension, alcohol abuse, and inherited bleeding problems. Also known as epistaxis.

nosebleed, treatment of   To stop a nosebleed, a person should pinch all the soft parts of the nose together between the thumb and index finger, and press firmly toward the face, compressing the pinched parts of the nose against the bones of the face. The person should hold the nose for at least 5 minutes and repeat as necessary until the nose has stopped bleeding, sitting quietly and keeping the head higher than the level of the heart (sitting up or lying with the head elevated). The person may also apply ice (crushed, in a plastic bag or washcloth) to the nose and cheeks.

nosocomial   Hospital-acquired. For example, a nosocomial infection is one that is caught in a hospital. Since antibiotics have come into common usage, bacteria that are resistant to them have also become common, especially in hospitals. As a result, there are now many nosocomial infections.

nostril   The external opening of the nose. The nostrils are also called the nares.

nostrum   **1** Formerly, a medicine of secret composition that was recommended by the person who concocted it, but with no scientific proof of its effectiveness. A patent medicine was a nostrum. **2** A worthless remedy. **3** In common usage, any questionable remedy or scheme for improving matters, a pet plan for accomplishing things, or a panacea.

NP   Nurse practitioner.

NPH   Normal pressure hydrocephalus.

NREM sleep   Non-rapid eye movement sleep, dreamless sleep. During NREM sleep, the brain waves seen on an electroencephalogram (EEG) are typically slow and of high voltage, the breathing and heart rate are slow and regular, the blood pressure is low, and the sleeper is relatively still. NREM sleep is divided into four stages of increasing depth, and the fourth and deepest stage eventually leads to REM sleep. About 80 percent of sleep is NREM sleep. See also *REM sleep; sleep.*

NS   Noonan syndrome.

NSAID   Nonsteroidal anti-inflammatory drug, a medication that is commonly prescribed or purchased over the counter to treat the inflammation associated with conditions such as arthritis, tendonitis, and bursitis. Examples of NSAIDs include aspirin, indomethacin (brand name: Indocin), ibuprofen (brand name: Motrin), naproxen (brand name: Naprosyn), piroxicam (brand name:

Feldene), and nabumetone (brand name: Relafen). The major side effects of NSAIDs are gastrointestinal problems. Some 10 to 50 percent of patients are unable to tolerate NSAID treatment because of these side effects, which include abdominal pain, diarrhea, bloating, heartburn, and upset stomach. Approximately 15 percent of patients on long-term NSAID treatment develop ulceration of the stomach and duodenum. Even though many of these patients with ulcers do not have symptoms, they are at risk of developing serious complications, such as bleeding or perforation of the stomach. The risk of serious complications is increased in elderly patients, in those with rheumatoid arthritis, in patients taking blood-thinning medications or cortisone medication, and in patients with heart disease or a history of bleeding ulcers.

NSE test Neuron-specific enolase test.

NTD Neural tube defect.

nuchal Referring to the back of the neck (nape). For example, nuchal rigidity is a stiff neck, sometimes a symptom of meningitis.

nuchal fold scan A prenatal ultrasound test that is done to screen for chromosome disorders such as Down syndrome and Turner syndrome. The scan measures the size of the space behind the neck of the fetus between 10 and 14 weeks of pregnancy and provides an index of the amount of fluid that has accumulated under the skin of the fetus. Also known as nuchal translucency test.

nucleic acid One of the family of large molecules that includes deoxyribonucleic acid (DNA) and ribonucleic acid (RNA). Nucleic acids were so named because they were first found in the nucleus of cells, but they have since been discovered to also exist outside the nucleus. See also *DNA; RNA.*

nucleosome A structure that is responsible in part for the compactness of a chromosome. Each nucleosome consists of a sequence of DNA wrapped around a core of histone, which is a type of protein.

nucleotide A subunit of DNA or RNA that consists of a nitrogenous base (A, G, T, or C in DNA; A, G, U, or C in RNA), a phosphate molecule, and a sugar molecule (deoxyribose in DNA, and ribose in RNA). Thousands of nucleotides are linked to form a DNA or an RNA molecule.

nucleus 1 In cell biology, the structure that houses the chromosomes. 2 In neuroanatomy, a group of nerve cells.

nullipara A woman who has not given birth to a viable child.

nummular eczema Coin-shaped patches of irritated skin that most commonly appear on the arms, back, buttocks, and lower legs and may be crusted, scaling, and extremely itchy.

nurse 1 A person who is trained, licensed, or skilled in nursing. 2 To breastfeed an infant.

nurse assistant A person who has completed a brief health care training program and who provides support services for RNs and LPNs. Also known as an orderly or, when certified by a state agency, a certified nurse aide (CNA).

nurse, licensed practical A nurse who has completed a 1- or 2-year training program in health care and has earned a state license. Abbreviated LPN. LPNs provide direct patient care for people with chronic illness, in nursing homes, hospitals, and home health care settings. They assist RNs in caring for acutely ill patients.

nurse practitioner A registered nurse (RN) who has completed an advanced training program in a medical specialty, such as pediatric care. Abbreviated NP. An NP may be a primary, direct health care provider, and can prescribe medications. Some NPs work in research rather than in direct patient care.

nurse, registered A nurse who has completed a 2- to 4-year degree program in nursing. Abbreviated RN. RNs provide direct patient care for acutely or chronically ill patients. RNs may further specialize in a particular area. For example, psychiatric nurses are RNs with special training in working with mentally ill patients, and trauma nurses work with physicians and surgeons to help patients in the emergency room of a hospital. Some RNs also work in health research.

nursing 1 A profession concerned with the provision of services that are essential to the maintenance and restoration of health. Nurses attend to the needs of sick people. Some nurses are licensed to directly diagnose and treat disease, and others work in medical research. 2 Breastfeeding.

nursing home A residential facility for people with chronic illness or disability, particularly older people who have mobility and eating problems. Also known as a convalescent home and long-term care facility.

nutraceutical A food or part of a food that allegedly provides medicinal or health benefits, including the prevention and treatment of disease. A nutraceutical may be a naturally nutrient-rich or medicinally active food, such as garlic or soybeans, or it may be a specific component of a food, such as the omega-3 fish oil that can be derived from salmon and other cold-water fish.

nutrition   **1** The science or practice of taking in and utilizing foods.   **2** A nourishing substance, such as nutritional solutions delivered to hospitalized patients via an intravenous (IV) or nasogastric (NG) tube.

nutritionist   **1** In a hospital or nursing home, a person who plans and/or formulates special meals for patients. The term can also be a euphemism for a cook who works in a medical facility but who does not have extensive training in special nutritional needs.   **2** In clinical practice, a specialist in nutrition. Nutritionists can help patients with special needs, allergies, health problems, or a desire for increased energy or weight change devise healthy diets. Some nutritionists in private practice are well trained, have degrees, and are licensed. Depending on state law, however, a person who uses the title might not be trained or licensed at all.

nvCJD   New variant Creutzfeldt-Jakob disease.

nyctanopia   Impaired vision in dim light and in the dark, due to impaired function of the rods in the retina. Nyctanopia is a classic finding with vitamin A deficiency. Also known as day sight, nocturnal amblyopia, and nyctalopia.

nyctophobia   Pathological fear of the dark.

nymph   A stage in the life cycle of certain arthropods, such as ticks and lice. The nymph stage is between the nit and the adult louse stages. A nymph louse looks like an adult but is smaller. Nymphs mature into adults about 7 days after hatching. To live, the nymph must feed on blood.

nystagmus   Rapid, rhythmic, repetitious, and involuntary eye movements. Nystagmus can be horizontal, vertical, or rotary. Whatever form it takes, nystagmus is an abnormal eye finding and a sign of disease within the eye or the nervous system.

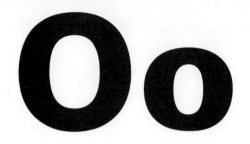

Oo

oat-cell lung cancer See *small-cell lung cancer.*

Oath of Hippocrates See *Hippocratic oath.*

Oath of Maimonides See *Daily Prayer of a Physician.*

OB **1** Obstetrician. **2** Obstetrics.

obese Overweight. People are considered to be obese if they are more than 20 percent over their ideal weight. That ideal weight must take into account the person's height, age, sex, and build. Obesity is often multifactorial, based on both genetic and behavioral factors. Accordingly, treatment of obesity usually requires more than just dietary changes. Exercise, counseling and support, and sometimes medication can supplement diet to help patients conquer weight problems. Extreme diets, on the other hand, can actually contribute to increased obesity. Obesity is a significant contributor to health problems. See also *obesity-related disease.*

obesity, endogenous A state of being overweight that is caused by malfunction of the hormonal or metabolic system.

obesity, exogenous A state of being overweight that is caused by consuming more food than the person's activity level warrants, leading to increased fat storage.

obesity, gynecoid A state of being overweight with fat distribution in a pattern that is generally characteristic of a woman, with the largest amount around the hips and thighs.

obesity, male A state of being overweight with fat distribution in a pattern that is generally characteristic of a man, with a prominent paunch.

obesity-related disease A disease for which obesity is a significant risk factor. Obesity increases the risk of developing a number of diseases, and it can be a diagnostic marker for others. Diseases related to obesity include type 2 (adult-onset) diabetes; high blood pressure (hypertension); stroke (cerebrovascular accident); heart attack (myocardial infarction); heart failure (congestive heart failure); certain forms of cancer, such as prostate and colon cancer; gallstones and gall bladder disease (cholecystitis); gout and gouty arthritis; osteoarthritis (degenerative arthritis) of the knees, hips, and lower back; sleep apnea; and Pickwickian syndrome.

OB/GYN Obstetrician/gynecologist.

objective lens See *lens, objective.*

observer variation Failure by the observer in a study or test to measure accurately, resulting in error.

obsessive-compulsive disorder An anxiety disorder that is characterized by obsessive thoughts and compulsive actions. Abbreviated OCD. The obsessive thoughts are unwanted ideas or impulses that repeatedly well up in the mind of the person with OCD. These thoughts are intrusive and unpleasant, and they produce a high degree of anxiety. In response to their obsessions, most people with OCD resort to repetitive behaviors called compulsions. The most common of these are washing and checking. Other compulsive behaviors include counting and endlessly rearranging objects in an effort to keep them in precise alignment with each other. Treatment includes behavioral therapy and medication, and a specific behavior therapy approach called exposure and response prevention is effective for many people with OCD. The neurotransmitter serotonin has been found to decrease the symptoms of OCD. Selective serotonin reuptake inhibitors (SSRIs) are therefore used to treat OCD. Among the drugs approved for treatment of OCD are clomipramine (brand name: Anafranil), fluoxetine (brand name: Prozac), fluvoxamine (brand name: Luvox), paroxetine (brand name: Paxil), and sertraline (brand name: Zoloft). More than 75 percent of patients are helped by these medications, which suggests that OCD has a neurobiological basis. OCD is different from obsessive-compulsive personality disorder, which is a personality disorder rather than an anxiety disorder.

obsessive-compulsive personality disorder A personality disorder that is characterized by pervasive preoccupation with orderliness, perfectionism, and interpersonal control. Abbreviated OCPD. OCPD may feature a preoccupation with details, rules, lists, order, organization, or schedules; perfectionism; excessive devotion to work to the exclusion of leisure activities and friendships; inability to discard worthless objects of no sentimental value; reluctance to delegate tasks or work with others unless everything is done a certain way; miserliness; rigidity; and stubbornness. OCPD is different from obsessive-compulsive disorder, which is a type of anxiety disorder. OCPD may require no treatment or may benefit from counseling.

obstetrical forceps An instrument that has two blades and a handle and is designed to aid in the vaginal delivery of a baby.

obstetrician   A physician who specializes in obstetrics.

obstetrician/gynecologist   An obstetrician who also specializes in treating diseases of the female reproductive organs. Abbreviated OB/GYN. Some OB/GYNs also provide general health care for women.

obstetrics   The art and science of managing pregnancy, labor, and the puerperium (the time after delivery).

obstruction, airway   See *airway obstruction.*

obstructive sleep apnea   See *sleep apnea, obstructive.*

obtunded   Mentally dulled. Head trauma may obtund a person.

occipital bone   The bone that forms the rear and rear bottom of the skull.

occiput   The back of the head.

occlude   **1** To close, obstruct, or prevent passage. For example, to occlude an artery is to block the flow of blood. **2** To bring together. For example, to occlude the teeth is to oppose the upper with the lower teeth, as for chewing.

occult   Hidden. For example, occult blood in the stool is hidden from the eye but can be detected by chemical tests.

occupational disease   A disease that is due to a factor in a person's work. For example, an occupational disease for coal miners is lung disease.

occupational medicine   The field of medicine that encompasses occupational diseases. Occupational medicine was founded in 1700 by the Italian physician Bernardino Ramazzini, who recognized the relationship between lead and antimony and the symptoms of poisoning in painters and other artisans exposed to them. Ramazzini also first recognized miners' lung disease.

occupational therapist   A person who is trained and licensed to design and deliver occupational therapy services. Abbreviated OT. See also *occupational therapy.*

occupational therapy   Therapy designed to help patients gain or relearn skills needed for activities of daily living, including self-care, handwriting and other school-related skills, and work-related skills. In occupational therapy, patients may do exercises, manipulate items to help develop normal hand motion, or learn to use assistive devices, among other activities. Abbreviated OT.

OCD   **1** Obsessive-compulsive disorder.   **2** Osteochondritis dissecans.

OCP   Oral contraceptive pill.

OCPD   Obsessive-compulsive personality disorder.

ocular   Having to do with the eye.

ocular lens   See *lens, ocular.*

oculomotor nerve   The third cranial nerve. The oculomotor nerve is responsible for the nerve supply to muscles around the eye, including the upper eyelid muscle, which raises the eyelid; the extraocular muscle, which moves the eye inward; and the pupillary muscle, which constricts the pupil. Paralysis of the oculomotor nerve results in a drooping eyelid (ptosis), deviation of the eyeball outward (and therefore double vision), and a dilated (wide-open) pupil.

OD   **1** Osteochondritis dissecans.   **2** Overdose.   **3** The right eye (oculus dexter), as opposed to OS (left eye).

off-label use   The practice of prescribing approved medications for conditions other than those indicated on the official medication label. In the US, the regulations of the Food and Drug Administration (FDA) permit physicians to prescribe medications for off-label use.

offspring   The progeny, or young, born to a person. In a larger sense, the offspring are collectively all the descendants, the brood, or the family. For example, the offspring of someone with a genetic (inherited) condition, such as Huntington's disease, are themselves at risk for the disease.

ointment   An oil-based preparation that is applied to the skin. Whereas an ointment has an oil base, a cream is water soluble.

olecranon   The bony tip of the elbow. The olecranon is the near end of the ulna, the bone in the forearm, and it forms the pointed portion of the elbow. The triceps muscle tendon of the back of the arm attaches to the olecranon. Disease can affect the olecranon. For example, inflammation of the tiny fluid-filled sac (bursa) at the tip of the elbow can occur; this is referred to as olecranon bursitis. A firm nodule can form at the tip of the elbow; it is referred to as an olecranon nodule and is sometimes found in gout or rheumatoid arthritis. Also known as the olecranon process of the ulna.

olfaction   The sense of smell.

olfactory apparatus   The whole system that is needed to have a sense of smell, including the nose and affiliated nerves.

olfactory nerve The nerve that carries impulses for the sense of smell from the nose to the brain. The olfactory nerve is the first cranial nerve.

oligohydramnios Too little amniotic fluid. The opposite of polyhydramnios: Too much amniotic fluid.

oligosaccharidosis One of a group of inherited metabolic disorders that are similar to the mucopolysaccharidoses. These conditions include aspartylglycosaminuria (AGU), fucosidosis, mannosidosis, and multiple sulfatase deficiency. Symptoms generally include deterioration of the nervous system. No treatment is available.

oligo- Prefix meaning just a few, or scanty, as in oligodactyly (having fewer than 10 fingers or 10 toes) and oliguria (less urination than normal).

oligodactyly Having fewer than the normal number of fingers or toes. Oligodactyly is the opposite of polydactyly.

oligodendrocyte A type of cell in the central nervous system. The oligodendrocytes surround and insulate the long fibers (axons) through which the nerves send electrical messages.

oligodendroglioma A rare, slow-growing brain tumor that begins in cells called oligodendrocytes, which provide support and nourishment for cells that transmit nerve impulses. Also known as oligodendroglial tumor.

oligohydramnios Very little amniotic fluid. Oligohydramnios often represents an underlying disease state in the mother or fetus.

oligomenorrhea Less menstrual blood flow than usual.

oligonucleotide A short DNA molecule that is composed of relatively few nucleotide bases.

oligonucleotide probe A short sequence of nucleotides that are synthesized to match a region where a mutation is known to occur and then used as a molecular probe to detect the mutation.

oligopeptide A molecule that is composed of a few amino acids linked to one another.

oligospermia Fewer sperm than usual. Azospermia, by contrast, means absolutely no sperm at all.

oliguria Less urination than normal.

Ollier's disease See *multiple enchondromatosis*.

omega-3 fatty acids A class of fatty acids found in fish oils, especially salmon and other cold-water fish, that acts to lower the levels of total cholesterol and LDL cholesterol in the blood. Omega-3 fish oil is considered a neutraceutical, a food that provides health benefits. Eating fish has been reported to protect against age-related macular degeneration, a common eye disease.

omentum A sheet of fat that is covered by peritoneum. The greater omentum is attached to the bottom edge of the stomach and hangs down in front of the intestines. Its other edge is attached to the transverse colon. The lesser omentum is attached to the top edge of the stomach and extends to the undersurface of the liver.

Ommaya reservoir A device that is implanted under the scalp to deliver anticancer drugs to the fluid surrounding the brain and spinal cord.

omphalo- Prefix indicating a relationship to the umbilicus (the navel). From the Greek word for the decorative boss protruding from the center of a Greek warrior's shield. The omphalos in the temple of Apollo at Delphi was a rounded conical stone; it was sacred and marked what the ancient Greeks believed to be the central point of the earth.

omphalocele A birth defect in which part of the intestine, covered only by a thin transparent membrane, protrudes outside the abdomen at the umbilicus. An omphalocele occurs due to a failure during embryonic development for a section of the intestines (the midgut) to return from outside the abdomen and reenter the abdomen as it should. The opening in the abdominal wall cannot close because to do so would pinch off part of the intestines. An omphalocele must be repaired with surgery.

onchocerciasis See *river blindness*.

oncogene A gene that had a normal role in the cell, has been altered by mutation, and may contribute to the growth of a tumor. See *proto-oncogene*.

oncologist A physician who specializes in the diagnosis and treatment of cancer. After a cancer diagnosis is made, it is the oncologist's role to explain the cancer diagnosis and the meaning of the disease stage to the patient; discuss various treatment options; recommend the best course of treatment; deliver optimal care; and improve quality of life both through curative therapy and palliative care with pain and symptom management.

oncology The field of medicine that is devoted to cancer. Clinical oncology consists of three primary disciplines: medical oncology (the treatment of cancer with medicine, including chemotherapy), surgical oncology (the surgical aspects of cancer including biopsy, staging, and surgical resection of tumors), and radiation oncology (the treatment of cancer with therapeutic radiation).

Ondine's curse   Failure of the central nervous system to control breathing while a person is asleep. People with Ondine's curse usually have no problem breathing while awake. With Ondine's curse, the voluntary control of ventilation that operates during waking hours is generally intact, but the involuntary (autonomic) control of respiration is impaired. The patient can have problems with the normal movement of the esophagus and the colon, and his or her heart rate may be abnormally slow. Some patients have downward slanting eyes, a small nose, a triangular-shape mouth, and ears that are low set and backward rotated. Also known as congenital central hypoventilation syndrome (CCHS), CCHS with Hirschsprung's disease, congenital failure of autonomic control, idiopathic central alveolar hypoventilation, and central sleep apnea with severe hypoventilation. In Greek mythology, Ondine (Undine) was a water sprite who was condemned to stay awake in order to breathe.

oneiric   Relating to dreams, dream-like. From the Greek *oneiros,* meaning "dream."

oneirophrenia   A hallucinatory (dream-like) state that is caused by such conditions as prolonged sleep deprivation, sensory isolation, and drug use.

onycho-   Prefix having to do with the nails, as in onychodystrophy (abnormal growth and development of nails).

onychodystrophy   Malformation of the nails.

onycholysis   Loosening of a nail from the nail bed, usually starting at the border of the nail. The nail tends to turn whitish or yellowish, reflecting the presence of air under it. The treatment is to trim the nail short, not to clean under the nail, and to be patient.

onychomycosis   Fungus infection of the nail bed under the fingernails or toenails. Onychomycosis makes the nails look white and opaque, thickened, and brittle. Older women (perhaps because estrogen deficiency may increase the risk of infection), and men and women with diabetes or disease of the small blood vessels (peripheral vascular disease) are at increased risk for onychomycosis. Artificial nails (acrylic nails or "wraps") increase the risk because the nail surface is usually abraded when an artificial nail is applied. If the emery board carries infection and water collects under the nail, it creates a moist, warm environment for fungal growth. Treatment includes avoiding artificial nails, using safer application techniques and only new artificial nails and emery boards for each customer, and using topical antifungal medication. Also known as nail fungus and tinea unguium.

onychomycosis, proximal white subungual   The rarest form of fungus infection of the fingernail or toenail. The proximal white subungual onychomycosis infection begins in the nail fold, the portion of the nail opposite the tip of the finger. Proximal white subungual onychomycosis is typically associated with HIV infection (AIDS), although it can follow injury to the nail. The most common fungus implicated is Trichophyton rubrum. Other causes include T. megninii, T. tonsiurans, T. mentagrophytes, T. schoenleinii, and Epidermophyton floccosum. Diagnosis is made via observation of infection in the portion of the nailbed closest to the hand and can be confirmed by seeing the fungus in a scraping of the tissue placed under a microscope. Proximal white subungual onychomycosis is treated with antifungal medications taken by mouth. Examples include itraconazole (brand name: Sporanox) and terbinafine (brand name: Lamisil).

onychoosteodysplasia   See *nail-patella syndrome.*

oo-   Prefix meaning egg or egg-related, as in oocyte (a female germ cell—an egg—in the process of development) and oophoritis (inflammation of the egg sac).

oocyte   A female germ cell in the process of development. The oocyte is produced in the ovary by an ancestral cell called an oogonium and gives rise to the ovum (the egg), which can be fertilized.

oogonium   An ancestral cell that gives rise to an oocyte.

oomphalomesenteric duct   See *yolk stalk.*

oophorectomy   The removal of one or both ovaries by surgery.

oophoritis   Inflammation of the ovary, or egg sac.

open fracture   See *fracture, compound.*

open reading frame   A portion of DNA that is available to be translated into a protein. In genetics, an open reading frame in DNA has no termination codon (no signal to stop reading the nucleotide sequence), and so may be translated into protein.

open wound   An injury that is exposed because of broken skin. An open wound is at high risk for infection.

opening, vaginal   The opening to the muscular canal that extends from the cervix to the outside of the body. In medicine, the vaginal opening is called the vestibule of the vagina.

operating room   A facility that is equipped for performing surgery. Abbreviated OR.

operation In medicine, a surgical procedure. Many operations are named after persons. They range from A to Z, from the Abbe operation (on the lip) to the Ziegler operation (on the eye).

operation, Blalock-Taussig See *Blalock-Taussig operation.*

operation, Macewen See *Macewen operation.*

ophthalmia Severe inflammation of the eye. Also known as ophthalmitis.

ophthalmia, sympathetic See *sympathetic ophthalmia.*

ophthalmic Pertaining to the eye. For example, an ophthalmic ointment is designed for the eye.

ophthalmic artery The artery that supplies blood to the eye and adjacent structures of the face. It arises from the internal carotid artery, which courses up from deep within the front of the neck. See also *artery.*

ophthalmic migraine See *migraine, ophthalmic.*

ophthalmic vein One of the paired veins that drain the orbital cavity that contains the eye. The superior ophthalmic vein arises at the inner angle of the orbit and follows the course of the ophthalmic artery into the cavernous sinus, a large channel of venous blood. The inferior ophthalmic vein arises from a venous network at the forepart of orbit and divides into two branches, one of which also ends in the cavernous sinus. See also *cavernous sinus; vein.*

ophthalmitis See *ophthalmia.*

ophthalmologist A physician (MD) who practices ophthalmology.

ophthalmology The art and science of eye medicine.

ophthalmopathy Any eye disease.

ophthalmoscope A lighted instrument that is used to examine the inside of the eye, including the retina and the optic nerve.

ophthalmoscopy Examination of the interior of the eye, including the lens, retina, and optic nerve, using an ophthalmoscope. Ophthalmoscopy can be indirect or direct. Indirect ophthalmoscopy, which is generally performed by an ophthalmologist, employs a headlamp device to shine a very bright light into the eye. Direct ophthalmoscopy is in more common usage by many health practitioners. The examiner uses a device the size of a flashlight to examine the eye. The device consists of a concave mirror and a battery-powered light (contained within the handle). The operator looks through a single monocular eyepiece into the patient's eye. The ophthalmoscope is equipped with a rotating disc of lenses to permit the eye to be examined at different depths and magnifications. The ophthalmoscope operator can better see into the eye by using one of a number of drugs to dilate the patient's pupil and enlarge the opening into the structures within the eye.

opiate A medication or an illegal drug that is derived from the opium poppy or that mimics the effect of an opiate (a synthetic opiate). Opiate drugs are narcotic sedatives that depress activity of the central nervous system, reduce pain, and induce sleep. Side effects may include oversedation, nausea, and constipation. Long-term use of opiates can produce addiction, and overuse can cause overdose and potentially death.

opioid **1** A synthetic narcotic that resembles the naturally occurring opiates. **2** Any substance that binds to or otherwise affects the opiate receptors on the surface of the cell. Opiate receptors are the cell-surface proteins to which opiates and opiods bind in order to cause their effects.

opisthotonos A great rigid spasm of the body, with the back fully arched and the heels and head bent back. Opisthotonos occurs in meningitis, especially in infants, due to irritation of the membranes surrounding the brain and spinal cord. It also occurs with depressed brain function and injury to the brain. Opisthotonos is an ominous neurologic sign.

opium An addictive narcotic drug that is derived from the unripe seedpods of the opium poppy. Preparations of opium were called laudanum. Derivatives of opium include paregoric (a drug used to treat diarrhea), morphine, and heroin. For centuries, opium was used as a painkiller in the Middle East and Asia. It gained great popularity in Europe and the European colonies in the 18th century and became a main ingredient in patent medicines that patients could easily obtain without prescriptions. Many people became addicted to opium. Wounded Civil War soldiers who were in pain often received morphine. By 1900, it is estimated that more than 200,000 people in the US were addicted to opium and its derivatives. In 1909, the US Congress passed a law prohibiting the manufacture and sale of opium.

opportunistic condition A condition that occurs especially or exclusively in persons with weak immune systems due, for example, to AIDS, cancer, or immunosuppressive drugs, such as corticosteroids or chemotherapy.

An opportunistic condition may be an infection, such as toxoplasmosis or cytomegalovirus (CMV), or a tumor, such as Kaposi sarcoma in AIDS. See also *opportunistic infection; opportunistic microorganism.*

opportunistic infection   An infection that occurs because a person's immune system is weakened. Opportunistic infections are a particular danger for people with immunodeficiency, such as AIDS. The HIV virus itself does not cause death, but the opportunistic infections that occur because of the effect of the virus on the immune system can be lethal. See also *opportunistic condition; opportunistic microorganism.*

opportunistic microorganism   A bacterium, virus, or fungus that takes advantage of certain opportunities to cause disease (opportunistic conditions). Opportunistic microorganisms are often ones that can lie dormant in body tissues for many years, such as the human herpesviruses, or that are extremely common but usually cause no symptoms of illness. When the immune system cannot raise an adequate response, these microorganisms are activated, begin to multiply, and soon overwhelm the body's weakened defenses. See also *opportunistic condition; opportunistic infection.*

optic   Having to do with vision.

optic glioma   See *glioma, optic.*

optic nerve   The second cranial nerve, which connects the eye to the brain. The optic nerve carries the impulses that are formed by the retina—the nerve layer that lines the back of the eye, senses light, and creates impulses. These impulses are dispatched through the optic nerve to the brain, which interprets them as images. Using an ophthalmoscope, one can easily see the head of the optic nerve. It is the only anatomic extension of the brain, and it is a part of the central nervous system rather than a peripheral nerve.

optic nerve pathways   The course of the chemical and electrical impulse from light stimulating the retina as it passes from the optic nerve to the vision center of the brain. The left and right branches of the optic nerves join behind the eyes, just in front of the pituitary gland, to form a cross-shaped structure called the optic chiasma. Within the optic chiasma, some of the nerve fibers cross. The fibers from the nasal (inside) half of each retina cross over, but those from the temporal (outside) half do not. Specifically, the fibers from the nasal half of the left eye and the temporal half of the right eye form the right optic tract; and the fibers from the nasal half of the right eye and the temporal half of the left form the left optic tract. The nerve fibers then continue along in the optic tracts.

Just before they reach the thalamus of the brain, a few of the nerve fibers leave to enter nerve nuclei that function in visual reflexes. Most of the nerve fibers enter the thalamus, forming a junction (synapse) in the back of the thalamus. From there the visual impulses enter nerve pathways called the optic radiations, which lead to the visual (sight) cortex of the occipital (back) lobes of the brain.

optic neuroma   A rare benign tumor of the optic nerve.

optician   A specialist in fitting eyeglasses and making lenses to correct vision problems. An optometrist performs eye examinations and writes prescriptions for corrective lenses; an optician fills that prescription.

optometrist   A practitioner who provides primary eye and vision care, performs eye examinations to detect vision problems, and prescribes corrective lenses to correct those problems. Some optometrists also make and fit eyeglasses, but many leave that job to opticians. An optometrist is a doctor of optometry (OD), not an MD. When an optometrist detects eye disease, the patient may be referred instead to an ophthalmologist, an MD who specializes in evaluating and treating diseases of the eye.

OPV   Oral polio vaccine. See *polio vaccine, oral.*

OR   Operating room.

oral   Having to do with the mouth. For example, an oral solution is a solution that is given by mouth.

oral cancer   Cancer within the mouth. Oral cancer is associated with smoking cigarettes and cigars as well as chewing tobacco. It is generally noticed as a painless growth on the inner cheek, gum, or tongue. Treatment options include surgical resection, radiation, and/or chemotherapy.

oral contraceptive   A birth control pill taken by mouth. Most oral contraceptives include both estrogen and progestogen. When given in certain amounts and at certain times in the menstrual cycle, these hormones prevent the ovary from releasing an egg for fertilization. Colloquially known as "the pill." See also *birth control; contraceptive.*

oral polio vaccine   See *polio vaccine, oral.*

oral rehydration solution   A specially designed liquid that contains water, glucose, and electrolytes and is given to treat dehydration. Abbreviated ORS.

oral rehydration therapy   The administration of special fluids by mouth to treat dehydration. Abbreviated ORS. See also *oral rehydration solution.*

oral surgeon A dentist who has special training in surgery to correct problems of the mouth and jaw.

oral-motor Relating to the muscles of the mouth and/or to movements of the mouth.

oral-motor apraxia of speech See *apraxia of speech.*

orbit In medicine, the bony cavity in which the eyeball sits.

orbital In anatomy, pertaining to the orbit, the bony cavity that contains the eyeball.

orbital ridge The bony ridge beneath the eyebrow.

orchidectomy The surgical removal of one or both testes.

orchiectomy Orchidectomy.

orchiopathy Any and all diseases of the testes.

orchiopexy Surgery to bring an undescended testicle down into the scrotum.

orchitis Inflammation of the testis. Causes of orchitis include mumps and other infections; diseases, such as polyarteritis nodosa; and injury.

organ A relatively independent part of the body that carries out one or more special functions. The organs include the eyes, ears, heart, lungs, and liver.

organic 1 A chemical compound that contains carbon. 2 Related to an organ. 3 Grown or prepared without the use of chemicals or pesticides, as in organic food.

organic brain syndrome Psychiatric or neurological symptoms that arise from damage to or disease in the brain. Also known as organic mental disorder.

organotherapy The use of extracts of animal glands or organs to treat disease. Pituitary extracts from pigs, for example, were used for many years to treat hormone disorders.

organs of reproduction, female See *female organs of reproduction.*

organs of reproduction, male See *male organs of reproduction.*

orgasm A series of muscle contractions in the genital region that is accompanied by sudden release of endorphins. Orgasm normally accompanies male ejaculation as a result of sexual stimulation, and it also occurs in females as a result of sexual stimulation.

orifice An opening. For example, the mouth is an orifice.

oromandibular dystonia A condition that affects the muscles of the jaw, lips, and tongue. The jaw may be pulled open or shut, and speech and swallowing can be difficult. Local injections of botulism toxin (Brand name: Botox) has been used as a treatment.

oropharynx The part of the throat that is at the back of the mouth, in contrast to the nasopharynx (the part of the throat that is behind the nose).

orphan disease A disease that has not been "adopted" by the pharmaceutical industry because it provides little financial incentive for the private sector to make and market new medications to treat or prevent it. An orphan disease may be a rare disease (according to US criteria, a disease that affects fewer than 200,000 people) or a common disease that has been ignored (such as tuberculosis, cholera, typhoid, and malaria) because it is far more prevalent in developing countries than in the developed world. The US Orphan Drug Act of 1983 offered tax incentives on clinical trials and 7 years of marketing exclusivity for drugs developed for conditions that occur only rarely in the US. Since then, more than 200 orphan drugs have been approved by the US Food and Drug Administration (FDA) and are on the market. Similar legislation has been adopted in Japan and Australia. In the year 2000, the European Union adopted "orphan medicinal products" legislation that is modeled on the US law but includes tropical diseases and other disorders that are prevalent only in the developing world. The EU law provides for 10 years of marketing exclusivity but no tax incentives (because there is no centralized EU taxation system).

orphan drug A drug that is designed to treat or prevent an orphan disease. See also *orphan disease.*

ORS Oral rehydration solution.

ORT Oral rehydration therapy.

ortho- Prefix meaning straight or erect, as in orthodontics (the straightening of the teeth) and orthostatic (in an upright posture).

orthodontic treatment The use of devices, such as dental braces, to move teeth or adjust underlying bone. The ideal age for starting orthodontic treatment is between 3 and 12 years. Teeth can be moved with removable appliances or with fixed braces. Crowding of teeth can require extraction. Retainers may be necessary long after dental braces are removed, especially with orthodontic treatment of adults. Temporomandibular joint

(TMJ) problems can be corrected with splinting or dental braces.

orthodontics　The dental specialty that is concerned with the diagnosis and treatment of dental deformities as well as irregularity in the relationship of the lower to the upper jaw.

orthomolecular medicine　1 A type of medicine that, according to biochemist Linus Pauling, is concerned with "the preservation of good health and the treatment of disease by varying the concentration in the human body of substances that are normally present in the body." The treatment of diabetes with the injection of insulin and the prevention of goiter with iodine are examples of orthomolecular medicine.　2 A form of alternative medicine in which practitioners try to prevent and cure disease by using specific doses of vitamins, amino acids, fatty acids, trace minerals, electrolytes, and other natural substances.

orthopaedics　See *orthopedics.*

orthopaedist　See *orthopedist.*

orthopedics　The branch of surgery that is broadly concerned with the skeletal system. Sometimes spelled orthopaedics.

orthopedist　An orthopedic surgeon, a physician who corrects congenital or functional abnormalities of the bones with surgery, casting, and bracing. Orthopedists also treat injuries to the bones. Sometimes spelled orthopaedist.

orthopnea　The inability to breathe easily except when sitting up straight or standing erect.

orthopod　Slang term for an orthopedist.

orthoscopic　Having correct vision, producing correct vision, free from optical distortion, or designed to correct distorted vision.

orthostatic hypotension　See *hypotension, orthostatic.*

OS　The left eye (oculus sinister), as opposed to the right eye (oculus dexter).

os sacrum　The large, heavy bone at the base of the spine. The os sacrum is symmetrical and roughly triangular in shape. The female sacrum is wider and less curved than the male sacrum, to permit easier childbearing.

Osgood-Schlatter disease　A condition that is characterized by inflammation and sometimes tearing of ligaments within the knee and lower leg. Osgood-Schlatter disease is caused by repetitive stress or tension on a part of the growth area of the upper tibia (the apophysis). It is characterized by inflammation of the patellar tendon and surrounding soft tissues at the point where the tendon attaches to the tibia. The disease may also be associated with an avulsion injury, in which the tendon is stretched so much that it tears away from the tibia and takes a fragment of bone with it. Osgood-Schlatter disease most commonly affects active young people, particularly boys between the ages of 10 and 15, who play games or sports that include frequent running and jumping. Treatment includes rest, casting if necessary, and sometimes surgery. See also *osteochondrosis.*

Osler node　One of the small, tender, transient nodules in the pads of fingers and toes and on the palms and soles. Osler nodes are a highly diagnostic sign of bacterial infection of the heart (subacute bacterial endocarditis).

Osler-Rendu-Weber syndrome　See *hereditary hemorrhagic telangectasia.*

osseous　Having to do with bone, consisting of bone, or resembling bone.

ossicle　Any small bone, such as the tiny bones within the human ear.

ossification　1 The normal process of bone growth. 2 Hardening, becoming bone-like.

ossify　To harden.

osteitis　Inflammation of the bone.

osteitis deformans　See *Paget's disease.*

osteitis fibrosa cystica　A condition that is associated with excessive parathyroid hormone production (hyperparathyroidism), in which bone tissue is gradually replaced by cysts and fibers. Treatment is directed toward the underlying parathyroid condition and relieving any bone pain.

osteo-　Prefix meaning bone, as in osteogenesis (the production of bone) and osteosarcoma (cancer arising in the bone).

osteoarthritis　See *arthritis, degenerative.*

osteoblastoma　A noncancerous tumor in bone tissue. Osteoblastomas are small and are seen most frequently in children and young adults. Symptoms include pain and bone-mass reduction. Treatment includes surgery, sometimes followed by chemotherapy.

osteochondritis dissecans　A condition in which a fragment of bone in a joint is deprived of blood and separates from the rest of the bone, causing soreness and making the joint give way. Diagnosis is made via X-ray.

Treatment usually involves casting, although if the fragment has detached completely, arthroscopic surgery may be necessary. Abbreviated OCD and OD.

osteochondroma An abnormal, solitary, benign growth of bone and cartilage, typically at the end of a long bone. Osteochondromas are usually discovered in persons 15 to 25 years of age. An osteochondroma is typically detected when the area around it is injured or when it becomes large.

osteochondromatosis A condition that is characterized by multiple benign tumors of cartilage, called osteochondromas, projecting from bone, most often from near the ends of long bones. In a small proportion of cases, an osteochondroma may become malignant. Also known as multiple exostoses. The condition can be hereditary, in which case it is called hereditary multiple exostoses (HMS).

osteochondrosis Any disease that affects the progress of bone growth by killing bone tissue. Osteochondrosis is seen only in children and teens whose bones are still growing.

osteoclasia Destruction and reabsorption of bone tissue, as occurs when broken bones heal.

osteoclasis The surgical destruction of bone tissue. Osteoclasis is performed to reconstruct a bone that is malformed, often a broken bone that healed improperly. The bone is broken and then reshaped with the aid of metal pins, casting, and bracing.

osteoclast A type of large bone cell that appears when bones are growing or need to be repaired. Osteoclasts may also appear abnormally. See also *osteoclastoma*.

osteoclastoma A tumor of the bone that begins in osteoclast cells, often osteoclasts that have formed abnormally. The tumor may be coated by new bony growth. An osteoclastoma causes pain, restricts movement, and is usually cancerous. Treatment involves surgery, usually followed by chemotherapy.

osteocyte A bone cell.

osteodystrophy A bone disorder that adversely affects bone growth. Osteodystrophy is most commonly caused by chronic kidney failure, but it can be inherited, such as in Albright hereditary osteodystrophy. Osteodystrophy can require treatment with vitamin D. See also *osteodystrophy, renal*.

osteodystrophy, renal A bone disorder that adversely affects bone growth and is caused by chronic kidney failure (renal disease). Osteodystrophy can require treatment with vitamin D. Also known as kidney osteodystrophy.

osteogenesis The production of bone.

osteogenesis, electrically stimulated A procedure that is used to stimulate bone growth. Electrically stimulated osteogenesis involves implanting electrodes in an area of bone and sending electrical current to them. Electrically stimulated osteogenesis may be used to jumpstart the healing process after a bone has been broken.

osteogenesis imperfecta A group of genetic diseases, all of which affect collagen in connective tissue in the body, and all of which result in fragile bones. The best known types of osteogenesis imperfecta are types I and II. Also known as brittle bone disease.

osteogenesis imperfecta congenita See *osteogenesis imperfecta type II*.

osteogenesis imperfecta tarda See *osteogenesis imperfecta type I*.

osteogenesis imperfecta type I An inherited, generalized connective-tissue disorder that features bone fragility and blue sclerae (bluish whites of the eyes). Osteogenesis imperfecta type I is the classic, mild form of brittle bone disease. It is inherited as a dominant trait, so one copy of the mutant gene is sufficient to cause the disease, and both males and females can be affected. It is characterized by fragile bones, the onset after birth of growth deficiency, abnormal teeth that look as if they have been sandblasted, thin skin, blue sclerae, and overly extensible joints. Ten percent of patients have their first fractures noted at birth, about 25 percent in the first year, about 50 percent in the preschool years, and the balance in the early school years. The risk of fractures decreases after adolescence. Common problems include the development of bowed legs, curvature of the spine (scoliosis and kyphosis), umbilical and inguinal hernias, and mild mitral valve prolapse. Hearing impairment begins in the third decade of life, due to otosclerosis, a disorder of the bones of the middle ear. Osteogenesis imperfecta type I results from mutations that impair the production of type I collagen, a key component of connective tissue. Such mutations have been identified in both the COL1A1 gene on chromosome 17 and the COL1A2 gene on chromosome 7. Also known as osteogenesis imperfecta tarda and Lobstein disease.

osteogenesis imperfecta type II An inherited connective-tissue disorder that features very severe bone fragility. Osteogenesis imperfecta type II is the lethal form of brittle bone disease. It is inherited as a recessive trait, so two copies of the mutant gene are needed to cause the disease. Both males and females can be affected. The disease is characterized by short-limb dwarfism, thin skin, a soft skull, unusually large fontanels (soft spots), blue sclerae (bluish whites of the eyes), small nose, low nasal bridge, inguinal hernia, and numerous bone fractures at birth. The limbs are bowed due to multiple fractures. Children with osteogenesis imperfecta type II are usually stillborn or die of respiratory failure in early infancy. The condition results from mutations that impair the production of type I collagen, a key component of connective tissue. Mutations have been identified in both the COL1A1 gene on chromosome 17 and the COL1A2 gene on chromosome 7. Also known as osteogenesis imperfecta congenita and Vrolik disease.

osteogenesis imperfecta with blue sclerae See *osteogenesis imperfecta type II.*

osteogenic sarcoma See *osteosarcoma.*

osteoid osteoma A benign tumor of bone tissue. Osteoid osteoma emerges most often in a person's teens or 20s and is found most frequently in the femur and in males. Symptoms include pain, mostly at night. Diagnosis is made via X-ray. Most cases do not require invasive treatment, but just the use of aspirin or nonaspirin analgesics to treat pain.

osteomalacia Softening of the bone. Osteomalacia may be caused by poor diet or inadequate absorption of calcium and other minerals needed to harden bones. Treatment includes dietary change and sometimes hormone supplements for postmenopausal women. See also *osteoporosis.*

osteomyelitis Inflammation of the bone due to infection, for example, by the bacteria salmonella or staphylococcus. Osteomyelitis is sometimes a complication of surgery or injury, although infection can also reach bone tissue through the bloodstream. Both the bone and the bone marrow may be infected. Symptoms include deep pain and muscle spasms in the area of inflammation, as well as fever. Treatment includes bed rest, use of antibiotics (usually injected locally), and sometimes surgery to remove dead bone tissue.

osteonecrosis See *avascular necrosis.*

osteopath An osteopathic physician; a Doctor of Osteopathy (DO). In most US states, osteopaths complete a course of study equivalent to that of an MD and are licensed to practice medicine. They may prescribe medication and perform surgery, and they often use techniques similar to those used in chiropractic and physical therapy.

osteopathy A system of therapy founded in the 19th century that is based on the concept that the body can formulate its own remedies against diseases when its parts are in a normal structural relationship, it has a normal environment, and it enjoys good nutrition. Although osteopathy takes a holistic approach to medical care, it also embraces modern medical knowledge, including use of medication, surgery, radiation, and chemotherapy when warranted. Osteopathy is particularly concerned with maintaining correct relationships between bones, muscles, and connective tissues. The practice of osteopathy often includes chiropractic-like adjustments of skeletal structures. Craniosacral therapy, a practice in which the bones and tissues of the head and neck are manipulated, also arose in osteopathy.

osteopenia Mild thinning of the bone mass. Osteopenia represents a low bone mass and is not as severe as osteoporosis. Osteopenia results when formation of new bone (osteoid synthesis) is not sufficient to offset normal bone loss (osteoid lysis). Diminished bone calcification, as visualized on plain X-ray film, is referred to as osteopenia, whether or not osteoporosis is present.

osteopetrosis A genetic disease that is characterized by abnormally dense thick bone. A severe autosomal recessive form of osteopetrosis can occur in infants and children, and a milder autosomal dominant form can occur in teens and adults. In the recessive form, the thickened bone obliterates the marrow cavity, causing anemia, and narrows the openings of the skull, causing compression of nerves to the ears and eyes, ultimately resulting in deafness and blindness. Fractures are common in both forms. Also known as marble bone disease.

osteoporosis Thinning of the bones, with reduction in bone mass, due to depletion of calcium and bone protein. Osteoporosis predisposes a person to fractures, which are often slow to heal and heal poorly. It is most common in older adults, particularly postmenopausal women, and in patients who take steroids or steroidal drugs. Unchecked osteoporosis can lead to changes in posture, physical abnormality (particularly the form of hunched back known colloquially as dowager's hump), and decreased mobility. Treatment of osteoporosis includes exercise (especially weight-bearing exercise that builds bone density), ensuring that the diet contain adequate calcium and other minerals needed to promote new bone growth, use of medications to improve bone density, and for postmenopausal women, use of estrogen or combination hormone supplements.

osteosarcoma A cancer of the bone that is most common in adolescents and young adults. Treatment involves surgery, usually followed by chemotherapy or radiation. The site of the tumor is the most important prognostic factor, because it determines whether the tumor can be surgically removed. Also known as osteogenic sarcoma.

osteotomy Taking out part or all of a bone, or cutting into or through bone.

osteotomy, block Surgical removal of a section of bone.

osteotomy, cuneiform Surgical removal of a triangular piece of bone.

osteotomy, displacement Surgical reconfiguration of a bone by changing its physical relationship to other bones.

ostomy An operation to create an opening from an area inside the body to the outside. An ostomy may be used to permit drainage of feces (colostomy) or urine (cystostomy) from the body when the normal route is missing or blocked. It can be permanent or temporary. See also *colostomy; enterostomy.*

OT 1 Occupational therapist. 2 Occupational therapy.

Otahara syndrome A seizure disorder that occurs within the first month of life. Otahara syndrome patients may have many different types of seizures. The patient's development is slowed, and the child can become progressively more impaired. Otahara syndrome is often due to underdevelopment of part of the brain, although it is occasionally due to a metabolic problem. A magnetic resonance imaging (MRI) scan can uncover brain underdevelopment; if none is found, metabolic testing should be done. Diagnosis is made via observation and electroencephalogram (EEG). Treatment includes use of antispasmodic medication and educational and physical services aimed at enhancing development. Also known as early infantile epileptic encephalopathy.

OTC Over-the-counter.

otitis Inflammation of the ear. See also *ear infection.*

otitis externa See *ear infection, external.*

oto- Prefix meaning ear, as in otology (the study and medical care of the ear) and otoplasty (plastic surgery to reshape the outer ear).

otolaryngologist See *ENT.*

otology The study and medical care of the ear.

otopharyngeal tube See *Eustachian tube.*

otoplasty Plastic surgery to reshape the outer ear.

otoscope An instrument for looking in the ear.

ounce 1 A measure of weight equal to 28.4 grams or $\frac{1}{16}$ pound. Abbreviated oz. An old saying states that an ounce of prevention is worth a pound of cure. 2 A measure of volume equal to 5 milliliters, 2 tablespoons, or $\frac{1}{8}$ cups.

outer ear See *ear, outer.*

outpatient A patient who is not hospitalized, but instead comes to a physician's office, clinic, or day surgery office for treatment.

outpatient care See *ambulatory care.*

output, cardiac See *cardiac output.*

ova Plural of ovum.

ovarian cancer See *cancer, ovarian.*

ovarian carcinoma See *cancer, ovarian.*

ovarian cyst See *cyst, ovarian.*

ovarian disease, polycystic See *Stein-Leventhal syndrome.*

ovarian teratoma An ovarian tumor that is usually benign and typically contains a diversity of tissues. An ovarian teratoma develops from a totipotential germ cell—a primary oocyte—that is retained within the ovary. Totipotential cells can give rise to all orders of cells that are necessary to form mature tissues and often recognizable structures, such as hair, bone, and sebaceous (oily) material, neural tissue, and teeth. Any of these tissues may be found in an ovarian teratoma. Such cysts may occur at any age, but the prime age of detection is in the childbearing years. Up to 15 percent of women with ovarian teratomas have them in both ovaries. These tumors can range in size from less than $\frac{1}{2}$ inch to about 17 inches in diameter. Ovarian teratomas can cause the ovary to twist, imperiling its blood supply and requiring emergency surgery. The larger the ovarian teratoma, the greater the risk of rupture. Spillage of its greasy contents can create problems, such as adhesions and pain. Although about 98 percent of ovarian teratomas are benign, the remaining fraction do become cancerous. Treatment of both benign and malignant ovarian teratomas involves surgical removal, which can be done via laparotomy (open surgery) or laparoscopy (with a scope). Also known as dermoid cyst of the ovary or simply dermoid. See also *cyst, ovarian; parthenogenesis.*

ovary The female gonad, one of a pair of reproductive glands in women. The ovaries are located in the pelvis, one on each side of the uterus. Each ovary is about the size and shape of an almond. The ovaries produce eggs (ova) and female hormones. During each monthly menstrual cycle, an egg is released from one ovary. The egg travels from the ovary through a fallopian tube to the uterus. The ovaries are the main source of female hormones, which control the development of female body characteristics, such as the breasts, body shape, and body hair. They also regulate the menstrual cycle and pregnancy.

ovary cyst, follicular   See *cyst of the ovary, follicular.*

ovary, dermoid cyst of the   See *ovarian teratoma.*

overgrowth   Excessive growth. Also sometimes called gigantism.

overgrowth syndrome   A condition with multiple features, most notably excessive growth. A number of overgrowth syndromes affect children, such as fragile X syndrome. Excessive growth of specific body parts is also a feature of a number of disorders, such as Beckwith-Wiedemann syndrome, in which there is macroglossia (a large tongue due to overgrowth of the tongue). Overactivity of the pituitary gland with overproduction of growth hormone causes overgrowth before adolescence and a distinctive pattern of overgrowth called acromegaly. See also *acromegaly; fragile X syndrome.*

overload, iron   See *excess iron.*

over-the-counter drug   A drug that is available without a prescription, in contrast to prescription drugs that require a physician's order. Abbreviated OTC.

overweight   See *obese.*

ovulation   The release of the ripe egg (ovum) from the ovary. The egg is released when the cavity surrounding it (the follicle) breaks open in response to a hormonal signal. Ovulation occurs around 14 or 15 days from the first day of the woman's last menstrual cycle. When ovulation occurs, the ovum moves into the Fallopian tube and becomes available for fertilization.

ovum   An egg within the ovary of the female. An ovum can combine with sperm to form a zygote.

oximetry   The process of determining the level of oxygenation in arterial blood, an important measure of whether the heart and lungs are working properly. Oximetry may be done continuously during certain medical treatments or surgery, or it may be done sporadically to monitor a patient's health.

oximetry catheter   See *catheter, oximetry.*

oxygen   The odorless gas that is present in the air and necessary to maintain life. Oxygen may be given in a medical setting, either to reduce the volume of other gases in the blood or as a vehicle for delivering anesthetics in gas form. It can also be delivered via nasal tubes, an oxygen mask, or an oxygen tent. Patients with lung disease or damage may need to use portable oxygen devices on a temporary or permanent basis.

oxygen chamber, hyperbaric   See *hyperbaric oxygen chamber.*

oxygen mask   A mask that covers the mouth and nose and is hooked up to an oxygen tank. It delivers oxygen directly to the patient.

oxygen tent   A tent-like device that is used in a medical setting to deliver high levels of oxygen to a bedridden patient. The tent covers the entire head and upper body, and oxygen is pumped in from a tank.

oxygenation   **1** The process of treating a patient with oxygen.   **2** The process of combining a medication or another substance with oxygen.

oxymetholone   A male hormone that stimulates production of the male hormone testosterone. Oxymetholone is sometimes given to treat hormonal imbalance in men or certain types of disease in both men and women.

oxytocin   A hormone made in the brain that plays a role in childbirth and lactation by causing muscles to contract in the uterus and in the mammary glands. Animal studies have shown that oxytocin also has a role in mating pairs becoming attached to one another (pair bonding), and protecting each other (mate guarding), as well as members of groups recognizing one another as part of the group (social memory). Oxytocin is a peptide (a compound consisting of two or more amino acids) that is secreted by the hypothalamus and transported to the posterior lobe of the pituitary gland at the base of the brain. See also *pituitary, posterior.*

oxyuris   A group of intestinal worms that includes pinworm.

oz.   Abbreviation for ounce.

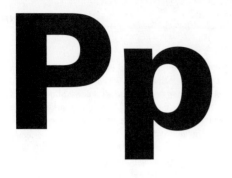

Pp

p **1** In biochemistry, protein. For example, p53 is a protein that is 53 kilodaltons in size. **2** In population genetics, the frequency of the more common of two different alternative (allelic) versions of a gene. (The frequency of the less common allele is q.) **3** In statistics, probability.

p arm of a chromosome The short arm of a chromosome. Each human chromosome has two arms—a short arm and a long arm. By international convention, the short arm is termed p, and the long arm is termed q. For example, if a gene is on 4p12, that gene is on the short arm of chromosome 4, in region 12. See also *chromosome.*

P-24 antibody An antibody that is created by B cells in the immune system to fight the P-24 antigen. The P-24 antibody attaches to the foreign protein and sends a signal to T-4 cells to attack it. The presence of P-24 antibodies is a good sign in cases of HIV infection. See also *HIV; P-24 antigen.*

P-24 antigen A protein that is found only in the HIV virus and is considered a trend marker. In cases of HIV infection, tests for the level of P-24 antigen may be done to measure the progression of AIDS. These tests always return a positive value. On one blood test, the Coulter test, a score of 11 or less is considered negative (no disease progression), and a higher score may mean that the infection is progressing. On the Highly Sensitive (HS) blood test, the level of P-24 antigen can be detected more specifically. See also *HIV; HS test; P-24 antibody.*

p53 A protein that is 53 kilodaltons in size and is produced by a tumor-suppressor gene. Like other tumor-suppressor genes, the p53 gene normally controls cell growth. If p53 is physically lost or functionally inactivated, cells can grow without restraint.

PA **1** Physician assistant. **2** Posteroanterior.

PA X-ray An X-ray picture in which the beams pass from back to front (posteroanterior), as opposed to an AP (anteroposterior) film, in which the rays pass through the body from front to back.

pacemaker A device or system that sends electrical impulses to the heart in order to set the heart rhythm. A pacemaker can be the natural pacemaker of the heart (the sinoatrial node) or it can be an electronic device that serves as an artificial pacemaker. See also *pacemaker, artificial; pacemaker, implantable; sinoatrial node.*

pacemaker, artificial An electronic device that uses electrical impulses to regulate the heart rhythm. A pacemaker may be external (located outside the body) or internal (implanted in the body). Although there are many different types of pacemakers, all are designed to treat bradycardia, a too-slow heart rate. Pacemakers may function continuously and stimulate the heart at a fixed rate or at an increased rate during exercise. A pacemaker can also be programmed to detect too long a pause between heartbeats and then stimulate the heart. See also *pacemaker, implantable.*

pacemaker, implantable A pacemaker in which the electrodes to the heart, the electronic circuitry, and the power supply are all implanted internally within the body. The implantable pacemaker was invented by Wilson Greatbatch in 1958. While building an oscillator to record heart sounds, Greatbatch installed a resistor with the wrong resistance, and it began to give off a steady electrical pulse. Greatbatch realized that the device could be used to regulate the heart, and he handcrafted the world's first implantable pacemaker. Greatbatch later invented the corrosion-free lithium battery to power the pacemaker.

pacemaker, internal See *pacemaker, implantable.*

pacemaker, natural See *sinoatrial node.*

pachyonychia congenita, Jadassohn-Lewandowski type See *pachyonychia congenita, type 1.*

pachyonychia congenita, type 1 An inherited condition that is characterized by abnormally thick, curved nails; thickening of the skin of the palms, soles, knees, and elbows; white plaques in the mouth; excessive sweating of the hands and feet; and the presence of erupted (visible) teeth at birth. This syndrome is inherited as an autosomal dominant trait. The gene that is responsible for type 1 pachyonychia congenita (named PD1) is on chromosome 12 in band 12q13, and a single copy of the PD1 gene is capable of causing the disease. The basic abnormality is a mutation in a gene for keratin, which is a primary constituent of nails, hair, and skin. Also known as elephant nails from birth, Jadassohn-Lewandowski syndrome, Jadassohn-Lewandowski type pachyonychia congenita, pachyonychia congenita with natal teeth, and type 1 pachyonychia congenita.

Paget's disease A chronic bone disorder that typically results in enlarged, deformed bones due to excessive breakdown and formation of bone tissue that can cause bones to weaken and may result in bone pain, arthritis, bony deformities, and fractures. Paget's disease generally occurs in persons over the age of 40 years. Men and women are affected equally. Because Paget's disease may be familial, after age 40, brothers, sisters, and children of someone with the disease may wish to have an alkaline phosphatase blood test every 2 or 3 years to screen for Paget's disease. Many people do not know they have Paget's disease because they have a mild form of the disease, with no symptoms. Sometimes, symptoms may be confused with those of arthritis or other disorders. Paget's disease may be diagnosed by using one or more of the following tests: X-rays, because bone in Paget's disease has a characteristic appearance; alkaline phosphatase tests, because an elevated level of alkaline phosphatase in the blood can be suggestive of Paget's disease; and bone scans. Treatment options include use of aspirin, other anti-inflammatory medications, pain medications, and medications that slow the rate of bone turnover, such as calcitonin and the bisphosphonates. The outlook with Paget's disease is generally good, particularly if treatment is given before major changes have occurred in the affected bones. Paget's disease occurs most frequently in the spine, skull, pelvis, thighs, and lower legs. In general, symptoms progress slowly, and the disease does not spread to normal bones. Treatment can control Paget's disease and lessen symptoms, but there is no cure. The goal of drug treatment is to control Paget's disease activity for as long a period of time as possible. The disease is named for the English surgeon Sir James Paget. Also known as osteitis deformans.

Paget's disease of the breast See *breast, Paget's disease of the.*

pain A sensation that can range from mild, localized discomfort to agony. Pain has both physical and emotional components. The physical part of pain results from nerve stimulation. Pain may be contained to a discrete area, as in an injury, or it may be more diffuse, as in disorders such as fibromyalgia. Pain is mediated by specific nerve fibers that carry the pain impulses to the brain. See also *pain management.*

pain, abdominal See *abdominal pain.*

pain, ankle See *ankle pain.*

pain, back Pain in any part of the back. Pain in the back can relate to the bony spine, discs between the vertebrae, ligaments around the spine and discs, spinal cord and nerves, muscles of the back, internal organs, or skin covering the back. Causes of back pain can include injury, overstress, or disease.

pain, chest See *chest pain.*

pain, elbow See *elbow pain.*

pain, knee Pain in the knee. Causes of knee pain include injury, degeneration, arthritis, infection (infrequently), and, rarely, bone tumors.

pain management The process of providing medical care that alleviates or reduces pain. Pain management is an extremely important part of health care because patients who are forced to remain in severe pain often become agitated and/or depressed and have poorer treatment outcomes than patients who do not remain in severe pain. Mild to moderate pain can usually be treated with analgesic medications, such as aspirin. For chronic or severe pain, opiates and other narcotics may be used, sometimes in concert with analgesics; with steroids or nonsteroidal anti-inflammatory drugs when the pain is related to inflammation; or with antidepressants, which can potentiate some pain medications without raising the actual dose of the drug and which affect the brain's perception of pain. Narcotics carry with them the potential for side effects and addiction. However, the risk of addiction is not normally a concern in the care of terminal patients. For hospitalized patients with severe pain, devices for self-administration of narcotics are frequently used. Other procedures can also be useful in pain management programs. For bedridden patients, simply changing position regularly or using pillows to support a more comfortable posture can be effective. Massage, acupuncture, acupressure, and biofeedback have also shown some validity for increased pain control in some patients.

pain, phantom limb Pain perceived to be located in the distribution of a previously removed extremity. See also *phantom limb syndrome.*

pain, phantom tooth See *phantom tooth pain.*

pain, shingles See *shingles.*

pains, growing See *growing pains.*

palate The roof of the mouth. The bony front portion is the hard palate, and the muscular back portion is the soft palate. See also *cleft palate.*

palate, cleft See *cleft palate.*

paleostriatum See *globus pallidus.*

palilalia See *palinphrasia.*

palindromic rheumatism A form of joint inflammation whereby the joints involved appear to change periodically from one region of the body to another and back again.

palinphrasia A speech disorder that is characterized by the repetition of words or phrases. Palinphrasia is encountered in autistic spectrum disorders and Tourette's syndrome. Also known as palilalia.

palladum See *globus pallidus.*

palliate To treat a disease partially and insofar as possible, but not cure it completely. See also *palliative care*.

palliation See *palliative care*.

palliative care 1 Medical or comfort care that reduces the severity of a disease or slows its progress rather than providing a cure. For incurable diseases, in cases where the cure is not recommended due to other health concerns, and when the patient does not want to pursue a cure, palliative care is the focus of treatment. For example, if surgery cannot be performed to remove a tumor, radiation treatment might be tried to reduce the tumor's rate of growth, and pain management could help the patient manage physical symptoms. 2 In a negative sense, provision of only perfunctory health care when a cure is possible.

palmar surface The palm or grasping side of the hand.

palpable Something that can be felt. For example, a palpable growth is one that can be detected by touch.

palpate To touch or feel. For example, a physician may palpate the liver's edge.

palpebra Medical term for eyelid. The plural is palpebrae.

palpebral fissure The opening for the eyes between the eyelids.

palpebral glands See *glands, Meibomian*.

palpitations Unpleasant sensations of irregular and/or forceful beating of the heart. In some patients with palpitations, no heart disease or abnormal heart rhythms can be found. In others, palpitations result from abnormal heart rhythms (arrhythmias).

palsy Paralysis, generally partial, whereby a local body area is incapable of voluntary movement. For example, Bell's palsy is localized paralysis of the muscles on one side of the face.

palsy, Bell's See *Bell's palsy*.

palsy, cerebral See *cerebral palsy*.

palsy, laryngeal See *laryngeal palsy*.

paludism See *malaria*.

panacea A universal remedy, a cure-all. The ancients sought—but never found—a panacea that would cure all disease.

pancolitis See *colitis, ulcerative*.

pancreas A spongy, tube-shaped organ that is about 6 inches long and is located in the back of the abdomen, behind the stomach. The head of the pancreas is on the right side of the abdomen. It is connected to the upper end of the small intestine. The narrow end of the pancreas, called the tail, extends to the left side of the body. The pancreas makes pancreatic juices and hormones, including insulin and secretin. Pancreatic juices contain enzymes that help digest food in the small intestine. Pancreatic hormones are active in the digestive system, blood, and possibly the brain. Both pancreatic enzymes and hormones are needed to keep the body working correctly. As pancreatic juices are made, they flow into the main pancreatic duct, which joins to the common bile duct, which connects the pancreas to the liver and the gallbladder and carries bile to the small intestine near the stomach. The pancreas is thus a compound gland in the sense that it is composed of both exocrine and endocrine tissues. The exocrine function of the pancreas involves the synthesis and secretion of pancreatic juices. The endocrine function resides in the million or so cellular islands (the islets of Langerhans) that are embedded between the exocrine units of the pancreas. Beta cells of the islets of Langerhans secrete insulin, which helps control carbohydrate metabolism. Alpha cells of the islets of Langerhans secrete glucagon, which counters the action of insulin.

pancreas, annular An abnormal ring of pancreatic tissue that encircles the duodenum and often causes intestinal obstruction.

pancreas, artificial A machine that constantly measures the level of glucose in the blood and, if that level is elevated, releases an appropriate amount of insulin into the bloodstream.

pancreatectomy A surgical procedure in which part or all of the pancreas is removed.

pancreatic Having to do with the pancreas.

pancreatic alpha cell See *alpha cell, pancreatic*.

pancreatic beta cell See *beta cell, pancreatic*.

pancreatic cancer See *cancer, pancreatic*.

pancreatic delta cell See *delta cell, pancreatic*.

pancreatic insufficiency Having not enough of the digestive enzymes that are normally secreted by the pancreas into the intestine. Pancreatic insufficiency is a hallmark of cystic fibrosis. See also *cystic fibrosis*.

pancreatic juice Fluids made by the pancreas that contain digestive enzymes.

pancreatitis Inflammation of the pancreas. Of the many causes of pancreatitis, the most common are alcohol consumption and gallstones. Other causes include medications (azathioprine, estrogen, thiazides, metronidazole, valproic acid, and tetracycline), trauma, abdominal surgery, abnormalities of the pancreas and intestine, and infections such as mumps. Acute pancreatitis usually begins with pain in the upper abdomen that may last for a few days. The pain may be sudden and intense, or it may begin as a mild pain that is aggravated by eating and slowly grows worse. The abdomen may be very tender. Other symptoms may include nausea, vomiting, and fever. The patient often feels and looks very sick. Chronic pancreatitis usually follows many years of alcohol abuse and may cause pain; malabsorption of food, leading to weight loss; and diabetes, if the insulin-producing cells of the pancreas (islet cells) are damaged.

pancytopenia A shortage of all types of blood cells. Pancytopenia can be caused by a side effect of many medications (such as azathioprine, methotrexate, and others) or diseases (such as lupus and bone marrow disorders). Treatment is directed toward the underlying cause and may be supplemented by medications that stimulate the bone marrow.

pancytopenia, Fanconi See *anemia, Fanconi.*

PANDAS Pediatric autoimmune disorders associated with streptococcus, the sudden onset of symptoms such as those of obsessive-compulsive disorder or Tourette's syndrome following infection with streptococcus bacteria. PANDAS is caused by an autoimmune reaction that affects the basal ganglia in the brain. If tics are seen in patients with PANDAS, they may or may not be choreaform, like those of Sydenham's chorea, a closely related condition that can follow a bout of rheumatic fever, which is caused by the streptococcus bacteria. Diagnosis is primarily made through observation, although a blood marker for the disorder has been identified. Treatment involves plasmapheresis and use of intravenous immunoglobulin, prophylactic antibiotics, and/or medication for specific symptoms. See also *obsessive-compulsive disorder; streptococcus; Tourette's syndrome.*

pandemic 1 An epidemic of disease that is very widespread, affecting a whole region, a continent, or the world. 2 Widely epidemic. For example, AIDS is currently pandemic in Africa.

pandiculation The act of stretching and yawning.

panencephalitis, subacute sclerosing See *subacute sclerosing panencephalitis.*

panic A sudden strong feeling of fear that prevents reasonable thought or action. The word comes from the name of the Greek woodland god Pan, who was a frightening figure—part human, part goat—and whose pet caprice was to terrify people who ventured into rural areas.

panic disorder An anxiety disorder that is characterized by sudden attacks of fear and panic. Panic attacks may occur without a known reason, but more frequently they are triggered by fear-producing events or thoughts, such as taking an elevator or driving. Symptoms of panic attacks include rapid heartbeat, strange chest sensations, shortness of breath, dizziness, tingling, and anxiousness. Hyperventilation, agitation, and withdrawal are common results. Panic disorder is believed to be due to an abnormal activation of the body's hormonal system, causing a sudden "fight or flight" response. Treatment involves cognitive behavioral therapy, using exposure to effect symptom reduction, and use of medication.

pantothenic acid Vitamin B5. See also Appendix C, "Vitamins."

Pap test A screening test for cervical cancer that involves the microscopic examination of cells collected from the cervix, smeared on a slide, and specially stained. A Pap test can reveal premalignant and malignant changes in the cells, as well as changes that are due to noncancerous conditions, such as inflammation. Named after the physician George Papanicolaou, who developed the test. Also known as Pap smear.

papilla, fungiform See *fungiform papillae.*

papillary muscle See *muscle, papillary.*

papillary tumor A tumor that is shaped like a small mushroom, with its "stem" attached to the inner lining of the bladder.

papilledema Swelling of the head of the optic nerve, a sign of increased pressure within the skull. The optic nerve head is the area where the optic nerve (the nerve that carries information from the retina to the brain) enters the eyeball. Papilledema is diagnosed through use of an ophthalmoscope. The optic nerve head is abnormally elevated in papilledema, almost always in both eyes. The causes of papilledema include swelling of the brain (as from encephalitis or trauma), tumors and other lesions that occupy space within the skull, increased production of cerebrospinal fluid (CSF), decreased resorption of CSF (due to meningitis, venous sinus thrombosis, or subarachnoid hemorrhage), obstruction of the ventricular system within the brain, hydrocephalus, craniosynostosis (premature closure of the sutures of the skull), and pseudotumor cerebri (increased pressure within the brain in the absence of a tumor). When papilledema is found, the patient requires immediate further evaluation and, if needed, intervention. Also known as a choked disk. See also *brain cancer; cerebrospinal fluid; craniosynostosis; encephalitis; hydrocephalus; meningitis; pseudotumor cerebri; ventricle, cerebral.*

papilloma A small solid benign tumor with a clear-cut border that projects above the surrounding tissue. A cutaneous papilloma is a skin tag. See also *skin tag.*

papilloma, intraductal See *intraductal papilloma.*

papilloma virus, human See *human papilloma virus.*

papillomatosis A disorder that is characterized by the growth of numerous papillomas (warts). For example, laryngeal papillomatosis is the presence of multiple papillomas on the vocal cords.

papillomatosis, juvenile laryngeal See *laryngeal papillomatosis, juvenile.*

papillomatosis, laryngeal See *laryngeal papillomatosis.*

papillomatosis, recurrent respiratory The appearance of numerous warty growths on the larynx or vocal cords, usually in children and young adults. A baby whose mother has vaginal warts can contract recurrent respiratory papillomatosis during birth. Treatment usually involves surgical excision. Recurrence is frequent, but remission may occur after several years.

papular Referring to papules.

papule A solid, rounded growth that is elevated from the skin. A papule is usually less than 1 cm (0.5 in.) across. Papules may open when scratched and become crusty and infected.

para Any woman who has given birth once or more. A woman who is para I (a primipara) has given birth once, a woman who is para II has given birth twice, and so on. Technically, for a pregnancy to count as a birth, it must last for at least 20 weeks (the midpoint of a full-term pregnancy) or yield an infant who weighs at least 500 grams, regardless of whether the infant is liveborn.

para- A prefix with many meanings, including alongside, beside, near, resembling, beyond, apart from, and abnormal, as in parathyroid glands (glands that are adjacent to the thyroid) and paraumbilical (alongside the umbilicus).

paracentesis The removal of fluid from a body cavity via a needle, a trocar, a cannula, or another hollow instrument. A paracentesis may be used for diagnosis or treatment, as, for example, in ascites, where there is free fluid in the abdominal (peritoneal) cavity. If the cause of the ascites is uncertain, diagnostic paracentesis is done in order to obtain fluid that can be examined. Therapeutic paracentesis may then be done to remove more fluid, as part of the plan of treatment. Paracentesis of the chest cavity is called a thoracentesis.

paracentric chromosome inversion See *chromosome inversion, pericentric.*

paradoxical embolism See *embolism, paradoxical.*

paraffin dip A treatment for the symptoms of joint and muscle conditions, such as arthritis, that involves applying melted mineral wax derived from petroleum to a body area. Paraffin dips can be especially helpful in relieving the pain and stiffness of arthritis involving the small joints of the hands. The hands are repeatedly dipped into the melted, warm wax, and the wax is allowed to cool and harden around the sore joints. The paraffin is then peeled off and can be remelted in the bath for repeated use. Also known as wax dip.

paralysis Loss of voluntary movement (motor function). Paralysis that affects only one muscle or limb is partial paralysis, also known as palsy; paralysis of all muscles is total paralysis, as may occur in cases of botulism.

paralysis agitans See *Parkinson's disease.*

paralysis, infantile See *polio.*

paralysis, laryngeal nerve See *laryngeal palsy.*

paralysis, stomach See *gastroparesis.*

paralytic ileus See *ileus.*

paraneoplastic syndrome A group of signs and symptoms caused by a substance that is produced by a tumor or in reaction to a tumor. Paraneoplastic syndrome can be due to a number of causes, including hormones or other biologically active products made by the tumor, blockade of the effect of a normal hormone, autoimmunity, immune-complex production, and immunosuppression. By definition, paraneoplastic syndrome is not produced by the primary tumor itself or by its metastases, nor is it caused by compression, infection, nutritional deficiency, or treatment of the tumor.

paraphilia One of several complex psychiatric disorders that are manifested as deviant sexual behavior. For example, in men, the most common forms are pedophilia (sexual behavior or attraction toward children) and exhibitionism (exposing one's body in a public setting). Other paraphilias include compulsive sexual behavior (nymphomania and priapism), sadism, masochism, fetishism, bestiality (zoophilia), and necrophilia. Treatment may include cognitive behavioral therapy, psychotherapy, behavior modification, use of antidepressant medications, and use of medications that alter hormone production, particularly of testosterone. However, the cause and treatment of paraphilia are poorly understood, and treatment is rarely effective. In addition, many professionals prefer not to pathologize sexual behavior that involves only willing adults, even if the behavior might be deemed deviant in mainstream society. In cases where the behavior is potentially criminal, as in pedophilia, treatment is usually delivered within the penal system.

paraphimosis   A condition in which the foreskin of the penis, once retracted, cannot return to its original location. The foreskin remains trapped behind the groove of the coronal sulcus, between the shaft and the glans. This causes blood to pool in the veins behind the entrapment, leading to swelling and severe pain. With lubrication, the foreskin can sometimes be reduced. This works only if the paraphimosis is discovered early, and it requires a short-acting general anesthetic or heavy sedation. Circumcision can prevent and cure paraphimosis.

paraquat lung   Lung disease caused by the contact herbicide paraquat, which selectively accumulates in the lungs and is highly toxic. When X-ray changes from paraquat are evident in the lungs, death is virtually certain. Paraquat lung is rare because the herbicide must be directly inhaled to cause the disease. Paraquat lung emerged as a health concern in the 1970s, when the US government sprayed paraquat aerially over some illegal marijuana fields. Some of the sprayed plants survived and were sold, causing paraquat lung in purchasers who smoked the product.

parasite   A plant or an animal organism that lives in or on another and takes its nourishment from that other organism. Parasitic diseases include infections that are due to protozoa, helminths, or arthropods. For example, malaria is caused by Plasmodium, a parasitic protozoa.

parasitemia   The presence of parasites in the blood. In malaria, a measure called the parasitemia index reflects the severity of the disease.

parasitic   Having to do with a parasite, as in a parasitic infection; or acting like a parasite by taking nourishment from another.

parasympathetic nervous system   The part of the involuntary nervous system that serves to slow the heart rate, increase intestinal and glandular activity, and relax the sphincter muscles. The parasympathetic nervous system, together with the sympathetic nervous system, constitutes the autonomic nervous system.

parathormone   A hormone that is made by the parathyroid gland and is critical to maintaining calcium and phosphorus balance. Deficiency of parathormone results in abnormally low calcium in the blood (hypocalcemia). Excessive parathormone leads to elevated calcium levels in the blood and calcium deposition in cartilage. Also known as parathyroid hormone and parathyrin.

parathyrin   See *parathormone.*

parathyroid gland   The gland that regulates calcium metabolism. The parathyroid gland is located behind the thyroid gland in the neck. It secretes a hormone called parathormone that is critical to the metabolism of calcium and phosphorus. Although the number of parathyroid glands can vary, most people have four. The parathyroid glands appear as a pair, one above the other, on each side of the thyroid gland, and they are plastered against the back of the thyroid gland. These glands are therefore at risk for being accidentally removed during thyroidectomy. See also *parathormone.*

parathyroid hormone   See *parathormone.*

parathyroids, hypoplasia of the thymus and   See *DiGeorge syndrome.*

parenteral   Not delivered via the intestinal tract. For example, parenteral nutrition is feeding that is delivered intravenously.

parenteral nutrition   Intravenous feeding. Also known as parenteral alimentation.

paresis   Incomplete paralysis or slight paralysis.

paresis, general   See *general paresis.*

paresthesia   An abnormal sensation of the body, such as numbness, tingling, or burning.

parietal bone   The bone on the side of the upper skull.

parietal lobes   A pair of lobes in the cerebral hemisphere that are involved in sensation, perception, memory, and integrating sensory input, primarily visual input.

parietal pericardium   The outer layer of the pericardium. See also *pericardium.*

Parkinson's disease   A slowly progressive neurologic disease that is characterized by a fixed inexpressive face, tremor at rest, slowing of voluntary movements, gait with short accelerating steps, peculiar posture and muscle weakness (caused by degeneration of an area of the brain called the basal ganglia), and low production of the neurotransmitter dopamine. Most patients are over 50, but at least 10 percent are under 40. Treatment involves use of medication, such as levodopa (brand name: Larodopa) and carbidopa (brand name: Sinemet). A surgically implanted device that helps control the shaking that accompanies Parkinson's disease has recently become available. In some cases, surgery on the globus pallidus or thalamus can be helpful. A rare early-onset form of Parkinson's disease is due to mutation in chromosome 9, whereas people with the more common late-onset form of the disease tend to have mutations in chromosome 17. From a genetic viewpoint it is now clear that Parkinson's disease is heterogeneous; that is, it is several diseases. Genes appear to be involved in all forms of Parkinson's disease. Also known as paralysis agitans and shaking palsy.

parotid gland One of the largest of the three major salivary glands. The parotid glands are located on the sides of the face in front of the ear, below the level of the ear, and behind the jawbone. See also *parotitis.*

parotitis Inflammation of the parotid glands, a classic feature of mumps.

paroxysmal atrial tachycardia Bouts of rapid, regular heart beating that originates in the upper chamber of the heart (atrium). Abbreviated PAT. PAT is caused by abnormalities in the atrioventricular (AV) node that lead to rapid firing of electrical impulses from the atrium that bypass the AV node under certain conditions, including excess alcohol consumption, stress, caffeine use, overactive thyroid or excessive thyroid hormone intake, and use of certain drugs. PAT is an example of an arrhythmia in which the abnormality is in the electrical system of the heart, while the heart muscle and valves may be normal.

parrot fever See *psittacosis.*

Parry disease See *goiter, toxic multinodular.*

parthenogenesis Development of a germ cell without fertilization. A form of nonsexual reproduction.

partial hysterectomy See *hysterectomy, partial.*

partial syndactyly See *syndactyly, partial.*

parturition See *labor.*

passage, nasal See *nasal passage.*

passive smoking Inhalation of smoke that comes from someone else smoking. Passive smoking appears to be associated with the same array of diseases as actual smoking, with an elevated risk of lung cancer and other diseases.

Pasteur, Louis A French chemist and biologist who invented pasteurization, developed the germ theory,

founded the field of bacteriology, and created the first vaccines against anthrax and rabies.

pasteurization A method of treating food by heating it to a certain point to kill disease-causing organisms but keep the flavor or quality of the food intact. Pasteurization is used with beer, milk, fruit juice, cheese, and egg products.

PAT Paroxysmal atrial tachycardia.

Patau syndrome See *trisomy 13 syndrome.*

patella See *kneecap.*

patellar Pertaining to the patella (kneecap).

patellectomy An operation to remove a shattered patella.

patellofemoral joint The joint formed by the kneecap (patella) and the femur. See also *knee.*

patellofemoral syndrome The most common cause of chronic knee pain, which characteristically results in vague discomfort of the inner knee area. Abbreviated PFS. PFS is aggravated by activity, such as running, jumping, climbing, or descending stairs, and also by prolonged sitting with the knees in a moderately bent position: the so-called "theater sign" of pain upon arising from a desk or theater seat. The knee may be mildly swollen. If chronic symptoms are ignored, the loss of quadriceps strength may cause the leg to "give out." PFS is caused by an abnormality in the way the kneecap slides over the lower end of the femur. Normally, the quadricep muscle pulls the kneecap over the end of the femur in a straight line. In PFS, the kneecap is pulled toward the outer side of the femur. This off-kilter path permits the underside of the kneecap to grate along the femur, leading to chronic inflammation and pain. Females are at greater risk than males for PFS. Knock-kneed and flat-footed runners, and persons with unusually shaped patellas, are also predisposed to PFS. Initial pain management involves icing, using anti-inflammatory drugs such as ibuprofen, and avoiding motions that irritate the kneecap. Treatment and rehabilitation are designed to create a straighter pathway for the patella to follow during quadriceps contraction. Selective strengthening of the inner portion of the quadriceps muscle helps normalize its tracking. Occasionally, bracing with patellar centering devices is required. Also known as chondromalacia patella, housemaid's knee, and secretary's knee.

patent **1** A legal device that gives exclusive control and possession of a device, an invention, or a procedure to an individual or a corporation. Before the commercialization of biomedical inventions, the word *patent* had no place in a medical dictionary. Now the patent is the foundation of the biotechnology industry. Health-related items that may be patented include medical devices, surgical procedures, medications, and even cell lines. **2** Open, unobstructed, or affording free passage. For example, the bowel can be patent, as opposed to obstructed.

patent ductus arteriosus See *ductus arteriosus.*

patho- A prefix meaning suffering or disease, as in pathogen (a disease agent) and pathology (the study of disease).

pathobiology The biology of disease.

pathogen An agent of disease. For example, Bacillus anthracis is the pathogen that causes anthrax.

pathogenesis The development of a disease and the chain of events leading to that disease.

pathogenetic Pertaining to genetic cause of a disease or condition. For example, BRCA 1 and BRCA2 are genes that, when mutated, are responsible for many cases of cancer of the breast. Therefore, these genes are pathogenetic.

pathogenic Capable of causing disease. For example, pathogenic E. coli are Escherishia coli bacteria that can make a person ill.

pathognomonic A sign or symptom that is so characteristic of a disease that it can be used to make a diagnosis. For example, Koplik spots in the mouth opposite the first and second upper molars are pathognomonic of measles.

pathologist A physician who identifies diseases and conditions by studying cells and tissues under a microscope.

pathology **1** The study of disease. **2** Incorrectly (but commonly), disease. For example, "The physician found no pathology" would mean the physician found no evidence of disease.

pathophysiology Deranged function in an individual or an organ due to a disease. For example, a pathophysiologic alteration is a change in function as distinguished from a structural defect.

-pathy Suffix indicating suffering or disease, as in neuropathy (disease of the nervous system).

Pavlovian conditioning A method to cause a reflex response or behavior by training with repetitive action. The Russian physiologist Ivan Petrovich Pavlov conditioned dogs to respond in what proved to be a predictable manner. For example, when he customarily rang a bell before feeding them, the dogs would begin to salivate whenever the bell rang. The principles of Pavlovian conditioning form the basis of much modern behavioral science.

PBC Primary biliary cirrhosis. See *cirrhosis, primary biliary.*

p.c. Post cibum. Abbreviation meaning after meals. See also Appendix A, "Prescription Abbreviations."

PCL Posterior cruciate ligament.

PCM Protein-calorie malnutrition. See *kwashiorkor.*

PCP Pneumocystis carinii pneumonia.

PCR Polymerase chain reaction.

PDA Patent ductus arteriosus. See *ductus arteriosus.*

PDR **1** *Physicians' Desk Reference.* **2** Postdelivery room, used as a staging room for the mother after delivering her baby in the delivery room.

pecs See *pectoral muscle.*

pectoral muscle One of the muscles of the front of the upper chest. The pectoral muscles are familiarly known as the pecs and are the muscles underneath the breasts. Pectoral muscles are used by the upper extremities to push objects in front of the body. For example, these are the muscles that are exercised in doing the bench press exercise.

pectoralis muscle absence with syndactyly See *Poland syndrome.*

pectus carinatum See *pigeon breast.*

pectus excavatum See *funnel chest.*

pediatric Pertaining to children.

pediatric arthritis See *arthritis in children.*

pediatric autoimmune disorders associated with streptococcus See *PANDAS.*

pediatric rheumatologist See *rheumatologist, pediatric.*

pediatrics The field of medicine that is concerned with the health of infants, children, and adolescents; their growth and development; and their opportunity to achieve full potential as adults.

pediculosis See *head lice.*

pediculus humanus capitis See *head lice.*

pedigree In medicine, a family health history that is diagrammed with a set of international symbols to indicate the individuals in the family, their gender, their relationships to one another, those with diseases, and other data. A pedigree is a basic tool of clinical genetics that is used to determine that a disease is genetic, track the transmission of the disease, and estimate risks to the patient, other family members, and the unborn from a genetic disease.

pedodontics Children's dentistry.

pedophilia Adult sexual fondness for and activity with children. Pedophilia is a form of paraphilia (deviant sexual behavior). If acted out, pedophilia is legally defined as sexual child abuse. Pedophilia includes fondling a child's genitals, intercourse, incest, rape, sodomy, exhibitionism, and commercial exploitation of children through prostitution or the production of pornographic materials. Pedophiles who have sexually abused children require intense psychological and pharmacological therapy prior to release into the community because of the high rate of repeat offenders. Treatment is rarely effective because the disorder is not yet well understood. The incidence of pedophilia has been markedly underestimated. It is essential that pedophilia be reported so that appropriate steps can be taken to protect the children involved and all other children.

peer review The process used by medical journals to screen articles that are submitted for publication. Peer-reviewed articles are scrutinized by members of the biomedical community before publication.

PEG Percutaneous endoscopic gastrostomy. See *gastrostomy, percutaneous endoscopic.*

pellagra Extreme niacin deficiency, characterized by a rash (dermatitis) on areas of the skin that are exposed to light, trauma and ulcerations within the mouth, diarrhea, mental disorientation (dementia), confusion, delusions, and depression. Pellagra can be fatal if untreated. Proper intake of niacin, a readily available B vitamin, both prevents and cures pellagra. See also *niacin.*

pelvic 1 Having to do with the pelvis. 2 Colloquially, a pelvic exam.

pelvic exam An examination of the organs of the female reproductive system. During a typical pelvic exam, a speculum is used to open the vagina so that the physician can see the uterine cervix. A sample of cells may be taken from the surface of the cervix for a Pap test, or a sample may be obtained for laboratory culture. During a pelvic exam, a physician feels the uterus (womb) and ovaries with the fingers to detect swellings or other abnormalities.

pelvic inflammatory disease Ascending infection of the upper female genital tract, usually caused by bacteria migrating upward from the urethra and cervix into the upper genital tract. Abbreviated PID. Many different organisms can cause PID, but most cases are associated with gonorrhea and chlamydial infections, two very common sexually transmitted diseases (STDs). Symptoms include fever, foul-smelling discharge, extreme pain, pain during intercourse, and bleeding. PID can scar the fallopian tubes, which can lead to infertility. Treatment involves use of antibiotics for the patient as well as all known sexual partners of the patient.

pelvis The lower part of the abdomen, located between the hip bones. Structures in the female pelvis include the uterus, vagina, ovaries, fallopian tubes, bladder, and rectum. Structures in the male pelvis include the bladder, rectum, testicles, and penis.

pelvis, android See *male pelvis.*

pelvis, female See *female pelvis.*

pelvis, gynecoid See *female pelvis.*

pelvis, male See *male pelvis.*

Pendred syndrome A genetic disease that is characterized by congenital deafness, abnormality of the bony labyrinth in the inner ear, and goiter. The congenital nerve deafness in Pendred syndrome is severe to profound. Abnormality of the labyrinth is evident on a CT scan of the temporal bone in the skull. In Pendred syndrome, the goiter is not present at birth but develops in early puberty or adulthood and is due to a defect in the making of thyroid hormone. However, the patient usually has a normal level of thyroid hormone in the blood due to compensated hypothyroidism. Other key features of the syndrome include defects in vestibular function, malformation of the balance portion of the ear (cochlea), swelling in the front of the neck due to the goiter, and mental retardation due to the congenital thyroid defect. Pendred syndrome is inherited in an autosomal recessive manner and is due to mutation in the SLC26A4 gene on chromosome 7q31, which encodes a protein called pendrin. Also known as deafness with goiter, goiter-deafness syndrome, and thyroid hormone organification defect IIb.

penetrance The likelihood that a given gene will result in disease. For example, if 50 percent of people with the neurofibromatosis (NF) gene develop the disease NF, the penetrance of the NF gene is 0.5, and if there is full penetrance with the gene for achondroplasia, 100 percent of people with that gene will develop achondroplasia.

penicillin Historically the most famous of antibiotics, which kills most bacteria and some other microorganisms by attacking and destroying their cell walls. Penicillin is not effective against viruses, however, and specific penicillin types may be needed for certain bacteria. The different varieties of penicillin include amoxicillin, ampicillin, bacampicillin, carbenicillin, cloxacillin, dicloxacillin, nafcillin, oxacillin, penicillin G, and penicillin V. See also *antibiotic.*

penicillin-resistant bacterium A bacterium that is unaffected by penicillin. Such organisms can often be killed by using sulfa drugs, combinations of several medications, or other tactics, but some resistant infections cannot be treated successfully. The rise of penicillin-resistant bacteria is due to overuse of penicillin drugs, including their ineffective but nonetheless frequent use against colds and viral infections.

penile Of or pertaining to the penis.

penis The external male sex organ. The penis contains two chambers, the corpora cavernosa, which run the length of the organ. These chambers are filled with spongy tissue and surrounded by a membrane called the tunica albuginea. The spongy tissue contains smooth muscles, fibrous tissues, spaces, veins, and arteries. The urethra, which is the channel for urine and ejaculate, runs along the underside of the corpora cavernosa. The urethra emerges at the glans, the rounded tip of the penis.

penis, cancer of the See *cancer, penis*

penis, erection of the See *erection, penile.*

penis, hypospadias of the See *hypospadias.*

penis, inflammation of the foreskin and glans See *balanoposthitis.*

penis, inflammation of the head of the See *balanitis.*

penis, small See *micropenis.*

peptic ulcer See *ulcer, peptic.*

percentile The percentage of individuals in a group who have achieved a certain quantity—such as height, weight, or head circumference—or a developmental milestone. For example, the fiftieth percentile for walking well is 12 months of age.

percutaneous Through the skin. For example, a percutaneous biopsy is a biopsy that is obtained by putting a needle through the skin in order to obtain tissue within the body for examination.

percutaneous endoscopic gastrostomy See *gastrostomy, percutaneous endoscopic.*

percutaneous nephrolithotripsy A technique for removing large, dense, and staghorn kidney stones. Abbreviated PNL. PNL is done via a port created by puncturing through the skin and into the kidney. This access port is then enlarged to about 0.4 centimeters (3/8 inches) in diameter. There is no surgical incision with PNL. PNL is done under anesthesia and with real-time, live X-ray control (fluoroscopy). Because X-rays are involved, a specialist in radiology, known as an interventional radiologist, may perform this part of the procedure. The urologist then inserts instruments into the kidney via the access port to break up the stone and to remove most of the debris from the stone.

percutaneous transluminal coronary angioplasty The use of a balloon-tipped catheter to enlarge a narrowed coronary artery. Abbreviated PTCA.

percutaneous umbilical blood sampling A procedure in which a needle is inserted through the mother's abdominal wall and then through the uterine wall. Abbreviated PUBS. In PUBS, blood can be withdrawn from the umbilical vein at the point where the umbilical cord inserts into the placenta. Blood may also be taken from the umbilical vein on its way to the fetal liver. PUBS is used both for prenatal diagnosis and prenatal treatment of a fetus.

peri- Prefix meaning around or about, as in pericardial (around the heart) and periaortic lymph nodes (lymph nodes around the aorta).

perianal Located around the anus, the opening of the rectum to the outside of the body.

perianal abscess A local accumulation of pus that forms next to the anus, causing tender swelling in that area and pain on defecation.

periaortic Around the aorta. For example, periaortic lymph nodes are lymph nodes around the aorta.

pericardial Referring to the pericardium, the sac of fibrous tissue that surrounds the heart.

pericardial effusion Too much fluid within the pericardium, which normally contains a small amount of serous, pale yellow fluid.

pericardial sac See *pericardium.*

pericardial tamponade See *tamponade, cardiac.*

pericarditis Inflammation of the lining around the heart (the pericardium) that causes chest pain and accumulation of fluid around the heart (pericardial effusion).

There are many causes of pericarditis, including infections, injury, radiation treatment, and diseases.

pericardium   The conical sac of fibrous tissue that surrounds the heart and the roots of the great blood vessels. The pericardium's outer coat (the parietal pericardium) is tough and thickened, loosely cloaks the heart, and is attached to the central part of the diaphragm and the back of the breastbone. Its inner coat (the visceral pericardium, or epicardium) is double, with one layer closely adherent to the heart and the other lining the inner surface of the outer coat. The intervening space between these layers is filled with pericardial fluid. This small amount of fluid acts as a lubricant to allow normal heart movement within the chest. Also known as pericardial sac. See also *pericarditis.*

pericardium, parietal   The tough, thickened outer layer of the pericardium. The parietal pericardium loosely cloaks the heart and is attached to the central part of the diaphragm and the back of the breastbone.

pericardium, visceral   The double inner layer of the pericardium. One layer of the visceral pericardium closely adheres to the heart, and the other lines the inner surface of the outer (parietal) pericardium. The intervening space is filled with pericardial fluid. Also known as epicardium.

pericentric chromosome inversion   See *chromosome inversion, pericentric.*

perichondrial   Having to do with the perichondrium, the membrane that surrounds cartilage.

perichondritis   Inflammation of the perichondrium.

perichondrium   A dense membrane that is composed of fibrous connective tissue that closely wraps all cartilage except the cartilage in joints, which is covered by a synovial membrane.

perichondroma   A benign tumor that arises from the perichondrium.

perimenopause   See *menopause transition.*

perinatal   Pertaining to the period immediately before and after birth. The perinatal period is defined in diverse ways. Depending on the definition, it starts at the 20th to 28th week of gestation and ends 1 to 4 weeks after birth.

perinatal transmission   See *vertical transmission.*

perinatalogist   An obstetrical subspecialist who is concerned with the care of the mother and fetus when there is a higher-than-normal risk of complications. Most perinatologist are obstetricians. A high-risk baby is often cared for by a perinatologist before birth and by a neonatologist after birth.

perinatalogy   A subspecialty of obstetrics that is concerned with the care of the mother and fetus when there is a higher-than-normal risk for complications.

perineal   Pertaining to the perineum.

perineal prostatectomy   An operation to remove the prostate gland through an incision made between the scrotum and the anus.

perineum   The area between the anus and the scrotum in the male and between the anus and the vulva in the female. See also *episiotomy.*

periodontal   Having to do with the gums and supporting structures of the teeth.

periodontal disease   A bacterial infection that destroys the attachment fibers and supporting bones that hold the teeth in the mouth. Left untreated, periodontal disease can lead to tooth loss. The main cause of periodontal disease is bacterial plaque, a sticky, colorless film that constantly forms on teeth.

periodontics   The branch of dentistry that is concerned with prevention, diagnosis, and treatment of diseases that affect the gums and supporting structures of the teeth.

periodontitis   Gum disease with inflammation of the gums. See also *periodontal disease.*

periosteal   Pertaining to the periosteum.

periosteoma   A benign tumor that arises from the periosteum. Also known as periostoma.

periosteum   A dense membrane composed of fibrous connective tissue that closely wraps all bone except that of the articulating surfaces in joints, which is covered by a synovial membrane.

periostitis   Inflammation of the periosteum.

periostoma   See *periosteoma.*

peripheral   Situated away from the center or being at or near the periphery, as opposed to central. For example, peripheral vision is the type of vision that allows a person to see objects that are not in the center of his or her visual field.

peripheral blood stem cell transplantation   See *stem cell harvest, peripheral blood.*

peripheral nervous system The portion of the nervous system that is outside the brain and spinal cord. Abbreviated PNS. The nerves in the PNS connect the central nervous system (CNS) to sensory organs, such as the eye and ear, and to other organs of the body, muscles, blood vessels, and glands. The peripheral nerves include the 12 cranial nerves, the spinal nerves and roots, and the autonomic nerves. The autonomic nerves are concerned with automatic functions of the body, specifically with the regulation of the heart muscle, the tiny muscles that line the walls of blood vessels, and glands.

peripheral neuropathy A problem with the functioning of the nerves outside the spinal cord. Symptoms of peripheral neuropathy may include numbness, weakness, burning pain (especially at night), and loss of reflexes.

peripheral T cells See *T cell, peripheral.*

peripheral vascular disease Atherosclerosis of the arteries of the extremities. Peripheral vascular disease can lead to pain in the legs when walking (claudication) that is relieved by resting. See also *atherosclerosis.*

periphery 1 The outside or surface of a structure or the portion outside the central region. 2 The circumference of a circle or another geometric figure.

peristalsis The rippling motion of muscles in the digestive tract. In the stomach, this motion mixes food with gastric juices, turning it into a thin liquid.

peritoneal Having to do with the peritoneum.

peritoneal dialysis A dialysis technique that uses the patient's own body tissues inside the abdominal cavity as a filter. A plastic tube called a dialysis catheter is placed through the abdominal wall, into the abdominal cavity. A special fluid is then flushed into the abdominal cavity and washed around the intestines. The intestinal walls act as a filter between this fluid and the bloodstream. By using different types of solutions, waste products and excess water can be removed from the body. This form of dialysis can be done either manually or by machine at home, thereby avoiding hospitalization or receiving dialysis treatment at a dialysis center.

peritoneum The membrane that lines the abdominal cavity and covers most of the abdominal organs.

peritonitis Inflammation of the peritoneum, the membrane that lines the inner wall of the abdomen and pelvis. Peritonitis can result from infection, as by bacteria or parasites; injury and bleeding; or diseases, such as systemic lupus erythematosus. See also *peritonitis, acute; peritonitis, chronic.*

peritonitis, acute Sudden inflammation of the peritoneum that results in abrupt abdominal pain (acute abdomen). The most serious causes of acute peritonitis include perforation of the esophagus, stomach, duodenum, gallbladder, bile duct, bowel, appendix, colon, rectum, and bladder; trauma; intestinal obstruction; pancreatitis; vascular catastrophes (mesenteric thrombosis or embolism); and as an infectious complication of peritoneal dialysis and pelvic inflammatory disease.

peritonitis, chronic Longstanding inflammation of the peritoneum. Causes of chronic peritonitis include repeated attacks of infection such as from pelvic inflammatory disease, foreign substances such as talc, and chronic infections within the abdomen such as tuberculosis.

peritonsillar abscess A collection of pus behind the tonsils that pushes one of the tonsils toward the uvula. A peritonsillar abscess is generally very painful and is usually associated with a decreased ability to open the mouth. If left untreated, the infection can spread deep in the neck, causing airway obstruction and life-threatening complications.

pernicious anemia See *anemia, pernicious.*

pernicious vomiting of pregnancy See *hyperemesis gravidarum.*

perspiration 1 The secretion of fluid by the sweat (sudoriferous) glands. These small, tubular glands are situated within the skin and in the subcutaneous tissue under it. They discharge fluid through tiny openings in the surface of the skin. Perspiration serves at least two purposes: It removes waste products such as urea and ammonia, and it cools the body as sweat evaporates. 2 The transparent, colorless, acidic fluid that is secreted by the sweat glands. Perspiration contains some fatty acids and mineral matter. Adult perspiration gains its characteristic odor from the waste products that are excreted. Also known as sweat.

Perthes disease See *Legg-Calvé-Perthes disease.*

pertussis A communicable, potentially deadly illness that is characterized by fits of coughing followed by a noisy, "whooping" indrawn breath. Pertussis is caused by the bacterium Bordetella pertussis. The illness is most likely to affect young children, but it sometimes appears in teenagers and adults, even those who have been previously immunized. When teenagers and adults get pertussis, it appears first as coughing spasms and then as a stubborn dry cough that lasts up to 8 weeks. Treatment involves supportive therapy (depending on the age of the patient this includes humidification of the air, cough suppressants, and pain medication). Young infants need hospitalization if the coughing becomes severe. Immunization with diphtheria-tetanus-pertussis (DTP) vaccine provides protection against pertussis, although that immunity may wear off with age. Also known as whooping cough. See also *DTP immunization; DTaP immunization.*

pervasive developmental disorder Abreviated PPD, one of a group of disorders characterized by delays in the development of multiple basic functions including socialization and communication. Parents may note symptoms as early as infancy and typically onset is prior to 3 years of age. Symptoms may include communication problems such as using and understanding language; difficulty relating to people, objects, and events; unusual play with toys and other objects; difficulty with changes in routine or familiar surroundings, and repetitive body movements or behavior patterns. Examples of PPD include autism, Asperger's syndrome, Rett's syndrome, and childhood disintegrative disorder. Children with PDD vary widely in abilities, intelligence, and behaviors. See *also autism; Asperger's syndrome; Rett's syndrome; childhood disintegrative disorder.*

pes Latin word meaning foot.

pes cavus A foot with an arch that is too high.

pes planus Flatfoot.

pest See *plague.*

pestilence 1 Originally, bubonic plague. See also *plague.* 2 Any epidemic disease that is highly contagious, infectious, virulent, and devastating.

pestis See *plague.*

PET scan Positron emission tomography scan, a highly specialized imaging technique that uses short-lived radioactive substances. This technique produces three-dimensional colored images. PET scanning provides information about the body's chemistry that is not available through other procedures. Unlike computerized tomography (CT) and magnetic resonance imaging (MRI), which look at anatomy or body form, PET studies metabolic activity or body function. PET scanning has been used primarily to evaluate problems of the heart and nervous system and to demonstrate the spread of cancer. In particular, PET scanning has been used to assess the benefit of coronary artery bypass surgery, identify causes of childhood seizures and adult dementia, and detect and grade tumors. PET scanning is very sensitive in detecting active tumor tissue, but it does not measure the size of a tumor. The radioisotope used in a PET scan is short-lived, and the amount of radiation exposure the patient receives

is about the same as that from two chest X-rays. Because the radiopharmaceutical contains a chemical that is commonly used by the body, PET scanning enables the physician to see the location of the metabolic process. For example, glucose combined with a radioisotope shows where glucose is being used in the brain, the heart muscle, or a growing tumor, etc.

petechiae Tiny red spots in the skin that do not blanch when pressed upon and that result from blood leaking from capillaries. The causes of petachiae include use of aspirin or other medications, allergic reactions, autoimmune disease, viral infection, thrombocythemia (an abnormally high platelet level), idiopathic thrombocytopenic purpura (ITP), leukemia and other bone marrow malignancies that can lower the number of platelets, chemotherapy and radiotherapy, and sepsis (bloodstream infection). Petechiae are often seen right after birth in newborns and after violent vomiting or coughing. A person with petechiae should see a physician because they may be of major consequence.

petit mal See *seizure, absence; seizure disorder.*

Peutz-Jeghers syndrome A genetic form of cancer that is characterized by freckle-like spots on the lips, mouth, and fingers and benign polyps in the intestines. Patients with Peutz-Jeghers syndrome are at increased risk for cancer of the esophagus, stomach, colon, rectum, breast, ovary, testis, and pancreas. The polyps may occur in any part of the gastrointestinal tract, but polyps in the jejunum (the middle portion of the small intestine) are a consistent feature of the disease. Intussusception (telescoping of the bowel) and intestinal bleeding are also common symptoms. Females with Peutz-Jeghers syndrome are at risk for sex cord tumors with annular tubules, a rare benign tumor of the ovary. Males may develop Sertoli cell tumors of the testes, which secrete estrogen and can lead to gynecomastia (male breast enlargement). Females can also have a malignancy of the cervix called adenoma malignum. Peutz-Jeghers syndrome is inherited in an autosomal dominant manner and is due to mutation in a gene on chromosome 19p13.3 called STK11 (serine/threonine-protein kinase 11). Half of patients with Peutz-Jeghers syndrome have affected parents and the other half have new mutations in the STK11 gene. Also known as polyps-and-spots syndrome.

PFS Patellofemoral syndrome.

PFT Pulmonary function test.

Ph See *Philadelphia chromosome.*

pH The symbol for the measure of the acidity or alkalinity of a solution. The pH number is from a scale where a pH of 7 is neutral, numbers less than a pH of 7 are increasingly more acidic, and numbers greater than a pH of 7 are increasingly more alkaline.

phacoemulsification A type of cataract surgery in which the lens with the cataract is broken up by ultrasound, irrigated, and suctioned out.

phage See *bacteriophage*.

phagocyte A cell that can engulf particles, such as bacteria and other microorganisms or foreign matter. The principal phagocytes include the neutrophils and monocytes, both of which are types of white blood cells.

phalanges The bones of the fingers and of the toes. There are generally three phalanges (distal, middle, proximal) for each digit except the thumbs and large toes. The singular of phalanges is phalanx.

phalanx See *phalanges*.

phantom limb syndrome The perception of sensations, often including pain, in an arm or leg long after the limb has been amputated. Phantom limb syndrome is relatively common in amputees, especially in the early months and years after limb loss.

phantom sensation A phenomenon that involves any of the senses that mimic the presence of sensory abilities that are no longer available. Phantom sensations are probably caused by abnormal firing of nerve impulses, although the mechanism for these sensations is not understood. For example, people who have lost much of their vision often experience visual phantoms. See also *phantom limb syndrome; phantom tooth pain*.

phantom tooth pain Persistent pain in an area from which a tooth has been extracted. Phantom tooth pain may last for months and can spread beyond the extraction site to other areas of the mouth.

phantom vision A phenomenon that involves seeing images after loss of eyesight.

pharmacist A professional who fills prescriptions and, in the case of a compounding pharmacist, makes them. Pharmacists are very familiar with medication ingredients, interactions, cautions, and hints.

pharmacogenetics The convergence of pharmacology and genetics, which deals with genetically determined responses to drugs. For example, after the administration of a muscle relaxant that is commonly used in surgery, a patient may remain incapable of breathing on his or her own for hours due to a genetically determined defect in metabolizing the muscle relaxant. The study of pharmacogenetics seeks to identify such patients and prevent the improper choice of that muscle relaxant. More prosaically,

pharmacogenetics can find out about common differences in the metabolism of medications among children, adults, and senior citizens; men and women; and people with various medical conditions.

pharmacologist A specialist in the science of medications. A pharmacologist is usually especially knowledgeable about new and obscure medications that may be needed for hard-to-treat or rare illnesses and about drug interactions and how to prevent them. Pharmacologists usually act as consultants to primary care physicians or specialists.

pharmacology 1 The study of concocting and using medications. 2 The study of drugs, their sources, their nature, and their properties.

pharmacopeia An official authoritative listing of medications. Some countries, such as the UK, establish official pharmacopeias, as do some medical groups and health maintenance organizations (HMOs).

pharmacy A location where prescription medications are sold. A pharmacy is constantly supervised by a licensed pharmacist.

pharmacy, compounding A place that both makes and sells prescription medications. A compounding pharmacy can often concoct drug formulas that are specially tailored to patients (for example, liquid versions of medications that are normally available only in pill form for patients who cannot swallow pills).

pharyngeal Having to do with the pharynx (throat).

pharyngitis Inflammation of the pharynx. Pharyngitis is a common cause of sore throat.

pharynx The hollow tube that is about 5 inches long and starts behind the nose and ends at the top of the trachea (windpipe) and esophagus. The pharynx serves as a vestibule or entryway for the trachea and esophagus.

phase, resting See *interphase*.

PhD Doctor of Philosophy. PhDs are involved in clinical care, as in clinical psychology; biomedical research, as in the Human Genome Project; health administration; teaching; and other areas of medicine.

Phe Phenylalanine.

phenocopy 1 An environmental condition that imitates a condition that is produced by a gene. 2 A person who has an environmental condition that mimics a condition that is produced by a gene.

phenomenon, Babinski See *Babinski reflex*.

phenomenon, phantom limb   See *phantom limb syndrome.*

phenomenon, Raynaud's   See *Raynaud's phenomenon.*

phenotype   The appearance of an individual, which results from the interaction of the person's genetic makeup and his or her environment. By contrast, the genotype is merely the genetic constitution (genome) of an individual. For example, if a child's genotype includes the gene for osteogenesis imperfecta (brittle bone disease), minimal trauma can cause fractures. The gene is the genotype, and the brittle bones themselves are the phenotype.

phenylalanine   An essential amino acid that is required in the human diet. Abbreviated phe. Most of the phe that is ingested is transformed (hydroxylated) to form tyrosine, which is used in protein synthesis. Too little phe does not permit normal physical and intellectual growth. Too much phe (as in PKU) is highly toxic to the brain. See also *phenylalanine hydroxylase deficiency; PKU; PKU, maternal.*

phenylalanine hydroxylase deficiency   The inherited inability to normally process the amino acid phenylalanine, due to partial or complete deficiency of the enzyme phenylalanine hydroxylase. This deficiency is caused by mutation in the PAH gene (which is on chromosome 12, in band 12q23.2). Phenylalanine hydroxylase deficiency causes a spectrum of disorders, including classic phenylketonuria (PKU), variant PKU, and non-PKU elevation of phenylalanine in the blood (non-PKU HPA). The decision about whether an individual needs to be on a low-phenylalanine diet is based on the person's blood level of phenylalanine (phe) rather on the precise condition that causes the elevated phe, because phe is toxic to the brain. Infants must avoid regular cow's milk formula or meat products. See also *PKU; PKU, maternal.*

phenylketonuria   See *PKU.*

phenylketonuria, maternal   See *PKU, maternal.*

pheresis   A procedure in which the blood is filtered and separated, and a portion is retained, with the remainder being returned to the individual. There are various types of pheresis. For example, in leukapheresis, the leukocytes (white blood cells) are removed; in platelet-pheresis, the thrombocytes (blood platelets) are removed; and in plasmapheresis, the liquid part of the blood (the plasma) is removed. See also *plasmapheresis.*

Philadelphia chromosome   Abbreviated Ph, the hallmark of chronic myeloid leukemia (CML), a small chromosome 22 that was shortchanged in a reciprocal exchange of material with chromosome 9. This translocation occurs in a cell in the bone marrow and causes CML. It is also found in a form of acute lymphoblastic leukemia (ALL). On a molecular level, the Philadelphia chromosome translocation results in the production of a large fusion protein. The malignant state is a consequence of this process. Understanding this process led to the development of the drug imatinib mesylate (brand name: Gleevec), the first in a new class of genetically targeted agents against leukemia.

philtrum   The area from below the nose to the upper lip. Normally the philtrum is grooved. In fetal alcohol syndrome, the philtrum is flat.

phimosis   A condition in which the foreskin of the penis is too tight to be pulled back to reveal the glans. This usually causes no problems and nothing needs be done. If phimosis causes obstruction of the urinary stream, meaturia (blood in the urine), or pain, this can be a urologic emergency and require surgery to relieve the phimosis. Circumcision prevents phimosis.

phlebitis   Inflammation of a vein. With phlebitis, there is infiltration of the walls of the vein and, usually, the formation of a clot (thrombus) in the vein (thrombophlebitis). Phlebitis in a leg, for example, causes the leg to swell with fluid (edema). The swollen leg feels stiff and painful. Phlebitis can be superficial and not very serious, or it can be deep and carry the potential for dislodging blood clots to the lungs.

phlebo-   Prefix meaning vein, as in phlebitis (inflammation of the veins) and phlebotomist (a person who draws blood from veins).

phlebotomist   A person who draws blood for diagnostic tests or to remove blood for treatment purposes.

phlebotomy   The field of obtaining blood from a vein. In the past, this was done by incising (cutting) a vein and just letting the blood flow into a container. Today phlebotomy is done more neatly by puncturing a vein with a needle. Phlebotomy may be done in order to obtain blood for diagnostic tests or to remove blood for treatment purposes (for example, to relieve iron overload in hemochromatosis).

phobia   An unreasonable sort of fear that can cause avoidance and panic. Phobias are a relatively common type of anxiety disorder. Examples of phobias are extreme fear of spiders, called arachnophobia, and fear of being outside, which is known as agoraphobia. Phobias can be treated with cognitive behavioral therapy, using exposure and fear-reduction techniques. In many cases, antianxiety or antidepressant medication proves helpful, especially during the early stages of therapy.

phobia, social See *social phobia.*

phocomelia A birth defect in which the hands and feet are attached to abbreviated arms and legs. The term comes from *phoco* (meaning "seal") and *melia* (meaning "limb"), to indicate that a limb is like a seal's flipper, as in exposure of the developing fetus to thalidomide. Phocomelia may also, in some cases, be genetic.

phosphatase, acid See *acid phosphatase.*

phosphatase, alkaline See *alkaline phosphatase.*

phosphate A form of phosphoric acid that may bind to other organic chemicals to form a variety of compounds. For example, calcium phosphate makes bones and teeth hard. See also *phosphorylation.*

phosphorus An essential element in the diet and a major component of bone.

phosphorylation A biochemical process that involves the addition of phosphate to an organic compound. Examples include the addition of phosphate to glucose to produce glucose monophosphate and the addition of phosphate to adenosine diphosphate (ADP) to form adenosine triphosphate (ATP). Phosphorylation is carried out through the action of enzymes known as phosphotransferases or kinases.

photochemotherapy See *photodynamic therapy.*

photodynamic therapy A form of treatment that uses a photosensitizing agent, administered by mouth or intravenously, which concentrates selectively in certain cells, followed by exposure of the involved tissue to a special light (such as laser or ultraviolet light), in order to destroy as much of the abnormal cells as possible. For example, photodynamic therapy is used to treat some forms of cancer and psoriasis. Also known as photochemotherapy.

photophobia Painful oversensitivity to light. For example, photophobia is often seen in measles and iritis. Keeping lights dim and rooms darkened is helpful when a patient has photophobia. Sunglasses may also help.

photorefractive keratectomy A kind of laser eye surgery that is designed to change the shape of the cornea, potentially eliminating or reducing the need for glasses or contact lenses. Abbreviated PRK. A laser is used to remove the outer layer of the cornea and flatten the cornea. The flattening of the cornea is intended to correct myopia (nearsightedness) and astigmatism (uneven curvature of the cornea that distorts vision). PRK is done in a physician's office, with anesthesia via numbing eyedrops. PRK takes about 1 minute to perform, and the patient heals in about 3 days. No eye patch need be worn after PRK.

photosensitivity Oversensitivity of skin to light. Photosensitivity can be a side effect of medications or result from diseases, such as lupus. Treatment depends on the severity of the reaction and the cause. Photosensitivity can be prevented by avoiding skin exposure to ultraviolet light.

phototherapy Treatment with light. For example, a newborn with jaundice may be put under special lights to help reduce the amount of bilirubin pigment in the skin.

phrenology The study of variations in the size, shape, and proportion of the cranium. Phrenology was a pseudoscience of the 18th and 19th centuries, based on the belief that a person's character could be learned by looking with care at the shape of the person's head and noting each and every bump and depression in the skull. The individual mental faculties were believed to be contained in neat compartments in the cerebral cortex, and the sizes of these faculties were supposed to be reflected by the configuration of the skull.

PHS Public Health Service. See *United States Public Health Service.*

physiatrist A physician who specializes in physical medicine and rehabilitation. Physiatrists specialize in restoring optimal function to people with injuries to the muscles, bones, tissues, or nervous system, such as stroke victims.

physical child abuse See *child abuse.*

physical map A map of the locations of identifiable landmarks on chromosomes. Physical distance between landmarks is measured in base pairs. The physical map differs from the genetic map, which is based purely on genetic linkage data. In the human genome, the lowest-resolution physical map is the banding patterns of the 24 different chromosomes. The highest-resolution physical map is the complete nucleotide sequence of all chromosomes.

physical therapist A person who is trained and certified by a state or accrediting body to design and implement physical therapy programs. Abbreviated PT. PTs may work in hospitals or clinics, in schools that provide assistance to special education students, or as independent practitioners.

physical therapy A branch of rehabilitative health that uses specially designed exercises and equipment to help patients regain or improve their physical abilities. Abbreviated PT. PT is appropriate for many types of patients, from infants born with musculoskeletal birth defects, to adults suffering from sciatica or the after effects of injury or surgery, to elderly poststroke patients.

physician A person who is trained in the art of healing. Contemporary physicians express their skills by combining art with science. In the UK, a physician is a specialist in internal or general medicine, whereas in the US a physician is any doctor of medicine. The term generally refers to a person who has earned a Doctor of Medicine (MD), Doctor of Osteopathy (DO), or Doctor of Naturopathy (ND) degree and who is accepted as a practitioner of medicine under the laws of the state, province, and/or nation in which he or she practices.

physician assistant A midlevel practitioner who is able to practice medicine under the auspices of a licensed physician (MD or DO). Abbreviated PA. Although the physician need not be present during the time the PA performs his or her duties, there must be a method of contact between the supervising physician and the PA at all times. The PA must be competent in the duties he or she is performing, and the physician for whom the PA is working must also be licensed and trained to perform the relevant duties. A PA has at least a bachelor's degree. Although there is not yet a requirement to hold a degree beyond the bachelor's level, the current trend in the US is for PAs to have a master's degree.

Physicians' Desk Reference A book that provides a guide to all the prescription drugs available in the US. Abbreviated PDR. PDR is a key reference to the US pharmacopeia and is published annually.

physiologic Something that is normal, that is due neither to anything pathologic nor significant in terms of causing illness. For example, physiologic jaundice is jaundice that is within normal limits.

physiologic amenorrhea See *amenorrhea, physiologic.*

physiologic jaundice Jaundice that is within normal limits. A newborn may have physiologic jaundice due to the release of the pigment bilirubin (from red blood cells) that the immature liver cannot process for excretion in the urine. Physiologic jaundice causes no illness and clears up in a few days.

physiology The study of how living organisms function, including such processes as nutrition, movement, and reproduction.

phytanic acid storage disease See *Refsum disease.*

phytochemical A plant compound that is thought to have health-protecting qualities. Also known as phytonutrient.

phytonutrient See *phytochemical.*

pia mater One of the meninges, the delicate innermost membrane that envelopes the brain and spinal cord. Known informally as the pia. See also *meninges.*

pianist's cramp A dystonia that affects the muscles of the hand and sometimes the forearm, and that only occurs when one plays the piano or another keyboard instrument. Similar focal dystonias have also been called writer's cramp, typist's cramp, musician's cramp, and golfer's cramp.

pica A craving for something that is not normally regarded as nutritive, such as dirt, clay, paper, or chalk. Pica is a classic clue to iron deficiency in children, and it may also occur with zinc deficiency. Pica is also seen as a symptom in several neurobiological disorders, including autism and Tourette's syndrome, and it is sometimes seen during pregnancy.

Pick disease A form of dementia that is characterized by a slowly progressive deterioration of social skills and changes in personality, along with impairment of intellect, memory, and language. The common symptoms include loss of memory, lack of spontaneity, difficulty in thinking or concentrating, and disturbances of speech. Other symptoms include gradual emotional dullness, loss of moral judgment, and progressive dementia. The age of onset may range from 20 to 80 but is often between 40 and 60. Pick disease is of unknown origin. The course ranges in duration from less than 2 years to more than 10 years. There is no treatment. Death is usually caused by infection that overwhelms the emaciated body. See also *dementia.*

Pickwickian syndrome A syndrome that is characterized by the combination of obesity, sleepiness, hypoventilation, and red face. The syndrome is named for the "fat and red-faced boy in a state of somnolency" whom Charles Dickens described in his novel *The Pickwick Papers.*

PID Pelvic inflammatory disease.

pigeon breast Having a prominent breastbone and chest. Also known as pectus carinatum.

pigment A substance that gives color to tissue. Pigments are responsible for the colors of skin, eyes, and hair.

pigmentation The coloring of the skin, hair, mucous membranes, and retina of the eye. Pigmentation is due to the deposition of the pigment melanin, which is produced by specialized cells called melanocytes. Other pigment-related terms include hyperpigmentation (too much pigment), hypopigmentation and underpigmentation (too little pigment), and depigmentation (loss of pigment).

piles See *hemorrhoids.*

pill, the See *oral contraceptive.*

piloerection Erection of the hair of the skin due to contraction of the tiny arrectores pilorum muscles that elevate the hair follicles above the rest of the skin and move the hair vertically, so the hair seems to "stand on end."

pilonidal cyst An abscess that occurs in the cleft between the buttocks. Pilonidal cysts are common in adolescence, often after long trips that involve sitting.

pimple An inflamed area with pus formation that results from an oil gland being infected with bacteria. Pimples are due to overactivity of the oil glands located at the base of the hair follicles, especially on the face, back, chest, and shoulders.

pineal gland A small gland that is located deep within the brain. This gland is believed to secrete melatonin, and it may therefore be part of the body's sleep-regulation apparatus.

pineal region tumor A brain tumor on or near the pineal gland. There are at least 17 types of pineal gland tumors, most of which are not cancerous but can nonetheless cause extreme distress. Pineal region tumors account for about 1 percent of brain tumors in adults and up to 8 percent of brain tumors in children. Symptoms include frozen upward gaze, hydrocephalus, and precocious puberty. Diagnosis is made via biopsy of affected tissue. Benign pineal tumors are treated with surgery; malignant tumors are usually treated with radiation followed by chemotherapy.

pinealoblastoma See *pineoblastoma.*

pinealocytoma See *pinealoma.*

pinealoma An uncommon slow-growing tumor of the pineal gland. Symptoms include hydrocephalus, paralysis of upward gaze, gait disturbances, and precocious puberty. Also known as a pinealocytoma and pineocytoma.

pineoblastoma A fast-growing brain tumor in the pineal gland that originates in neuroepithelial cells. This malignancy is one of the primitive neuroectodermal tumors (PNETs). Also known as pinealoblastoma.

pineocytoma See *pinealoma.*

pinguecula A yellow spot on the white of the eye, usually toward the inside of the eye, that is associated with aging. A pinguecula looks fatty and is due to an accumulation of connective tissue. Also known as pinguicula.

pinguicula See *pinguecula.*

pinkeye See *conjunctivitis.*

pinna 1 The ear. 2 The part of the ear that projects like a wing from the head.

pinworm infestation An infestation of the intestinal tract by small, white pinworms (Enterobius vermicularis). Pinworms are about the length of a staple, and they live for the most part within the human rectum. While a pinworm-infested person is asleep, female pinworms leave the intestines through the anus and deposit eggs on the skin around the anus. Most symptoms of pinworms are mild, such as anal itching, disturbed sleep, and irritability. If the infection is heavy, however, symptoms may include loss of appetite, restlessness, and insomnia. Pinworm is the most common worm infection in the US. School-age children have the highest rates of pinworm infestation, followed in frequency by preschoolers. Pinworms spread easily in daycare centers, schools, and homes. Within a few hours of being deposited on the skin around the anus, pinworm eggs become capable of infesting another person. They can survive up to 2 weeks on clothing, bedding, or other objects. If pinworms are suspected, transparent adhesive tape or a pinworm paddle supplied by a health care provider is applied to the anal region. The eggs adhere to the sticky tape or paddle and are identified via examination under a microscope. The test should be done as soon as the patient wakes up in the morning because bathing or having a bowel movement may remove eggs. Also known as enterobiasis. Treatment requires antibiotics.

piriformis muscle See *muscle, piriformus.*

piriformis syndrome Irritation of the sciatic nerve that is caused by compression of the nerve within the buttock by the piriformis muscle. Typically, the pain of piriformis syndrome is increased by contraction of the piriformis muscle, prolonged sitting, or direct pressure applied to the muscle. Buttock pain is common. Piriformis syndrome can cause difficulty walking due to pain in the buttock and lower extremity. Piriformis syndrome is one of the causes of sciatica. A physician can often detect tenderness of the piriformis muscle during a rectal examination. Piriformis syndrome is treated with rest and measures to reduce inflammation of the muscle and its tendon. Treatments include piriformis stretching exercises, physical therapy, use of anti-inflammatory medications, and use of pain medications. With persistent symptoms, further treatment can include local injection of anesthetic and cortisone medication. Rarely, surgery is performed to relieve the pressure. During surgical operations, the piriformis muscle can be thinned, elongated, divided, or removed.

pit, ear See *ear pit.*

pit, preauricular See *ear pit.*

pituitary 1 Pertaining to the pituitary gland or its hormonal secretions. 2 The pituitary gland.

pituitary adenoma A benign tumor of the pituitary gland, the master gland that controls other glands and influences numerous body functions, including growth. Although a pituitary adenoma itself is not cancerous, it may affect pituitary function and therefore may need to be removed. See also *pituitary gland; gigantism, pituitary.*

pituitary, anterior The front portion of the pituitary gland. Hormones secreted by the anterior pituitary influence growth, sexual development, skin pigmentation, thyroid function, and adrenocortical function. These influences are exerted through the effects of pituitary hormones on other endocrine glands, except in the case of growth hormone, which acts directly on cells. The effects of underfunction of the anterior pituitary include dwarfism in childhood and decrease in all other endocrine gland functions that are normally under the control of the anterior pituitary (except the parathyroid glands). The results of overfunction of the anterior pituitary include gigantism in children and acromegaly in adults. See also *acromegaly; dwarfism, pituitary; gigantism, pituitary.*

pituitary dwarfism See *dwarfism, pituitary.*

pituitary gigantism See *gigantism, pituitary.*

pituitary gland The main endocrine gland, which produces hormones that control other glands and many body functions, including growth. The pituitary is really two glands: the anterior pituitary and the posterior pituitary. Also known as simply the pituitary. See also *pituitary, anterior; pituitary, posterior.*

pituitary, posterior The back portion of the pituitary gland. The posterior pituitary secretes the hormone oxytocin, which increases uterine contractions and antidiuretic hormone (ADH), which increases reabsorption of water by the tubules of the kidney. Underproduction of ADH results in diabetes insipidus, which is characterized by inability to concentrate the urine and, consequently, excess urination, leading potentially to dehydration. See also *antidiuretic hormone; diabetes insipidus; oxytocin.*

PKD Polycystic kidney disease.

PKU Phenylketonuria, a metabolic disease that is due to the inherited inability to metabolize (process) the essential amino acid phenylalanine. The biochemical basis of PKU is complete or near-complete deficiency of the enzyme phenylalanine hydroxylase. Newborns in many countries are now routinely screened for PKU via a blood test. Treatment of PKU involves a special diet that is low in phenylalanine. No regular cow's milk formula or meat are allowed. The goal is to normalize the levels of phenylalanine and tyrosine in the blood to prevent brain damage. Failure or lack of treatment results in profound irreversible mental retardation, microcephaly, epilepsy, and behavior problems. If an appropriate diet is not followed closely, especially during childhood, some impairment is inevitable. PKU is inherited in an autosomal recessive manner, as are lesser degrees of phenylalanine hydroxylase deficiency. See also *Guthrie test; phenylalanine hydroxylase deficiency; PKU, maternal.*

PKU, maternal The disease phenylketonuria (PKU) in a pregnant woman whose high blood levels of phenylalanine (phe) are dangerous to a developing fetus. High phe can damage a baby before birth. A woman with PKU who has gone off the special PKU diet (which is low in phe) should resume it, ideally prior to conception. During pregnancy, the woman must be on the diet and have her blood phe levels carefully monitored. If the mother's PKU is not controlled, the fetus (which may not have PKU) is at high risk for congenital heart disease, growth retardation, microcephaly, and mental retardation. See also *phenylalanine hydroxylase deficiency; PKU.*

PKU, variant A form of phenylalanine hydroxylase deficiency that is more mild than classic PKU and typically causes less intellectual impairment.

placebo A sugar pill or any other inactive substance that is given instead of medication. In a controlled clinical trial, one group may be given a medication and another group a placebo, to learn whether a difference in treatment response is due to the medication, the power of suggestion, or other factors. See also *placebo response.*

placebo response A positive medical response to taking a placebo, as if it were an active medication. Up to one-third of patients given a placebo may have a placebo response, responding with a reduction in symptoms, depending on the condition. Although this phenomenon is often believed to be due to patients believing their symptoms have improved when in fact they have not, evidence is beginning to emerge that actual physiological changes—and even side effects—can result from believing that one is receiving medical treatment.

placenta A temporary organ that joins the mother and fetus, transferring oxygen and nutrients from the mother to the fetus and permitting the release of carbon dioxide and waste products from the fetus. The placenta is roughly disk-shaped, and at full term it measures about 7 inches in diameter and slightly less than 2 inches thick. The upper surface of the placenta is smooth, and the under surface is rough. The placenta is rich in blood vessels. The placenta is expelled with the fetal membranes during the birth process; together, these structures form the afterbirth.

placenta, accessory A condition in which there is an extra placenta that is separate from the main placenta. Also known as a succenturiate or supernumerary placenta.

placenta accreta The abnormal adherence of the chorion (chorionic villi) to the myometrium. Normally there is tissue intervening between the chorionic villi and the myometrium, but in placenta accreta, these vascular processes of the chorion grow directly in the myometrium. Placenta accreta can progress into placenta percreta.

placenta, low See *placenta previa.*

placenta percreta A condition in which the placenta invades the uterine wall. In placenta percreta, the vascular processes of the chorion (chorionic villi), a fetal membrane that enters into the formation of the placenta, may invade the full thickness of the myometrium. This can cause an incomplete rupture of the uterus. The chorionic villi can go right on through both the myometrium and the outside covering of the uterus (serosa), causing complete and catastrophic rupture of the uterus.

placenta previa A condition in which the placenta is implanted near the outlet of the uterus, so that at the time of delivery the placenta precedes the baby. Placenta previa can cause painless bleeding in the last trimester of pregnancy, and it may be a reason to perform a C-section. Also known as low placenta.

placenta, succenturiate See *placenta, accessory.*

placenta, supernumerary See *placenta, accessory.*

placental chorioangioma A benign vascular (blood vessel) tumor of the placenta. Large chorioangiomas can cause complications, including excess amniotic fluid (polyhydramnios), maternal and fetal clotting problems (coagulopathies), premature delivery, toxemia, fetal heart failure, and hydrops (excess fluid) that affect the fetus. Chorioangiomas probably act as peripheral shunts between arteries and veins, leading to progressive heart failure of the fetus. Labor is usually induced when the fetus is viable. Fetal blood transfusion has also been used in fetuses that are found to be anemic. Alcohol injection into the placental chorioangioma is being tried as a new method of treatment.

placental dystocia Difficulty in delivering the placenta. A number of techniques may be tried to overcome placental dystocia, including changing position, massage, nursing the newborn baby to induce uterine contractions, and in some cases using medications that induce uterine contractions.

placental stage of labor The part of labor that lasts from the birth of the baby until the placenta and fetal membranes are delivered. Also known as third stage of labor.

plague An infectious disease that is caused by the bacterium Yersinia pestis, which mainly infects rats and other rodents. Fleas function as the prime vectors for carrying Y. pestis from one species to another: The fleas bite the rodents that are infected with Y. pestis, and then they bite people and so transmit the disease. Transmission of the plague to people can also occur if people eat infected animals, such as squirrels. When someone has the plague, he or she can transmit it to another person via aerosol droplets. The plague has been responsible for devastating epidemics. The disease occurs at a consistent but low level (endemically) in many countries, including the US. It can now be easily treated with antibiotics, if it is caught early enough. The General Accounting Office, the investigative arm of the US Congress, considers plague to be a "possible, but not likely" biologic threat for terrorism, because it is difficult to acquire a suitable strain of Y. pestis and to weaponize and distribute it. Seed stock is difficult to acquire and to process and heat, and disinfectants and sunlight render it harmless. Also known as pest and pestis. See also *bubonic plague; plague, bubonic; plague, black.*

plague, bubonic See *bubonic plague.*

Plague, Great See *Great Plague.*

plague, sylvatic A type of plague that is spread by ground squirrels and other wild rodents. Sylvatic plague is sometimes seen in the western portion of the US.

plantar Having to do with the sole of the foot.

plantar fasciitis See *fasciitis, plantar.*

plantar response See *Babinski reflex.*

plantar wart See *wart, plantar.*

plaque **1** The white, semihardened substance that forms on the teeth as a result of bacterial action on food particles and provides an ideal environment for dental caries (cavities). Plaque should be removed with daily brushing and flossing and with regular dental cleanings. **2** A semihardened accumulation of substances, including cholesterol, on the inner walls of blood vessels that can lead to blood clot formation, heart attacks, and strokes. These risks can be reduced by maintaining normal blood cholesterol. **3** In dermatology, a small area of skin that appears different from the surrounding skin and is raised.

plaque, skin A broad, raised area on the skin. A skin plaque is broader than it is high.

plasma The liquid part of the blood and lymphatic fluid, which makes up about half of the volume of blood. Plasma is devoid of cells and, unlike serum, has not clotted. Blood plasma contains antibodies and other proteins. It is taken from donors and made into medications for a variety of blood-related conditions.

plasma cell A type of white blood cell that produces and secretes antibodies. A plasma cell is a fully differentiated, mature lymphocyte in the B cell lineage. As with most cell types, plasma cells can mutate to give rise to cancer. Plasma cell malignancies include plasmacytoma, multiple myeloma, Waldenstrom macroglobulinemia, and plasma cell leukemia. Also known as plasmacyte.

plasma donation The donation or sale of blood plasma for use in medical or other products. Unlike blood donors, most plasma donors in the US are paid. The procedure is done in a walk-in facility, where whole blood is taken through an IV needle and separated into plasma and blood cells. The blood cells are then returned to the donor intravenously. As long as the IV needles are disposable and not reused, there is no danger of infection for plasma donors.

plasmacyte See *plasma cell.*

plasmacytoma Cancer of the plasma cells (white blood cells that produce antibodies) that may turn into multiple myeloma.

plasmapheresis A procedure in which whole blood is taken from a person and separated into plasma and blood cells; the plasma is removed and replaced with another solution, such as saline solution, albumin, or specially prepared donor plasma; and the reconstituted solution is then returned to the patient. Plasmapheresis is increasingly being used to treat autoimmune disorders, such as lupus, multiple sclerosis, and PANDAS. When the plasma is removed, it takes with it the antibodies that have been developed against self-tissue, hopefully stopping the attack on the patient's own body. Plasmapheresis carries with it the same risks as any intravenous procedure but is otherwise generally safe. The risk of infection increases with the use of donor plasma, which may carry viral particles, despite screening procedures. Plasmapheresis is done in a clinical or hospital setting. Topical numbing cream may be used to reduce discomfort.

Plasmodium The genus of the class of Sporazoa that includes the parasite that causes malaria. Plasmodium is a type of protozoa, a single-celled organism that is able to divide only within a host cell. The main types of Plasmodium are P. falciparum, the species that causes falciparum malaria, the most dangerous type of malaria; P. malariae, the species that causes quartan malaria; P. ovale, a species found primarily in east and central Africa that causes ovale malaria; and P. vivax, the species that causes vivax malaria, which tends to be milder than falciparum malaria.

plastic surgeon A surgeon who specializes in reducing scarring or disfigurement that may occur as a result of accidents, birth defects, or treatment for diseases, such as melanoma. Many plastic surgeons also perform cosmetic surgery that is unrelated to medical conditions, such as rhinoplasty to change the shape of the nose.

plastic surgery A surgical specialty that is dedicated to reconstruction of facial and body defects due to birth disorders, trauma, burns, and disease. Plastic surgery is also involved with the enhancement of the appearance of a person through such operations as facelift, rhinoplasty, breast augmentation, and liposuction.

plasticity, brain See *brain plasticity.*

platelet An irregular, disc-shaped element of blood that assists in blood clotting. During normal blood clotting, platelets group together (aggregate). Although platelets are often classified as blood cells, they are actually fragments of large cells called megakaryocytes. Also known as thrombocyte. See also *blood cell.*

platelet count The calculated number of platelets in a volume of blood, usually expressed as platelets per cubic millimeter (cmm) of whole blood. Platelets are the smallest cell-like structures in the blood and are important for blood clotting and plugging damaged blood vessels. Platelet counts are usually done by laboratory machines that also count other blood elements such as white and red cells. Platelets can also be counted with the help of a microscope. Normal platelet counts are in the range of 150,000 to 400,000 per microliter (that is, 150 to 400 multiplied by 109 per liter). These values many vary slightly among different laboratories.

pleiotropic Producing or having multiple effects from a single gene. For example, the Marfan gene is pleiotropic, potentially causing such diverse effects as long fingers and toes (arachnodactyly), dislocation of the lens of the eye, and dissecting aneurysm of the aorta.

pleomorphic Many-formed. For example, a pleomorphic tumor would be a gowth that is composed of different types of tissues. Also known as protean.

plethoric Florid, red-faced. Persons with polycythemia vera commonly have plethoric facial appearance.

pleura One of the two membranes around the lungs. These two membranes are called the visceral and parietal pleurae. The visceral pleura envelops the lung, and the parietal pleura lines the inner chest wall. There is normally a small quantity (about 3 to 4 teaspoons) of fluid that is spread thinly between the visceral and parietal pleurae. The fluid acts as a lubricant between the two membranes.

pleural effusion   See *effusion, pleural.*

pleural space   The tiny area between the two pleurae, which is normally filled with a small amount of fluid. See also *effusion, pleural.*

pleurisy   Inflammation of the pleurae, the membranes surrounding the lungs. Symptoms include pain in the chest, chest tenderness, cough, and shortness of breath. The chest pain is very distinctive. It is sharp and aggravated by breathing. A physician can often hear the friction generated by the rubbing of the two inflamed layers of pleurae with each breath. The causes of pleurisy include lung infections, collagen vascular diseases such as lupus and rheumatoid arthritis, cancer of the lung or pleura, heart failure, pulmonary embolism (blood clot in the lungs), obstruction of lymph channels, trauma such as rib fractures, drugs such as Dilantin, pancreatitis, and cirrhosis of the liver. Removal of pleural fluid, when present, with a needle and syringe is key in diagnosing the cause of pleurisy and can also relieve the pain and shortness of breath associated with pleurisy. If the fluid is infected, treatment involves use of antibiotics and drainage of the fluid. If there is pus inside the pleural space, a chest drainage tube is inserted. In severe cases, in which there are large amounts of pus and scar tissue (adhesions), there may be a need for decortication (opening the pleural space and removing portions of one or two ribs in order to clear scar tissue and remove pus and debris). Also known as pleuritis.

pleuritis   See *pleurisy.*

pleurodesis   A procedure that causes the membranes around the lungs to stick together and prevents the buildup of fluid in the space between the membranes (pleural space). Pleurodesis is done in cases of severe recurrent pleural effusions (outpourings of fluid around the lungs) to prevent the reaccumulation of the fluid. During pleurodesis, an irritant (such as bleomycin, tetracycline, or talc powder) is instilled inside the pleural space in order to create inflammation that tacks the two pleura together. This procedure thereby permanently obliterates the space between the pleura and prevents the reaccumulation of fluid.

pleurodynia   See *Bornholm disease.*

plumbism   See *lead poisoning.*

Plummer disease   See *goiter, toxic multinodular.*

PMR   Polymyalgia rheumatica.

PMS   Premenstrual syndrome.

pneumatic larynx   A device that uses air to produce sound, helping a person whose larynx has been removed to talk.

pneumo-   Prefix pertaining to breathing, respiration, the lungs, pneumonia, or air, as in pneumonectomy (an operation to remove an entire lung or part of a lung) and pneumonia (inflammation of one or both lungs).

pneumococcal immunization   A vaccine that prevents one of the most common and severe forms of pneumonia, the form that is caused by Streptococcus pneumoniae (pneumococcus bacterium). This vaccine has long been offered to people over 55 years of age, people who have had their spleens removed, those with ongoing lung problems (such as chronic obstructive pulmonary disease) and asthma or other chronic diseases, including those that involve the heart and kidneys. Pneumococcal immunization is now recommended for use in all children 23 months of age and younger. The vaccine is also recommended for all children 24 to 59 months of age who are at especially high risk of invasive pneumococcal infection, including children with sickle cell disease or human immunodeficiency virus (HIV) and other children who are immunocompromised.

pneumococcal pneumonia immunization   A vaccine that prevents one of the most common and severe forms of pneumonia. Pneumococcal pneumonia immunization is usually given only once in a lifetime, usually after the age of 55, to someone with ongoing lung problems such as chronic obstructive pulmonary disease or asthma, or to persons with other chronic diseases, including those involving the heart and kidneys. This vaccination is rarely given to children.

pneumococcus   See *Streptococcus pneumoniae.*

pneumoconiosis   Inflammation and irritation caused by deposition of dust or other particulate matter in the lungs. Pneumoconiosis usually occurs in workers in certain occupations and in people who live in areas that have a great deal of particulate matter in the air. Types of pneumoconiosis range from nearly harmless forms to destructive or fatal conditions, such as asbestosis and silicosis.

pneumoconiosis, coal miner's   See *black lung disease.*

pneumocystis carinii pneumonia   A parasitic infection of the lungs that is particularly common and life threatening in premature or malnourished infants and in immunosuppressed persons. Abbreviated PCP. PCP causes fever, cough, shortness of breath, and bluish extremities. Untreated, it leads to dense areas of lung inflammation, low blood oxygen levels, and death. Preventive treatment is available to prevent PCP in persons who are at increased risk.

pneumomediastinum Free air in the space between the lungs (mediastinum), which may give rise to pneumothorax or pneumopericardium and compromise the lungs or heart.

pneumonectomy An operation to remove an entire lung or part of a lung.

pneumonia Inflammation of one or both lungs, with dense areas of lung inflammation. Pneumonia is frequently but not always due to infection. The infection may be bacterial, viral, fungal, or parasitic. Symptoms may include fever, chills, cough with sputum production, chest pain, and shortness of breath. Pneumonia is suggested by the symptoms and confirmed by chest X-ray testing. Treatment includes antibiotics.

pneumonia, aspiration Inflammation of the lungs due to the sucking in of food particles or fluids into the lungs (aspiration).

pneumonia, bilateral See *pneumonia, double.*

pneumonia, double Pneumonia in both lungs. Also known as bilateral pneumonia.

pneumonia, giant cell A deadly but fortunately rare complication of measles that tends to strike children who are immunodeficient from leukemia or AIDS. The lung tissue shows multinucleated giant cells lining the alveoli (air sacs) of the lungs. Also known as Hecht's pneumonia, named for the early 20th-century Austrian pathologist Victor Hecht.

pneumonitis, radiation Inflammation of the lungs that results from radiation. Radiation pneumonitis typically occurs after radiation treatments for cancer within the chest or breast. Radiation pneumonitis usually manifests itself 2 weeks to 6 months after completion of radiation therapy. Symptoms include shortness of breath upon activity, cough, and fever. Radiation pneumonitis is frequently discovered serendipitously, as an incidental finding on a chest X-ray in patients who have no symptoms. If radiation pneumonitis persists, it can lead to scarring of the lungs, referred to as radiation fibrosis. Radiation fibrosis typically occurs 1 year after the completion of radiation treatments. Radiation pneumonitis is often reversible with medications that reduce inflammation, such as cortisone drugs. Radiation fibrosis, however, is usually irreversible. See also *fibrosis, radiation.*

pneumopericardium Air or other gas in the sac surrounding the heart (pericardium).

pneumothorax Free air in the chest outside the lung. Pneumothorax can occur spontaneously, follow a fractured rib, occur in the wake of chest surgery, or be deliberately induced in order to collapse the lung.

PNL Percutaneous nephrolithotripsy.

PNS Peripheral nervous system.

p.o. Per os. Abbreviation meaning by mouth, orally. See also Appendix A, "Prescription Abbreviations."

podiatrist A specialist in the diagnosis and care of foot disorders, including their medical and surgical treatment.

poikiloderma Extra pigmentation of the skin that demonstrates a variety of shades and is associated with widened capillaries (telangiectasia) in the affected area.

poikiloderma congenita See *Rothmund-Thomson syndrome.*

point, McBurney See *McBurney point.*

point mutation A single nucleotide base change in DNA. For example, a point mutation is the cause of sickle cell disease.

poison Any substance that can cause severe distress or death if ingested, breathed in, or absorbed through the skin. Many substances that normally cause no problems, including water and most vitamins, can be poisonous if taken in excessive quantity. Poison treatment depends on the substance: If there are treatment instructions on the substance's container and the container contained no other item, one should follow those directions immediately. It is important to contact the nearest poison control center with concerns about possible poison ingestion.

poison control center A special information center set up to inform people about how to respond to potential poisoning. These centers maintain databases of poisons and appropriate emergency treatment. Local poison control centers should be listed with other community-service numbers in the front of the telephone book, and they can also be reached immediately through any telephone operator.

poison ivy Skin inflammation that results from contact with the poison ivy vine. Chemicals produced by this vine cause an immune reaction, producing redness, itching, and blistering of the skin. Treatment involves use of topical medication, such as calamine lotion.

poison oak Skin inflammation that results from contact with the poison oak plant. Chemicals produced by this plant cause an immune reaction, producing redness, itching, and blistering of the skin. Treatment involves use of topical medication, such as calamine lotion.

poisoning Taking a substance that is injurious to health or can cause death. Poisoning is still a major hazard to children, despite child-resistant packaging and dose-limits per container. See also *poison; Poison control center.*

poisoning, silver See *argyria.*

Poland syndrome A unique pattern of one-sided malformations that is characterized by a defect of the chest muscle (pectoralis) on one side of the body and webbing and shortening of the fingers (cutaneous syndactyly) on the hand on the same side. The serratus anterior and latissimus dorsi muscles may also be absent, as may be the armpit hair. In girls, the breast on the affected side is also usually absent. Usually the child is otherwise normal, although on rare occasions Poland syndrome is associated with more severe finger and arm involvement or with vertebral or kidney problems. Intelligence is not impaired. Poland syndrome is not common, affecting 1 child in about 20,000. Poland syndrome occurs three times more frequently in boys than in girls. Its cause is uncertain, although diminished blood flow through the subclavian artery that goes to the fetal arm has been blamed. The disorder is currently considered a nonspecific developmental field defect, occurring at about the sixth week of fetal development. The syndrome occurs sporadically and does not appear to run in families. Treatment may include reconstructive surgery, and bioengineered cartilage may be implanted to help give the chest a more normal look. Also known as absence of the pectoralis muscle with syndactyly.

polio An acute and sometimes devastating viral disease that can take several different forms. Humans are the only natural hosts for poliovirus. The virus enters the mouth and multiplies in lymphoid tissues in the pharynx and intestine. Small numbers of virus particles enter the blood and go to other sites, where the virus multiplies more extensively. Another round of virus in the bloodstream leads to invasion of the spinal cord and brain, the target sites struck by the virus. When the central nervous system (CNS) is inflamed, the anterior horn cells of the spinal cord and the brainstem are especially affected. Polio is a minor illness in 80 to 90 percent of clinical infections; this is termed the abortive type of polio. Abortive polio appears chiefly in young children and does not involve the CNS. Symptoms are slight fever, malaise, headache, sore throat, and vomiting 3 to 5 days after exposure. Recovery occurs in 24 to 72 hours. As a major illness, polio may or may not cause paralysis. Symptoms usually appear without prior illness, particularly in older children and adults, 7 to 14 days after exposure. Symptoms are fever, severe headache, stiff neck and back, deep muscle pain, and sometimes areas of increased or altered sensation. There may be no further progression from this type of illness, which is similar to viral meningitis, or there may be loss of tendon reflexes and weakness or paralysis of muscle groups. Recovery is complete with the abortive and nonparalytic forms of polio, although a set of symptoms known as postpolio syndrome may appear many years later. In paralytic polio, about 50 percent of patients recover, with no residual paralysis; about 25 percent are left with mild disabilities, and the remaining 25 percent of patients have severe permanent disability. The greatest return of muscle function occurs in the first 6 months, but improvement may continue for up to 2 years. Physical therapy is the most important part of treatment of paralytic polio during convalescence. The ideal strategy with polio is clearly to prevent it by immunizing against poliovirus. Also known as infantile paralysis and poliomyelitis. See also *postpolio syndrome.*

polio, abortive A minor form of infection with poliovirus that accounts for 80 to 90 percent of clinically apparent cases of polio in the US, chiefly in young children. The usual symptoms—slight fever, malaise, headache, sore throat, and vomiting—emerge 3 to 5 days after exposure to the virus. Full recovery occurs in 24 to 72 hours. Abortive polio does not involve the nervous system or cause permanent disabilities of any kind.

polio immunization One of the two polio vaccines that are available: oral polio vaccine (OPV) and inactivated polio vaccine (IPV). OPV is the preferred vaccine for most children. As its name suggests, it is given by mouth. Infants and children should be given four doses of OPV. The doses are given at 2 months, 4 months, 6 to 18 months, and 4 to 6 years of age. Persons who are allergic to eggs or the drugs neomycin or streptomycin should receive OPV, not the injectable IPV. Conversely, IPV should be given if the vaccine recipient is on long-term steroid (cortisone) therapy, has cancer, or is on chemotherapy, or if a household member has AIDS or is an unimmunized adult. IPV is given as a shot in the arm or leg.

polio vaccine, inactivated A vaccine that is made from a suspension of poliovirus types I, II, and III that are grown in monkey kidney cell tissue culture and inactivated (killed) with formalin. Abbreviated IPV. IPV is given by injection. It does not give long-lasting protection against polio and so requires booster shots. IPV has been largely superseded by the oral polio vaccine. In the US, IPV is now reserved for the immunization of immunologically deficient patients and for the primary immunization of unimmunized at-risk adults. IPV is also known as the Salk vaccine and, formerly, the polio vaccine. IPV was developed by the US microbiologist Jonas E. Salk, who inoculated volunteers with his vaccine in 1952 and in

1953 published the results in the *Journal of the American Medical Association*. Nationwide testing of IPV was carried out in 1955. IPV was the first polio vaccine available.

polio vaccine, killed See *polio vaccine, inactivated.*

polio vaccine, live See *polio vaccine, oral.*

polio vaccine, oral A vaccine that contains live attenuated (weakened) poliovirus types I, II, and III that are grown in monkey kidney cell tissue culture. Abbreviated OPV. OPV is now used for the routine immunization of children against polio. OPV induces long-lasting immunity and does not require a booster; OPV should not be given to immunodeficient persons or to their close contacts. Also known as Sabin vaccine, for US microbiologist Albert B. Sabin, who first gave volunteers his vaccine in 1955. By 1957–1959, the vaccine was in use in the Soviet and Eastern Bloc. The first US trial was not until 1960. The OPV developed by Sabin is in standard use today.

polio vaccine, Sabin See *polio vaccine, oral.*

polio vaccine, Salk See *polio vaccine, inactivated.*

poliomyelitis See *polio.*

pollen Small, light, dry protein particles from trees, grasses, flowers, and weeds that may be spread by the wind. Pollen particles are usually the male sex cells of a plant, and they are smaller than the tip of a pin. Pollen is a potent stimulator of allergic responses. It lodges in the mucous membranes that line the nose and in other parts of the respiratory tract, causing irritation and histamine reactions.

pollex The thumb.

poly- Prefix meaning much or many, as in polycystic (characterized by many cysts).

poly A short form for polymorphonuclear leukocyte, a type of white blood cell.

polyarteritis nodosa An autoimmune disease that is characterized by spontaneous inflammation of the arteries (arteritis) and can affect any organ of the body. Polyarteritis nodosa most commonly affects muscles, joints, intestines, nerves, kidneys, and skin. Inflammation of the arteries can lead to inadequate blood supply and permanent damage to organs. Typically, polyarteritis nodosa is treated with medications that suppress the immune system, such as prednisone and cyclophosphamide.

polyarticular Involving many joints, as opposed to monoarticular (affecting just one joint).

polycystic kidney disease An inherited disorder that is characterized by the development of innumerable cysts in the kidneys that are filled with fluid and replace much of the mass of the kidneys. The cysts eventually reduce kidney function, leading to kidney failure. Abbreviated PKD. PKD can be diagnosed via ultrasound imaging and via CAT or MRI scan. Treatment involves managing pain and treating infections, high blood pressure, and kidney failure. There are two major forms of PKD—autosomal dominant and autosomal recessive—that differ in many respects. See also *polycystic kidney disease, autosomal dominant; polycystic kidney disease, autosomal recessive.*

polycystic kidney disease, adult See *polycystic kidney disease, autosomal dominant.*

polycystic kidney disease, autosomal dominant A late-onset systemic disorder that is characterized by the progressive development of innumerable cysts in the kidneys, causing hypertension, renal pain, and renal insufficiency (kidney failure). Other features of the disease are cysts in other organs, such as the liver and pancreas, intracranial aneurysms, dilatation (widening) and dissection of the aorta, mitral valve prolapse, and abdominal wall hernias. Half of patients have end-stage renal disease by age 60. The disease is due to mutations in the PKD1 gene on chromosome 16 or, less often, in the PKD2 gene on chromosome 4. Also known as adult polycystic kidney disease.

polycystic kidney disease, autosomal recessive An early-onset disorder that is characterized by the presence of innumerable cysts in the kidneys and enlarged kidneys that can usually be detected via ultrasound before birth or in the neonatal period. Some cases are diagnosed later in childhood. Underdevelopment of the lungs—due to inadequate amniotic fluid caused by kidney failure before birth—is a major cause of disease and death in the newborn period. Children who live beyond the first year of life tend to develop kidney failure in the first decade of life and need kidney transplants. The gene for the disease is on chromosome 6. Also known as infantile polycystic kidney disease.

polycystic kidney disease, infantile See *polycystic kidney disease, autosomal recessive.*

polycystic ovarian disease See *Stein-Leventhal syndrome.*

polycythemia Too many red blood cells. The opposite of polycythemia is anemia. Polycythemia exists when the hemoglobin, red blood cell (RBC) count, and total RBC volume are all above normal. Polycythemia can lead to heart failure, stroke, and other medical problems when severe. Treatment can involve bloodletting. See *polycythemia vera.*

polycythemia vera   Overproduction of red blood cells due to bone marrow disease (myeloproferative disorder). Abbreviated PV. PV tends to evolve into acute leukemia or myelofibrosis, in which the marrow is replaced by scar tissue. For a diagnosis of PV, there must be polycythemia. See also *polycythemia.*

polydactyly   More than the normal number of fingers or toes. The opposite of polydactyly is oligodactyly. See also *hexadactyly.*

polydipsia   Constant, excessive drinking as a result of thirst. Polydipsia occurs in untreated or poorly controlled diabetes mellitus.

polygenes   Many genes. For example, eye color is polygenically controlled because many genes are involved in the determination of eye color.

polygenic disease   A genetic disorder that is caused by the combined action of more than one gene. Examples of polygenic conditions include hypertension, coronary heart disease, and diabetes. Because such disorders depend on the simultaneous presence of several genes, they are not inherited as simply as are single-gene diseases.

polyhydramnios   Too much amniotic fluid. The opposite of polyhydramnios is oligohydramnios.

polymerase chain reaction   A key technique in molecular genetics that permits the analysis of any short sequence of DNA or RNA without having to clone it. Abbreviated PCR. PCR is used to amplify selected sections of DNA in only a few hours. The PCR technique has innumerable uses, from diagnosing genetic diseases to DNA fingerprinting. PCR has become an essential tool for biologists, forensics labs, and scientists who want to study genetic material.

polymerase, DNA   See *DNA polymerase.*

polymerase, RNA   See *RNA polymerase.*

polymorphonuclear leukocyte   See *leukocyte, polymorphonuclear.*

polymyalgia rheumatica   A disorder of the muscles and joints that is characterized by pain and stiffness that affect both sides of the body and involves the shoulders, arms, neck, and buttock areas. Abbreviated PMR. PMR generally affects persons who are over the age of 50 years. Blood testing in a person with PMR usually shows a significantly elevated sedimentation rate. PMR is characteristically very responsive to treatment with low doses of cortisone-related medications, such as prednisone.

polymyositis   An inflammatory disease of muscle that begins when white blood cells spontaneously invade muscles, especially those closest to the trunk or torso. This immune activity results in muscle pain, tenderness, and weakness. Blood testing in a person with polymyositis shows significantly elevated creatinine phosphokinase levels. The diagnosis is further suggested by electromyogram testing and confirmed with muscle biopsy. Treatment of polymyositis requires high doses of cortisone-related medications, such as prednisone, and immune suppression with medications, such as methotrexate and cyclophosphamide.

polyneuritis, acute idiopathic   See *Guillain-Barre syndrome.*

polyostotic fibrous dysplasia   A genetic disorder that is characterized by bone, skin pigmentation, and hormonal problems, with premature sexual development. Polyostotic fibrous dysplasia refers specifically to the replacement of multiple areas of bone by fibrous tissue, which may cause fractures and deformity of the legs, arms, and skull. A patient with polyostotic fibrous dysplasia has flat areas of increased skin pigment called café au lait spots. The hormonal problems related to polyostotic fibrous dysplasia include early puberty (with premature menstrual bleeding and development of breasts and pubic hair), thyroid abnormalities, and an increased rate of growth. Polyostotic fibrous dysplasia is usually caused by mosaicism for a mutation in the gene guanine nucleotide binding protein, alpha stimulating activity polypeptide 1. Also known as McCune-Albright syndrome.

polyp   A mass of tissue that develops on the inside wall of a hollow organ, such as the colon.

polypapilloma tropicum   See *yaws.*

polyploid   Having three or more full sets of chromosomes. For example, a polyploid brain tumor cell might have 69 or 92 chromosomes.

polyps-and-spots syndrome   See *Peutz-Jeghers syndrome.*

polypsis of the colon   See *familial adenomatous polyposis.*

polysomnography   Electronic monitoring of a sleeping patient to look for abnormalities in sleep patterns and/or brain waves. Polysomnography correlates electroencephalogram readings with observation of the patient. Usually, respiration, oxygen saturation, body position, and other factors are also measured during polysomnography. See also *sleep apnea; sleep apnea, central; sleep apnea, obstructive; sleep disorders.*

polysomy Y syndrome   See *XYY syndrome.*

popliteal Referring to the back of the knee. For example, the popliteal fossa is the hollow behind the knee.

popliteal fossa The hollow behind the knee.

popliteal pterygium syndrome An inherited condition that is characterized by a web (pterygium) behind the knee. Facial abnormalities in popliteal pterygium syndrome are cleft palate (with or without cleft lip), pits in the lower lip, and fibrous bands in the mouth. Genital abnormalities in popliteal pterygium syndrome are underdevelopment of the labia majora, malformation of the scrotum, and failure of the testes to descend into the scrotum. Patients have an extensive web running from behind the knee down to the heel, malformed toenails, and webbed toes. The disorder is inherited in an autosomal dominant manner and is due to mutation of the interferon regulatory factor 6 gene. Also known as facio-genitopopliteal syndrome.

pork tapeworm See *Taenia solium.*

porphyria One of a variety of hereditary diseases that are characterized by increased formation and excretion of chemicals called porphyrins. Attacks may range from mild to severe. Besides having abdominal and nerve pain, the patient may suffer rapid heartbeat, mania, muscle cramps, muscle weakness, breathing problems, hallucinations, and coma. Acute attacks are often precipitated by the use of certain drugs, such as barbiturates, sulphonamides, and birth control pills; alcohol use; hormonal changes during menstruation or pregnancy; dieting or fasting; and infections. Treatment involves following a high-carbohydrate diet and avoiding precipitating factors. One type of porphyria, acute intermittent porphyria, may have affected members of the House of Hanover in England, including "Mad" King George. The king may not have been mad, but rather may have suffered attacks of porphyria.

portal vein A large vein formed by the union of the splenic and superior mesenteric veins. The portal vein conveys venous blood to the liver for detoxification before the blood is returned to circulation via the hepatic veins.

port-wine stain A mark on the skin whose rich, rubyred color resembles that of port wine. Due to an abnormal aggregation of capillaries, a port-wine stain is a type of hemangioma. It can occur on the face as a sign of Sturge-Weber syndrome. See also *Sturge-Weber syndrome.*

positive, false See *false positive.*

positron emission tomography See *PET scan.*

post- Prefix meaning after.

posterior The back. The opposite of posterior is anterior. See also Appendix B, "Anatomic Orientation Terms."

posterior cruciate ligament The cross-shaped ligament that crosses behind the anterior cruciate ligament and within the knee joint. Abbreviated PCL. See also *knee.*

posterior pituitary See *pituitary, posterior.*

posteroanterior In anatomy, from back to front. Abbreviated PA. For example, a chest X-ray taken with the chest against the film plate and the X-ray machine behind the patient is a PA view. The opposite of posteroanterior is anteroposterior (AP). See also Appendix B, "Anatomic Orientation Terms."

postherpetic neuralgia See *neuralgia, postherpetic.*

posthitis Inflammation of the foreskin of the penis. In an uncircumcised male, posthitis usually occurs together with balanitis, inflammation of the glans, as balanoposthitis. Circumcision prevents and cures posthitis. See also *balanitis; balanoposthitis.*

postmature infant A baby born 7 days or more after the usual 40 weeks of gestation. See also *postterm infant.*

postmenopausal After menopause, especially the period of time after a woman has experienced 12 consecutive months without menstruation.

postnasal drip Mucous accumulation in the back of the nose and throat that leads to or gives the sensation of mucus dripping down from the back of the nose. Postnasal drip is one of the most common consequences of sinusitis, nasal allergies, and the common cold.

postop Short for postoperative; after a surgical operation. to the opposite of postop is preop.

postpolio muscular atrophy Muscle wasting that occurs years after the acute polio episode has resolved as part of postpolio syndrome. Abbreviated PPMA. See also *postpolio syndrome.*

postpolio syndrome A constellation of symptoms and signs that appear 20 to 40 years after the initial polio infection and at least 10 years after what was thought to be recovery from polio. Abbreviated PPS. It is estimated that 1.63 million people in the US were struck by polio in the epidemics of the 1940s, '50s, and early '60s, and that 440,000 of the survivors suffer the effects of PPS. The typical features of PPS include unaccustomed weakness, muscle fatigue (and sometimes central fatigue), pain, breathing and/or swallowing difficulties, sleep disorders, muscle twitching, and gastrointestinal problems. The muscle problems in PPS can occur in previously affected muscles or in muscles that were thought not to be affected at the onset of polio. The onset of PPS is usually gradual, but it is sometimes abrupt, with major loss of function suffered over several months or a couple years. This process often seems to start after some physical or emotional trauma, an illness, or an accident. Complications of PPS may include neuropathies, nerve entrapments, arthritis, scoliosis, osteoporosis, and sometimes postpolio muscular atrophy. Diagnosis is made via history, via clinical findings, and by ruling out other diseases that may mimic PPS. There are no specific tests to provide unquestionable confirmation of the diagnosis of PPS. The general rule is that those who were most seriously affected by poliovirus at initial onset and made the best recovery come to suffer the worst PPS symptoms years later. No clear-cut cause for PPS has been found. There is known to be a failure at the neuromuscular junction. There is also known to be impairment in the production of certain hormones and neurotransmitters, but whether these changes are the cause of PPS or its effect is unknown. Polio survivors tend to be hard-driving, type-A personalities, as compared to nondisabled control subjects—and the more driven polio survivors tend to have more PPS symptoms. Treatment may include slowing down to conserve strength and energy. Musculoskeletal problems can sometimes be helped with anti-inflammatory or pain medications, with or without surgical procedures. See also *polio.*

postremission therapy   Chemotherapy to kill leukemia cells that survive after remission-induction therapy.

post-term infant   A baby born 14 days or more after the usual 40 weeks of gestation, as calculated from the mother's last menstrual period. This is an important calculation because if delivery is delayed 3 weeks beyond term, the possibility of infant mortality skyrockets to 3 times its normal rate.

post-traumatic stress disorder   A psychological disorder that develops in some individuals who have had major traumatic experiences, such as those who have experienced serious accidents, survived or witnessed violent crimes, or been through wars. Abbreviated PTSD. Typically a person with PTSD is emotionally numb at first but later has symptoms that may include depression, excessive irritability, guilt for having survived if others were injured or died, recurrent nightmares, flashbacks to the traumatic scene, and overreactions to sudden noises. PTSD was known as shell shock during World War I and battle fatigue during World War II.

postulates, Koch   See *Koch postulates.*

postural   Pertaining to the posture or position of the body, the attitude or carriage of the body as a whole, or

the position of the limbs (the arms and legs). See also *hypotension, orthostatic.*

postural hypotension   See *hypotension, orthostatic.*

potassium   The major positive ion (cation) found inside cells. The chemical notation for potassium is K+. The proper level of potassium is essential for normal cell function. An abnormal increase of potassium (hyperkalemia) or decrease of potassium (hypokalemia) can profoundly affect the nervous system and heart, and when extreme, can be fatal. The normal blood potassium level is 3.5–5.0 milliEquivalents/liter (mEq/L), or 3.5 international units.

Pott's disease   See *tuberculous diskitis.*

pouch of Douglas   An extension of the peritoneal cavity between the rectum and the back wall of the uterus. Also known as the rectouterine pouch.

pouch, rectouterine   See *pouch of Douglas.*

pound   A measure of weight that is equal to 16 ounces or, metrically, 453.6 grams. Abbreviated lb.

power of attorney, durable   See *durable power of attorney.*

PPMA   Postpolio muscular atrophy.

PPS   Postpolio syndrome.

Prader-Willi syndrome   A syndrome that is characterized by severe hypotonia (floppiness), poor sucking and feeding problems in early infancy, and, later in infancy, excessive eating that, if unchecked, leads gradually to huge obesity. Abbreviated PWS. All children with PWS show developmental delay and mild to moderate mental retardation with multiple learning disabilities. Small gonads are present in both females (with small labia minora and clitoris) and males (with underdeveloped scrotum and nondescent of the testes). Short stature and small hands and feet are common. The basic cause of PWS is extraordinary: It is due to absence of the paternally contributed region on chromosome 15q11–15q13. The child can have two copies of chromosome region 15q11–15q13, but if both are from the mother (a phenomenon called maternal disomy), the child still has PWS because of lack of the region from the father. When the maternally contributed region 15q11–15q13 is missing, the result is a different disease, called Angelman syndrome. There is currently no specific treatment or cure for PWS. Parents are advised to limit consumption of high-calorie foods and to use techniques such as special education, speech therapy, and physical therapy to maximize the child's potential. Severe psychiatric illness is common in adults with PWS. Those with psychotic illness have a double maternal copy of 15q11–15q13, suggesting that genes in this region are important in causing psychotic illness.

Prayer of Maimonides   See *Daily Prayer of a Physician.*

pre-   Prefix meaning before.

preauricular tag   See *ear tag.*

preauricular pit   See *ear pit*

precancerous   Pertaining to something that is not yet cancerous but appears to be on its way to becoming a cancer. See also *premalignant.*

preclinical study   A study to test a drug, a procedure, or another medical treatment in animals. The aim of a preclinical study is to collect data in support of the safety of the new treatment. Preclinical studies are required before clinical trials in humans can be started.

precocious   Unusually early development of intellectual powers, speech, physical traits, and so on.

precocious puberty   The onset of secondary sexual characteristics, such as breast buds in girls, growth of the penis and thinning of the scrotum in boys, and the appearance of pubic hair in both sexes, before the normal age of puberty. There is much normal variation in the age of puberty, but precocious puberty is generally defined as onset before the age of 8 in girls and 9 in boys.

preconceptual   Referring to before conception. For example, preconceptual counseling is the interchange of information prior to pregnancy.

preconceptual counseling   The interchange of information prior to pregnancy. Preconceptual counseling usually occurs for pregnancy planning and care, but sometimes it takes the form of genetic counseling. See also *genetic counseling.*

preeclampsia   A condition that is characterized by a sharp rise in blood pressure during the third trimester of pregnancy. Hypertension may be accompanied by swollen ankles, irritability, and kidney problems, as evidenced by protein in the urine. Although preeclampsia is relatively common, occurring in about 5 percent of all pregnancies and more frequently in first pregnancies than in others, it can be a sign of serious problems. It may indicate that the placenta is detaching from the uterus, for example. In some cases, untreated preeclampsia can progress to eclampsia, a life-threatening situation for both the mother and the fetus. Treatment involves bed rest and sometimes medication. If treatment is ineffective, induced birth or a

C-section may have to be considered. See also *eclampsia; HELLP syndrome.*

preemie   See *premature baby.*

pregnancy   The state of carrying a developing embryo or fetus within the female body. Pregnancy can be indicated by positive results on an over-the-counter urine test and confirmed through a blood test, an ultrasound, detection of fetal heartbeat, or an X-ray. Pregnancy lasts for about 40 weeks, measured from the date of the woman's last menstrual period. It is conventionally divided into three trimesters, each roughly 3 months long. The most important tasks of basic fetal cell differentiation occur during the first trimester, so any harm done to the fetus during this period is most likely to result in miscarriage or serious disability. There is little to no chance that a first-trimester fetus can survive outside the womb, even with the best hospital care; its systems are simply too undeveloped. This stage truly ends with the phenomenon of quickening, the mother's first perception of fetal movement. In the first trimester, some women experience morning sickness. The breasts also begin to prepare for nursing, and painful soreness from hardening milk glands may occur. As the pregnancy progresses, the mother may experience many physical and emotional changes, ranging from increased moodiness to darkening of the skin in various areas. During the second trimester, the fetus undergoes a remarkable series of developments. Its physical parts become fully distinct and at least somewhat operational. With the best medical care, a second-trimester fetus born prematurely has at least some chance of survival, although developmental delays and other problems may emerge later. As the fetus grows in size, the mother's pregnant state begins to be obvious. In the third trimester, the fetus enters the final stage of preparation for birth. It increases rapidly in weight, as does the mother. As the end of the pregnancy nears, there may be discomfort as the fetus moves into position in the woman's lower abdomen. Swelling of the ankles, back pain, and balance problems are sometimes experienced during this time. Most women are able to go about their usual activities, including nonimpact exercise and work, until the very last days or weeks of pregnancy. During the final days, some women feel too much discomfort to continue at a full pace, although others report greatly increased energy just before the birth. Pregnancy ends when the birth process begins. See also *acute fatty liver of pregnancy; birth; birth defect; conception; eclampsia; ectopic pregnancy; fetal alcohol effect; fetal alcohol syndrome; HELLP syndrome; hyperemesis gravidarum; preeclampsia; pregnancy, tubal; prenatal care; prenatal development; teratogen.*

pregnancy, acute fatty liver of   See *acute fatty liver of pregnancy.*

pregnancy, alcohol during   See *fetal alcohol syndrome; fetal alcohol effect.*

pregnancy, drugs during   See *teratogen.*

pregnancy, ectopic   See *ectopic pregnancy.*

pregnancy, extrauterine   See *ectopic pregnancy.*

pregnancy, molar   See *hydatidiform mole.*

pregnancy, pernicious vomiting of   See *hyperemesis gravidarum.*

pregnancy planning   Planning that addresses issues that may affect a woman's ability to carry a child to term, such as nutrition, vitamins, body weight, exercise, potentially harmful medications and illnesses, immunizations, and genetic counseling. A woman who plans to become pregnant should make lifestyle choices for optimal health before the planned conception. See also *birth control; family planning.*

pregnancy, tubal   An ectopic pregnancy that takes place in a fallopian tube. Tubal pregnancies are due to the inability of the fertilized egg to make its way through the fallopian tube into the uterus. Most tubal pregnancies occur in women 35 to 44 years of age. Tubal pregnancies account for 95 percent of all ectopic pregnancies. See also *ectopic pregnancy.*

preleukemia   See *myelodysplastic syndrome.*

premalignant   Pertaining to tissue that is not yet malignant but is poised to become malignant. Appropriate clinical and laboratory studies are designed to detect premalignant tissue while it is still in a premalignant stage. A battery of techniques are available to remove or kill the tissue, thereby preventing the development of cancer. The proper treatment method depends on the particular premalignant tissue involved. Examples of premalignant growths include polyps in the colon, actinic keratosis of the skin, dysplasia of the cervix, metaplasia of the lung, and leukoplakia (white patches in the mouth)

premature aging disorder   A condition that causes a person to appear far older than their actual age. See *progeria; Werner syndrome.*

premature baby   A baby who is born before 37 weeks of gestation have passed since the mother's last menstrual period. A premature baby who is born very close to its due date may suffer few, if any, consequences. The earlier in development that birth takes place, the greater the likelihood that life-support systems will be needed and the greater the risk for birth defects and death. Colloquially known as a preemie. See also *pregnancy; premature birth.*

premature birth   Birth before 37 weeks of gestation have passed. Premature birth carries increased risks the farther it occurs from the 37-week goal. Many procedures are available to prevent premature birth, from bed rest to medications. If premature birth is medically necessary or inevitable, however, it may be accomplished via C-section to limit stress on the fetus. See also *pregnancy; premature baby.*

premature contraction of the heart   A single heartbeat that occurs earlier than normal. This phenomenon can be within normal limits, or it may represent a medically significant arrhythmia.

premature ventricular contraction   Contraction of the lower chambers of the heart, the ventricles, that occurs earlier than usual because of abnormal electrical activity of the ventricles. Abbreviated PVC. The premature contraction is followed by a pause as the heart's electrical system resets itself; the contraction following the pause is usually more forceful than normal. These more forceful contractions are frequently perceived as palpitations.

premenstrual syndrome   A combination of physical and mood disturbances that occur in the last half of a woman's menstrual cycle, after ovulation, and normally end with the onset of the menstrual flow. Abbreviated PMS. Physical features of PMS include breast tenderness and bloating. Psychological changes include anger and depression. Monthly chemical changes may be responsible for PMS. These chemical changes may involve sex hormones, neurotransmitters, and opioid peptides. PMS can be mimicked and must be distinguished from other disorders. The most helpful diagnostic tool for PMS is a menstrual diary. Treatment of PMS includes exercise, dietary changes, emotional support of family and friends, and medications, including diuretics, pain killers, oral contraceptives, drugs that suppress ovarian function, and antidepressants.

prenatal care   Health care that a pregnant woman receives from an obstetrician or a midwife. Services needed include dietary and lifestyle advice, weighing to ensure proper weight gain, and examination for problems of pregnancy such as edema and preeclampsia. In cases where complications are likely, such as pregnancy after age 40 or in a women with diabetes, prenatal care may be sought from an experienced specialist.

prenatal development   The process of growth and development within the womb, in which a single-cell zygote (the cell formed by the combination of a sperm and an egg) becomes an embryo, a fetus, and then a baby. The first 2 weeks of development involve simple cell multiplication. This tiny mass of cells then adheres to the inside wall of the uterus. The next 3 weeks see intense cell differentiation, as the cell mass divides into separate primitive systems. At the end of 8 weeks, the embryo takes on a roughly human shape and is called a fetus. For the next 20 weeks the fetus's primitive circulatory, nervous, pulmonary, and other systems become more mature, and the fetus begins to move its limbs. At 28 weeks, fat begins to accumulate under the skin, toenails and fingernails appear, and downy hair sprouts on the body and scalp. The fetus may open its eyes periodically. For the remaining weeks of development, the fetus continues to gain weight, and its internal systems reach full development.

prenatal diagnosis Diagnosis before birth. Methods for prenatal diagnosis include ultrasound of the uterus, placenta, and/or developing fetus; chorionic villus sampling (CVS) to obtain tissue for chromosome or biochemical analysis; and amniocentesis to obtain amniotic fluid for the analysis of chromosomes, enzymes, or DNA. A growing number of birth defects and diseases can be diagnosed prenatally and in some cases treated before birth. Also known as antenatal diagnosis.

preop Short for preoperative; before a surgical operation. The opposite of preop is postop.

prepuce See *foreskin.*

prepuce, inflammation of the See *posthitis.*

presbyopia The loss of the eye's ability to change focus to see near objects due to advancing age. Presbyopia is said to be due to the lens becoming less elastic with age. The first sign of presbyopia is often the need to hold reading material farther away. See *eye.*

prescription A physician's order for the preparation and administration of a drug or device for a patient. A prescription has several parts, including the superscription, or heading, with the symbol R or Rx, which stands for the word "recipe" (Latin for "to take"); the inscription, which contains the names and quantities of the ingredients; the subscription, or directions for compounding the drug; and the signature, often preceded by the sign s., which stands for "signa" (Latin for "mark"), giving the directions to be marked on the container. See also Appendix A, "Prescription Abbreviations."

prescription drug A drug requiring a prescription, as opposed to an over-the-counter (OTC) drug, which can be purchased without a prescription.

presentation, breech See *breech birth.*

presentation, footling See *footling birth.*

presentation, vertex See *vertex birth.*

pressure, high blood See *hypertension.*

pressure, intraocular See *intraocular pressure.*

pressure, low blood See *hypotension.*

preventive medicine Medical practices that are designed to avert and avoid disease. For example, screening for hypertension and treating it before it causes disease is good preventive medicine. Preventive medicine takes a proactive approach to patient care.

priapism Abnormally persistent erection of the penis in the absence of desire. Treatments include medications, anesthesia, and drainage of blood from the penis.

primary amenorrhea See *amenorrhea.*

primary biliary cirrhosis See *cirrhosis, primary biliary.*

primary care A patient's main source for regular medical care, ideally providing continuity and integration of health care services. All family physicians, and most pediatricians and internists, are in primary care. The aims of primary care are to provide the patient with a broad spectrum of preventive and curative care over a period of time and to coordinate all the care that the patient receives.

primary care provider In insurance parlance, a physician who is chosen by or assigned to a patient and both provides primary care and acts as a gatekeeper to control access to other medical services.

primary dentition See *primary teeth.*

primary HIV infection See *HIV infection, primary.*

primary sclerosing cholangitis A chronic disorder of the liver in which the ducts carrying bile from the liver to the intestine, and often the ducts carrying bile within the liver, become inflamed, thickened, scarred (sclerotic), and obstructed. This relentlessly progressive process can in time destroy the bile ducts and lead to cirrhosis. Abbreviated PSC. PSC can occur by itself or in association with other diseases, including inflammatory bowel disease, especially with ulcerative colitis; certain uncommon diseases, such as multifocal fibrosclerosis syndrome, Riedel struma, and pseudotumor of the orbit; and AIDS. Changes in the biliary tract are quite common in AIDS and are very much like those in PSC; however, in AIDS the changes in the biliary tract are probably due to infection with mycoplasma, cytomegalovirus, or other agents. PSC often triggers jaundice (yellowing), pruritus (generalized itching all over the body), upper abdominal pain, and infection. Later on, PSC progresses to cirrhosis of the liver and liver failure, creating a need for liver transplantation. Diagnosis is made via clinical observation and routine laboratory tests and is confirmed through demonstration of thickened bile ducts, using special radiologic tests called cholangiography. Treatment includes cholestyramine to diminish itching, antibiotics for infection, vitamin D and calcium to prevent bone loss (osteoporosis), sometimes balloon dilatation or surgery for obstructed ducts, and liver transplantation when necessary and possible. The prognosis depends on the age of the person, the degree of jaundice, the stage of PSC found via liver biopsy, and the size of the spleen. Most patients die within 10 years of diagnosis unless a liver transplant is performed. Also known as idiopathic sclerosing cholangitis.

primary teeth The first 20 teeth, which are shed and replaced by permanent teeth. The first primary tooth comes in (erupts) at about 6 months of age, and the last erupts at around 2½ years. Replacement with permanent teeth usually begins at about age 6. Also known as baby teeth, milk teeth, primary dentition, temporary teeth, and deciduous teeth.

primum non nocere See *first do no harm.*

principal joints of the body See *joints of the body, principal.*

Prinzmetal angina See *angina, Prinzmetal.*

prion A disease-causing agent that is neither bacterial nor fungal nor viral and that contains no genetic material. A prion is a protein that occurs normally in a harmless form. When it is folded into an aberrant shape, a normal prion turns into a rogue agent. It then co-opts other normal prions to become rogue prions. Prions have been held responsible for a number of degenerative brain diseases, including mad cow disease, Creutzfeldt-Jakob disease, fatal familial insomnia, kuru, an unusual form of hereditary dementia known as Gertsmann-Straeussler-Scheinker disease, and possibly some cases of Alzheimer's disease.

private mutation A rare gene mutation that is usually found only in a single family or a small population. A private mutation is like a privately printed book, it mutated and was passed in a few family members, but not to future generations.

PRK Photorefractive keratectomy.

p.r.n. Pro re nata. Abbreviation meaning as needed. See also Appendix A, "Prescription Abbreviations."

pro- A prefix (from both Greek and Latin) with many meanings, including before, in front of, preceding, on behalf of, in place of, and the same as.

pro 1 Professional. 2 Prothrombin.

pro time Prothrombin time.

probability The likelihood that something will happen. For example, a probability of less than .05 indicates that the likelihood of something occurring by chance alone is less than 5 in 100, or 5 percent. This level of probability is usually taken as the level of biologic significance, so a higher incidence may be considered meaningful. Abbreviated p.

proband The family member through whom a family's medical history comes to attention. For example, a proband might be a baby with Down syndrome. The proband may also be called the index case, propositus (if male), or proposita (if female).

probe 1 In surgery, a slender, flexible rod with a blunt end that is used to explore. For example, a probe might explore an opening to see where it goes. 2 In molecular genetics, a labeled bit of DNA or RNA that is used to find its complementary sequence or to locate a particular clone.

probiotic A substance that appears to replenish or support the growth of helpful bacteria in the intestinal tract. The most common probiotic is acidophilus, which is present in yogurt, in acidophilus milk, and in supplements. As the name indicates, probiotics have been developed to counter one unfortunate effect of treatment with antibiotics: the decimation of helpful intestinal bacteria along with disease-causing bacteria. See also *acidophilus.*

process In anatomy, a projection from a structure. For example, the process of the mandible is the part of the lower jaw that projects forward.

proclivity An inclination or a predisposition toward something, especially a strong inherent inclination toward something objectionable. For example, a patient might be said to have a proclivity toward alcohol.

proctitis Inflammation of the rectum. Proctitis may be due to a considerable number of causes, including infectious agents and ulcerative colitis. Infectious proctitis is often due to agents such as Chlamydia trachomatis, Neisseria gonorrheae, and herpes simplex virus, all of which can be acquired during anoreceptive intercourse. Proctitis is also a hallmark of ulcerative colitis, in which case it may be accompanied by intermittent rectal bleeding, crampy abdominal pain, and diarrhea.

proctitis, ulcerative Ulcerative colitis that is limited to the rectum. See also *colitis, ulcerative; proctitis.*

proctology A medical specialty that deals with disorders of the rectum and anus.

proctosigmoidoscopy An examination of the rectum and the lower part of the colon, using a thin, lighted instrument called a sigmoidoscope.

product, gene See *gene product*.

progeria A rare genetic disorder that causes premature aging in children. The classic type of progeria is Hutchinson-Gilford progeria syndrome, which is characterized by dwarfism, baldness, pinched nose, small face and small jaw relative to the head size, delayed tooth formation, aged-looking skin, stiffness of joints, hip dislocations, arteriosclerosis, and heart disease. Children with progeria have a remarkably similar appearance to one another. At present, there is no cure or specific treatment. Progeria is due to an autosomal dominant mutation. A diagnosis of progeria can be confirmed because a chemical (hyaluronic acid) is elevated in the urine, as it is in Werner syndrome, which is sometimes called progeria of the adult. See also *Werner syndrome*.

progesterone A female hormone, the principal hormone that prepares the uterus to receive and sustain fertilized eggs.

progesterone receptor test A lab test that is used to determine whether breast cancer cells have progesterone receptors. If the cells have progesterone receptors, they may depend on progesterone for growth and usually respond to hormone therapy. Breast cancer cells that do not have progesterone receptors do not need the hormone progesterone to grow and usually do not respond to hormone therapy.

prognathism An overly prominent jaw. Prognathism may cause no problems or be associated with dental problems. Prognathism is characteristic of some diseases, such as acromegaly.

prognosis The forecast of the probable outcome or course of a disease; the patient's chance of recovery.

prognostic Pertaining to the prognosis, the outlook for the patient.

progressive Increasing in scope or severity, advancing, or going forward. For example, a disease that is progressive is going from bad to worse.

prokaryote A cell that lacks a discrete nucleus and other special subcellular compartments. Bacteria and viruses are prokaryotes. Humans are not prokaryotes, but rather eukaryotes.

prominent vertebra The seventh cervical (neck) vertebra, which has a long spinous process that projects out from the back of its vertebral body.

promoter In molecular biology, a site on DNA to which the enzyme RNA polymerase can bind to initiate the transcription of DNA into RNA.

pronation Rotation of the arm or leg inward. In the case of the arm, the palm of the hand faces posteriorly when it is pronated. See also Appendix B, "Anatomic Orientation Terms."

prone With the front or ventral surface downward (lying face down), as opposed to supine. See also Appendix B, "Anatomic Orientation Terms."

pronucleus A cell nucleus with a haploid (halved) set of chromosomes—23 chromosomes in humans—that results from division (meiosis) of a germ cell. The male pronucleus is the sperm nucleus after it has entered the ovum at fertilization but before fusion with the female pronucleus. Similarly, the female pronucleus is the nucleus of the ovum before fusion with the male pronucleus.

prophylactic **1** A medication or treatment given to prevent development of disease. **2** A drug or device for preventing pregnancy, particularly a condom.

prophylactic cranial irradiation Radiation therapy to the head that is intended to prevent cancer from spreading to the brain.

prophylaxis The prevention of disease.

propositus See *proband*.

propriception The ability to sense stimuli arising within the body. Even if a person is blindfolded, he or she knows through propriception if an arm is above the head or hanging by the side of the body. The sense of propriception is disturbed in many neurological disorders. It can sometimes be improved through the use of sensory integration therapy, a type of specialized occupational therapy. See also *sensory integration*.

prostaglandin A hormone-like substance that participates in a wide range of body functions such as the contraction and relaxation of smooth muscle, the dilation and constriction of blood vessels, control of blood pressure, modulation of inflammation, and production of the normal protective mucus lining of the stomach. Prostaglandins are derived from a chemical called arachidonic acid.

prostate See *prostate gland*.

prostate acid phosphatase An enzyme that is produced by the prostate gland that is elevated in some patients with prostate cancer.

prostate cancer See *cancer, prostate*.

prostate enlargement Overgrowth of the prostate gland, usually due to a common, benign, and very treatable condition known as benign prostatic hyperplasia (BPH).

Far fewer cases of prostate enlargement are due to prostate cancer, but men over age 30 should have regular prostate examinations to detect developing prostate cancer as early as possible. See also *digital rectal exam; prostate cancer; prostate gland; prostate specific antigen test; prostatic hyperplasia, benign.*

prostate gland   A gland in the male reproductive system that is located just below the bladder. It surrounds part of the urethra, the canal that empties the bladder. The prostate gland helps to control urination, and it forms part of the content of semen. Also known as simply the prostate.

prostate, nodular hyperplasia of the   See *benign prostatic hyperplasia.*

prostate specific antigen test   A test that is used to screen for cancer of the prostate and to monitor treatment. Prostate specific antigen (PSA) is a protein that is produced by the prostate gland. Although most PSA is carried out of the body in semen, a very small amount escapes into the bloodstream. The PSA test is done on blood. PSA in blood can be by itself as free PSA, or it can join with other substances in the blood as bound PSA. Total PSA is the sum of free and bound forms. The PSA value that is used most frequently as the highest normal level is 4 ng/mL (nanograms per milliliter). However, because the prostate gland generally increases in size and produces more PSA with increasing age, it is normal to have lower levels in young men and higher levels in older men. Age-specific PSA levels are as follows: 2.5 ng/mL for ages 40 to 49, 3.5 ng/mL for ages 50 to 59, 4.5 ng/mL for ages 60 to 69, and 6.5 ng/mL for ages 70 and older. The use of age-specific PSA ranges for the detection of prostate cancer is controversial. Not all studies have agreed that this is better than simply using a level of 4 ng/mL as the highest normal value. An abnormal result on a PSA test indicates the need for additional testing if it is being used as a screening measure. Levels above 4 ng/mL but less than 10 ng/mL are suspicious. However, most men who have this level of abnormality actually do not have prostate cancer. As levels increase above 10 ng/mL, the probability of prostate cancer increases dramatically. When the PSA test is used as a monitoring test following therapy, an abnormal result indicates recurrence of prostate cancer. PSA is not specific to prostate cancer. Other diseases can cause elevated PSA. The most frequent is benign prostatic hypertrophy (BPH), an increase in the size of the prostate that typically occurs with aging. Infection of the prostate gland (prostatitis) is another relatively common cause of elevated PSA. Other conditions that can increase PSA include ischemia, infarction, urethral instrumentation, urinary retention, and prostate biopsy. Also, a small proportion of prostate cancers do not produce a detectable increase in blood PSA, even with advanced disease. Many

early cancers do not produce enough PSA to cause a significantly abnormal blood level. It is therefore important not to rely only on blood PSA testing. The most useful additional test is a physical prostate exam known as the digital rectal exam. See also *digital rectal exam; prostate cancer; prostate gland; prostatic hyperplasia, benign.*

prostatectomy   Surgical removal of the prostate gland. Prostatectomy can be done through an incision in the abdomen or through the urethra (transurethral resection).

prostatectomy, retropubic   Surgical removal of the prostate gland through an incision in the abdomen. Retropubic prostatectomy is a treatment option for some forms of prostate cancer.

prostatic hyperplasia, benign   See *benign prostatic hyperplasia.*

prostatic hypertrophy, benign   See *benign prostatic hyperplasia.*

prostatitis   Inflammation of the prostate gland. Prostatitis can result from infection or certain diseases, such as reactive arthritis.

prostatitis, bacterial   Inflammation of the prostate gland due to bacterial infection. Symptoms of bacterial prostatitis include chills, fever, pain in the lower back and genital area, body aches, testicular pain, burning or painful urination, and the frequent and urgent need to urinate. In bacterial prostatitis, the urinary tract is infected, as evidenced by the presence of white blood cells and bacteria in the urine. Acute bacterial prostatitis is treated with antibiotics. In chronic bacterial prostatitis, a defect in the prostate gland is the focal point for the persistent infection. Effective treatment of chronic bacterial prostatitis requires identification and correction of this defect before antibiotics can be effective.

prosthesis   An artificial replacement of a part of the body, such as a tooth, a facial bone, the palate, or a joint. A prosthesis may be removable, as in the case of most prosthetic legs or a prosthetic breast form used after mastectomy. A person who uses a removable prosthesis—for example, an artificial hand—may want to have more than one available for different types of tasks. Other types of prosthetic devices, such as artificial hips or teeth, are permanently implanted. With advances in medical science, a few experimental prostheses have been integrated with body tissues, including the nervous system. These highly advanced devices can respond to commands from the central nervous system, more closely approximating normal movement and utility than older prostheses.

prosthetics   The art and science of developing artificial replacements for body parts. Depending on the type of prosthesis, prosthetics may be built and fitted/implanted in a hospital (as in the case of an artificial knee joint) or by an outside specialist. Postmastectomy prosthetics, for example, may be purchased and fitted by specialized lingerie shops.

prosthodontist A dentist with special training in making replacements for missing teeth or other structures of the oral cavity, to restore the patient's appearance, comfort, and/or health.

protease An enzyme that can split a protein into the peptides from which it was originally created.

protease inhibitor An agent that can keep a protease from splitting a protein into peptides. Protease inhibitors include saquinavir (brand names: Invirase, Fortovase) and ritonavir (brand name: Norvir) and are used primarily in HIV/AIDS treatment. They are taken as part of a two- or three-drug cocktail, accompanied by one or more nucleoside antiviral drugs. These treatments are capable of lowering the level of HIV virus in the blood until it cannot be measured with current tools. Side effects associated with protease inhibitors include lipodystrophy syndrome, in which the face, arms, and legs become thin due to loss of subcutaneous fat; the skin becomes dry; weight loss occurs; and abnormal deposits of fat occur. Some new strains of HIV may be resistant to protease inhibitors.

protein One of the three nutrients used as energy sources (calories) by the body. Proteins are essential components of the muscle, skin, and bones. Proteins and carbohydrates each provide 4 calories of energy per gram, whereas fats provide 9 calories per gram.

protein C A vitamin K–dependent protein in plasma that enters into the cascade of biochemical events and leads to the formation of clots.

protein C deficiency A condition that results in thrombotic (clotting) disease and excess platelets, with recurrent inflammation of the vein that occurs when a clot forms (thrombophlebitis). The clot can break loose and travel through the bloodstream (thromboembolism) to the lungs, causing a pulmonary embolism; to the brain, causing a stroke (cerebrovascular accident); to the heart, causing a heart attack; to the skin, causing purpura fulminans; or to the adrenal gland, causing hemorrhage with abdominal pain, abnormally low blood pressure, and salt loss. Protein C deficiency is due to possession of one gene in chromosome band 2q13–2q14. The possession of two such genes (homozygosity) is usually lethal.

protein, C-reactive See *C-reactive protein*.

protein, G See *G protein*.

protein malnutrition See *kwashiorkor*.

protein-calorie malnutrition See *kwashiorkor*.

protein-losing enteropathy A condition in which plasma protein is lost excessively to the intestine. Protein-losing enteropathy can be due to diverse causes, including gluten enteropathy, extensive ulceration of the intestine, intestinal lymphatic blockage, or infiltration of leukemic cells into the intestinal wall. Treatment can involve special diets and vitamin supplementation.

proteins, acute-phase See *acute-phase protein*.

proteinuria See *albuminuria*.

Proteus syndrome A disturbance of cell growth that causes benign tumors under the skin; overgrowth of the body, often more on one side than the other (hemihypertrophy); and overgrowth of fingers (macrodactyly). John Merrick, the 19th-century Englishman known as the "elephant man," is thought to have had Proteus syndrome. No specific treatment is available.

prothrombin A coagulation (clotting) factor that is needed for the normal clotting of blood. A cascade of biochemical events leads to the formation of the final clot. In this cascade, prothrombin is a precursor to thrombin. Also known as thrombinogen and simply pro. See also *prothrombin time*.

prothrombin time A test that is done to gauge the integrity of part of the clotting process. Prothrombin time is commonly used to monitor the accuracy of blood-thinning treatment (anticoagulation) with drugs such as warfarin (brand names: Coumadin, Panwarfin, Sofarin). It measures the time needed for clot formation after thromboplastin and calcium are added to plasma. Familiarly known as pro time.

proto-oncogene A normal gene that, when altered by mutation, becomes an oncogene that can contribute to cancer. See *oncogene*.

protozoa A parasitic single-celled organism that can divide only within a host organism. For example, malaria is caused by the protozoa Plasmodium.

proximal Toward the beginning, the nearer (or nearest) distant of two (or more) items. For example, the proximal end of the femur is part of the hip joint, and the shoulder is proximal to the elbow. The opposite of proximal is distal. See also Appendix B, "Anatomic Orientation Terms."

proximal white subungual onychomycosis See *onychomycosis, proximal white subungual*.

proxy, health care See *health care proxy.*

pruritic Itchy. For example, a scab may be pruritic.

pruritus See *itching.*

pruritus ani See *anal itching.*

PSA Prostate specific antigen. See *prostate specific antigen test.*

PSC Primary sclerosing cholangitis.

pseudo- Prefix indicating a medical condition that resembles another condition but appears to have different causes, as in pseudoseizure (a seizure-like episode that may not show up as unusual electrical activity in the brain).

pseudodementia A severe form of depression that results from a progressive brain disorder in which cognitive changes mimic those of dementia.

pseudogout Inflammation of the joints that is caused by deposits of calcium pyrophosphate crystals, resulting in arthritis, most commonly of the knees, wrists, shoulders, hips, and ankles. Pseudogout usually affects only one or a few joints at a time. True gout is due to a different type of crystal, which is formed by the precipitation of uric acid.

pseudo-Hurler polydystrophy See *mucolipidosis III.*

pseudomembranous colitis See *colitis, pseudomembranous.*

Pseudomonas pseudomallei A bacterium that causes an infectious illness called melioidosis.

pseudo-obstruction, intestinal See *intestinal pseudo-obstruction.*

pseudo-obstruction, myopathic Intestinal pseudo-obstruction that is caused by damage to muscle cells in the walls of the bowel.

pseudo-obstruction, neuropathic Intestinal pseudo-obstruction that is caused by damage to nerve cells in the walls of the bowel.

pseudoparalysis, spastic See *Creutzfeldt-Jakob disease.*

pseudotumor cerebri Increased pressure within the brain in the absence of a tumor. Pseudotumor cerebri can cause headache, ringing in the ears, double vision, loss of visual accuracy, and even complete blindness. It is most common in young to middle-aged women. Although its cause is usually not known, pseudotumor cerebri is sometimes linked to use of tetracycline, nalidixic acid, nitrofurantoin, phenytoin, lithium, or amiodarone, or overuse of vitamin A. Diagnosis is made via brain imaging and lumbar puncture. Drugs to reduce cerebrospinal fluid production or hyperosmotic drugs may be used to reduce fluid buildup. Excess cerebrospinal fluid may be removed with repeated spinal taps, shunting, or a type of surgery called optic nerve sheath fenestration that allows the excess fluid to escape. Steroids may be prescribed to reduce swelling of brain tissue. Also known as benign intracranial hypertension.

pseudoxanthoma elasticum A disorder that is characterized by degeneration of elastic fibers and tiny areas of calcification in the skin, back of the eyes (retinae), and blood vessels. Abbreviated PXE. PXE can be inherited as an autosomal dominant or autosomal recessive trait, and it can occur sporadically in the absence of a family history of the disease. Small yellow-white raised areas appear in the skin folds in the second or third decades of life, on the neck, armpits, and other areas that bend a great deal (flexure areas). A physician may see abnormalities in the back of the eye called angioid streaks, tiny breaks in the elastin-filled tissue that can lead to blindness. The patient's heart can be affected by atherosclerosis and mitral valve prolapse. Small blood vessels are abnormally fragile because the blood-vessel walls contain elastin. This can lead to abnormal bleeding in the bowel and, very rarely, the uterus. Impairment of circulation to the legs can lead to pains in the legs while walking (claudication). The dominant and recessive forms of PXE as well as the sporadic cases of PXE are all caused by mutations in the ABCC6 gene, located on chromosome 16p13.1

psittacosis An infectious disease that is due to a bacterium (Chlamydia psittaci) contracted from psittacine birds, especially caged birds such as parrots, parakeets, and lovebirds. It is also seen in turkey-processing plants. C. psittaci enters the human body by inhalation of air that contains it, or through a bite from an infected bird. The incubation period is 1 to 3 weeks. Signs and symptoms include fever and chills, ill feeling (malaise), loss of appetite, cough, and shortness of breath. Diagnosis is made by finding the bacterium in the patient's blood or sputum. Treatment involves use of antibiotics, such as tetracycline. With early diagnosis and proper treatment, the disease is usually over in 1 to 2 weeks. To avoid psittacosis, one should avoid dust from bird feathers and cage contents and not handle sick birds. Also known as parrot fever.

psoas Two muscles of the lower back. There are two psoas muscles on each side of the back. The larger of the two is called the psoas major and the smaller the psoas minor. The psoas major originates at the spine, around the bottom of the rib cage, and runs down to the thigh-bone (the femur). The psoas major acts to flex the hip. The psoas minor also originates at the spine, around the bottom of the rib cage, but it runs down to the bony pelvis. The psoas minor acts to flex the lower (lumbar) spine.

psoriasis A reddish, scaly rash that is often located over the surfaces of the elbows, knees, and scalp, and around or in the ears, navel, genitals, or buttocks. Approximately 10 to 15 percent of patients with psoriasis develop joint inflammation (inflammatory arthritis). Psoriasis is caused by the body making too many skin cells, and in some cases it is believed to be an autoimmune condition. Treatment options include use of topical steroid creams, use of tar soap preparations, and exposure to ultraviolet light. See also *psoriasis, guttate; psoriasis, pustular; psoriatic arthritis.*

psoriasis, guttate A type of psoriasis that is character-ized by red, scaly patches of inflamed skin on all parts of the body. Guttate psoriasis can be associated with lung infection. See *psoriasis.*

psoriasis, pustular A type of recurring psoriasis that is characterized by the appearance of pus-filled pimples and sores in clusters. Pustular psoriasis can be intensely painful, and hospitalization may be necessary.

psoriatic arthritis Joint inflammation that is associ-ated with psoriasis. Psoriatic arthritis is a potentially destructive and deforming form of arthritis that affects approximately 10 percent of persons with psoriasis.

psyche The mind.

psychiatrist A physician (MD) who specializes in the prevention, diagnosis, and treatment of mental illness. A psychiatrist must receive additional training and serve a supervised residency in his or her specialty. He or she may also have additional training in a psychiatric specialty, such as child psychiatry or neuropsychiatry. Psychiatrists can prescribe medication, which psychologists cannot do.

psychiatry The medical specialty that is concerned with the prevention, diagnosis, and treatment of mental illness.

psychogenic Caused by the mind or emotions.

psychological child abuse See *child abuse, emotional.*

psychological imprinting See *imprinting, psychological.*

psychologist A professional who specializes in the diag-nosis and treatment of diseases of the brain, emotional

disturbance, and behavior problems. Psychologists use talk therapy as treatment; a person must see a psychiatrist or another medical doctor to be treated with medication. A psychologist may have a master's degree (MA) or doc-torate (PhD) in psychology. Psychologists may also have other qualifications, including board certification and additional training in a type of therapy.

psychosis A thought disorder in which perception of reality is grossly impaired. Symptoms can include seeing, hearing, smelling, or tasting things that are not there; paranoia; and delusional thoughts. Depending on the condition underlying the psychotic symptoms, symptoms may be constant or they may come and go. Psychosis can occur as a result of brain injury or disease, and it is seen particularly in schizophrenia and bipolar disorders. Psychotic symptoms can occur as a result of drug use, but that is not true psychosis. Diagnosis is made via observa-tion and interview. Treatment involves use of neuroleptic medication, either the newer, safer, atypical neuroleptics such as risperadone (brand name: Risperdal) or the older neuroleptics such as haloperidol (brand name: Haldol). In cases that do not respond to medication, elec-troshock therapy (ECT) is sometimes helpful.

psychosis, ICU See *ICU psychosis.*

psychosomatic illness A situation in which the mind influences the body to create or complicate an illness.

PTCA Percutaneous transluminal coronary angioplasty.

pterygium A wing-like triangular membrane. Although a pterygium can be anywhere, including behind the knee, it commonly refers to a winglet of the conjunctiva. This pterygium may extend across the white of the eye, toward the inner corner of the eye. It is caused by prolonged exposure of the eyes to wind and weather, or it can be an inherited disorder caused by a single gene. A pterygium can be removed with surgical procedures including laser treatment.

ptosis Downward displacement. For example, ptosis of the eyelids is drooping of the eyelids.

ptosis of the eyelids, congenital See *congenital ptosis of the eyelids.*

pubarche The age at which pubic hair first appears, puberty.

puberty Adolescence, the period in which the human body first becomes capable of reproduction. The timing of the development of puberty is variable and involves many factors including genetic, nutritional, environmen-tal, and social factors.

pubic lice Parasitic insects found in the genital area of humans. Pubic lice are usually spread through sexual contact. Rarely, infestation can be spread through contact with an infested person's bed linens, towels, or clothes. A common misbelief is that infestation can be spread by sitting on a toilet seat. This is not likely because lice cannot live long away from a warm human body. Also, lice do not have feet that are designed to walk or hold on to smooth surfaces such as toilet seats. Infection in a young child or teenager may indicate sexual activity or sexual abuse. Pubic lice are generally found in the genital area on pubic hair but may occasionally be found on other coarse body hair, such as hair on the legs, armpit, mustache, beard, eyebrows, and eyelashes. Infestations in young children are usually on the eyebrows or eyelashes. Lice found on the head are not pubic lice; they are head lice. Animals do not get or spread pubic lice. The key symptom of pubic lice is itching in the genital area. Nits (lice eggs) or crawling lice may be seen. Pubic lice are treated with a 1 percent permethrin or pyrethrin lice shampoo. Such products are available without a prescription at drug stores. A prescription medication, called Lindane (1 percent), is also available. Also known as crabs.

pubic symphysis The joint between the pubic bones at the front of the pelvis.

pubis The front center portion of the pelvis.

public health **1** Medicine that is concerned with the health of the community as a whole. Community health. **2** In common usage, a facility or a government agency that provides low-income or free health care.

Public Health Service, United States See *United States Public Health Service.*

PUBS Percutaneous umbilical blood sampling.

pueperal fever See *childbed fever.*

pueperium The time immediately after the delivery of a baby.

pulmonary Having to do with the lungs.

pulmonary edema Fluid in the lungs.

pulmonary embolism Sudden closure of a pulmonary artery or one of its branches, caused by a blood-borne clot or foreign material that plugs the vessel.

pulmonary embolus A blood clot within the lung's pulmonary artery that causes an embolism. In the case of a pulmonary embolus, the embolus, a clot or foreign material, has been carried through the blood into the pulmonary artery or one of its branches, plugging the vessel.

pulmonary fibrosis Scarring throughout the lungs that can be caused by many conditions, such as sarcoidosis, hypersensitivity pneumonitis, asbestosis, and certain medications. Pulmonary fibrosis can also occur without an identifiable cause, in which case it is referred to as idiopathic pulmonary fibrosis. Symptoms include shortness of breath, coughing, and diminished exercise tolerance. Treatment involves use of corticosteroids (such as prednisone) and/or other medications that suppress the body's immune system. The goal of treatment is to decrease lung inflammation and subsequent scarring. Responses to treatment vary. Toxicity and side effects of treatment can be serious. Therefore, patients with pulmonary fibrosis are generally cared for by lung specialists.

pulmonary function test A test that is designed to measure how well the lungs are working. Abbreviated PFT. PFTs gauge how the lungs are expanding and contracting (when a person inhales and exhales) and measure the efficiency of the exchange of oxygen and carbon dioxide between the blood and the air within the lungs.

pulmonary hypertension See *hypertension, pulmonary.*

pulmonary insufficiency A condition in which the valve between the right ventricle of the heart and the pulmonary artery is incompetent in its performance, allowing blood to slosh back from the pulmonary artery into the right ventricle.

pulmonary stenosis A condition in which the pulmonary valve is too tight, so that the flow of blood from the right ventricle of the heart into the pulmonary artery is impeded. This means that the right ventricle must pump harder than normal to overcome the obstruction. If the stenosis is severe in a baby, the infant may become blue (cyanotic). Older children often have no symptoms with pulmonary stenosis. Treatment is necessary if the pressure in the right ventricle is higher than normal. The obstruction can usually be relieved by a procedure called balloon valvuloplasty or by open-heart surgery during which the stenotic valve is opened. The outlook after either procedure is favorable.

pulmonary stenosis, peripheral, with cholestasis See *Alagille syndrome.*

pulmonary syndrome, hantavirus See *hantavirus pulmonary syndrome.*

pulmonary valve One of the four valves in the heart, which stands at the opening from the right ventricle in the pulmonary artery trunk. The pulmonary valve moves blood toward the lungs and keeps it from sloshing back from the pulmonary artery into the heart.

pulmonary vein One of four vessels that carry aerated blood from the lungs to the left atrium of the heart. The pulmonary veins are the only veins that carry bright-red oxygenated blood.

pulse The rhythmic dilation of an artery that results from beating of the heart. Pulse is often measured by feeling the arteries of the wrist or neck.

pulse, Corrigan See *Corrigan pulse.*

pulse rate A measure of the number of pulsations in the radial artery each minute. Pulse rate is usually taken at the wrist or neck.

pulse, water-hammer See *Corrigan pulse.*

pump-oxygenator See *heart-lung machine.*

punch biopsy A biopsy that is performed by using a punch, an instrument for cutting and removing a disk of tissue. For example, a punch biopsy of the skin may be done to make a diagnosis of skin cancer.

puncture, ear See *ear puncture.*

puncture, lumbar See *lumbar puncture.*

puncture wound An injury that is caused by a pointed object that pierces or penetrates the skin. Any puncture wound through athletic shoes (as with a nail) has a high risk of infection because the foam in athletic shoes can harbor the bacteria Pseudomonas. Puncture wounds also carry a danger of tetanus.

pupil The opening of the iris. The pupil may appear to open (dilate) and close (constrict), but it is really the iris that is the prime mover; the pupil is merely the absence of iris. The pupil determines how much light is let into the eye. Both pupils are usually of equal size. If they are not, the condition is called anisocoria.

purine One of the two classes of bases in DNA and RNA. The purine bases are guanine (G) and adenine (A). Uric acid, the offending substance in gout, is a purine end product. See also *pyrimidine.*

purpura Hemorrhage (bleeding) into the surface of the skin. The area of skin with purpura is greater than 3 millimeters in diameter. The appearance of an individual area of purpura varies with the duration of the lesions. Early purpura is red and becomes darker, then purple, and brown-yellow as it fades.

purpura, acute thrombocytopenic See *acute thrombocytopenic purpura.*

purpura, anaphylactoid See *anaphylactoid purpura.*

purpura, Henoch-Schonlein See *anaphylactoid purpura.*

purpura, thrombotic thrombocytopenic See *thrombotic thrombocytopenic purpura.*

pus A thick, whitish-yellow fluid that results from the accumulation of white blood cells, liquefied tissue, and cellular debris. Pus is commonly a sign of infection or foreign material in the body.

pustulosis A highly inflammatory skin condition that results in large, fluid-filled, blister-like areas (pustules). Pustulosis typically occurs on the palms of the hands and/or the soles of the feet. The skin of these areas peels and flakes (exfoliates).

PV Polycythemia vera.

PVC Premature ventricular contraction.

PWS Prader-Willi syndrome.

PXE Pseudoxanthoma elasticum.

pyarthrosis See *arthritis, septic.*

pycnodysostosis An inherited disorder of bone that causes short stature and abnormally dense brittle bones. Pycnodysostosis is due to a defect in the enzyme cathepsin K. Sometimes spelled pyknodysostosis. The French artist Toulouse-Lautrec is thought to have had this disease. No specific treatment is available.

pyelo See *pyelonephritis.*

pyelogram An X-ray study of the kidneys, especially showing the pelvis (urine-collecting basin), and the ureter.

pyelonephritis Bacterial infection of the kidneys. Pyelonephritis can be acute or chronic, and it is most often due to the ascent of bacteria from the bladder up the ureters to infect the kidneys. Symptoms include flank (side) pain, fever, shaking chills, sometimes foul-smelling urine, frequent and urgent need to urinate, and general malaise. Tenderness is elicited by gently tapping over the kidney with a fist (percussion). Diagnosis is made via urinalysis, which reveals white blood cells and bacteria in the urine. Usually there is also an increase in circulating white cells in the blood. Treatment involves use of appropriate antibiotics. Often called simply pyelo.

pyloric stenosis Narrowing (stenosis) of the outlet of the stomach so that food cannot pass easily from it into the duodenum. Pyloric stenosis results in feeding problems and projectile vomiting. The obstruction can be corrected with a relatively simple surgical procedure.

pylorus The outlet of the stomach.

pyoderma gangrenosum An ulcerating condition of skin that results in heaped borders with a typical appearance. Pyoderma gangrenosum appears to be mediated by the immune system, but the exact cause is unknown. The lesion usually begins as a soft nodule on the skin that then ulcerates. The ulcer enlarges, and the skin at the edge is purple-red. The ulcers can become quite large. Pyoderma gangrenosum is associated with several other diseases, including ulcerative colitis, Crohn's disease, rheumatoid arthritis, leukemia, and cryoglobulinemia. Pyoderma gangrenosum is usually responsive to corticosteroids.

pyogenic arthritis   Purulent arthritis with pus as a result of infection within the joint. See *arthritis, septic.*

pyrexia   See *fever.*

pyrimidine   One of the two classes of bases in DNA and RNA. The pyrimidine bases in DNA are thymine (T) and cytosine (C), and the pyrimidine bases in RNA are thymine (T) and uracil (U). See also *purine.*

pyuria   Pus in the urine. Pyuria is a sign of inflammation, often related to infection.

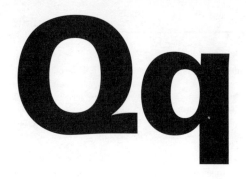

q arm of a chromosome The long arm of a chromosome. All human chromosomes have 2 arms—a short arm and a long arm. By international convention, the short arm is termed p, and the long arm of the chromosome is termed q. For example, if a gene is on 3q12, that gene is on chromosome 3, on its long arm, in region 12.

Q fever An infectious disease whose symptoms include fever, headache, malaise, and pneumonia (interstitial pneumonitis), but not rash. The Q stands for Query because the cause of the disease was long a question mark. It is now known to be due to the bacterium Coxiella burnetii. Q fever is a zoonotic disease and is contracted from cattle, sheep, and goats. Most patients recover within several months without treatment, but 1 to 2 percent of people with acute Q fever die of the disease. Chronic Q fever, characterized by infection that persists for more than 6 months, is uncommon but is an even more serious disease. Patients who have had acute Q fever may develop the chronic form as soon as 1 year after or as long as 20 years after initial infection. A grave complication of chronic Q fever is endocarditis, generally involving the aortic heart valves and less commonly the mitral valve. Transplant recipients, patients with cancer, and patients with chronic kidney disease are at high risk of developing chronic Q fever. There has been concern about Q fever as a possible weapon for bioterrorism, in part because the C. burnetii bacterium is stable and can persist for months on wood or in sand.

q.d. Seen on a prescription, one per day. Also known as quotid. See Appendix A, "Prescription Abbreviations."

q.h. On a prescription, every hour. See Appendix A, "Prescription Abbreviations."

q.2h. On a prescription, every 2 hours. See Appendix A, "Prescription Abbreviations."

q.3h. On a prescription, every 3 hours. See Appendix A, "Prescription Abbreviations."

q.i.d. On a prescription, four times daily. See Appendix A, "Prescription Abbreviations."

q.n.s. On a lab report, insufficient quantity of sample.

QRS complex The deflections in an electrocardiograph (EKG) tracing that represent the ventricular activity of the heart.

q.s. On a prescription, as needed. See Appendix A, "Prescription Abbreviations."

QT syndrome, long See *long QT syndrome*.

quack 1 A practitioner who suggests for prevention or treatment of disease substances or devices that are known to be ineffective. 2 Someone who pretends to be able to diagnose or heal people but is unqualified and incompetent.

quackery Deliberate misrepresentation of the ability of a substance, a device, or a person to prevent or treat disease.

quadrant A quarter. For example, the liver is in the right upper quadrant of the abdomen.

quadriceps 1 Any four-headed muscle. 2 The large muscle of the thigh that comes down the bone of the upper leg (femur) and over the kneecap (patella), and then anchors into the top of the big bone in the lower leg (tibia). The function of the quadriceps is to straighten (extend) the leg. Also known as musculus quadriceps femoris and quad.

quadriparesis Weakness of all four limbs, both arms and both legs, as from muscular dystrophy.

quadriplegia Paralysis of all four limbs, both arms and both legs, as from a high spinal cord accident or stroke.

qualitative Having to do with quality, in contrast to quantitative, which pertains strictly to quantity. The results of a qualitative analysis may vary from those of a quantitative analysis, even if the same event or procedure is being examined. See also *quantitative*.

quality of life The patient's ability to enjoy normal life activities. Quality of life is an important consideration in medical care. Some medical treatments can seriously impair quality of life without providing appreciable benefit, whereas others greatly enhance quality of life.

quantitative Having to do with quantity or with the amount. See also *qualitative*.

quarantine A period of isolation decreed to control the spread of infectious disease. Before the era of antibiotics and other medications, quarantine was one of the few available means for halting the spread of infectious diseases.

quasi- Prefix meaning seemingly, as in quasidominant (seemingly dominant).

Queensland tick typhus See *typhus, Queensland tick*.

quickening The moment during pregnancy when the baby is first felt to move.

quiescent Inactive, resting. For example, tuberculosis can be a quiescent (inactive) infection.

quinacrine An antimalarial drug and, in cytogenetics, a fluorescent dye used to stain chromosomes. The Y chromosome stains brilliantly with quinacrine. See also *malaria; plasmodium.*

quinidine A medication (brand name: Cardioquin, Quinaglute, Quinalan, Quinidex, Quinora) that is prescribed to treat abnormal heart rhythms. Quinidine is derived from the same botanical source as quinine. Side effects may include nausea and diarrhea. Quinidine interacts with a number of other medications, particularly over-the-counter cold and cough remedies. Therefore, one should talk with a physician before taking any other drug at the same time as quinidine. See also *quinine.*

quinine An antimalarial agent. Quinine takes its name from the Peruvian Indian word for "bark of the tree," referring to the cinchona tree from which quinine was obtained. Until World War I, quinine was the only effective treatment for malaria. In fact, quinine was the first chemical compound to be successfully used to treat an infectious disease. See also *malaria; plasmodium.*

quinsy See *peritonsillar abscess.*

Quintan fever See *trench fever.*

quotid See *q.d.*

quotidian Recurring each day, as in a fever that returns every day.

quotient The result of mathematical division. For example, an intelligence quotient (IQ) can be derived from dividing a person's mental age as determined by the Stanford-Binet test by the person's chronological age and multiplying by 100. For example, if a 6-year-old child scores at the 8-year-old level, the IQ is $(8/6) \times 100 = 133$.

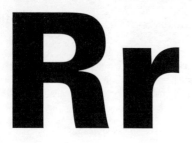

R **1** Respiration. For example, a medical chart note of "R20" is shorthand for 20 respirations (breaths) per minute. **2** Right. A medical chart note of a burn on the "R digit 5" places the burn on the right little finger or toe. **3** Roentgen. **4** In chemistry, a radical. **5** On a prescription, recipe, which is Latin for "to take." Also known as Rx.

rabies A potentially fatal viral infection that attacks the central nervous system. Rabies is carried by wild animals (particularly bats and raccoons) and finds its way to humans by many routes. Most cases of rabies can be traced to animal bites, but cases have been documented in which the virus was inhaled in bat caves, contracted in lab accidents, or received from transplanted donor tissue. Symptoms include fever, aching muscles, and headache, potentially progressing to inflammation of the brain, confusion, seizures, paralysis, coma, and death. There is no cure for rabies after it has settled in the brain, so immediate emergency care for any suspicious animal contact is imperative. Rabies immunoglobulin shots, antibiotics, and rabies vaccine may be used immediately after contact with a suspected rabies carrier. To prevent rabies, pets should be vaccinated against the virus, and people should avoid contact with wild or unknown animals. A human rabies vaccine is available, but it is recommended only for those in high-risk occupations (such as game wardens, zookeepers, and animal control officers).

racemose A descriptive term for something that is in a cluster or bunch. For example, a racemose aneurysm is an aneurysm that looks like a bunch of grapes.

rad Radiation absorbed dose, a measurement for a dose of ionizing radiation.

radial **1** Pertaining to the radius, the smaller bone in the forearm. The radial artery is so named because of its proximity to the radius. **2** Pertaining to the radius of a circle. **3** Spreading from a central point. A radial keratotomy, for instance, is an eye operation in which incisions are made in the cornea that resemble the spokes in a wheel.

radial aplasia-thrombocytopenia syndrome See *TAR syndrome.*

radial artery A major artery that emerges through the neck of the radius in the crook of the elbow and sends out 12 branches to various areas of the forearm, wrist, and hand.

radiate To spread out from a central area. For example, sciatic pain may radiate outward from the lower back.

radiation **1** Rays of energy. Gamma rays and X-rays are two types of radiation that are often used in medicine. **2** The use of energy waves to diagnose or treat disease.

radiation fibrosis See *fibrosis, radiation.*

radiation menopause See *menopause, induced.*

radiation oncologist A specialist in the use of radiation therapy as a treatment for cancer.

radiation oncology The medical specialty that is involved in the use of radiation (X-rays, gamma rays, or electrons) to treat cancer.

radiation pneumonitis See *pneumonitis, radiation.*

radiation, seed See *radiation therapy, interstitial.*

radiation therapy The use of high-energy rays to damage cancer cells, stopping them from growing and dividing. Like surgery, radiation therapy is a local treatment that affects cancer cells only in the treated area. Radiation can come from a machine (external radiation) or from a small container of radioactive material implanted directly into or near a tumor (internal radiation). Some patients receive both kinds of radiation therapy. External radiation therapy is usually given on an outpatient basis in a hospital or clinic, 5 days per week for several weeks. Patients are not radioactive during or after the treatment. For internal radiation therapy, the patient stays in the hospital for a few days. The implant may be temporary or permanent. Because the level of radiation is highest during the hospital stay and this might place nearby persons at risk, patients may not be able to have visitors or may have visitors only for a short time. After an implant is removed, there is no radioactivity in the body. The amount of radiation in a permanent implant goes down to a safe level before the patient leaves the hospital. Side effects of radiation therapy depend on the treatment dose and the part of the body treated. The most common side effects of radiation are fatigue, skin reactions (such as a rash or redness) in the treated area, and loss of appetite. Radiation therapy can cause inflammation of tissues and organs in and around the body site that is radiated. Radiation therapy can also cause a decrease in the number of white blood cells. Although the side effects of radiation therapy can be unpleasant, they can usually be treated or controlled. Furthermore, in most cases, they are not permanent.

radiation therapy, external Radiation therapy in which the source of radiation is a machine outside the body.

radiation therapy, internal Radiation therapy in which a small container of radioactive material is implanted in the body, in or near the cancerous tumor.

radiation therapy, interstitial A form of radiotherapy in which tiny radioactive "seeds" are permanently implanted directly in the affected tissue with a needle-like instrument. Interstitial radiation therapy has shown particular promise in treating prostate cancer.

radiation therapy, stereotactic The use of a number of precisely aimed beams of ionizing radiation, each coming from a different direction and meeting at a specific point, to deliver radiation treatment to that spot.

radical dissection Removal of not affected tissue as well as nearby tissue that may be covertly affected.

radical, free See *free radical.*

radical mastectomy See *mastectomy, radical.*

radical neck dissection Often called a "radical neck," a surgical procedure that involves the removal of a tumor from the neck with an additional margin of seemingly normal tissue of at least 2 cm together with the removal of the lymph nodes from the neck.

radiculitis See *radiculopathy.*

radiculopathy Any disease of the spinal nerve roots and spinal nerves. Radiculopathy is characterized by pain that seems to radiate from the spine, extending outward to cause symptoms away from the source of the spinal nerve root irritation. Causes of radiculopathy include deformities of the discs between the vertebrae. Patients with diabetes can be affected by a curious form of radiculopathy that may be caused by inadequate blood supply to the spinal nerve roots. Also known as radiculitis.

radioactive Emitting energy waves due to decaying atomic nuclei. Radioactive substances are used in medicine as tracers for diagnosis and in treatment to kill cancerous cells.

radioactive iodine A version (isotope) of the chemical element iodine that is radioactive. Abbreviated RAI. RAI is used in diagnostic tests as well as in radiotherapy of the thyroid. For hyperthyroidism, RAI is administered in capsule form on a one-time basis. It directly radiates thyroid tissues, thereby destroying them. It takes 8 to 12 weeks for the thyroid to become euthyroid (normal) after treatment. The majority of patients undergoing this treatment eventually become hypothyroid, which is easily treated using thyroid hormones (levothyroxine). RAI should not be used during pregnancy and breastfeeding. See also *Graves disease.*

radioactive tracer A radioactive molecule that can be sent through the body's circulatory or urinary system, with its progress followed by a radiation-sensitive machine.

radioallergosorbent test See *RAST.*

radiograph In medicine, an X-ray or a film produced through X-ray.

radiography Film records (radiographs) of internal structures of the body. Radiography is made possible by X-rays passing through the body to act on a specially sensitized film.

radioimmunoassay A very sensitive, specific laboratory test (assay) that uses radiolabeled and unlabeled substances in an immunological (antibody-antigen) reaction.

radioinsensitive Not sensitive to X-rays and other forms of radiant energy. For example, if a tumor is radioinsensitive, it cannot be successfully attacked by using radiation therapy. The opposite of radioinsensitive is radiosensitive.

radioisotope A version of a chemical element that has an unstable nucleus and emits radiation during its decay to a stable form. Radioisotopes have important uses in medical diagnosis, treatment, and research.

radiologic Having to do with radiology.

radiologist A physician who specializes in radiology, the branch of medicine that uses radiation for the diagnosis and treatment of disease. Like other physicians, a radiologist must have graduated from an accredited medical or osteopathy school, passed a licensing examination, and completed a residency. Radiologists are usually board certified (that is, they have taken and passed an examination and thus are approved to practice in the field of radiology). A radiologist can subspecialize and become, for example, a radiation oncologist or an interventional radiologist. See also *radiation oncologist; radiologist, interventional.*

radiologist, interventional A radiologic subspecialist who uses fluoroscopy, computerized axial tomography (CT), and ultrasound to guide wires and catheters for performing procedures such as biopsies, draining fluids, inserting catheters, and dilating or stenting narrowed ducts or vessels. See also *radiology, interventional.*

radiology The science of radiation, both ionizing radiation such as X-rays and nonionizing radiation such as ultrasound, and of how it can be applied to the diagnosis and treatment of disease. Also known as roentgenology.

radiology, interventional The use of image guidance methods to gain access to the deepest interior of most organs and organ systems. Through a galaxy of techniques, interventional radiologists can treat certain conditions through the skin (percutaneously) that might otherwise require surgery. Interventional radiology includes the use of balloons, catheters, microcatheters, stents, therapeutic embolization (deliberately clogging up a blood vessel), and more. The specialty of interventional radiology overlaps with other surgical arenas, including interventional cardiology, vascular surgery, endoscopy, laparoscopy, and other minimally invasive techniques, such as biopsies. Specialists performing interventional radiology procedures today include not only radiologists but also other types of physicians, such as general surgeons, vascular surgeons, cardiologists, gastroenterologists, gynecologists, and urologists.

radiolucent Permeable to one or another form of radiation, such as X-rays. Radiolucent objects do not block radiation but let it pass. Plastic is usually radiolucent. The opposite of radiolucent is radiopaque.

radionuclide scan An exam that produces pictures (scans) of internal parts of the body. The patient is given an injection or swallows a small amount of radioactive material. A machine called a scanner then measures the radioactivity in certain organs.

radiopaque Opaque to one or another form of radiation, such as X-rays. Radiopaque objects block radiation rather than allow it to pass through. Metal, for instance, is radiopaque, so metal objects that a patient may have swallowed are visible on X-rays. Radiopaque dyes are used in radiology to enhance X-ray pictures of internal anatomic structures. For example, an intravenous pyelogram (IVP) is an X-ray study of the kidneys that highlights the renal pelvis and the ureters. The opposite of radiopaque is radiolucent.

radiosensitive Sensitive to X-rays and other forms of radiant energy. For example, if a tumor is radiosensitive, it is potentially treatable with radiation therapy. The opposite of radiosensitive is radioinsensitive.

radiotherapy See *radiation therapy*.

radium The radioactive element discovered by Marie and Pierre Curie in 1898. Since the radium discovery, many radioactive isotopes have been used for both the diagnosis and the treatment of diseases.

radius The smaller of the two bones on the thumb's side of the forearm. (The larger bone in the forearm is the ulna.)

radon A radioactive element that is formed, as a gas, during the breakdown of radium. The Surgeon General has declared radon exposure to be the second leading cause of lung cancer deaths in the United States, after smoking. Exposure to natural radon is estimated to be responsible for 7,000 to 30,000 lung cancer deaths each year in the US. Radon gas continuously seeps into the air from uranium- and radium-bearing soil and rock. Well water can be contaminated with radon and may carry radon into a house through the water pipes. There are several radon testing devices on the market.

Raeder syndrome See *cluster headache*.

ragweed Any of several weedy composite herbs that produce a pollen to which many people are allergic. Of all allergy sufferers in the US, 75 percent are allergic to ragweed.

RAI Radioactive iodine.

rale An abnormal lung sound that can be heard through a stethoscope. Rales may be sibilant (whistling), dry (crackling), or wet (sloshy), depending on the amount and density of fluid refluxing back and forth in the air passages.

Ramsey Hunt syndrome A herpesvirus infection of the geniculate nerve ganglion, which causes paralysis of the facial muscles on the same side of the face as the infection. It is usually associated with an unusual rash (composed of vesicles, or tiny water-filled bumps, in the skin) in or around the ear and sometimes on the roof of the mouth. Ramsey Hunt syndrome is commonly more painful and more debilitating than Bell's palsy. Treatment with steroids and antiviral agents, such as acyclovir (brand name: Zovirax) may improve recovery and lessen pain.

ramus In anatomy, a branch, such as a branch of a blood vessel or nerve. For example, the ramus acetabularis arteriae circumflexae femoris medialis is the branch of an artery that goes to the socket of the hip joint. The plural of ramus is rami.

ramus of the mandible One of the two prominent, projecting back parts of the horseshoe-shaped lower jaw bone.

random Determined solely by chance.

random mating Totally haphazard mating, with no regard to the genetic makeup (genotype) of the mate, so that any sperm has an equal chance of fertilizing any egg. Random mating rarely, if ever, occurs, but the concept is important in population genetics. Also known as panmixus.

random sample A test group that is selected solely by chance.

range In medicine and statistics, the difference between the lowest and highest numeric values. For example, if five premature infants are born, weighing 2, 3, 4, 5, and 6 pounds, respectively, the range of their birth weights is 2 to 6 pounds.

range of motion The full movement potential of a joint, usually its range of flexion and extension. For example, a knee might lack 10 degrees of full extension due to an injury.

range, normal See *normal range.*

rapid eye movement sleep See *REM sleep.*

rash Breaking out (eruption) of the skin. A rash can be caused by an underlying medical condition, hormonal cycles, allergies, or contact with irritating substances. Treatment depends on the underlying cause of the rash. Medically, a rash is referred to as an exanthem.

Rasmussen syndrome A rare brain disorder that is caused by inflammation of brain cells in one hemisphere. Rasmussen syndrome, whose cause is unknown, features seizures that can be difficult or impossible to control with medication, and it eventually results in brain shrinkage (atrophy). Treatment is surgery, if possible. The inflammation seems to stop of its own accord eventually, but the damage done is irreversible.

RAST Radioallergosorbent test, an allergy test that is done on a sample of blood. RAST is used to check for allergic sensitivity to specific substances.

rat-flea typhus See *typhus, murine.*

rattlesnake bite A poisonous bite from a member of the pit viper family. All rattlesnakes are venomous and secrete poisonous venom, and they are the main culprit in deaths from snakebites in the US. Emergency treatment is essential: With proper care, rattlesnake bites are rarely fatal. The affected body part should be kept immobile and below the level of the heart, and the bite victim should be taken to the nearest hospital. A tourniquet or bandage should not be used, and no one should attempt to suction out the wound by mouth. Treatment includes use of antivenom and care for the puncture wound itself and any symptoms that emerge, such as respiratory distress. See also *snakebite.*

Raynaud's disease A condition that results in discoloration of the skin on the fingers and/or toes when a person is exposed to changes in temperature or to emotional events. Raynaud's disease, also known as primary Raynaud's phenomenon, can accompany other diseases; when it does, it is called Raynaud's phenomenon or secondary Raynaud's phenomenon. The skin discoloration occurs because an abnormal spasm of the blood vessels causes a diminished blood supply. Initially, the digits

involved turn white because of diminished blood supply, and then they turn blue because of prolonged lack of oxygen. Finally, the blood vessels reopen, causing flushing that turns the digits red.

Raynaud's phenomenon A condition that results in discoloration of fingers and/or toes when a person is exposed to changes in temperature or emotional events and that occurs with a number of conditions, including rheumatic diseases such as scleroderma, rheumatoid arthritis, and systemic lupus erythematosus; hormone imbalance, including hypothyroidism and carcinoid imbalances; trauma, such as from frostbite or the use of vibrating tools; medications, particularly propranolol (brand name: Inderal), estrogens, nicotine, and bleomycin; and, uncommonly, cancer. When the discoloration occurs alone, it is called Raynaud's disease. See also *Raynaud's disease.*

reabsorption Being absorbed again. For example, the kidney selectively reabsorbs substances it has already secreted into the renal tubules, such as glucose, protein, and sodium. These reabsorbed substances are returned to the blood.

reaction kinetics The rate of change in a biochemical (or other) reaction.

reactive arthritis A chronic form of inflammatory arthritis that combines arthritis, inflammation of the eyes (conjunctivitis), and inflammation of the genital, urinary, or gastrointestinal systems. Reiter syndrome is a systemic rheumatic disease, meaning that it can and does affect organs as well as joints. It can cause inflammation in many areas, including the eyes, mouth, lungs, kidneys, heart, and skin. See also *arthritis; arthritis, Reiter; keratodermia blennorrhagicum.*

reading frame One of the three possible ways to read a nucleotide sequence in DNA, depending on whether reading starts with the first, second, or third base in a triplet.

reading frame, open A reading frame in DNA that has no termination codon (no signal to stop reading the nucleotide sequence). An open reading frame can be translated into protein.

reading retardation Impaired ability to read. Reading retardation may reflect mental retardation, cultural deprivation, or learning disability. See also *dyslexia.*

reagent A substance that is used to produce a chemical reaction that allows researchers to detect, measure, produce, or change other substances.

rebound The reversal of response upon withdrawal of a stimulus.

rebound effect The production of increased negative symptoms when the effect of a drug has passed or the patient no longer responds to the drug. If a drug produces a rebound effect, the condition it was used to treat may come back even stronger when the drug is discontinued or loses effectiveness.

recalcitrant Stubborn. For example, a recalcitrant case of pneumonia stubbornly resists treatment.

recent memory See *memory, short-term.*

receptor 1 In cell biology, a structure on the surface of a cell or inside a cell that selectively receives and binds a specific substance. For example, there are insulin receptors and low-density lipoprotein (LDL) receptors. 2 In neurology, the terminal of a sensory nerve that receives and responds to stimuli.

receptor, chemokine See *chemokine receptor.*

receptor, visual The layer of rods and cones, the visual cells, of the retina.

recessive A genetic trait that appears only in individuals who have received two copies of a mutant gene, one copy from each parent. The individuals with a double dose of the mutated gene are called homozygotes. Their parents, each with a single dose of the mutated gene, appear normal and are called heterozygotes, or gene carriers. There are two types of recessive diseases—autosomal recessive and X-linked recessive—that describe different patterns of inheritance. The opposite of recessive is dominant. See also *autosomal recessive; dominant; X-linked recessive.*

recessive, autosomal See *autosomal recessive.*

recessive, X-linked See *X-linked recessive.*

recipient In medicine, someone who is given something, such as a blood transfusion or an organ transplant, that is derived from another person (the donor).

recombinant A person with a new combination of genes, a combination not present in either parent, due to parental recombination of those genes.

recombinant clone A clone that contains recombinant DNA.

recombinant DNA molecules A combination of DNA molecules of different origin that are joined using recombinant DNA technology.

recombinant DNA technology A series of procedures that are used to join together (recombine) DNA segments.

A recombinant DNA molecule is constructed from segments of two or more different DNA molecules. Under certain conditions, a recombinant DNA molecule can enter a cell and replicate there, either on its own or after it has been integrated into a chromosome.

recombination The trading of fragments of genetic material between chromosomes before the egg and sperm cells are created. Key features of recombination include the point-to-point association of paired chromosomes (synapsis), followed by the visible exchange of segments (crossing over) at X-shaped crosspoints (chiasmata). Recombination is the principal way of creating genetic diversity between generations. By shuffling the genetic deck of cards, recombination ensures that children are dealt a different genetic hand than their parents.

Recombivax-HB A vaccine that stimulates the body's immune system to produce antibodies against the hepatitis B virus. See also *hepatitis B; hepatitis B immunization.*

recrudescence Reappearance, as of a rash or arthritis.

rectal 1 Having to do with the rectum. 2 Informally, digital rectal exam.

rectal cancer See *cancer, rectal.*

rectal exam, digital See *digital rectal exam.*

rectouterine pouch See *pouch of Douglas.*

rectum The last 6 to 8 inches of the large intestine. The rectum stores solid waste until it leaves the body through the anus.

rectus See *rectus abdominis.*

rectus abdominis A large muscle in the front of the abdomen that assists in regular breathing movements, supports the muscles of the spine while a person lifts something, and keeps the intestines and other abdominal organs in place.

recuperate To recover health and strength. Also known as convalesce.

recur To occur again; to return. For example, a symptom, sign, or disease can recur.

recurrence The return of a sign, symptom, or disease after a remission. The reappearance of cancer cells at the same site or in another location is, unfortunately, a familiar form of recurrence.

recurrence risk In medical genetics, the chance that an inherited disease that is present in a family will recur in that family, affecting another person or persons. Recurrence risk is the chance that a disease will strike again.

recurrent Appearing or occurring again. For example, a recurrent fever is a fever that has returned after an intermission, a recrudescent fever.

recurrent aural vertigo See *Ménière's disease.*

recurrent laryngeal nerve See *laryngeal nerve, recurrent.*

recurrent respiratory papillomatosis See *laryngeal papillomatosis.*

red blood cell See *erythrocyte.*

red cell See *erythrocyte.*

red cell count The number of red blood cells in a volume of blood. The normal range varies slightly between laboratories, but is generally in the range 4.2–5.9 million cells/cmm. Red cell count can be expressed in international units as (4.2–5.9)×1,012 cells per liter. Also known as erythrocyte count.

red-green colorblindness A form of colorblindness in which red and green are perceived as being identical. Red-green colorblindness is the most common type of colorblindness. It is inherited in an X-linked recessive manner and affects 6 percent of males. Also known as deutan colorblindness, deuteranopia, and Daltonism. The chemist and physicist John Dalton gave the first recognized account of red-green colorblindness (in himself and his brother) in 1798. See also *colorblindness.*

reduction division The first cell division in meiosis, the process by which germ cells are formed. In reduction division, the chromosome number is reduced from diploid (46 chromosomes) to haploid (23 chromosomes). Also known as first meiotic division and first meiosis.

Reed-Sternberg cell A type of cell that appears in patients with Hodgkin's disease and is a hallmark of Hodgkin's disease. The number of these cells increases as the disease advances. See also *Hodgkin's disease.*

referral The recommendation of a medical or paramedical professional. If one gets a referral to ophthalmology, for example, the person is being sent to the eye doctor. In health maintenance organizations (HMOs) and other managed-care schemes, a referral is usually necessary in order to see any practitioner or specialist other than the primary care physician (PCP) and have the service covered. The referral is obtained from the PCP, who may require a telephone or office consultation first.

The term *referral* can pertain both to the act of sending a patient to another physician or therapist and to the actual paper authorizing the visit.

reflex An involuntary reaction. For example, the corneal reflex is the blink that occurs upon irritation of the eye.

reflex, Babinski See *Babinski reflex.*

reflex sympathetic dystrophy syndrome A condition that features a group of typical symptoms, including pain (often perceived as burning pain), tenderness, and swelling of an extremity. Reflex sympathetic dystrophy syndrome is associated with varying degrees of sweating, warmth and/or coolness, flushing, discoloration, and shiny skin.

reflux See *gastroesophageal reflux disease.*

reflux laryngitis See *laryngitis, reflux.*

refraction In opthalmology, the bending of light that takes place within the human eye. Refractive errors include nearsightedness (myopia), farsightedness (hyperopia), and astigmatism. Lenses can be used to control the amount of refraction and correct those errors.

refractory Not yielding, or not yielding readily, to treatment.

refractory anemia See *anemia, refractory.*

Refsum disease A genetic disorder that affects the metabolism of the fatty acid phytanic acid. When phytanic acid accumulates, it causes a number of progressive problems, including inflammation of numerous nerves (polyneuritis), diminishing vision due to retinitis pigmentosa, and wobbliness (ataxia) caused by damage to the cerebellar portion of the brain. Refsum disease is caused by mutations in the PAHX gene on chromosome 10 that encodes the enzyme phytanoyl-CoA hydroxylase (PAHX). Also known as phytanic acid storage disease.

regenerate To reproduce or renew something that was lost. For example, after an injury, the liver has the capacity to regenerate.

regimen A plan or a regulated course, such as a diet, exercise, or treatment, that is designed to give a good result. A low-salt diet is one type of dietary regimen.

regional enteritis See *Crohn's disease.*

regional lymphadenitis See *cat scratch fever.*

registry A collection of information. A registry is usually organized so that the data in it can be analyzed. For example, analysis of data in a tumor registry maintained at a hospital may show a rise in lung cancer among women.

regress To return or go back, particularly to return to a pattern of behavior or level of skill characteristic of a younger age. For example, if a 3-year-old child begins to regress by losing the ability to control his bowels or speak, that is a cause for medical concern.

regulatory gene A gene that regulates the expression of other genes.

regurgitation A backward flowing. For example, vomiting is a regurgitation of food from the stomach, and the sloshing of blood back into the heart when a heart valve is incompetent is a regurgitation of blood.

rehab An abbreviation for rehabilitation.

rehabilitation The process of helping a person who has suffered an illness or injury restore lost skills and so regain maximum self-sufficiency. For example, rehabilitation work after a stroke may help the patient walk and speak clearly again.

rehydrate To restore lost water to the body tissues and fluids. Prompt rehydration is imperative whenever dehydration occurs, whether from diarrhea, exposure, lack of drinking water, or medication use. Rehydration can occur orally or via IV administration of fluids.

Reiter syndrome See *reactive arthritis*.

rejection In transplantation biology, the refusal to accept transplanted cells, tissues, or organs. For example, a transplanted kidney may be rejected.

relapse The return of signs and symptoms of a disease after a remission.

relaxant Something that relaxes, relieves, or reduces tension. For example, a muscle relaxant is often administered during abdominal surgery to relax the diaphragm and keep it from moving during the surgery.

relaxin A hormone that is produced during pregnancy that facilitates the birth process by causing a softening and lengthening of the cervix and the pubic symphysis (the place where the pubic bones come together). Relaxin also inhibits contractions of the uterus and may play a role in determining the timing of delivery. Relaxin works by simultaneously decreasing collagen production and increasing collagen breakdown to loosen the ligaments. A synthetic form of relaxin is being studied for use in treating scleroderma (a connective tissue disease that causes the skin to become tight and thick), improving the skin condition, mobility, and function.

release, carpal tunnel See *carpal tunnel release*.

rem In radiation, an international unit of X-ray or gamma-ray radiation adjusted for the atomic makeup of the human body.

REM Rapid eye movement of the eyes during sleep. During REM sleep, the eyeballs appear to flick around under the closed eyelids. See *REM sleep*.

REM sleep The portion of sleep during which rapid eye movements (REMs) occur. Dreams occur during REM sleep, and people typically have three to five periods of REM sleep per night. These periods occur at intervals of 1 to 2 hours and can vary in length from 5 minutes to over an hour. REM sleep is also characterized by rapid, low-voltage brain waves that are detectable on an electroencephalogram (EEG) recording; irregular breathing and heart rate; and involuntary muscle jerks. See also *NREM sleep*.

remedy Something that consistently helps treat or cure a disease.

remission Disappearance of the signs and symptoms of cancer or other disease. A remission can be temporary or permanent.

remission induction chemotherapy See *induction therapy*.

remote telesurgery A surgical procedure that is carried out from a great distance, thanks to advances in computer and robotic technology and their application to surgery.

renal Having to do with the kidney. For example, renal cancer is cancer of the kidneys.

renal aneurysm An aneurysm that involves the renal artery, the main artery to the kidney.

renal artery stenosis Narrowing of the major artery to the kidney that can lead to seriously elevated blood pressure. Common causes of renal artery stenosis include atherosclerosis and thickening of the muscular wall (fibromuscular dysplasia) of the renal artery.

renal calculus See *kidney stones*.

renal cancer See *cancer, kidney*.

renal capsule The fibrous connective tissue that surrounds each kidney.

renal cell carcinoma   See *cancer, renal cell.*

renal osteodystrophy   See *osteodystrophy, renal.*

renal pelvis   The area at the center of the kidney. Urine collects in the renal pelvis and is funneled into the ureter.

renal stone   See *kidney stones.*

renal transplant   See *kidney transplant.*

renal tubule   A small structure in the kidney that filters blood and produces urine.

renal vein thrombosis   A blood clot in the major vein that drains blood from the kidney.

Rendu-Osler-Weber syndrome   See *hereditary hemorrhagic telangectasia.*

rep   **1** Slang for a pharmaceutical company representative.   **2** Roentgen equivalent physical, a unit of absorbed radiation approximately equivalent to one roentgen.

repair, DNA   See *DNA repair.*

reperfusion   The restoration of blood flow to an organ or to tissue. After a heart attack, an immediate goal is to quickly open blocked arteries and reperfuse the heart muscles. Early reperfusion minimizes the extent of heart muscle damage and preserves the pumping function of the heart.

repetitive stress injury   An injury that occurs due to recurrent overuse or improper use. One of the best-known repetitive stress injuries is carpal tunnel syndrome, which often results from the trauma of highly repetitive work such as that of supermarket checkers, assembly-line workers, typists, word processors, accountants, and writers.

replacement therapy, estrogen   See *estrogen replacement therapy.*

replacement therapy, hormone   See *hormone replacement therapy.*

replication   A turning back, repetition, duplication, or reproduction. See also *DNA replication.*

replication, DNA   See *DNA replication.*

reproduction   The production of offspring. Reproduction need not be sexual; for example, yeast can reproduce by budding.

reproductive cell   An egg or a sperm. Each mature reproductive cell is haploid, meaning that it has a single

set of 23 chromosomes and so contains half the usual amount of DNA.

reproductive cloning   Cloning designed to create new individuals, in contrast to the goal of therapeutic cloning. This idea has stirred great controversy and has met with almost uniform disapproval. See also *therapeutic cloning.*

reproductive system   In women, the organs that are directly involved in producing eggs and in conceiving and carrying babies; in men, the organs directly involved in creating, storing, and delivering sperm to fertilize an egg.

research, controlled   A study that compares results from a treated group and a control group. The control group may receive no treatment, a placebo, or a different treatment. See also *blinded study; double-blinded study.*

resection   Surgical removal of part of an organ.

reservoir, Ommaya   A device that is implanted under the scalp to deliver anticancer drugs to the fluid surrounding the brain and spinal cord.

resident   In medicine, a physician who has finished medical school and is receiving training in a specialized area, such as surgery, internal medicine, pathology, or radiology. Board certification in all medical and surgical specialties requires the satisfactory completion of a residency program.

residual disease   A disease that has not been fully eradicated.

resin, bile acid   See *bile acid resin.*

resistance   Opposition to something, or the ability to withstand something. For example, some forms of the staphylococcus bacterium are resistant to treatment with antibiotics.

resistance, antibiotic   See *antibiotic resistance.*

resistance, pulmonary   Opposition of the respiratory system to air flow.

resistance, vascular   Opposition to the flow of blood by a blood vessel.

resolution   In genetics, the degree of molecular detail on a physical map of DNA. Resolution may range from low to high.

resorb   To absorb again, to lose substance. For example, some of a tooth may be resorbed.

resorption The process of losing substance. For example, when bone is surgically reshaped, it undergoes both new formation and resorption.

respiration The act of inhaling and exhaling air in order to exchange oxygen for carbon dioxide.

respiratory Having to do with respiration.

respiratory distress syndrome, acute See *acute respiratory distress syndrome.*

respiratory failure Inability of the lungs to perform their basic task of gas exchange, the transfer of oxygen from inhaled air into the blood and the transfer of carbon dioxide from the blood into exhaled air. Respiratory failure occurs because of the failure of the exchange of oxygen and carbon dioxide in tiny air sacs in the lung (alveoli), failure of the brain centers that control breathing, or failure of the muscles required to expand the lungs that can cause respiratory failure. Many different medical conditions can lead to respiratory failure, including asthma, emphysema, chronic obstructive lung disease, surgery (on the abdomen, heart, or lungs), overdose of sleeping pills or other depressant drugs, premature birth, multiple physical injuries (as in auto accidents), extensive burns, muscle disease, nerve disease, profuse bleeding, near drowning, heart failure, severe infection, and extreme obesity.

respiratory papillomatosis, recurrent See *laryngeal papillomatosis.*

respiratory rate The number of breaths per minute or, more formally, the number of movements indicative of inspiration and expiration per unit time. In practice, the respiratory rate is usually determined by counting the number of times the chest rises or falls per minute. The aim of measuring respiratory rate is to determine whether the respirations are normal, abnormally fast (tachypnea), abnormally slow (bradypnea), or nonexistent (apnea).

respiratory syncytial virus A virus that causes mild respiratory infections, colds, and coughs in adults and can produce severe respiratory problems, including bronchitis and pneumonia, in young children and anyone with compromised immune, cardiac, or pulmonary systems. Abbreviated RSV. RSV is spread via respiratory secretions and is highly contagious. Infections usually occur during annual community outbreaks, often lasting 4 to 6 months, during the late fall, winter, or early spring. RSV typically features fever, prominent nasal secretions, and congestion coupled with wheezing for 1 to 2 weeks. Having immunity against RSV requires having a continuous, solid level of antibodies against the virus. There is particular concern about RSV occurring in premature babies, because their immune systems lack maturity and antibodies. There is no RSV vaccine.

respiratory system The organs that are involved in breathing, including the nose, throat, larynx, trachea, bronchi, and lungs. Also known as the respiratory tree.

respiratory therapy Exercises and treatments that help patients recover lung function, such as after surgery.

resting phase See *interphase.*

restless leg syndrome An uncomfortable (creeping, crawling, tingling, pulling, twitching, tearing, aching, throbbing, prickling, or grabbing) sensation in the calves that occurs while sitting or while lying down. The result is an uncontrollable urge to relieve the uncomfortable sensation by moving the legs. Restless leg syndrome is a common cause of painful legs. The leg pain typically eases with motion of the legs and becomes more noticeable at rest, worsens during the early evening or later at night, and may cause insomnia.

retardation, mental See *mental retardation.*

retardation, reading See *reading retardation.*

retina The nerve layer that lines the back of the eye, senses light, and creates impulses that travel through the optic nerve to the brain. A small area called the macula in the retina contains special light-sensitive cells that allow the clear perception of fine details. The retina is filled with tiny blood vessels. See also *eye.*

retinal vasculitis Inflammation of the tiny blood vessels of the retina. Retinal vasculitis ranges in severity from mild to severe. Damage to the blood vessels of the retina can cause minimal, partial, or even complete blindness. Retinal vasculitis by itself is painless, but many of the diseases that cause it can also cause painful inflammation elsewhere, such as in the joints. Signs of retinal vasculitis can be observed by a physician using an ophthalmoscope. Further definition of the blood vessel condition can be determined with a special X-ray dye test (angiogram) of the retina. Diseases that cause retinal vasculitis include Behcet's syndrome, systemic lupus erythematosus, antiphospholipid antibody syndrome, systemic necrotizing vasculitis, Wegener's granulomatosus, Takayasu's vasculitis, and giant cell arteritis. Treatment typically involves use of high doses of cortisone-related medications, such as prednisone. In addition, some related diseases require immunosuppression with medication, such as cyclosporine, chlorambucil, and cyclophosphamide.

retinitis pigmentosa A group of inherited disorders in which abnormalities of the photoreceptors (the rods and cones) of the retina lead to progressive visual loss. Abbreviated RP. People with RP first experience defective dark adaptation (night blindness), then constriction of the visual field (tunnel vision), and eventually, late in the course of the disease, loss of central vision. RP may be inherited in an autosomal dominant, autosomal recessive, or X-linked recessive manner or as a mitochondrial disorder. RP can occur alone or as part of a syndrome involving other abnormalities. More than 30 different genes are known to cause nonsyndromic RP (RP alone). Usher syndrome, which is RP and deafness, is a form of syndromic RP.

retinitis pigmentosa and deafness See *Usher syndrome.*

retinoblastoma A malignant eye tumor in children, usually under age 5, that arises in cells in the developing retina that contain cancer-predisposing mutations in both copies of the gene RB1. Abbreviated RB. The most common sign of RB is a white pupillary reflex to light (leukocoria). Strabismus (lazy eye) is the second most common sign. There are two forms of RB: hereditary and sporadic. The inherited form of RB is usually present at birth as multiple tumors in both eyes. It is due to the transmission of an RB1 germline mutation followed by an acquired somatic RB1 mutation. The sporadic form of retinoblastoma has later onset and typically leads to a single tumor in only one eye. It is due to acquired mutations in both RB1 genes. Patients with hereditary RB are at increased risk of developing tumors outside the eye, including pinealomas (in the pineal gland of the brain), osteosarcomas, soft tissue sarcomas, and melanomas. When RB is detected at an early stage, it can sometimes be treated locally but often requires removal of the eye (enucleation). Early diagnosis and treatment of RB and RB-related tumors reduces morbidity and increases longevity.

retinoic acid syndrome A disorder due to the cancer treatment retinoic acid that is characterized by fever, difficulty breathing, chest pain, lung infiltrates, fluid around the lungs and heart, and hypoxia (lack of oxygen). The syndrome occurs within the first 3 weeks of retinoic acid treatment for malignancy and involves the adhesion (sticking) of the malignant cells to the pulmonary blood vessels. Steroids and chemotherapy can be used to treat retinoic acid syndrome. About 10 percent of patients with the syndrome die.

retinol Vitamin A. See also Appendix C, "Vitamins."

retrograde intrarenal surgery A procedure for performing surgery within the kidney by using a viewing tube called a fiber-optic endoscope. Abbreviated RIRS. In RIRS, the scope is placed through the urethra into the bladder and then through the ureter, into the urine-collecting part of the kidney. The scope is thus moved in a retrograde direction—up the urinary tract system, through which urine normally flows outward—to a position within the kidney (intrarenal). RIRS may be done to remove a stone. The stone can be seen through the scope, manipulated or crushed by an ultrasound probe, evaporated by a laser probe, or grabbed with small forceps. RIRS is performed by a specialist, a urologist with special expertise in RIRS (endourologist). The procedure is usually done under general or spinal anesthesia. The advantages of RIRS over open surgery include a quicker solution of the problem, the elimination of prolonged pain after surgery, and much faster recovery. Also known as kidney scoping.

retropubic prostatectomy Surgical removal of the prostate through an incision in the abdomen.

retrosternal Behind the sternum (breastbone).

retrovirus A virus that is composed not of DNA but of RNA. Retroviruses have an enzyme, called reverse transcriptase, that gives them the unique property of transcribing their RNA into DNA. The retroviral DNA can then integrate into the chromosomal DNA of the host cell, to be expressed there. HIV is a retrovirus.

Rett syndrome A neurological disease that affects girls only and is one of the most common causes of mental retardation in females. Girls with the syndrome show normal development during the first 6 to 18 months of life, followed first by a period of stagnation and then by rapid regression in motor and language skills. The hallmark of Rett syndrome is the loss of purposeful hand use and its replacement with stereotyped hand wringing. Screaming fits and inconsolable crying are common. Other key features include loss of speech, behavior reminiscent of autism, panic-like attacks, bruxism (grinding of teeth), rigid gait, tremors, intermittent hyperventilation, and microcephaly (small head). Seizures occur in about half of cases. Girls with Rett syndrome typically survive into adulthood but are at risk of sudden death due to a heart conduction problem—an abnormally long QT interval. Rett syndrome is an X-linked dominant trait and is due to mutation in the MECP2 gene on the X chromosome (in band Xq28). The vast majority of cases are sporadic and result from a new mutation in the girl with Rett syndrome or inheritance of the mutation from a parent who has somatic or germline mosaicism with the MECP2 mutation in only some of his or her cells. Atypical Rett syndrome with MECP2 mutations has been found in patients previously diagnosed with autism, mild learning disability, and mental retardation with spasticity or tremor. Males with MECP2 mutation suffer severe brain disease and die before their first birthday. See also *autism; long QT syndrome; X-linked dominant.*

reversal of organs, total Complete transposition of the thoracic and abdominal organs from right to left, placing the heart in the right side of the chest, and so on.

Organs appear as if in mirror image when examined or X-rayed. Total reversal of organs has been estimated to occur in about 1 in 6,000 to 8,000 births. It also occurs in a rare, abnormal congenital condition called Kartagener syndrome. Also known as situs inversus totalis. See also *dextrocardia; Kartagener syndrome.*

reverse genetics In molecular genetics, identifying genes purely on the basis of their position in the genome, with no knowledge whatsoever of the gene product. In classic genetics, the traditional approach was to find a gene product and then try to identify the gene itself. Also known as positional cloning.

reverse transcriptase An enzyme that permits DNA to be made, using RNA as the template. A retrovirus, such as the HIV virus, can propagate itself by converting its RNA into DNA with reverse transcriptase.

Reye's syndrome A sudden and sometimes fatal disease of the brain (encephalopathy) that is accompanied by degeneration of the liver. Reye's syndrome usually occurs in children between the ages of 4 and 12, comes after infection with chickenpox (varicella) or an influenza-type illness, and is associated with taking medications that contain aspirin. A child with Reye's syndrome first tends to be unusually quiet, lethargic (stuporous), and sleepy. Vomiting may occur. In the second stage, the lethargy deepens, and the child becomes confused, combative, and delirious. This stage is followed by decreasing consciousness, coma, seizures, and eventually death. Early diagnosis and control of the increased intracranial pressure can prevent death or brain damage. Preventing Reye's syndrome is a good reason to have a child immunized against chickenpox. It is also why physicians no longer recommend giving children aspirin for fever or for any other reason.

RF Rheumatoid factor.

Rh factor An antigen found in the red blood cells of most people. Those who have Rh factor are said to be Rh positive (Rh+), and those who do not are Rh negative (Rh-). Blood used in transfusions must match donors for Rh status as well as for ABO blood group because Rh- patients will develop anemia if given R+ blood. Rh typing is also important during abortion, miscarriage, pregnancy, and birth, as mother and fetus may not be Rh compatible. Rh stands for rhesus monkeys, in whose blood this antigen was first found. See also *Rh incompatibility; RhoGAM.*

Rh incompatibility A difference in Rh blood group types between an Rh- mother and her Rh+ baby that leads to hemolytic disease of the newborn. See also *hemolytic disease of the newborn.*

rhabdomyolysis A condition in which skeletal muscle is broken down, releasing muscle enzymes and electrolytes from inside the muscle cells. Risks of rhabdomyolysis include muscle breakdown and kidney failure because the cellular component myoglobin is toxic to the kidneys. Rhabdomyolysis is relatively uncommon, but it most often occurs as the result of extensive muscle damage as, for example, in crush injury or electrical shock. Drugs or toxins, particularly some the cholesterol-lowering medications, may cause this disorder. Underlying diseases that can also lead to rhabdomyolysis include collagen vascular diseases, such as systemic lupus erythematosus.

rhabdomyosarcoma A fast-growing malignancy of muscle that mainly affects children (more than 60 percent of cases are diagnosed before age 10) but can occur at any age. Treatment includes surgery, radiotherapy, chemotherapy, and, most often, a combination of these modes of treatment. For example, the surgeon may remove as much tumor as possible and then have the patient undergo several weeks of chemotherapy, possibly followed by radiation therapy, and then more chemotherapy. The outlook depends on a number of factors, including the original location of the tumor.

rhabdomyosarcoma, embryonal See *sarcoma botryoides.*

rheumatic fever An illness that occurs in the wake of a streptococcus infection (strep throat, or related condition) or scarlet fever, primarily in children. Symptoms include fever, pain in the joints, nausea, stomach cramps, and vomiting. Rheumatic fever can cause long-lasting effects in the joints, heart, brain, and skin. Rheumatic fever may be followed by Sydenham's chorea and by symptoms characteristic of obsessive-compulsive disorder or a tic disorder. Treatment usually involves use of prophylactic antibiotics, as reoccurrence is common and can cause further damage to body tissues. See also *Sydenham's chorea.*

rheumatic heart disease Heart damage caused by rheumatic fever. Treatment involves prevention of reinfection with streptococcus and use of medications to treat any heart complications, as needed.

rheumatism An older term used to describe a number of painful conditions of muscles, tendons, joints, and bones. Rheumatic conditions have been classified as localized (confined to a specific location, such as bursitis and tendonitis), regional (in a larger region, such as chest wall pain), or generalized (affecting many and diverse parts of the body, as in fibromyalgia). Rheumatic diseases and conditions are characterized by symptoms involving the musculoskeletal system; many also feature immune system abnormalities.

rheumatism, psychogenic Rheumatism in which the patient reports inconsistent pains of muscles and joints that do not correspond to true anatomy and physiology.

The patient is felt to have underlying psychological causes for these symptoms.

rheumatism, regional Rheumatism in a larger region, such as chest wall pain, temporomandibular joint pain, and myofascial pain syndrome pain.

rheumatoid arthritis See *arthritis, rheumatoid.*

rheumatoid arthritis, systemic-onset juvenile See *arthritis, systemic-onset juvenile rheumatoid.*

rheumatoid factor An antibody that is measurable in the blood. Measures of rheumatoid factor are commonly taken with a blood test and used to diagnose rheumatoid arthritis. Rheumatoid factor is present in about 80 percent of adults, and a much lower proportion of children, who have rheumatoid arthritis. It is also present in patients with other connective-tissue diseases, such as systemic lupus erythematosus, and in some patients with infectious diseases, such as infectious hepatitis.

rheumatoid nodule A firm lump in the skin of a patient with rheumatoid arthritis. Rheumatoid nodules usually occur at pressure points of the body, most commonly the elbows.

rheumatologist A specialist in the treatment of rheumatic illnesses, especially forms of arthritis. Classic rheumatology training includes 4 years of medical school, 1 year of internship in internal medicine, 2 years of internal medicine residency, and 2 years of rheumatology fellowship. There is a subspecialty board for rheumatology certification, the American College of Rheumatology, which can offer board certification to approved rheumatologists. See also *rheumatologist, pediatric; rheumatology.*

rheumatologist, pediatric A rheumatologist who specializes in caring for children with rheumatic diseases. Pediatric rheumatologists are pediatricians who have completed an additional 2 to 3 years of specialized training in pediatric rheumatology and are usually board certified in pediatric rheumatology. They have special interests in unexplained rash, fever, arthritis, anemia, weakness, weight loss, fatigue, muscle pain, autoimmune disease, and anorexia.

rheumatology A subspecialty of internal medicine that involves the nonsurgical evaluation and treatment of rheumatic diseases and conditions.

rhinitis Irritation of the nose.

rhinitis, acute Inflammation of the nose that occurs for only a few days. Typically, acute rhinitis is caused by a virus (a cold). If rhinitis continues longer than a week, it is probably bacterial.

rhinitis, allergic See *allergic rhinitis.*

rhinitis, allergic, perennial See *allergic rhinitis, perennial.*

rhinitis, allergic, seasonal See *allergic rhinitis, seasonal.*

rhinitis, chronic Inflammation of the nose that lasts for weeks to months. Chronic rhinitis may be caused by bacterial infection, allergy, nasal irritants, structural issues, or physiological problems.

rhinitis, vasomotor Inflammation of the nose due to abnormal neuronal (nerve) control of the blood vessels in the nose. Vasomotor rhinitis is not an allergic reaction as is allergic rhinitis. It is brought on by irritation of the nose, frequently by cool temperatures.

rhinophyma A condition characterized by a bulbous, enlarged red nose and puffy cheeks. There may also be thick bumps on the lower half of the nose and the nearby cheek areas. Rhinophyma occurs mainly in men, and it is a complication of the common skin disease rosacea. Rhinophyma is best treated with surgery. The excess tissue is removed with a scalpel or a laser, or via electrosurgery. Dermabrasion can help improve the final look of the tissue. See also *rosacea.*

rhinoplasty Plastic surgery on the nose, known familiarly as a nose job. Rhinoplasty is a facial cosmetic procedure that is usually performed to enhance the appearance of the nose. During this type of rhinoplasty, the nasal cartilage and bones are modified, or tissue is added. Rhinoplasty is also performed to repair nasal fractures and other structural problems. In these cases, the goal is to restore preinjury appearance or to create a normal appearance.

rhinorrhea See *nose, runny.*

RhoGAM RhO(D) immune globulin, an injectable drug that is used to protect an Rh+ fetus from antibodies in an Rh- mother's blood and to prevent Rh allergy in the mother.

rhythm method See *natural family planning.*

rib One of the 12 paired arches of bone that form the skeletal structure of the chest wall (the rib cage). The ribs attach to the vertebrae of the spine in the back. The 12 pairs of ribs consist of 7 pairs of ribs that attach to the sternum in the front and are known as true, or sternal, ribs; and 5 pairs of lower ribs that do not connect directly to the sternum and are known as false ribs. The upper 3 false ribs connect to the costal cartilages of the ribs just above them. The last 2 false ribs usually have no anchor in front and are known as floating, fluctuating, or vertebral ribs.

rib, cervical An extra rib that arises from the seventh cervical vertebra. It is located above the normal first rib.

A cervical rib is present in only about 1 in 200 people. It may cause pinching of nearby nerves or arteries, in which case it sometimes is removed surgically.

rib, false See *false rib.*

rib, floating See *false rib.*

rib, fluctuating See *false rib.*

rib, sternal See *true rib.*

rib, true See *true rib.*

rib, vertebral See *false rib.*

ribonucleic acid A nucleic acid that is similar to DNA but contains ribose rather than deoxyribose. Abbreviated RNA. RNA, in fact, can form upon a DNA template. The several classes of RNA molecules play important roles in protein synthesis and other cell activities. See also *messenger RNA; RNA, ribosomal; RNA, transfer.*

ribosome A tiny structure in the cytoplasm of a cell (outside the nucleus) that functions as the protein factory for the cell.

rickets A disease of infants and children that disturbs normal bone formation (ossification), leading to failure to mineralize bone. Rickets softens bone, producing osteomalacia, and permits marked bending and distortion of bones. Other features of rickets include softness of the infant's skull (craniotabes), enlargement of the front end of the ribs (creating the "rachitic rosary"), thickening of the wrists and ankles, lateral curving of the spine (scoliosis), abnormal forward–backward curving of the spine (kyphosis and lumbar lordosis), and deforming and narrowing of the pelvis, which in females interferes later with vaginal childbirth. As the child begins to walk, the weight on the soft shafts of the legs results in knock-knees or, more often, bowlegs. The deformities of the spine, pelvis, and legs reduce height, leading to short stature. The spinal deformities also impair posture and gait. Until the first third of the 20th century, rickets was usually due to lack of direct exposure to sunlight or to lack of vitamin D, calcium, and phosphorus. Sunlight provides the necessary ultraviolet (UV) rays, and thanks to improved diets, vitamin D supplements, and enriched food products, nutritional rickets has become relatively rare in industrialized nations. It still occurs sometimes in breastfed babies whose mothers are underexposed to sunlight, and in dark-skinned babies who are not given vitamin D supplements. In developing countries, vitamin D–deficiency rickets continues to be a problem. Rickets in North America and Europe is usually now due to other causes, such as disorders that create vitamin D deficiency by interfering with the absorption of vitamin D through the intestines; diseases of the liver, kidney, or other organs that impair the normal metabolic conversion and activation of vitamin D; and conditions that disrupt the normal balance in the body between calcium and phosphorus.

rickets, celiac Rickets caused by failure of the intestines to absorb calcium and fat from foods. See also *celiac sprue.*

rickets, hypophosphatemic A genetic form of rickets that is characterized by low blood phosphate level (hypophosphatemia), defective intestinal absorption of phosphate, and unresponsiveness to vitamin D. The basic problem in hypophosphatemic rickets is decreased resorption of phosphate by the tubules in the kidney. Females typically have less severe disease than males. Two different types of the disorder are inherited in an X-linked dominant manner. Type I is treated with oral phosphate and calcitriol, and it generally responds well. Type II is treated with oral phosphate alone and responds poorly. Also known as vitamin D–resistant rickets. See also *rickets.*

rickets, renal Rickets-like bone malformations that are caused by prolonged inflammation of the kidneys.

rickets, vitamin D–resistant See *rickets, hypophosphatemic.*

Rickettsia A member of genus Rickettsia, a family of microorganisms that, like viruses, require other living cells for growth, but also resemble bacteria in that they use oxygen, have metabolic enzymes and cell walls, and are susceptible to antibiotics. Rickettsiae cause a series of diseases, including Rocky Mountain spotted fever, typhus, and trench fever. See also *rickettsial diseases.*

rickettsial diseases Infectious diseases caused by Rickettsiae that fall into four groups: typhus, including epidemic typhus, Brill-Zinsser disease, murine (endemic) typhus, and scrub typhus; spotted fever, including Rocky Mountain spotted fever, Eastern tick-borne rickettsiosis, and rickettsialpox; Q fever; and trench fever.

rickettsialpox A mild infectious disease first observed in New York City that is caused by Rickettsia akari and is transmitted from its mouse host by chigger or adult mite bites. Features include fever, a dark spot that becomes a small ulcer at the site of the bite, swollen glands (satellite lymphadenopathy) near the site of the bite, and a raised, blistering (vesicular) rash. Treatment is with antibiotics.

rickettsiosis Infection with Rickettsia, a genus of bacteria that is transmitted by lice, mites, ticks, and fleas.

rickettsiosis, North Asian tick-borne One of the tick-borne rickettsial diseases of the eastern hemisphere, similar to but less severe than Rocky Mountain spotted fever. Symptoms include fever, a small ulcer (eschar) at the site of the tick bite, swollen glands near the site of the bite (satellite lymphadenopathy), and a red, raised (maculopapular) rash.

right heart   See *heart, right.*

right ventricle   See *ventricle, right.*

ring chromosome   A structurally abnormal chromosome in which the end of each chromosome arm has been lost and the broken arms have been reunited to form a ring. A ring chromosome is denoted by the symbol r.

ring, intrastromal corneal   See *intrastromal corneal ring.*

ringworm   See *tinea barbae.*

ringworm of the nails   See *onychomycosis.*

RIRS   Retrograde intrarenal surgery.

risk factor   Something that increases a person's chances of developing a disease. For example, cigarette smoking is a risk factor for lung cancer and obesity is a risk factor for heart disease.

risk, obesity-related   See *obesity-related disease.*

risk of recurrence   See *recurrence risk.*

ritonavir   A medication (brand name: Norvir) in the protease inhibitor family that is used to treat HIV infection (AIDS). See also *protease inhibitor.*

Ritter disease   See *staphylococcal scalded skin syndrome.*

river blindness   A disease caused by a parasitic worm (Onchocerca volvulus) that is transmitted by biting blackflies that breed in fast-flowing rivers. The adult worms can live for up to 15 years in nodules beneath the skin and in the muscles of infected persons, where they produce millions of worm embryos (microfilariae) that invade the skin and other tissues, including the eyes, causing blindness. The drug ivermectin (brand name: Stromectol), taken in a single oral dose administered once a year, prevents the accumulation of microfilariae in persons at risk. Treatment is with antibiotics that can kill the adult worms in the body. Also known as onchocerciasis.

RLL   Right lower lobe, the lower-right lobe of the lung.

RLQ   Right lower quadrant, the lower-right quarter of the abdomen.

RML   Right middle lobe, the middle-right lobe of the lung.

RMSF   Rocky Mountain spotted fever.

RN   Registered nurse. See *nurse, registered.*

RNA   Ribonucleic acid.

RNA editing   The process by which messenger RNA (mRNA) is modified (edited) after it is synthesized before it is translated into protein.

RNA interference   The process by which the introduction of double-stranded RNA into a cell interferes with the expression of genes. Abbreviated RNAi.

RNA, messenger   See *messenger RNA.*

RNA polymerase   The enzyme that makes the very large molecule RNA, by joining together many smaller molecules, using DNA as a template.

RNA, ribosomal   A component of ribosomes that functions as a nonspecific site for making polypeptides. Abbreviated rRNA. See also *ribosome.*

RNA, transfer   The form of the biochemical ribonucleic acid that brings (transfers) activated amino acids into position along the messenger RNA template. Abbreviated tRNA.

RNAi   RNA interference.

Rochalimaea quintana   See *Bartonella quintana.*

Rocky Mountain spotted fever   An acute febrile (feverish) disease that was initially recognized in the Rocky Mountain states. Abbreviated RMSF. RMSF is caused by Rickettsia rickettsii, transmitted by hard-shelled (ixodid) ticks, and occurs only in the Western hemisphere. Anyone frequenting tick-infested areas is at risk for RMSF. Onset of symptoms is abrupt, with headache, high fever, chills, muscle pain, and then a rash. The rickettsiae grow within damaged cells lining blood vessels, which may become blocked by clots. Blood vessel inflammation (vasculitis) is widespread in a person with RMSF. Early recognition of RMSF and prompt antibiotic treatment is important to prevent death. Also known as spotted fever, tick fever, and tick typhus.

rod   A specialized light-sensitive cell (photoreceptor) in the retina that provides side vision and the ability to see objects in dim light (night vision). See also *cone cell.*

roentgen   An international unit of X-ray or gamma-ray radiation.

roentgenology   See *radiology.*

rooting reflex   A reflex that is seen in normal newborn babies, who automatically turn the face toward the stimulus and make sucking (rooting) motions with the mouth when the cheek or lip is touched. The rooting reflex helps to ensure successful breastfeeding.

Rorschach test A common psychological test that involves using inkblots that show enigmatic and highly ambiguous shapes. Ten standardized blots are shown, one at a time, to a person, and the person's responses are recorded, to determine what the person perceives about the inkblots.

rosacea A chronic skin disease that causes persistent redness over the areas of the face and nose that normally blush: mainly the forehead, the chin, and the lower half of the nose. The tiny blood vessels in these areas enlarge (dilate) and become more visible through the skin, appearing like tiny red lines (telangiectasias). Pimples that look like teenage acne can occur. Rosacea occurs most often between the ages of 30 and 50, especially in people with fair skin. It affects both sexes. Although it tends to occur more common in women than in men, it is often worse in men. When rosacea first develops, it may come and go. However, in time the skin fails to return to its normal color, and the enlarged blood vessels and pimples arrive. Rosacea rarely reverses itself, and it worsens if untreated. Untreated rosacea can cause a condition called rhinophyma, characterized by a bulbous, enlarged red nose and puffy cheeks. There may also be thick bumps on the lower half of the nose and the nearby cheek areas. About half of all people with rosacea feel burning and grittiness of the eyes (conjunctivitis). If this is not treated, the complications of what is called rosacea keratitis may impair vision. Rosacea can be treated but not cured. Topical antibiotics such as metronidazole, and oral antibiotics such as tetracycline, are often used. Short-term topical cortisone (steroid) preparations of the right strength may also be used to reduce local inflammation. Over-the-counter medications for acne can irritate the skin in rosacea, however. Avoiding smoking and food and drink that cause flushing (such as spicy food, hot beverages, and alcoholic drinks) helps minimize the blood vessel enlargement. Limiting exposure to sunlight and to extreme hot and cold temperatures also helps relieve rosacea. Rubbing the face tends to irritate the reddened skin. Some cosmetics and hair sprays may aggravate redness and swelling. Facial products such as soap, moisturizers, and sunscreens should be free of alcohol and other irritating ingredients. Moisturizers should be applied very gently after any topical medication has dried. Outdoors, sunscreens with an SPF of 15 or higher are needed. The telangiectasias can be covered with cosmetics, or they can be treated with a small electric needle, a laser, or surgery to close off the dilated blood vessels. See also *rhinophyma*.

roseola See *measles*.

rotator cuff A group of four tendons that stabilize the shoulder joint. Each of these tendons hooks up to a muscle that moves the shoulder in a specific direction. The four muscles whose tendons form the rotator cuff are the subscapularis muscle, which moves the arm by turning it inward (internal rotation); the supraspinatus muscle, which is responsible for elevating the arm and moving it away from the body; the infraspinatus muscle, which assists the lifting of the arm during outward turning (external rotation) of the arm; and the teres minor muscle, which also helps in the outward turning (external rotation) of the arm. Damage to the rotator cuff is one of the most common causes of shoulder pain.

rotator cuff disease Damage to the rotator cuff that can be due to trauma, as from falling and injuring the shoulder; overuse in sports, particularly those that involve repetitive overhead motions; inflammation, as from tendonitis, bursitis, or arthritis of the shoulder; or degeneration, as from aging. The main symptom of rotator cuff disease is shoulder pain of gradual or sudden onset, typically located to the front and side of the shoulder and increasing when the shoulder is moved away from the body. A person with torn rotator cuff tendons may not be able to hold the arm up because of pain. With very severe tears, the arm falls because of weakness; this is called the positive drop sign. Diagnosis is made via observation and can be confirmed with X-rays showing bony injuries; an arthrogram in which contrast dye is injected into the shoulder joint to detect leakage out of the injured rotator cuff; or a magnetic resonance imaging (MRI) scan, which can provide more information than either an X-ray or an arthrogram. Treatment depends on severity. Mild rotator cuff disease is treated with application of ice, rest, and use of anti-inflammatory medications, such as ibuprofen. A patient with persistent pain and motion limitation may benefit from a cortisone injection in the rotator cuff and from doing exercises that are specifically designed to strengthen the rotator cuff. More severe rotator cuff disease may require arthroscopic or open surgical repair. Subacromial decompression, the removal of a small portion of the bone (acromion) that overlies the rotator cuff, can relieve pressure on the rotator cuff and promote healing. Very severe, complete full-thickness rotator cuff tears require surgery to mend the torn rotator cuff. Without treatment, including exercise, the outlook is not very good. Scarring around the shoulder (adhesive capsulitis) can lead to marked limitation of range of shoulder motion, a condition called a frozen shoulder. Some patients never recover full use of the shoulder joint.

rotavirus A leading cause of severe winter diarrhea in young children. Abbreviated RV. Each year RV leads to an estimated 500,000 physician visits and 50,000 hospital admissions in the US. Almost everyone catches RV before entering school, but, with rehydration and good nutrition, nearly all recover fully. However, in poor countries it is estimated that there are at least 600,000 deaths of children under age 5 from RV diarrhea and dehydration. Aside from causing acute infantile gastroenteritis and diarrhea in young children, RV is typically accompanied by low-grade fever. Immunization of infants with a vaccine against RV was halted in 1999 because of deaths due to bowel obstruction (from intussusception of the bowel) following vaccination, which prompted the manufacturer to withdraw the vaccine from the market.

Rothmund-Thomson syndrome A hereditary disease that is characterized by progressive degeneration (atrophy); effects on multiple parts of the body, including skin (premature aging, excess pigmentation, dilated blood vessels), eyes (juvenile cataract), nose (depressed nasal bridge), teeth (maldeveloped), skeletal system (congenital bone defects), hair (abnormal), gonads (underdevelopment), limbs (soft tissue contractures), growth (short stature), and blood (anemia); and a tendency to develop the bone cancer osteogenic sarcoma. Abbreviated RTS. RTS is inherited as an autosomal recessive trait. A child born to two parents with the RTS gene stands a 25 percent chance of receiving both RTS genes and the disease. RTS is caused by mutations in the RECQL4 gene on chromosome 8. This gene encodes a DNA helicase, an enzyme that promotes DNA unwinding, which permits many basic cellular processes to take place. Also known as poikiloderma congenita and poikiloderma atrophicans with cataract.

roundworm A type of parasitic worm that hatches in the intestines and lives there. The eggs of the roundworm usually enter the body through contaminated water or food or on fingers placed in the mouth after the hands have touched a contaminated object. Symptoms of roundworm infections include fatigue, weight loss, irritability, poor appetite, abdominal pain, and diarrhea. Treatment with medication results in a cure in about a week. Without treatment, anemia and malnutrition can develop. An example of a roundworm is Trichuris trichiura, also known as the human whipworm. This worm is found worldwide, but infections are most frequent in areas with tropical weather and poor sanitation practices, and among children. Presently, some 800 million people are infected. Infection with T. trichiura is not foreign to the US; it occurs in the southern US.

RPR test Rapid plasma reagin test. See *syphilis test, RPR.*

rRNA Ribosomal RNA. See *RNA, ribosomal.*

RSV **1** Respiratory syncytial virus. **2** Rous sarcoma virus, a virus that is the cause of a serious form of soft tissue cancer called sarcoma.

RTS Rothmund-Thomson syndrome.

RU-486 The French abortion pill, which has been used in combination with another drug called misoprostol to terminate pregnancy at an early stage. A woman using RU-486 can be no more than 7 weeks pregnant. The drug has 95 percent effectiveness. About 5 percent of women using RU-486 in early pregnancy need additional medical intervention due to incomplete abortion. Also known as mifepristone.

rubella German measles, a contagious viral disease caused by human papilloma virus 77 (HPV-77). Symptoms of rubella include upper respiratory tract infection, fever, swollen lymph glands, and a rash with small spots. Exposure of a pregnant woman to rubella can infect and damage the baby. Fetal rubella syndrome is the main reason for rubella immunization. See also *rubella syndrome, fetal.*

rubella immunization See *MMR.*

rubella syndrome, fetal A constellation of abnormalities caused by infection of a mother with the rubella (German measles) virus before the birth of her baby. The syndrome is characterized by mental retardation and multiple birth defects, including abnormally small head, cataracts, glaucoma, abnormally small eyes, and cardiovascular malformations. Deafness is common. After birth the child may develop diabetes due to gradual destruction of the pancreas by the rubella virus. The child has a 50 percent risk of being born with the congenital rubella syndrome (a syndrome of multiple birth defects), if the mother is infected with rubella in the first trimester of pregnancy. Risks still exist with infection in the second trimester. The virus persists throughout pregnancy, is still present at birth, and continues to be shed by the infected child for many months after birth. Even if a child born with rubella looks normal, the child can be contagious and infect caregivers.

rubeola See *measles.*

RUL Right upper lobe, the upper-right lobe of the lung.

runny nose See *nose, runny.*

rupture, uterine See *uterine rupture.*

ruptured spleen See *spleen, ruptured.*

RUQ Right upper quadrant, the upper-right quarter of the abdomen.

RV Rotavirus.

Rx **1** On a prescription, abbreviation for "recipe" (Latin for "to take"). See also Appendix A, "Prescription Abbreviations." **2** In a pharmacological catalog, an indicator that one will need a prescription to buy a listed item.

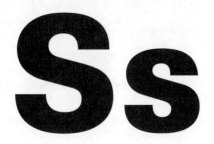

S1–S5 Symbols that represent the five thoracic vertebrae.

SA node Sinoatrial node.

Sabin vaccine See *polio vaccine, oral.*

sac, egg See *ovary.*

sac, pericardial See *pericardium.*

saccular Being like a small pouch. For example, the alveolar saccules are little air pouches within the lungs.

saccular aneurysm See *aneurysm, saccular.*

sacral Referring to the sacrum. For example, sacral agenesis is absence of all or part of the sacrum.

sacral agenesis Absence of all or part of the sacrum. See also *caudal regression syndrome; sacrum.*

sacral vertebrae The five vertebral bones situated between the lumbar vertebrae and the coccyx (tailbone). By adulthood, the sacral vertebrae are normally fused to form the sacrum. The sacral vertebrae are represented by the symbols S1 through S5. See also *vertebra; vertebral column.*

sacrum The large heavy bone at the base of the spine that is made up of the fused sacral vertebrae. In the vertebral column, the sacrum is situated between the lumbar vertebrae and the coccyx (tailbone). It is triangular in shape and forms the back wall of the pelvis. The female sacrum is wider and less curved than the male sacrum. From the Latin *os sacrum,* meaning "sacred bone" because it was used in sacrifice. See also *pelvis; sacral vertebrae; vertebral column.*

SAD Seasonal affective disorder.

safe sex Sexual practices that do not involve the exchange of bodily fluids, including blood, sperm, vaginal secretions, and saliva, to avoid AIDS and other sexually transmitted diseases. The term *safe sex* is generally used to mean sex without penetration or sex using condoms and Nonoxynol-9 spermicide and/or vaginal dams, with consistency. In reality, *safer sex* is a better term than *safe sex.*

sagittal A vertical plane passing through the standing body from front to back. The median plane that splits the body into left and right halves. See also Appendix B, "Anatomic Orientation Terms."

sagittal sinus A large vein that runs on the top of the skull from front to back and then splits to carry blood from the brain toward the heart.

saline **1** Relating to salt (sodium chloride). **2** Salty, containing salt. **3** A salt solution, often adjusted to the normal salinity of the human body. Saline solutions are commonly used in medicine as fluid replacements to treat or prevent dehydration. Certain concentrations of both sodium and chloride in the blood are essential for normal body functions.

salivary gland A gland in the mouth that produces saliva. The salivary glands can become inflamed, as in Sjogren's syndrome and mumps.

Salk vaccine See *polio vaccine, inactivated.*

salmon patch A small flat patch of pink or red (salmon-colored) skin, most commonly found on the forehead between the eyebrows (called an angel's kiss), on the eyelids, or on the nape of the neck (called a stork bite). Salmon patches are seen in 30 to 40 percent of newborns and are usually most noticeable when the baby cries. A salmon patch is a collection of capillaries. Salmon patches are of no consequence and tend to disappear in time.

Salmonella A group of bacteria that cause typhoid fever and other illnesses, including food poisoning, gastroenteritis, and enteric fever from contaminated food products. See also *food poisoning; Salmonellosis.*

salmonellosis Infection with bacteria belonging to the genus Salmonella. Salmonellosis is particularly dangerous for people with immunodeficiency diseases and sickle cell disease. Symptoms usually begin within 12 to 24 hours after exposure and may include stomach cramps, diarrhea, fever, and sometimes vomiting. Diagnosis can be confirmed via examination of a stool sample for Salmonella bacteria. Most people exposed to Salmonella feel fine within a few days and do not require treatment other than extra fluids. Some need antibiotics, and a few need hospitalization. See also *food poisoning.*

salpingo-oophorectomy Removal of the fallopian tubes and ovaries. See also *hysterectomy.*

salt **1** Sodium chloride. Table salt. Certain concentrations of both sodium and chloride in the blood are essential for normal body functions. Sodium ingestion can elevate the blood pressure, aggravate heart failure, or cause fluid retention in persons who are so inclined. **2** An ionic crystalline compound.

Salter-Harris fracture See *fracture, Salter-Harris.*

salvage therapy   A final treatment for people who are not responsive to or cannot tolerate other available therapies for a particular condition.

sample, random   See *random sample.*

Sandhoff disease   A genetic disorder with symptoms that are very similar to those of Tay-Sachs disease (TSD) and that is characterized by accumulation of fatty material called GM2 ganglioside in the nerve cells of the brain. Symptoms begin around 6 months of age, with motor weakness, and progress to include difficulties with swallowing and breathing. Death usually occurs by age 3. Sandhoff disease is an autosomal recessive disorder caused by a mutation to chromosome 5. Unlike TSD, it is most common in the non-Jewish population. See also *Tay-Sachs disease.*

Sanfilippo syndrome   The most common disorder of mucopolysaccharide metabolism, a syndrome in which the onset of clinical abnormalities occurs between ages 2 and 6, with mild coarsening of the facial features (but normal clear corneas), mild stiffening of the joints, slowing of growth, and intellectual deterioration that results in severe mental retardation. On a biochemical level, Sanfilippo syndrome is characterized by the excess excretion of heparin sulfate in the urine and the accumulation of mucopolysaccharides in the central nervous system and other tissues. On the genetic level, there are four types of Sanfilippo syndrome (types A, B, C, and D), each due to deficiency of a different enzyme. All four types are inherited in an autosomal recessive manner and result in identical clinical syndromes. Also known as mucopolysaccharidosis type III (MPS III).

sanguine   **1** Having a ruddy (reddish) complexion. **2** Cheerful, hopeful, confident, optimistic, or impulsive.

saphenous vein   One of the two saphenous veins—the great and the small saphenous veins—that serve as the principal veins running near the surface of the leg. The saphenous veins carry deoxygenated blood from the feet and legs toward the heart. See also *saphenous vein, great; saphenous vein, small.*

saphenous vein, great   The larger of the two saphenous veins, which runs from the foot all the way up to the saphenous opening, an oval aperture in the broad fascia of the thigh. The great saphenous vein passes through this fibrous membrane. Also known as large saphenous vein.

saphenous vein, large   See *saphenous vein, great.*

saphenous vein, small   The smaller of the two saphenous veins, which runs behind the outer malleolus (the protuberance on the outside of the ankle joint), comes up the back of the leg, and joins the popliteal vein in the space behind the knee (popliteal space). See also *saphenous vein.*

SAPHO syndrome   Synovitis, acne, pustulosis, hyperostosis, and osteitis syndrome, which involves symptoms including warmth, tenderness, pain, swelling, and stiffness of involved joints (arthritis); fluid-filled blister-like areas (pustules), typically on the palms of the hands and/or the soles of the feet, and peeling and flaking of skin in those areas; abnormal, excessive growth of bone, frequently at the points of the bone where tendons attach; and inflammation of the sacroiliac joints (sacroiliitis), as well as inflammation of the spine (spondylitis), leading to stiffness and pain of the neck and back. SAPHO syndrome is thought to be related to other arthritic conditions that typically affect the spine, including ankylosing spondylitis and reactive arthritis.

Sapphism   See *lesbianism.*

sarcoidosis   A disease of unknown origin that causes small lumps (granulomas) due to chronic inflammation in body tissues. Sarcoidosis can appear in almost any body organ, but it most often starts in the lungs or lymph nodes. It can also affect the eyes, liver, and skin; and less often it affects the spleen, bones, joints, skeletal muscles, heart, and central nervous system. In the majority of cases, the granulomas clear up with or without treatment. In cases where the granulomas do not heal and disappear, the tissues tend to remain inflamed and become scarred.

sarcoma   One of a group of tumors that usually arise from connective tissue. Most sarcomas are malignant. Many types are named after the type of cell, tissue, or structure involved. See also *angiosarcoma; chondrosarcoma; fibrosarcoma; liposarcoma; osteosarcoma; rhabdomyosarcoma; sarcoma botryoides; sarcoma, Ewing; Kaposi sarcoma; sarcoma, soft-tissue; sarcoma, synovial.*

sarcoma botryoides   A malignancy of the cervix, vagina, or bladder in infants and young children that arises from embryonal rhabdomyoblasts (ancestral muscle cells). The tumor resembles a bunch of grapes. It has a generally good prognosis. Treatment includes conservative surgery followed by chemotherapy. Also known as embryonal rhabdomyosarcoma. See also *rhabdomyosarcoma; sarcoma; sarcoma, soft-tissue.*

sarcoma, Ewing   A tumor that arises in a primitive nerve cell within bone or soft tissue and affects children and adolescents, especially between ages 10 and 20. Ewing sarcoma usually appears in the large bones of the arms and legs and the flat bones of the pelvis, spine, and ribs. The tumor may metastasize to bone, lung, or bone marrow. Ewing sarcoma is the second most common type of bone tumor (after osteosarcoma) in children and adolescents. Treatment usually includes chemotherapy and radiation therapy. The tumor typically responds to radiation. Surgery may be done to remove the primary (original) tumor or metastases. Survival is much better with a localized tumor (particularly if the tumor is below the elbow or midcalf) than with a tumor that has spread. The primitive nerve cell from which Ewing sarcoma arises also gives rise to a number of tumors, known as the Ewing family of tumors, which include Ewing sarcoma of bone, extraosseus (nonbone) Ewing sarcoma, primitive neuroectodermal tumor (PNET), and Askin tumor (PNET of the chest wall). Most Ewing family tumors have a translocation between chromosomes 11 and 22 that results in the fusion of the EWS gene on chromosome 22 with the transcription factor gene FLI1 on chromosome 11, leading to the production of a chimeric (fusion) protein. The remaining tumors in the Ewing family engage the EWS gene in other translocations that lead to formation of chimeric proteins. In all cases the chimeric protein is oncogenic; that is, it is responsible for the malignancy.

sarcoma, Kaposi   See *Kaposi sarcoma.*

sarcoma, osteogenic   See *osteosarcoma.*

sarcoma, soft-tissue   A sarcoma that begins in the muscle, fat, fibrous tissue, blood vessels, or other supporting tissue of the body. See also *sarcoma.*

sarcoma, synovial   A malignant sarcoma of soft tissue that arises near, but not in, a joint. Synovial sarcomas most often occur in adolescents or young adults, are typically slow-growing, and may escape notice until they become painful. They occur mainly in the arms and legs, near large joints, especially the knees. Although the tumor is called synovial sarcoma, it has never been shown to arise from synovial cells (the cells that line a joint). The cell of origin is not known. The diagnosis of synovial sarcoma can be suspected via X-ray or imaging, made via biopsy, and confirmed via cytogenetic studies that show a translocation (an exchange of material) between the X chromosome and chromosome 18, termed t(X;18) (p11.2;q11.2), in the tumor cells. The key treatment is surgery to remove the entire tumor, nearby muscle, and lymph nodes. Radiation, chemotherapy, or a combination of treatment methods may follow surgery. The tumor tends to recur locally and to involve local lymph nodes. Distant spread (metastasis) occurs in half of cases, sometimes many years after the initial diagnosis. Also known as synoviosarcoma.

SARS See *severe acute respiratory syndrome.*

sartorius muscle   The long band of muscle that stretches from the calf to the pelvis. It moves the thigh and, by extension, the leg.

saturated fat   A fat that is solid at room temperature and comes chiefly from animal food products. Some examples of saturated fat are butter, lard, meat fat, solid shortening, palm oil, and coconut oil. Saturated fat tends to raise the level of cholesterol in the blood.

sawbones   Slang for a physician, especially a surgeon, and in particular an orthopedic surgeon.

scabicide   A medication that is used to treat scabies. Examples include permethrin cream, lindane, or crotamiton lotion and cream. Sulfur in petrolatum (10%) is one of few effective scabicidal treatments that may be used safely without fear of toxicity in very small children and in pregnant women. See also *scabies; scabies, keratotic.*

scabies   Infestation of the skin by the human itch mite Sarcaptes scabies. The initial symptom of scabies are red, raised bumps that are intensely itchy. A magnifying glass reveals short, wavy lines of red skin, which are the burrows made by the mites. Treatment involves use of several scabicide medications. See also *scabicide.*

scabies, keratotic   A severe form of scabies that is caused by delaying treatment of the initial infestation. Keratotic scabies is characterized by mite-filled lesions covered with scabs. These lesions often become infected with bacteria such as staphylococcus. Keratotic scabies is most common in people with immune-system problems, including AIDS, diabetes, and lupus. Also known as crusted scabies.

scalded skin syndrome   See *staphylococcal scalded skin syndrome.*

scan   **1** Data or an image obtained from the examination of organs or regions of the body by gathering information with a sensing device.   **2** To examine or view with a sensing instrument or imaging machine.

scapula   The flat triangular bone at the back of the shoulder. Also known as shoulder blade and wingbone. See also *subscapular; subscapularis muscle.*

scarlatina   See *scarlet fever.*

scarlet fever   A skin condition that is due to a streptococcal sore throat or any other streptococcal infection. The group A streptococcal bacteria produce a toxin that causes a scarlet rash that initially appears on the neck and chest, then spreads over the body, and lasts around 3 days. As the rash fades, desquamation (peeling) may occur around the fingertips, toes, and groin area. Scarlet fever is usually not a serious illness when treated promptly with antibiotics such as penicillin. However, untreated streptococcal infection can cause kidney inflammation (glomerulonephritis) and rheumatic fever. Also known as scarlatina.

SCFE   Slipped capital femoral epiphysis.

Scheuermann's disease   A skeletal disease that usually begins in adolescence and results in a hunched back. Treatment with casting and a back brace is successful if undertaken early. Also known as juvenile kyphosis and curvature of the spine.

schistosomiasis   See *bilharzia.*

schizoaffective disorder   A mood disorder that is coupled with some symptoms that resemble those of schizophrenia, particularly loss of personality (flat affect) and social withdrawal.

schizoid   Having symptoms similar to those of schizophrenia.

schizophrenia   One of several brain diseases whose symptoms may include loss of personality (flat affect), agitation, catatonia, confusion, psychosis, unusual behavior, and social withdrawal. The illness usually begins in early adulthood. The cause of schizophrenia is not known, but there appear to be both genetic (inherited) and environmental components to the disease. Schizophrenia is not caused by abuse or poor parenting practices. Treatment involves use of neuroleptic medication and supportive interpersonal therapy. The prognosis is fairly good, with two-thirds of those diagnosed recovering significantly.

schizophrenia, childhood   The onset of schizophrenia before adulthood. This condition is very rare in young children, but it occurs with more frequency in the teenage years. Autism was once known as childhood schizophrenia, but it is a completely different disorder. See also *autism; childhood disintegrative disorder; developmental disorder; schizophrenia.*

schizotypal personality disorder   A personality type that is characterized by unusual patterns of speech and behavior and by social withdrawal. See also *Asperger syndrome.*

Schmorl's node   An upward and downward protrusion (pushing into) of a spinal disk's soft tissue into the bony tissue of the adjacent vertebrae. Schmorl's nodes, which are common, especially with minor degeneration of the aging spine, are detectable via X-ray as spine abnormalities. Schmorl's nodes are most common in the middle and lower spine. Schmorl's nodes usually cause no symptoms, but they reflect that "wear and tear" of the spine has occurred over time.

sciatic nerve   The largest nerve in the body, which begins from nerve roots in the lumbar spinal cord in the low back (sacrum) and extends through the buttock area, sending nerve endings down through the legs and knees. See also *sciatica.*

sciatica   Pain that results from irritation of the sciatic nerve and is typically felt at the back of the thigh. Although sciatica can result from a herniated disc pressing directly on the nerve, any cause of irritation or inflammation of this nerve can reproduce the painful symptoms of sciatica. Diagnosis is made via observation of symptoms, physical and nerve tests, and sometimes X-ray or magnetic resonance imaging (MRI), if a herniated disk is suspected. Treatment options include avoiding movements that further irritate the condition, use of medication, physical therapy, and sometimes surgery.

science, cognitive   See *cognitive science.*

scintigraphy   A diagnostic test in which a two-dimensional picture of a body radiation source is obtained through the use of radioisotopes. For example, scintigraphy of the biliary system (cholescintigraphy) is done to diagnose obstruction of the bile ducts by a gallstone, a tumor, or another problem; disease of the gallbladder; and bile leaks. For cholescintigraphy, a radioactive chemical is injected intravenously into the patient. The chemical is removed from the blood by the liver and secreted into the bile that the liver makes. The chemical then goes everywhere that the bile goes: into the bile ducts, the gallbladder, and the intestine. By placing over the abdomen a camera that senses radioactivity, a picture of the liver, bile ducts, and gallbladder can be obtained that corresponds to where the radioactivity is within the bile-filled liver, ducts, and gallbladder.

scintimammography   A scintigraphic imaging technique that uses the radioisotope technetium tetrofosmin (Tc-99 tetrofosmin) to detect breast cancer. Scintimammography can sometimes work better than standard mammography in situations where there is considerable uncertainty, as in women who have especially dense breast tissue.

sclera   The tough white outer coat that covers the surface of the eyeball. The sclera covers the back five-sixths of the eyeball. The sclera is continuous in the front of the eye with the cornea and in the back of the eye with the external sheath of the optic nerve. The plural is sclerae. See also *scleritis.*

sclerencephaly   Scarring and shrinkage of the substance of the brain. Sclerencephaly occurs because of chronic inflammation of the brain matter.

scleritis   Inflammation of the sclera. Scleritis causes local pain and can cause vision loss. Scleritis can occur with diseases such as rheumatoid arthritis, Wegener's granulomatosis, and lupus. Treatment may include use of anti-inflammatory and cortisone-related medications taken by mouth, intravenously, or injected into the eye.

sclerodactyly   Localized thickening and tightness of the skin of the fingers or toes. Sclerodactyly is commonly

ROR

associated with atrophy of the underlying soft tissues. Sclerodactyly is a characteristic feature of scleroderma.

scleroderma A disease of connective tissue that causes scar tissue (fibrosis) to form in the skin and sometimes also in other organs of the body. Scleroderma is classified into diffuse and limited forms. Diffuse scleroderma affects many internal and external areas of the body, including the skin of the entire body, the bowels, and the lungs. Limited scleroderma affects only certain body sections. The CREST syndrome is the most common limited form of scleroderma. CREST stands for

- **C** Calcinosis (the formation of tiny deposits of calcium in the skin)
- **R** Raynaud phenomenon (spasms of the tiny artery vessels that supply blood to the fingers, toes, nose, tongue, or ears)
- **E** Esophagus (esophageal involvement by the scleroderma)
- **S** Sclerodactyly (localized thickening and tightness of the skin of the fingers or toes)
- **T** Telangiectasias (dilated capillaries that form tiny red areas, frequently on the face, on the hands, and in the mouth, behind the lips)

The cause of scleroderma is unknown. There is some evidence that genes play at least a partial role in causing the disease. The immune system plays a central role in the disease process. It is not unusual to find other autoimmune diseases in families of scleroderma patients. The treatment of scleroderma is directed toward the particular organ system that is causing symptoms. The disease occurs more frequently in females than in males.

sclerosing cholangitis See *primary sclerosing cholangitis.*

sclerosing panencephalitis, subacute See *subacute sclerosing panencephalitis.*

sclerosis Localized hardening of skin. Sclerosis is generally caused by underlying diseases, such as diabetes and scleroderma. Treatment is directed toward the cause.

sclerosis, multiple See *multiple sclerosis.*

scoliosis Lateral (sideways) curving of the spine. The degree of scoliosis may range from mild to severe. Of every 1,000 children, 3 to 5 develop spinal curvature that is considered severe enough to need treatment. Adolescent idiopathic (of unknown cause) scoliosis is the most common type and appears after the age of 10, commonly in teens. Girls are more likely than boys to have this type of scoliosis. Scoliosis can run in families, so a child who has a parent, brother, or sister with idiopathic scoliosis should be checked regularly for this condition.

Severe scoliosis may require treatment that includes bracing, casting , surgical correction, and/or physical therapy.

scoliosis, acquired Lateral (sideways) curving of the spine that is neither present at birth nor results from a condition that is present at birth.

scoliosis, congenital Lateral (sideways) curving of the spine that is present at birth or is due to a condition that is present at birth. The condition may, for example, be a neuromuscular abnormality or be due to a malformation of the vertebral column.

scoliosis, functional Lateral (sideways) curving in a structurally normal spine. For example, functional scoliosis can be caused by pain on one side of the back that results in splinting. Also known as nonstructural scoliosis.

scoliosis, idiopathic Lateral (sideways) curving of the spine whose cause is unknown.

scoliosis, structural A fixed lateral (sideways) curve of the spine. The causes of structural scoliosis include cerebral palsy, polio, muscular dystrophy, Marfan syndrome, infections of the spine, and tumors of the spine. Structural scoliosis is different from functional scoliosis, in which the spine appears to have a lateral curve (scoliosis) but is structurally normal.

score, Apgar See *Apgar score.*

scrape An abrasion or cut that is caused by something rubbing roughly against the skin. To treat a scrape, one should wash the area with soap and water and keep it clean and dry. Alcohol, hydrogen peroxide, and iodine can delay healing and should be avoided. If a person with a scrape thinks he or she might need stitches, the person should seek medical care as any delay can increase the rate of wound infection. Redness, swelling, increased pain, and pus indicate infection that requires professional care.

scratch test for allergy See *allergy skin test.*

scrofula Tuberculosis of the lymph nodes in the neck. Also known in the past as the King's evil. See also *tuberculosis.*

scrotum A pouch of skin that contains the testes, epididymides, and lower portions of the spermatic cords.

scrub typhus See *typhus, scrub.*

scurvy A disorder that is caused by lack of vitamin C. Symptoms include anemia; soft, bleeding gums; and bumps under the skin near muscles. Scurvy in early childhood can cause musculoskeletal problems. Treatment involves including foods that are high in vitamin C in the diet and taking vitamin C supplements if necessary.

seasonal affective disorder   Depression that tends to occur (and recur) as the days grow shorter in the fall and winter. Affected persons may react adversely to decreasing amounts of light or colder temperatures, which affect the production of neurotransmitters in the brain. Also known as winter blues, winter depression, and hibernation reaction. Abbreviated SAD.

sebaceous cyst   See *cyst, sebaceous.*

sebaceous gland   See *gland, sebaceous.*

seborrhea   See *dandruff.*

seborrheic keratosis   See *keratosis, seborrheic.*

sebum   An oily secretion of the sebaceous glands that helps to preserve the flexibility of the hair and retain moisture in the skin. Sebum is also secreted by the Meibomian glands of the eyes. See also *gland, Meibomian.*

Seckel syndrome   An inherited form of dwarfism that features a small bird-like head, a receding forehead, large eyes, low ears, prominent beak-like protrusion of the nose, and small chin. Defects of bones in the arms and legs, dislocations of the elbow and hip, and inability to straighten the knees are common in Seckel syndrome. In boys with Seckel syndrome, the testes often fail to descend into the scrotum. About half of patients with Seckel syndrome have IQs below 50. The syndrome is inherited in an autosomal recessive manner. It can be due to genes on chromosomes 3 and 18. Also known as bird-headed dwarfism, microcephalic primordial dwarfism, nanocephalic dwarfism, and Seckel-type dwarfism. See also *dwarfism.*

second cranial nerve   See *optic nerve.*

second stage of labor   The part of labor that lasts from the full dilatation of the cervix until the baby is completely out of the birth canal. Also known as the stage of expulsion. See also *labor.*

secondary amenorrhea   See *amenorrhea, secondary.*

secondhand smoke   Smoke that comes from the burning end of a cigarette or that is exhaled by smokers. Inhalation of secondhand smoke is called involuntary or passive smoking. It can cause the same illnesses that actually smoking cigarettes causes. If someone in a person's house or restaurant or office smokes, that person is getting the same effects as the smoker because he or she can get lung cancer and the other deadly diseases associated with smoking. Also known as environmental tobacco smoke (ETS).

secretary's knee   See *patellofemoral syndrome.*

secretin   A hormone that is made by glands in the small intestine and that stimulates pancreatic secretion and may

have other effects as well. Secretin is often administered as part of the endoscopy process. In 1999, several research centers began studies on using secretin as a treatment for autism. Commercially available secretin is either porcine (from pigs) or a synthesized form of human secretin.

section   **1** In anatomy, a slice of tissue. A biopsy obtained via surgery is usually sectioned (sliced), and these sections are inspected under a microscope.   **2** In obstetrics, short for caesarean section. **3** In surgery, the division of tissue during an operation.

section, caesarean   See *caesarean section.*

section, cross   See *cross-section.*

section, longitudinal   See *longitudinal section.*

section, lower segment caesarean   See *caesarean section, lower segment.*

sedative   A drug that calms a patient, easing agitation and permitting sleep. Sedatives generally work by modulating signals within the central nervous system. If sedatives are misused or accidentally combined, as in the case of combining prescription sedatives with alcohol, they can dangerously depress important signals that are needed to maintain heart and lung function. Most sedatives also have addictive potential. For these reasons, sedatives should be used under supervision and only as necessary.

sedimentation rate   A blood test that detects and monitors inflammation in the body. Abbreviated sed rate. The sed rate measures the rate at which red blood cells in a test tube separate from blood serum over time, becoming sediment at the bottom of the test tube. The sed rate increases as inflammation increases. The sed rate can also become elevated in diseases that feature the production of abnormal proteins, such as multiple myeloma. Also known as erythrocyte sedimentation rate, or ESR.

Segawa dystonia   See *dopa-responsive dystonia.*

seizure   Uncontrolled electrical activity in the brain that may produce a physical convulsion, minor physical signs, thought disturbances, or a combination of symptoms. The type of symptoms and seizures experienced depend on where the abnormal electrical activity takes place in the brain, what its root cause is, and such factors as the patient's age and general state of health. Seizures can be caused by head injuries, brain tumors, lead poisoning, maldevelopment of the brain, genetic and infectious illnesses, and fevers. In half of patients with seizures, no cause can yet be found. See also *epilepsy; seizure disorder.*

seizure, absence   A seizure that takes the form of a staring spell: The person suddenly seems to be "absent." There is a brief loss of awareness, which can be accompanied by blinking or mouth twitching. Absence seizures have a very characteristic appearance on an EEG. Also known as petit mal seizure.

seizure, atonic A seizure in which the person suddenly loses muscle tone and cannot sit or stand upright. Also known as drop attack and drop seizure.

seizure, complex partial A form of partial seizure during which the person loses awareness. The patient does not actually become unconscious, and he or she may carry out actions as complex as walking, talking, or driving. The patient may have physical, sensory, and thought disturbances. When the seizure ends, the patient has no memory of those actions. See also *seizure, partial; fugue state.*

seizure disorder One of a great many medical conditions that are characterized by episodes of uncontrolled electrical activity in the brain (seizures). Some seizure disorders are hereditary, and others are caused by birth defects or environmental hazards, such as lead poisoning. Seizure disorders are more likely to develop in patients who have other neurological disorders, psychiatric conditions, or immune system problems than in others. In some cases, uncontrolled seizures can cause brain damage, lowered intelligence, and permanent mental and physical impairment. Diagnosis is made via observation, neurological examination, electroencephalogram (EEG), and in some cases, more advanced brain-imaging techniques. Treatment usually involves use of medication, although in difficult cases a special diet (ketogenic diet) or brain surgery may be tried. See also *epilepsy; seizure.*

seizure, drop See *seizure, atonic.*

seizure, febrile A convulsion that occurs in association with a fever. Febrile seizures are common in infants and young children and are usually of no lasting importance.

seizure, focal See *seizure, partial.*

seizure, grand mal See *seizure, tonic-clonic.*

seizure, Jacksonian A form of seizure that involves brief alterations in movement, sensation, or nerve function that is caused by abnormal electrical activity in a localized area of the brain. Jacksonian seizures typically cause no change in awareness or alertness. They are transient, fleeting, and ephemeral.

seizure, local See *seizure, partial.*

seizure, myoclonic A seizure that is characterized by jerking (myoclonic) movements of a muscle or muscle group, without loss of consciousness.

seizure, partial A seizure that affects only one part of the brain. Symptoms depend on which part of the brain is affected: One part of the body, or multiple body parts

confined to one side of the body, may start to twitch uncontrollably. Partial seizures may involve head turning, eye movements, lip smacking, mouth movements, drooling, rhythmic muscle contractions in a part of the body, apparently purposeful movements, abnormal numbness, tingling, and a crawling sensation over the skin. Partial seizures can also include sensory disturbances, such as smelling or hearing things that are not there or having a sudden flood of emotions. Although the patient may feel confused, consciousness is not lost. Also known as focal seizure and local seizure. See also *seizure, complex partial.*

seizure, petit mal See *seizure, absence.*

seizure, tonic-clonic The most obvious type of seizure, which has two parts: the tonic phase (in which the body becomes rigid) and the clonic phase (in which there is uncontrolled jerking). Tonic-clonic seizures may or may not be preceded by auras, and they are often followed by headache, confusion, and sleep. They may last for mere seconds or continue for several minutes. If a tonic-clonic seizure does not resolve or if such seizures follow each other in rapid succession, the patient needs emergency help. The patient could be in a life-threatening state known as status epilepticus. Also known as grand mal seizure. See also *status epilepticus.*

selective estrogen-receptor modulator A designer estrogen that possesses some, but not all, of the actions of estrogen. For example, raloxifene (brand name: Evista) prevents bone loss and lowers serum cholesterol as estrogen does, but unlike estrogen, it does not stimulate the endometrial lining of the uterus. Abbreviated SERM. See also *designer estrogen.*

selective mutism An inability to speak in certain situations. See also *apraxia; autism; elective mutism; mutism; social phobia.*

selective serotonin reuptake inhibitor See *SSRI.*

selenium An essential mineral that is a component of an antioxidant enzyme, glutathione reductase, that is key in tissue respiration. The National Academy of Sciences recommends 70 mg per day of selenium for men and 55 mg per day for women. Food sources of selenium include seafoods; some meats, such as kidney and liver; and some grains and seeds. Too much selenium may cause reversible balding and changes in the nails, give a garlic odor to the breath, and cause intestinal distress, weakness, and slowed mental functioning. Deficiency of selenium causes Keshan disease.

selenium deficiency See *deficiency, selenium.*

seminal vesicle One of two structures that are about 5 cm long and are located behind the bladder and above the prostate gland. The seminal vesicles contribute fluid to the ejaculate.

senile keratosis　See *keratosis, actinic.*

sensory　Relating to sensation, to the perception of a stimulus, to the voyage made by incoming nerve impulses from the sense organs to the nerve centersor to the senses themselves.

sensory integration　A form of occupational therapy in which special exercises are used to strengthen the patient's sense of touch (tactile), sense of balance (vestibular), and sense of where the body and its parts are in space (proprioceptive). Sensory integration appears to be effective for helping patients with movement disorders or severe under- or oversensitivity to sensory input. See also *occupational therapy.*

sentinel lymph node　See *lymph node, sentinel.*

sentinel-lymph-node biopsy　See *biopsy, sentinel-lymph-node.*

sepsis　The presence of bacteria (bacteremia), other infectious organisms, or toxins created by infectious organisms in the blood or in other tissues of the body. Sepsis may be associated with clinical symptoms of systemic illness, such as fever, chills, malaise, low blood pressure, and mental-status changes. Sepsis can be a serious situation, a life-threatening disease that calls for urgent and comprehensive care. Treatment depends on the type of infection but usually begins with antibiotics or similar medications. Also known as blood poisoning and septicemia.

sepsis, neonatal　A serious blood bacterial infection in an infant less than 4 weeks of age. Babies with sepsis may be listless, overly sleepy, floppy, weak, and very pale. Treatment involves urgent antibiotics and intravenous fluids.

septal defect, atrial　See *atrial septal defect.*

septal defect, ventricular　See *ventricular septal defect.*

septate　Divided. For example, a septate uterus is one that is divided.

septate vagina　See *vagina, septate.*

septic　Infected, or denoting infection. For example, septic shock is shock that is caused by infection.

septic arthritis　See *arthritis, septic.*

septic bursitis　See *bursitis, septic.*

septicemia　See *sepsis.*

septorhinoplasty　A surgical procedure that is done on the nose and the nasal septum to remove any internal obstructions that may be blocking breathing through the nose. See also *rhinoplasty.*

septum　A dividing wall or enclosure. For example, the septum of the nose is the thin cartilage that divides the left and right chambers of the nose from each other.

septum, atrial　The wall between the right and left atria (the upper chambers) of the heart. Also known as interatrial septum.

septum, cardiac　The dividing wall between the right and left sides of the heart. The portion of the septum that separates the right and left atria of the heart is termed the atrial (or interatrial) septum. The portion of the septum that lies between the right and left ventricles of the heart is called the ventricular (or interventricular) septum. Also known as heart septum.

septum, heart　See *septum, cardiac.*

septum, interatrial　See *septum, atrial.*

septum, interventricular　See *septum, ventricular.*

septum, nasal　The dividing wall that runs down the middle of the nose, creating two nasal passages, each ending in a nostril.

septum, ventricular　The wall between the two lower chambers (ventricles) of the heart. Also known as interventricular septum.

sequencing　Determining the order of nucleotides (base sequences) in a DNA or RNA molecule, or determining the order of amino acids in a protein.

SERM　Selective estrogen-receptor modulator.

seroconversion　The development of detectable antibodies in the blood that are directed against an infectious agent. Antibodies do not usually develop until some time after the initial exposure to the agent. Following seroconversion, a person tests positive for the antibody when given tests that are based on the presence of antibodies, such as ELISA.

serositis　Inflammation of the serous tissues of the body (the tissues that line the lungs, heart, abdomen, and inner abdominal organs).

serotonin　A neurotransmitter that is involved in the transmission of nerve impulses. Serotonin can trigger the release of substances in the blood vessels of the brain that in turn cause the pain of migraine. Serotonin is also key to mood regulation; pain perception; gastrointestinal function, including perception of hunger and satiety; and other physical functions.

serotype   The kind of microorganism that is characterized, through serologic typing of its surface, by recognizable antigens.

serous tissue   The tissue that lines the lungs, heart, abdomen, and inner abdominal organs. Serous tissue acts as a protective lining by providing a lubricating fluid that reduces friction forces between internal organs.

serum   **1** The clear liquid that can be separated from clotted blood. Serum differs from plasma, the liquid portion of normal unclotted blood, which contains the red cells, white cells, and platelets. The clot makes the difference between serum and plasma.   **2** Any normal or pathological fluid that resembles serum, as, for example, the fluid in a blister.

serum glutamic oxaloacetic transaminase   See *aspartate aminotransferase.*

serum glutamic pyruvic transaminase   See *alanine aminotransferase.*

serum hepatitis   See *hepatitis B.*

sesamoid bone   A little bone that is embedded in a joint capsule or tendon. For example, the kneecap (patella) is a sesamoid bone.

seven-day measles   See *measles.*

seventh cranial nerve   See *facial nerve.*

seventh cranial nerve paralysis   See *Bell's palsy.*

Sever condition   See *apophysitis calcaneus.*

severe acute respiratory syndrome   Abbreviated SARS. A serious, sometimes fatal, form of pneumonia due to a novel coronavirus. SARS first appeared in an outbreak late in 2002.

severe congenital neutropenia   A genetic disorder of the bone marrow that is evident at birth and characterized by a lack of neutrophils (white blood cells that are important in fighting infection). Children with severe congenital neutropenia suffer from frequent bacterial (but not viral or fungal) infections. They are also at increased risk for acute myelogenous leukemia (AML) and myelodysplasia. Autosomal dominant and sporadic forms of severe congenital neutropenia are caused by mutation in the neutrophil elastase gene (ELA2) on chromosome 19. There is an X-linked recessive form of severe congenital neutropenia in males that is caused by mutation in the WAS gene (which is also mutant in Wiskott-Aldrich syndrome). Treatment of severe congenital neutropenia involves use of recombinant human granulocyte colony–stimulating factor (GCSF). GCSF elevates the neutrophil count, helps resolve preexisting infections, diminishes the number of new infections, and results in significant improvements in survival and quality of life. Patients treated with GCSF may nonetheless develop leukemia or myelodysplastic syndrome. Also known as Kostmann disease and infantile genetic agranulocytosis.

sex chromosome   See *chromosome, sex.*

sexual child abuse   See *child abuse, sexual.*

sexually transmitted disease   Any disease that is transmitted via sexual contact; is caused by microorganisms that survive on the skin or mucous membranes of the genital area; or is transmitted via semen, vaginal secretions, or blood during intercourse. Abbreviated STD. Because the genital area provides a moist, warm environment that is especially conducive to the proliferation of bacteria, viruses, and yeasts, a great many diseases can be transmitted sexually. STDs include AIDS, chlamydia, genital herpes, genital warts, gonorrhea, syphilis, yeast infections, human papilloma virus, and some forms of hepatitis. Also known as a venereal disease. See also *sexually transmitted disease in men; sexually transmitted disease in women.*

sexually transmitted disease in men   Sexually transmitted disease (STD) as it affects men. Men can contract all the known STDs but may have no symptoms or have different symptoms than women do. For example, most men who have chlamydia have no symptoms at all but can easily pass the infection on to their sexual partners. The only sure protection against STDs is sexual abstinence. For sexually active men, the use of nonpenetrative sex practices (safe sex), condoms, dental dams, and spermicide with Nonoxynol-9 spermicide offer some protection.

sexually transmitted disease in women   Sexually transmitted disease (STD) as it affects women. Women can contract all the known STDs but may have no symptoms or have different symptoms than men do. For example, women infected with gonorrhea may not have any symptoms but may have a severe pelvic infection later, and they can pass the disease on to their sexual partners. Women can transmit STDs to their babies before, at, or after birth.

SGA   Small for gestational age.

SGOT   Serum glutamic oxaloacetic transaminase. See *aspartate aminotransferase.*

SGPT   Serum glutamic pyruvic transaminase. See *alanine aminotransferase.*

shaken baby syndrome   Characteristic injuries caused by violently shaking an infant. Shaken baby syndrome has distinctive features, including hemorrhage (bleeding) into the retina, hemorrhage and swelling of the brain, and patterned bruising and fractures (breaks) of the child's ribs or bones where they have been twisted from the shaking. Shaken baby syndrome is the most common cause of infant death due to head injuries and one of the most serious kinds of child abuse.

shaking palsy   See *Parkinson's disease.*

sharp   Medical slang for a needle or a similar pointed object.

shell shock   See *post-traumatic stress disorder.*

shigella   A group of bacteria that normally inhabit the intestinal tract and can cause infantile gastroenteritis, summer diarrhea of childhood (a common cause of death for children in the mid-19th century), and various forms of dysentery, including epidemic and opportunistic bacillary dysentery.

shigellosis   Epidemic and opportunistic (causes disease when the immune system is suppressed) dysentery that is due to infection with shigella bacteria. Shigellosis causes intestinal pain and diarrhea, with mucus and blood in the stool. It is especially common in tropical countries but frequently occurs elsewhere. It is a particular hazard for people with AIDS or other immunodeficiency states. Treatment is with antibiotics against the shigella bacteria.

shin splint   An inflammatory condition of the front part of the tibia (the big bone in the leg) that results from overuse, as, for example, from running too much on hard roads or sidewalks. Shin splints are due to injury to the posterior peroneal tendon, ligaments, and adjacent tissues in the front (anterior) of the leg. The pain from shin splints is usually noticed early in exercise, then it lessens, and then it reappears later, during running or other activity. Characteristically, the pain is dull at first but intensifies with continuing trauma. Shin splints may make running extremely difficult. Treatment involves a multifaceted approach of "relative rest" and stretching exercises to restore the person to a pain-free state.

shinbone   See *tibia.*

shinbone fever   See *trench fever.*

shingles   An acute infection caused by the virus herpes zoster, which also causes chickenpox. Shingles usually emerges in adulthood after exposure to chickenpox or reactivation of the chickenpox virus, which can remain latent in body tissues for years, until the immune system is weakened. Treatment involves use of antiviral medication and pain medication. Shingles can be an extraordinarily painful condition that involves inflammation of sensory nerves. Shingles typically causes a localized pain in the area of involvement of shingles with inflammation of the nerves of sensation. When such pain persists beyond 1

month, it is referred to as postherpetic neuralgia. Shingles pain can be severe and debilitating, and it occurs primarily in persons over age 50. Shingles pain can be reduced by a number of medications. Tricyclic antidepressant medications such as amitriptyline (brand name: Elavil) and antiseizure medications such as gabapentin (brand name: Neurontin) have been used. Capsaicin cream, a derivative of hot chili peppers, can be used topically after all blisters have healed. Acupuncture and electric nerve stimulation through the skin can be helpful for some patients. See also *neuralgia, postherpetic.*

shock   In medicine, a critical condition that is brought on by a sudden drop in blood flow through the body. The circulatory system fails to maintain adequate blood flow, sharply curtailing the delivery of oxygen and nutrients to vital organs. It also compromises the kidneys and so curtails the removal of wastes from the body. Shock can be due to a number of different mechanisms, including not enough blood volume and not enough output of blood by the heart. The signs and symptoms of shock include low blood pressure (hypotension); overbreathing (hyperventilation); a weak, rapid pulse; cold, clammy, grayish-bluish (cyanotic) skin; decreased urine flow (oliguria); and a sense of great anxiety and foreboding, confusion, and sometimes combativeness. Shock, which is a major medical emergency, is common after serious injury. Emergency care for shock involves keeping the patient warm and giving fluids by mouth or, if necessary, intravenously.

shock, anaphylactic   See *anaphylactic shock.*

shock, cardiogenic   Shock due to low blood output by the heart, most often seen in conjunction with heart failure or heart attack (myocardial infarction). In cardiogenic shock, the heart fails to pump blood effectively. For example, a heart attack (myocardial infarction) can cause an abnormal, ineffectual heartbeat (arrhythmia) with very slow, rapid, or irregular contractions of the heart, impairing the heart's ability to pump blood and lowering the volume of blood going to vital organs. Cardiogenic shock can also be due to drugs that reduce heart function or an abnormally low level of oxygen in the blood (hypoxemia) that may be caused, for instance, by lung disease. Whatever the cause of cardiogenic shock, the blood vessels constrict, and adrenaline-like substances are secreted into the bloodstream, increasing the heart rate. Treatment of cardiogenic shock is aimed at improving the heart's function. Cardiogenic shock is extremely serious. The mortality rate is over 80 percent.

shock, diabetic   See *diabetic shock.*

shock, electric   See *electric shock.*

shock, hemorrhagic Shock due to serious loss of blood. Symptoms include dizziness and loss of consciousness. Treatment includes intravenous fluids and blood transfusion. See also *shock, hypovolemic.*

shock, hypovolemic Shock due to a decrease in blood volume from bleeding, loss of blood plasma through severe burns, or dehydration. Symptoms include dizziness and loss of consciousness. This is the most frequent cause of shock. The primary treatment for hypovolemic shock is prompt intravenous administration of fluid and blood transfusion if necessary. See also *shock, secondary.*

shock, insulin See *insulin shock.*

shock, psychological See *post-traumatic stress disorder.*

shock, septic Shock caused by bloodstream infection. Symptoms include dizziness and loss of consciousness. Treatment includes intravenous fluids and antibiotics. See also *sepsis.*

shock, shell See *post-traumatic stress disorder.*

shock, spinal Shock caused by injury to the spinal cord. Symptoms include numbness, tingling, loss of feeling sensation, dizziness and loss of consciousness.

shock treatment See *electroconvulsive therapy.*

shock, vasogenic Shock caused by widening of the blood vessels, usually from medication. Symptoms include dizziness and loss of consciousness. Treatment includes lying supine, discontinuing the offending medication (if present), and fluid administration.

short arm of a chromosome See *p arm of a chromosome.*

short-term memory See *memory, short-term.*

shot, allergy See *allergy desensitization.*

shot, flu See *influenza vaccine.*

shoulder A structure that is made up of two main bones: the scapula (shoulder blade) and the humerus (the long bone of the upper arm). The end of the scapula, called the glenoid, is a socket into which the head of the humerus fits, forming a flexible ball-and-socket joint. The scapula is an unusually shaped bone. It extends up and around the shoulder joint at the rear to create a roof called the acromion, and it extends around the shoulder joint at the front to constitute the coracoid process. See also *shoulder joint.*

shoulder blade See *scapula.*

shoulder bursitis See *bursitis, shoulder.*

shoulder, frozen See *frozen shoulder.*

shoulder joint The flexible ball-and-socket joint that is formed by the junction of the humerus and the scapula. The shoulder joint is cushioned by cartilage that covers the face of the glenoid socket and the head of the humerus. The joint is stabilized by a ring of fibrous cartilage (labrum) around the glenoid socket. Ligaments connect the bones of the shoulder, and tendons join these bones to surrounding muscles. The biceps tendon attaches the biceps muscle to the shoulder and helps stabilize the joint. Four short muscles that originate on the scapula pass around the shoulder, where their tendons fuse together to form the rotator cuff. See also *shoulder.*

show, bloody See *bloody show.*

Shulman syndrome See *eosinophilic fasciitis.*

shunt **1** To move a body fluid, such as cerebrospinal fluid, from one place to another. **2** A vessel (tube) that is used as a passageway to transport fluid from one body area to another. For example, a spinal shunt carries cerebrospinal fluid from a ventricle in the brain to another area of the body. A shunt may be placed to relieve pressure due to hydrocephalus, for example.

shunt, ventriculoatrial A shunt that is used to drain fluid from the cerebral ventricle into the right atrium of the heart.

shunt, ventriculoperitoneal A shunt that is used to drain fluid from the cerebral ventricle into the abdomen.

shunt, ventriculopleural A shunt that is used to drain fluid from the cerebral ventricle into the chest cavity.

Siamese twins Identical (monozygotic) twins that do not separate fully from one another but remain partially united due to the incomplete division of one fertilized ovum. Such twins are known medically as conjoined twins. Conjoined twins are popularly known as Siamese twins after Chang and Eng, the celebrated conjoined Chinese twins born in Siam (Thailand) in the early 19th century. Depending on the anatomy of the union, surgical procedures can be done that separate conjoined twins.

sibling A brother or sister.

sibship The relationship between the children born to a set of parents.

sicca syndrome See *Sjogren's syndrome.*

sick sinus syndrome A condition that features symptoms including dizziness, confusion, fainting, and heart failure that is due to a problem with the sinoatrial node

(SA node) of the heart, which acts as the body's natural pacemaker. If the SA node is not functioning normally, the patient has an abnormally slow heart rate (bradycardia). This can cause poor pumping by the heart, which can impair the circulation. Diagnosis is usually made via electrocardiogram (EKG). Treatment includes use of medications, such as calcium antagonists.

sickle cell anemia   See *anemia, sickle cell.*

sickle cell disease   See *anemia, sickle cell.*

sickle cell trait   The condition in which a person has only one copy of the gene for sickle cell (and is called a sickle heterozygote) but does not have sickle cell disease (which requires two copies of the sickle cell gene). If two people with sickle cell trait mate and have children together, each of their children has a 25 percent chance of having sickle cell disease.

sickle hemoglobin   See *hemoglobin S.*

sickness, altitude   See *altitude sickness.*

sickness, motion   See *motion sickness.*

sickness, mountain   See *altitude sickness.*

side effect   **1** Problems that occur when treatment goes beyond the desired effect. An example is hemorrhage due to the use of too much anticoagulant (bloodthinner). **2** Problems that occur in addition to the desired therapeutic effect. For example, the common side effects of cancer treatment include fatigue, nausea, vomiting, decreased blood cell counts, hair loss, and mouth sores.

SIDS   Sudden infant death syndrome.

sig   Signature.

sight, day   See *nyctanopia.*

sigmoid   In human anatomy, the lower colon (the lower portion of the large bowel). *Sigmoid* is short for *sigmoid colon.* From the Greek letter sigma. which is shaped like a C. *Sigmoid* also means curved in two directions like the letter S. For example, a sigmoid curve is an S-shaped curve.

sigmoidoscope   A lighted instrument that is used to view the inside of the lower colon.

sigmoidoscopy   A procedure in which a physician inserts a viewing tube (sigmoidoscope) into the rectum for the purpose of inspecting the lower colon and rectum. If an abnormal area is detected, a biopsy can be performed.

sign   Any objective evidence of disease, as opposed to a symptom, which is, by nature, subjective. For example,

gross blood in the stool is a sign of disease; it is evidence that can be recognized by the patient, physician, nurse, or someone else. Abdominal pain is a symptom; it is something only the patient can perceive.

signature   **1** The part of the prescription that contains the physician's directions to the patient. For example, the signature might say "take twice daily with food." Also known as sig.   **2** The outward appearance of a natural object, which was once taken as a token of its special properties. This ancient doctrine of signatures led some to conclude that the walnut, which looks something like a tiny brain, could be used to heal brain problems; the liverwort plant, which has a three-lobed liver-like leaf, was useful in treating liver disease; and so on. Not many physicians accept such fanciful ideas today.

SIL   Squamous intraepithelial lesion.

silver   A metal that is used in some medications and in many natural remedies. Used in the past in silver amalgam for filling cavities in teeth. Silver has antibiotic properties. However, overuse of silver or use of products containing silver by people with certain health conditions can result in silver poisoning (argyria). See also *argyria.*

silver poisoning   See *argyria.*

single gene disease   See *disease, single gene.*

singultus   See *hiccup.*

sinoatrial node   The heart's natural pacemaker, one of the major elements in the cardiac conduction system, the system that controls the heart rate. Abbreviated SA node. The SA node consists of a cluster of cells that are situated in the upper part of the wall of the heart's right atrium, where the electrical impulses are generated. An electrical signal generated by the SA node moves from cell to cell, down through the heart, until it reaches the atrioventricular (AV) node, a cluster of cells situated in the center of the heart, between the atria and ventricles. The AV node serves as a gate, slowing the electrical current before the signal is permitted to pass down to the ventricles. This delay ensures that the atria have a chance to fully contract before the ventricles are stimulated. After passing the AV node, the electrical current travels to the ventricles along special fibers embedded in the walls of the lower part of the heart. The autonomic nervous system controls the firing of the SA node to trigger the start of this cardiac cycle. The autonomic nervous system can transmit a message quickly to the SA node, so it in turn can increase the heart rate to twice the normal rate within only 3 to 5 seconds. This rapid response is important during exercise, when the heart has to increase its beating speed to keep up with the body's heightened demand for oxygen. Also known as sinus node.

sinus 1 An air-filled cavity in a dense portion of a skull bone. The sinuses decrease the weight of the skull. The sinuses are formed in four right-left pairs. The frontal sinuses are positioned behind the forehead, while the maxillary sinuses are behind the cheeks. The sphenoid and ethmoid sinuses are deeper in the skull behind the eyes and maxillary sinuses. The sinuses are lined by mucous-secreting cells. Air enters the sinuses through small openings in the bone called ostia. If an ostium is blocked, air cannot pass into the sinus and likewise mucous cannot drain out. See also *sinusits.* 2 A channel permitting the passage of blood or lymph fluid that is not a blood or lymphatic vessel, such as the sinuses of the placenta. 3 A tract or fistula leading to a cavity which may be filled with pus.

sinus barotrauma See *aerosinusitis.*

sinus, cavernous See *cavernous sinus.*

sinus headache See *headache, sinus.*

sinus node See *sinoatrial node.*

sinus rhythm The normal regular rhythm of the heart that is set by the sinoatrial (or sinus) node, which is located in the wall of the right atrium (the right upper chamber of the heart). Normal electrical impulses of the heart start there and are transmitted to the atria and down to the ventricles (the lower chambers of the heart). The lack of normal sinus rhythm is an arrhythmia (abnormal heart rhythm). Sinus arrhythmia refers to the normal increase in heart rate that occurs during inspiration (breathing in). It is a normal response and is more accentuated in children than in adults. See also *sinus tachycardia.*

sinus tachycardia Fast heartbeat (tachycardia) that occurs because of overly rapid firing by the sinoatrial node. Sinus tachycardia is usually a rapid contraction of a normal heart in response to a condition, drug, or disease, such as pain, fever, excessive thyroid hormone, exertion, excitement, low blood oxygen level (hypoxia), or stimulant drugs, such as caffeine, cocaine, and amphetamines. However, in some cases sinus tachycardia can be a sign of heart failure, heart valve disease, or other illness.

sinusitis Inflammation of the lining membrane in any of the hollow areas (sinuses) of the skull around the nose. Sinusitis may be caused by anything that interferes with air-flow into the sinuses and the drainage of mucous out of the sinuses. The sinus openings, called ostia, may be obstructed by swelling of the tissue lining the ostia and adjacent nasal passage tissue; for example, from colds, allergies, and tissue irritants (nasal sprays, cocaine, cigarette smoke). Less commonly, sinuses can become obstructed by tumors or growths. Stagnated mucous then provides a perfect environment for bacterial infection.

The common symptoms of sinusitis include headache, facial tenderness or pain, fever, cloudy, discolored nasal drainage, a feeling of nasal stuffiness, sore throat, and cough. Acute sinusitis is usually treated with antibiotic therapy. Chronic forms of sinusitis require long courses of antibiotics and may require a sinus drainage procedure.

situational syncope See *syncope, situational.*

situs inversus totalis See *reversal of organs, total.*

sixth cranial nerve See *abducent nerve.*

sixth disease See *measles.*

Sjogren's syndrome An autoimmune disease that classically combines dry eyes, dry mouth, and another disease of the connective tissues, commonly rheumatoid arthritis, but sometimes lupus, scleroderma, polymyositis, or another autoimmune condition. Sjogren's syndrome is an inflammatory disease of glands and other tissues of the body. Inflammation of the glands that produce tears (lacrimal glands) leads to decreased tears and dry eyes. Inflammation of the glands that produce saliva in the mouth (salivary glands, including the parotid glands) leads to dry mouth. Sjogren's syndrome can consequently be complicated by infections of the eyes, breathing passages, and mouth. About 90 percent of Sjogren's syndrome patients are female, usually middle aged or older. Diagnostic clues include the presence of antibodies that are directed against a variety of body tissues (autoantibodies). Diagnosis can be made via biopsy of an affected gland. Treatment is directed toward the particular areas of the body involved and to complications, such as infection. Also known as keratoconjunctivitis sicca and sicca syndrome.

skeletal Pertaining to the skeleton, the bones of the body that collectively provide the frame for the body.

skeletal dysplasia One of a large contingent of genetic diseases in which the bony skeleton forms abnormally during fetal development. Achondroplasia is one form of skeletal dysplasia.

skeletal muscle Along with smooth and cardiac muscle, one of the types of muscle tissue in the body. Skeletal muscle represents the majority of muscle tissue. It is the type of muscle that powers movement of the skeleton, as in walking and lifting.

skeleton The framework of the body, which is composed of 206 bones. See also *bones of the arm, wrist, and hand; bones of the head; bones of the leg, ankle, and foot; bones of the trunk.*

skin The body's outer covering, which protects against heat and light, injury, and infection. Skin regulates body temperature and stores water, fat, and vitamin D. The skin, which weighs about 6 pounds, is the body's largest organ. It is made up of two main layers: the epidermis and the dermis. The outer layer of the skin (epidermis) is mostly made up of flat, scale-like cells called squamous cells. Under the squamous cells are round cells called basal cells. The deepest part of the epidermis also contains melanocytes, cells that produce melanin, which gives the skin its color. The inner layer of skin (dermis) contains blood and lymph vessels, hair follicles, and glands that produce sweat, which helps regulate body temperature, and sebum, an oily substance that helps keep the skin from drying out. Sweat and sebum reach the skin's surface through tiny openings called pores.

skin biopsy   Removal of a piece of skin for the purpose of diagnostic examination. Skin biopsy is most frequently done to diagnose skin growths, such as moles, or skin conditions, such as rashes. Different skin biopsy techniques are used in different situations. A shave biopsy takes a thin slice and can be used to remove superficial lesions. A punch biopsy takes a core and can be used to remove small lesions and to diagnose rashes and other conditions. Excisional biopsies are generally larger and deeper than shave and punch biopsies, and they are used to completely remove an abnormal area of skin (lesion), such as a skin cancer.

skin cancer   See *cancer, skin.*

skin graft   Skin used to cover an area where the patient's skin has been lost due to a burn, an injury, or surgery. The most effective skin grafts involve moving the patient's own skin from one part of the body to another. The second most effective type are skin grafts between identical twins. Beyond these two procedures, there is a strong chance that the body will reject the new skin, although the graft may protect the body and give the body time to grow new skin of its own.

skin graft, allogenic   A graft using skin from another person (not an identical twin). Also known as skin allograft.

skin graft, autologous   A graft using the patient's own skin. Also known as autogenic skin graft.

skin graft, composite   A graft technique in which both the patient's own skin and donor skin are used together.

skin graft, full-thickness   A graft technique in which sheets of skin containing both the epidermis and the dermis are used. For example, a full-thickness skin graft might be used to repair a severe burn wound.

skin graft, mesh   A graft technique in which multiple pieces of skin are carefully arranged to cover an area. This technique is used most frequently when a large area needs to be protected, as after a severe burn over a large area.

skin graft, pedicle   A graft technique in which a piece of skin from a nearby area remains attached at one of its corners, while the main part of the piece is reattached over the area that needs to be covered.

skin graft, pinch   A graft technique in which very small squares of skin are attached to the area that needs to be covered, in hopes that they will start to grow and cover the area.

skin graft, porcine   A skin graft in which pig skin is used. Like grafts from human donors, porcine grafts are usually just a short-term protective measure.

skin graft, split-thickness   A graft technique in which sheets of skin containing the epidermis and part of the dermis are used. This graft might be used when only portions of the skin have been injured, such as after a scraping injury.

skin plaque   See *plaque, skin.*

skin, scalded, syndrome   See *staphylococcal scalded skin syndrome.*

skin tag   A small tag of skin that may be squat (sessile) or on a stalk (a peduncle). Skin tags commonly occur on the eyelids, neck, armpits, upper chest, and groin. This tiny benign tumor of the skin usually causes no symptoms unless it is repeatedly irritated as, for example, by a collar. Treatment may involve freezing the skin tag with liquid nitrogen or cutting off the skin tag with a scalpel or scissors if the skin tag is irritating or cosmetically unwanted. Also known as acrochordon and cutaneous papilloma.

skin test for allergy   See *allergy skin test.*

skin test for immunity   A method of evaluating whether a person has developed an immune response to a certain infection. A substance is injected into the deep layer of the skin (dermis) and causes a reaction if the immune system recognizes it. One of the most common skin tests is the tuberculin test, which reveals whether a person has been exposed to tuberculosis. The injection is placed on the inside of the forearm, and a positive reaction results in a raised, firm area of skin at the injection site within 2 days.

skull   A collection of bones that encase the brain and give form to the head and face. These bones include the frontal, parietal, occipital, temporal, sphenoid, ethmoid, zygomatic, maxilla, nasal, vomer, palatine, inferior concha, and mandible. See also *bones of the head.*

slanted ear   See *ear, slanted.*

SLE   Systemic lupus erythematosus. See *lupus erythematosus, systemic.*

sleep The body's rest cycle. Sleep is triggered by a complex group of hormones that respond to cues from the body itself and the environment. About 80 percent of sleep is dreamless and is known as non-rapid eye movement (NREM) sleep. During NREM sleep, the breathing and heart rate are slow and regular, the blood pressure is low, and the sleeper is relatively still. NREM sleep is divided into four stages of increasing depth of sleep: Level 1 sleep is a transition period between sleep and wakefulness; Level 2 sleep features significant slowing of heartbeat and breathing and makes up about 50 percent of all sleep; and Levels 3 and 4 (delta) sleep are marked by very slow respiration and heartbeat. Level 4 sleep leads to rapid eye movement (REM) sleep, also known as Level 5 sleep. Dreams occur during three to five periods of REM sleep each night. REM sleep occurs at intervals of 1 to 2 hours and is variable in length. REM sleep is characterized by irregular breathing and heart rate and involuntary muscle jerks. Most adults need around 8 hours of sleep on a regular schedule to function well, although some require less and others more. Children, particularly teenagers, often need 9 or 10 hours for optimal functioning. See also *NREM sleep; REM sleep.*

sleep apnea Temporary stoppage of breathing during sleep, often resulting in daytime sleepiness. Treatment depends on the type of sleep apnea present. Sleep apnea is classified as obstructive or central. Sleep apnea that is associated with air passage obstruction may require losing excessive weight, avoiding alcohol and sedatives, sleeping on one side, medications to relieve nasal congestion, a breathing device, or surgical procedures. Central sleep apnea is uncommon and caused by problems in the brain that impair the signals to breathe and can require mechanical ventilation. See also *sleep apnea, central; sleep apnea, obstructive; sleep disorder.*

sleep apnea, central Brief interruptions of breathing during sleep caused by failure of the brain to send the appropriate signals to the breathing muscles to initiate respiration. Central sleep apnea is less common than obstructive sleep apnea and can require mechanical ventilation. See also *sleep apnea, obstructive.*

sleep apnea, obstructive Brief interruptions of breathing during sleep caused by physical obstruction to the flow of air. The air cannot flow through the nose or mouth, although efforts to breathe are made. The basic problem may be blockage in the mouth or nose. Sleep apnea that is associated with air passage obstruction may require losing excessive weight, avoiding alcohol and sedatives, sleeping on one side, medications to relieve nasal congestion, a breathing device, or surgical procedures. See also *sleep apnea, central.*

sleep disorder Any disorder that affects, disrupts, or involves sleep. The most common sleep disorder is snoring, although it is usually not medically significant. Insomnia, sleep apnea, restless leg syndrome, and sleepwalking are also sleep disorders. Many large medical centers have diagnostic and treatment facilities dedicated to diagnosing and treating sleep disorders. See also *sleep apnea; sleepwalking; snoring.*

sleep, non-rapid eye movement See *NREM sleep.*

sleep, NREM See *NREM sleep.*

sleep, rapid eye movement See *REM sleep.*

sleep, REM See *REM sleep.*

sleepwalking Purposeful moving, usually but not always including walking, while in a deep stage of sleep. Sleepwalking occurs most frequently in children, particularly boys. Sedatives tend to exacerbate rather than cure sleepwalking. The best measures are preventive: Ensure that the sleepwalker is in a safe room for walking and cannot accidentally fall through an open window or down stairs. Some types of sleepwalking are related to seizure disorders, bipolar disorders, and other neurological conditions, but most cases are transitory and due to unknown causes. Also known as somnambulism.

slipped capital femoral epiphysis A condition in which the growth plate of the femur is pushed out of position, causing hip pain, stiff gait, and sometimes knee pain. Abbreviated SCFE. SCFE is most common in overweight teenagers. Treatment involves orthopedic surgery to bring the bone back into alignment.

slipped disk See *herniated disk.*

slow virus A virus that has a long incubation period before the onset of a very gradual progressive disease. Typically, the diseases caused by slow viruses affect the central nervous system and are associated with a variety of nervous system symptoms while having a characteristically protracted, progressive clinical course.

sludge, biliary See *biliary sludge.*

small for gestational age In a full-term infant, weighing 2,500 g or less at birth. Abbreviated SGA. Infants who are SGA are considered to have intrauterine growth retardation, given their gestational age. By contrast, an infant may weigh 2,500 g or less simply because of prematurity.

small intestine See *intestine, small.*

small-cell lung cancer A type of lung cancer in which the cancerous cells are smaller than those in the other common forms of lung cancer (non-small-cell lung cancer). Small-cell lung cancer cells look like oats when examined under the microscope. Also known as oat-cell lung cancer. See also *non-small-cell lung cancer.*

smallpox A highly contagious and frequently fatal viral disease that is characterized by a biphasic fever and a distinctive skin rash that leaves pock marks in its wake. Because of its high case-fatality rates and transmissibility and because people haven't been vaccinated against it in years, smallpox now represents a serious bioterrorist threat. The disease is caused by the variola virus. The incubation period is about 12 days (range: 7–17 days) following exposure. Initial symptoms include high fever, fatigue, headaches, and backaches. A characteristic rash, most prominent on the face, arms, and legs, follows in 2 to 3 days. The rash starts with flat red lesions that evolve in 2 to 3 days. Lesions become pus filled and begin to crust early in the second week. Scabs develop and then separate and fall off after about 3 to 4 weeks. The majority of patients with smallpox recover, but death occurs in up to 30 percent of cases. Smallpox is spread from one person to another via infected saliva droplets that expose a susceptible person who has face-to-face contact with the ill person. Persons with smallpox are most infectious during the first week of illness because that is when the largest amount of virus is present in saliva. However, some risk of transmission lasts until all scabs have fallen off. Also known as variola.

smallpox vaccine A vaccine that contains a live virus called vaccinia that is used to prevent smallpox. The vaccine does not contain the variola virus that causes smallpox, but exposes the immune system to proteins that look like the virus so that an immune response occurs. Through the use of the vaccine, smallpox was eliminated from causing human infection in the world in 1977. Routine vaccination against smallpox ended in 1972. The level of immunity among persons who were vaccinated before 1972 is uncertain. In people exposed to smallpox who are not immune to the disease, the vaccine can lessen the severity of or even prevent the illness if given within 4 days of exposure.

smear, Pap See *Pap test.*

smell The sense that provides information about an object's scent, often giving clues to the palatability of food, the safety of air, and other matters. The organs of smell are made up of patches of tissue called the olfactory membranes that are each about the size of a postage stamp. These membranes are located in a pair of clefts just under the bridge of the nose. Most air breathed in normally flows through the nose, but only a small part reaches the olfactory clefts—just enough to get a response to an odor. When a person sniffs to detect a smell, air moves faster through the nose, increasing the flow to the olfactory clefts and carrying more odor to these sensory organs.

smoldering leukemia See *leukemia, smoldering.*

smooth muscle Along with skeletal and cardiac muscle, one of the types of muscle tissue in the body. Smooth muscle generally forms the supporting tissue of blood vessels and hollow internal organs, such as the stomach, intestine, and bladder. It is considered smooth because it does not have the microscopic lines (the striations) seen in the other two types of muscle.

snake stick See *Aesculapius.*

snakebite The bite of a snake, whether poisonous or not. Most snakes are not poisonous, but their bites can nonetheless cause painful puncture wounds that require treatment. If a snakebite victim knows a snake was poisonous, or if the person did not see or recognize the snake, he or she should immediately seek emergency treatment. The affected part should be kept immobile and below the level of the heart, and the bite victim should be taken to the nearest hospital. A tourniquet or bandage should not be used on a snakebite, and no one should attempt to suction out the wound by mouth. Treatment involves use of antivenom and care for the puncture wound itself and any symptoms that emerge, such as respiratory distress. See also *rattlesnake bite.*

Snellen chart See *chart, Snellen.*

snoring A sound created by vibrations of the uvula and soft palate during sleep. During normal breathing, air passing through the throat en route to the lungs travels by the tongue, soft palate, uvula, and tonsils. When a person is awake, the muscles in the back of the throat tighten to hold these structures in place and prevent them from collapsing and vibrating in the airway. Sometimes snoring can be a sign of obstructive sleep apnea or have repairable physical causes, in which case medical treatment may be necessary. Otherwise, patients who snore may want to try different sleep positions, nose clips, or similar steps to prevent unwanted snoring. See also *sleep apnea, obstructive; somnoplasty.*

social phobia A paralyzing fear of interacting with others. Symptoms include excessive blushing, sweating, trembling, rapid heartbeat, muscle tension, nausea, and extreme anxiety. Social phobia can occur in very young children or emerge at a later age. It can be disabling to a person's work and social and family relationships. Many people with social phobia have trouble reaching their educational and professional goals or even maintaining employment. They may depend on others financially and try to relieve anxiety by using alcohol and drugs. In extreme cases, a person with social phobia may begin to avoid all social situations and become housebound. Treatment options include using medications and cognitive-behavioral therapy, which employs exposure and response prevention. Medications for social phobias include antidepressants called selective serotonin reuptake inhibitors (SSRIs) and monoamine oxidase inhibitors (MAOIs), as well as high-potency benzodi-azepenes. People with the specific form of social phobia called performance phobia may be helped with drugs called beta blockers.

social worker   A health professional who assists individuals and families with social or emotional issues. Within the medical system, a social worker might help insured families who need medical care find help; work with grieving parents, spouses, or other family members; provide individual therapy; or help patients find resources to meet their needs for personal and community support. A social worker may have a BA or a master's in social work (MSW).

socialization   The learning process a child goes through as he or she learns how to interact appropriately with other people.

socialized medicine   A medical system like that of a socialist country, in which medical facilities and payments are under government, rather than private, control. Most industrialized nations, including the US, have medical systems under some combination of state and private control. For examples, socialized medicine is practiced in Canada and Britain.

sodium   The major positive ion (cation) in the fluid surrounding cells in the body. The chemical notation for sodium is Na+. When sodium is combined with chloride, the resulting substance is a crystal called table salt. Excess sodium (such as from fast food) is largely excreted in the urine, but too much salt in the diet tends to increase the blood pressure. Too much or too little sodium in the blood (called hypernatremia or hyponatremia respectively) can cause cells to malfunction, and extremes can be fatal. Normal blood sodium level is 135–145 milliEquivalents/liter (mEq/L) or 135–145 millimoles/liter (mmol/L) in international units.

soft palate   The muscular part of the roof of the mouth. The soft palate is directly behind the hard palate, and it lacks bone.

solar keratosis   See *keratosis, actinic.*

somatization   The normal, unconscious process by which psychological distress is expressed as physical symptoms. For example, a person with clinical depression may complain of stomach pains that prove to have no physical cause. Counseling can be helpful to overcome somatization.

somatostatin   A hormone that is widely distributed throughout the body, especially in the hypothalamus and pancreas, that acts as an important regulator of endocrine and nervous system function by inhibiting the secretion of

several other hormones such as growth hormone, insulin, and gastrin.

somatotropin   A growth that is produced by the anterior pituitary (the front part of the pituitary gland). Somatotropin acts by stimulating the release of another hormone called somatomedin by the liver, thereby causing growth to occur. Somatotropin is given to children with pituitary dwarfism (short stature due to underfunction of the anterior pituitary) to help them grow. Somatotropin is a polypeptide that contains 191 amino acids. Also known as somatropin.

somatropin   See *somatotropin.*

somnambulism   See *sleepwalking.*

somnolent   Sleepy or tending to cause sleep. From the Latin work *somnus,* meaning "sleep."

somnoplasty   A surgical treatment for snoring in which heat energy is used to remove tissues of the uvula and soft palate. Somnoplasty is usually done as an office procedure with local anesthesia. It is not indicated for the treatment of sleep apnea. See also *snoring.*

space, pleural   See *pleural space.*

span, memory   See *memory span.*

spasm   A brief, automatic jerking movement. A muscle spasm can be quite painful, with the muscle clenching tightly. A spasm of the coronary artery can cause the pain of angina. Spasms in various types of tissue may be caused by stress, medication, and overexercise.

spasm, coronary artery   See *coronary artery spasm.*

spasmodic dysphonia   See *dysphonia, spasmodic.*

spastic colitis   See *irritable bowel syndrome.*

spastic dysphonia   See *dystonia, laryngeal.*

spasticity   See *hypertonia.*

specific developmental disorder   See *developmental disorder, specific.*

specific-pathogen free   A term that is applied to animals reared for use in laboratory experiments which indicates that the animals are known to be free of germs that can cause disease. Abbreviated SPF.

speckled iris   See *Brushfield spot.*

SPECT scan   Single photon emission computed tomography scan, a nuclear medicine procedure in which a gamma camera rotates around the patient to produce images from many angles, which a computer then uses to form a tomographic (cross-sectional) image.

speculum An instrument that is used to widen the opening of the vagina so that the cervix is more easily visible.

speech, apraxia of See *apraxia of speech.*

speech disorder A disorder of the ability to produce normal speech. Speech disorders may affect articulation (phonetic or phonological disorders), fluency (stuttering or cluttering), and/or voice (tone, pitch, volume, or speed). Most speech disorders have their roots in oral-motor abnormalities, although some involve language-processing problems. A speech pathologist can diagnose speech disorders by testing the individual. See also *aphasia; apraxia of speech; articulation disorder; cluttering; stuttering.*

speech dyspraxia See *dyspraxia of speech.*

speech therapist See *speech-language pathologist.*

speech therapy The treatment of speech and communication disorders. The approach used depends on the disorder. Speech therapy may include physical exercises to strengthen the muscles used in speech (oral-motor work), speech drills to improve clarity, or sound production practice to improve articulation. See also *communication disorder; speech disorder; speech–language pathologist.*

speech–language pathologist A specialist who evaluates and treats people with communication and swallowing problems. Abbreviated SLP. An SLP has an MA or doctorate in a specialty, as well as a Certificate of Clinical Competence (CCC) earned by working under supervision. In some states a state license is also required. Formerly known as speech therapist. See also *speech therapy.*

sperm The male sex cell (gamete). The sperm has an oval head that contains its genetic matter, and it is propelled by a flagellating tail. A sperm is carried into the female reproductive tract within the semen (ejaculate). If the sperm is able to travel up into a fallopian tube, it must then break through the cell wall of the egg (the female gamete, or ovum) to fertilize the egg and form a zygote. This formation process is called fertilization. See also *fertilization; ovulation; ovum.*

spermatic cord A group of structures that go through the inguinal canal to the testis. These structures include the vas deferens, arteries, veins, lymphatic vessels, and nerves.

SPF 1 Sun protection factor. 2 Specific-pathogen free.

spherocytosis, hereditary A genetic disorder of the red blood cell membrane that is characterized by anemia, jaundice, and enlargement of the spleen (splenomegaly). Abbreviated HS. In HS, the red cells are smaller, rounder, and more fragile than normal. They have a spherical shape rather than the biconcave-disk shape of normal red cells. These rotund red cells (spherocytes) are osmotically fragile and less flexible than normal red cells, and they tend to get trapped in narrow blood passages, particularly in the spleen. If this occurs, they break up (hemolyze) where they have lodged, leading to hemolytic anemia. The clogging of the spleen with red cells almost invariably causes splenomegaly. The breakup of the red cells releases hemoglobin, and the heme part gives rise to bilirubin, the pigment of jaundice. This excess bilirubin leads to the formation of gallstones, even in childhood. Often patients with HS also have iron overload due to the excess destruction of iron-rich red cells. HS often appears in infancy or early childhood, causing anemia and jaundice. The bone marrow has to work extra hard to make more red cells, so if in the course of an ordinary viral illness the bone marrow stops making red cells, the anemia can quickly become profound; this is termed an aplastic crisis. HS is due to a deficiency of a blood cell membrane protein called erythrocytic ankyrin (ankyrin-R, ankyrin-1, or ANK1). Diagnosis is made via laboratory study of the blood, which shows evidence not only of many and distinctively shaped spherocytes but also increased numbers of young red blood cells (reticulocytes). HS is most common in people of northern European descent. The HS gene, which codes for production of ANK1, has been mapped to chromosome 8 in band 8p11.2. It is a dominant trait, so any child of a person with HS has a 50 percent chance of inheriting the gene and the disorder. Treatment involves removing the spleen (splenectomy). Although the red cell defect persists after splenectomy, the hemolysis ceases. However, because splenectomy puts young children at increased risk for overwhelming bloodstream infection (sepsis), particularly with the pneumococcus bacteria, it is usually postponed, if possible, until age 3. Before having a splenectomy, anyone with HS should have the pneumococcal vaccine. Persons with HS or another cause of brisk, ongoing hemolysis should take supplemental folic acid. The prognosis after splenectomy is for a normal life and a normal life expectancy. Also known as congenital hemolytic jaundice, severe atypical spherocytosis, spherocytosis type II, ankyrin deficiency, erythrocyte ankyrin deficiency, ankyrin-R deficiency, and ankyrin1 deficiency.

sphincter A muscle that surrounds and, by its contraction, closes a normal opening such as that from the intestinal tract or the urinary tract. Damage to the anal and urethral sphincters can cause fecal and urinary incontinence, respectively. Sphincters tend to be ring-like and, when contracted, to constrict the opening. From the Greek for "that which constricts."

sphingolipidosis One of a group of hereditary diseases that involve overproduction or accumulation of fatty substances called sphingolipids in the brain and nervous system. See also *Anderson-Fabry disease; Gaucher disease; GM1-gangliosidosis, histiocytosis, lipid; Krabbe disease; leukodystrophy; Tay-Sachs disease; Sandhoff disease.*

sphingomyelinosis See *histiocytosis, lipid.*

sphygmomanometer An instrument for measuring blood pressure, particularly in arteries. The two basic types of sphygmomanometers are the mercury column and the gauge with a dial face. The sphygmomanometer in most frequent use today consists of a gauge attached to a rubber cuff that is wrapped around the upper arm and is inflated to constrict the arteries. A blood pressure reading consists of two numbers: systolic and diastolic. Systolic refers to systole, the phase when the heart pumps blood out into the aorta. Diastolic refers to diastole, the resting period when the heart refills with blood. At each heartbeat, the blood pressure is raised to the systolic level, and, between beats, it drops to the diastolic level. With the cuff inflated with air, a stethoscope is placed over an artery (the brachial artery) in the crook of the arm. As the air in the cuff is released, the pressure reading when the first sound is heard through the stethoscope marks the systolic pressure. As the release of air from the cuff continues, a point is reached when the sound diminishes and then is no longer heard. The pressure at which the last sound is heard marks the diastolic pressure. The blood pressure reading might show the systolic and diastolic pressures to be, for example, 120 and 78mm of mercury (Hg), respectively. This is usually written 120/78 and said to be "120 over 78." Blood pressure readings vary depending on age and many other factors. Children and adults with smaller- or larger-than-average-sized arms may need special-sized pressure cuffs. See also *blood pressure; hypertension; hypotension.*

spider bite A bite from a spider. Bites from most spiders are irritating but not poisonous. Localized reddening and swelling are not unusual and should pass within a few days. A few spiders are poisonous, notably the black widow and brown recluse (brown fiddler) in the US. Bites from these spiders require emergency treatment, especially for children.

spider telangiectasia See *spider vein.*

spider vein A group of widened veins that can be seen through the surface of the skin. The wheel-and-spokes shape of the veins resembles a spider. Also known as spider telangiectasia.

spina bifida A major birth defect and a type of neural tube defect that involves an opening in the vertebral column caused by the failure of the neural tube to close properly during embryonic development. (The neural tube is the structure in the developing embryo that gives rise to the brain and spinal cord.) Because of the defect in the spine, part of the spinal cord is exposed and protrudes as a meningomyelocele. People with spina bifida often have neurological deficits below the level of the lesion and can suffer from bladder and bowel incontinence, limited mobility (due to paralysis of the legs), and learning problems. The risk of spina bifida varies according to country, ethnic group, and socioeconomic status. In the US as a whole, spina bifida occurs in 1 in every 1,000 to 2,000 births. The risk of spina bifida and other neural tube defects, such as anencephaly, can be significantly decreased if women take ample folic acid before conception and during pregnancy.

spina bifida cystica See *meningomyelocele.*

spina bifida occulta A bony defect in the vertebral column that causes a cleft in that column. The cleft remains covered by skin. Treatment is usually not required.

spinal column See *vertebral column.*

spinal cord The major column of nerve tissue that is connected to the brain and lies within the vertebral canal and from which the spinal nerves emerge. Thirty-one pairs of spinal nerves originate in the spinal cord: 8 cervical, 12 thoracic, 5 lumbar, 5 sacral, and 1 coccygeal. The spinal cord and the brain constitute the central nervous system. The spinal cord consists of nerve fibers that transmit impulses to and from the brain. Like the brain, the spinal cord is covered by three connective-tissue envelopes called the meninges. The space between the outer and middle envelopes is filled with cerebrospinal fluid (CSF), a clear colorless fluid that cushions the spinal cord against jarring shock. Also known simply as the cord.

spinal nerve One of the nerves that originates in the spinal cord. There are 31 pairs of spinal nerves: 8 cervical nerves, 12 thoracic nerves, 5 lumbar nerves, 5 sacral nerves, and 1 coccygeal nerve.

spinal stenosis Narrowing of the spinal canal. Spinal stenosis is most commonly caused by degeneration of the discs between the vertebrae. The result is compression of the nerve roots or spinal cord by bony spurs or soft tissues, such as discs, in the spinal canal. This most commonly occurs in the low back (lumbar spine) but can also occur in the neck (cervical spine) and less frequently in the upper back (thoracic spine). The symptoms of spinal stenosis vary depending on the location on the nerve tissues being irritated and the degree of irritation. The neck being affected can result in unusual sensations in the arms and/or poor leg function and incontinence. When the low back is affected, the classic symptom is pain that radiates down both legs while walking and is relieved by resting (pseudoclaudication). Persistent mechanical irritation of the nerves to the leg can have long-term consequences. If symptoms of spinal stenosis are mild, conservative measures designed to relieve the nerve irritation are taken, such as using medications to relieve inflammation, using mechanical supports, and doing back exercises. Anti-inflammatory medications can be given to reduce the swelling of tissues (disc or other local soft tissues) that are pressing against the nerves. When symptoms are severe, persistent, and intolerable, surgical resection of the bone and soft tissues that are impinging on the nerves and/or spinal cord can be helpful.

spinal tap See *lumbar puncture.*

spine **1** The column of bone known as the vertebral column that surrounds and protects the spinal cord. The spine can be categorized according to the level of the body: cervical spine (neck), thoracic spine (upper and middle back), and lumbar spine (lower back). See also *vertebral column.* **2** Any short prominence of bone. For example, the spines of the vertebrae protrude at the base of the back of the neck and in the middle of the back. These spines protect the spinal cord from injury from behind.

spiral CAT scan A specialized computerized axial tomography (CAT) scan technique that involves continuous movement of the patient through the scanner with the ability to scan faster and with high definition of internal structures. Spiral CAT scanning permits greater visualization of blood vessels and internal tissues, such as those within the chest cavity, than regular CAT scanning. This form of scanning is particularly helpful in the rapid evaluation of severe trauma injuries, such as those sustained in automobile accidents. Also known as helical CAT scan. See also *CAT scan.*

spiral fracture See *fracture, torsion.*

spirochete A microscopic bacterial organism in the Spirochaeta family that has a worm-like, spiral-shaped form and wiggles vigorously when viewed under a microscope. Treponema pallidum, the cause of syphilis, is a particularly well-known spirochete.

spleen An organ that is located in the upper-left part of the abdomen, not far from the stomach, that produces lymphoctes, which are important elements in the immune system. The spleen is the largest lymphatic organ in the body. The spleen also filters blood, serves as a major reservoir for blood, and destroys blood cells that are aged (or abnormal, as in the case of sickle cells).

spleen, ruptured Rupture of the capsule of the spleen that is a potential catastrophe and requires immediate medical and surgical attention. Splenic rupture permits large amounts of blood to leak into the abdominal cavity, and it is severely painful and life threatening. Shock, and

ultimately death, can result. Patients typically require immediate surgery. Rupture of a normal spleen can be caused by trauma, such as an accident. If an individual's spleen is enlarged, as is frequent in mononucleosis, most physicians will not allow major contact sports or other activities because injury to the abdomen could be catastrophic.

splenectomy An operation to remove the spleen.

splenic artery A large and critically important artery within the abdomen that arises from a branch off the aorta called the celiac trunk. The splenic artery supplies blood not only to the spleen but also to the esophagus, stomach, duodenum, liver, and pancreas. See also *aorta; artery.*

splenic fever See *anthrax.*

splenomegaly Abnormal enlargement of the spleen. Splenomegaly is a sign of an underlying condition, such as severe liver disease, leukemia, or mononucleosis. Patients with splenomegaly should avoid activities that risk trauma to the abdomen, including contact sports, because of risk of bleeding from the injured spleen.

split personality See *dissociation; dissociative disorder.*

spondylitis Inflammation of one or more of the vertebrae of the spine. Diffuse inflammation of the spine is seen, for example, in the disease ankylosing spondylitis. Localized spondylitis is seen with infections of a certain area of the spine, such as in Pott's disease (tuberculosis of the spine).

spondylitis, ankylosing See *ankylosing spondylitis.*

spondylolisthesis Forward movement of one vertebra in relationship to an adjacent vertebra.

spondylolysis The breaking down (dissolution) of a portion of a vertebra. The affected portion of the vertebra is a bone segment called the pars interarticularis, which can separate. Spondylolysis can be a cause of abnormal movement of the spine (spondylolisthesis) and lead to localized back pain.

spondylosis Degeneration of the disc spaces between the vertebrae. Spondylosis is common with aging and affects virtually everyone to some degree after the age of 60 years. When severe, it can cause local pain and decreased range of motion of the spine, requiring pain and/or antiinflammatory medications.

spongy degeneration of the central nervous system See *Canavan disease.*

spontaneous abortion See *miscarriage.*

sporadic Occurring upon occasion or in a scattered, isolated, or seemingly random way.

sporotrichosis An infection caused by the fungus Sporothrix schenckii, typically involving the skin. Persons handling thorny plants, sphagnum moss, or baled hay are at increased risk of developing sporotrichosis. The first sign is usually a small painless bump resembling an insect bite. The bump can be red, pink, or purple in color, and it usually appears on the finger, hand, or arm, where the fungus first entered through a break on the skin. This is followed by one or more additional bumps that open and may look like boils. Eventually, the bumps turn into open hollowed-out sores (ulcerations) that are very slow to heal. The infection can also spread to other areas of the body. Treatment is with antibiotics.

spot, Brushfield See *Brushfield spot.*

spots in front of the eyes See *floaters.*

spots, Koplik See *Koplik spots.*

sprain An injury to a ligament that results from overuse or trauma. The treatment of a sprain involves applying ice packs, resting and elevating the involved joint, and using anti-inflammatory medications. Depending on the severity and location of the sprain, support bracing can help. Local cortisone injections are sometimes given for persistent inflammation. Activity may be resumed gradually. Ice application after activity can reduce or prevent recurrent inflammation. Occasionally, supportive bracing can prevent reinjury. In severe sprains, orthopedic surgical repair is performed.

spreading melanoma, superficial See *melanoma, superficial spreading.*

sprue, nontropical See *celiac sprue.*

spur, heel See *calcaneal spur.*

sputum Mucous material from the lungs that is produced (brought up) by coughing.

squamous cell A flat cell that looks like a fish scale. Squamous cells make up most of the outer layer of the skin (epidermis). They also line the hollow organs of the body and the passages of the respiratory and digestive tracts.

squamous cell carcinoma See *carcinoma, squamous cell.*

squamous cell carcinoma in situ See *carcinoma in situ, squamous cell.*

squamous intraepithelial lesion Abnormal growth of squamous cells on the surface of the cervix, such as obtained from a PAP smear. The changes in the cells are described as low grade or high grade, depending on how much of the cervix is affected and how abnormal the cells are. Abbreviated SIL.

SSPE Subacute sclerosing panencephalitis.

SSRI Selective serotonin reuptake inhibitor, one of a family of antidepressant medications (brand names: Celexa, Luvox, Paxil, Prozac, Zoloft) that affect the neurotransmitter serotonin.

St. Anthony's fire One of several conditions characterized by intense inflammation of the skin, such as from erysipelas or ergotism. Erysipelas is a type of spreading hot, bright-red strep skin infection. Ergotism is an intensely painful burning sensation in the limbs and extremities caused by ergotamines from a fungus (Claviceps purpurea) that can contaminate rye and wheat. The fungus produces the ergotamines, which constrict blood vessels and cause the muscle of the uterus to contract. In excess, ergotamines are highly toxic and cause symptoms such as hallucinations, severe gastrointestinal upset, and a type of dry gangrene. Chronic ergot poisoning (ergotism) was rife during the Middle Ages due to the consumption of contaminated rye.

St. John's wort A flowering plant, Hypericum perforatum, also known as Perforate St. John's wort, that has long been believed to have medicinal qualities. There is, in fact, some evidence that St. John's wort may be useful in diminishing depression. Sun sensitivity, fatigue, stomach upset, and allergic reactions are among the side effects that have been reported in people taking St. John's wort. It is recommended that fair-skinned persons be particularly careful while in the sun. This herb should be avoided in combination with other medications that can affect sun sensitivity, such as tetracycline (brand name: Achromycin), sulfa-containing medications, and piroxicam (brand name: Feldene). St. John's wort can also cause headaches, sweating, and agitation when used in combination with serotonin reuptake inhibitor medications, such as fluoxetine (brand name: Prozac) and paroxetine (brand name: Paxil).

staff of Aesculapius See *Aesculapius.*

stage **1** A distinct phase in the course of a disease (or any biological process). **2** The extent of a cancer, and especially whether the disease has spread from the original site to other parts of the body. See also *staging.*

stage of dilation See *first stage of labor.*

stage of expulsion See *second stage of labor.*

staging   Doing exams and tests to learn the extent of a cancer, especially whether it has spread from its original site to other parts of the body. The following stage numbers are typically used in staging:

- **Stage I**   Cancer cells are found only on the surface of the affected organ or area.

- **Stage II**   Cancer cells are found in the deeper tissues of the organ or area and have spread.

- **Stage III**   Cancer cells are found in even deeper tissues and have spread to nearby lymph nodes or other nearby area.

- **Stage IV**   Cancer cells are found throughout the organ or area and in nearby lymph nodes and/or have spread to other parts of the body.

staph   See *staphylococcus.*

staph infection   See *staphylococcal infection.*

staphylococcal infection   Infection with one of the staphylococcal bacteria. Staphylococcal infection can cause pus-filled abscesses on the skin or internal organs and can migrate through the blood to infect the heart, meninges, and other areas. Treatment involves use of antibiotics and drainage of abscesses, as necessary. Also known as staph infection. See also *staphylococcal scalded skin syndrome; staphylococcus.*

staphylococcal scalded skin syndrome   An infection of the skin with group II staphylococcus aureus bacteria. The bacteria release toxins, causing inflamed, scaling skin that looks as though it has been burned. Abbreviated SSSS. SSSS is more common in children than in adults, but it is more likely to cause death when it does occur in adults. Rehydration and use of intravenous antibiotics are the most common treatments. Steroids worsen the condition and should not be used. See also *staphylococcus.*

staphylococcus   A group of bacteria that cause a multitude of diseases. Under a microscope, staphylococcus bacteria are round and bunched together. They can cause illness directly by infection or indirectly through products they make, such as the toxins responsible for food poisoning and toxic shock syndrome. The best-known member of the staphylococcus family is staphylococcus aureus. Staphylococci are the main culprits in hospital-acquired infections, and they cause thousands of deaths every year. Also known as staph.

staphylococcus, antibiotic-resistant   A form of staphylococcus bacteria that is unaffected by certain antibiotics. Antibiotic-resistant staphylococcus is a growing problem, particularly in hospitals, where staph infections can run rampant. Treatment involves using "super-antibiotics" when possible, although this type of infection can prove to be untreatable and deadly.

startle disease   See *hyperexplexia.*

startle reflex   A reflex seen in normal infants in response to a loud noise. The infant makes a sudden body movement, bringing the legs and arms toward the chest.

stasis   A stoppage or slowdown in the flow of blood or other body fluid, such as lymph. For example, a stasis ulcer is an ulcer that develops in an area in which the circulation is sluggish and the venous return (the return of venous blood toward the heart) is poor. A common location for stasis ulcers is the ankle.

STAT   A common medical abbreviation for urgent or rush. From the Latin word *statum,* meaning "immediately."

state, hypercoagulable   See *hypercoagulable state.*

statin   A class of drugs that lower cholesterol. The following statins are on the market in the US: lovastatin (brand name: Mevacor), simvastatin (brand name: Zocor), pravastatin (brand name: Pravachol), fluvastatin (brand name: Lescol), and atorvastatin (brand name: Lipitor). The major effect of the statins is that they lower LDL cholesterol levels; in fact, they lower LDL-cholesterol more than any other type of drugs. Statins inhibit an enzyme, HMG-CoA reductase, that controls the rate of cholesterol production in the body. This slows the production of cholesterol. They also increase the liver's ability to remove the LDL cholesterol already in the blood. Studies have reported 20 to 60 percent lower LDL cholesterol levels in patients on these drugs, as well as modest increases in HDL cholesterol and reduced triglyceride levels. Such reductions should prevent many heart attacks and deaths due to heart disease. Statins are usually given in a single dose at the evening meal or at bedtime, taking advantage of the fact that the body makes more cholesterol at night than during the day. Results should be seen after several weeks, with a maximum effect in 4 to 6 weeks. Serious side effects are rare, but a few patients experience upset stomach, gas, constipation, and abdominal pain or cramps. These symptoms are usually mild to moderate in severity, and they generally go away as the body adjusts. Rarely, patients on statins develop liver blood test abnormalities or muscle soreness, pain, and weakness as side effects of muscle problems.

status epilepticus   An epileptic seizure that lasts more than 30 minutes or a constant or near-constant state of having seizures. Status epilepticus is a health crisis and requires immediate treatment with antiseizure medications. See also *epilepsy; seizure disorder.*

STD   Sexually transmitted disease.

STDs in men See *sexually transmitted disease in men.*

STDs in women See *sexually transmitted disease in women.*

Stein-Leventhal syndrome A hormonal problem, also known as polycystic ovarian disease, that causes women to have symptoms that include irregular or no menstruation, acne, obesity, and excess hair growth. Women with Stein-Leventhal syndrome do not ovulate (release an egg for fertilization) every month. They are at an increased risk for high blood pressure, diabetes, heart disease, and cancer of the uterus (endometrial cancer). Much of this risk can be reversed with exercise and weight loss. Medication is generally prescribed to induce regular menstruation, thereby reducing the cancer risk. For acne and excess hair growth, the diuretic medication spironolactone (brand name: Aldactazide) can help. Clomiphene (brand name: Clomid) can be used to induce ovulation if pregnancy is desired. A type of surgery called a wedge resection, in which a piece of the ovary is removed, seems to help some women. The cause of Stein-Leventhal syndrome is unknown, but the ovaries of women with Stein-Leventhal syndrome contain a number of small cysts.

stem cell One of the human body's master cells, with the ability to grow into any one of the body's more than 200 cell types. Stem cells are unspecialized (undifferentiated) cells that are characteristically of the same family type (lineage). They retain the ability to divide throughout life and give rise to cells that can become highly specialized and take the place of cells that die or are lost. Stem cells contribute to the body's ability to renew and repair its tissues. Unlike mature cells, which are permanently committed to their fate, stem cells can both renew themselves and create new cells of whatever tissue they belong to (and other tissues). Bone marrow stem cells, for example, are the most primitive cells in the marrow. From them all the various types of blood cells are descended. Bone marrow stem cell transfusions (or transplants) were originally given to replace various types of blood cells.

stem cell harvest Obtaining stem cells for use in cancer or other treatment. Usually the cells are removed from the patient's own bone marrow. This procedure typically involves the use of a general anesthetic and an overnight hospital stay. Small cuts are made over the bones of the pelvis to allow entrance for the large needles used to puncture the bones and draw out marrow. The marrow is frozen for later use. In some situations, stem cells are removed from a closely genetically matched donor. Umbilical cords have been saved as a future source of stem cells for the baby.

stem cell harvest, peripheral blood A technique for obtaining stem cells from the patient's blood for use in bone marrow transplantation. The stem cells are lured out of the bone marrow with a special regimen of drugs. The blood is then filtered through a machine, and the stem cells are skimmed off. They can be used right away or stored in liquid nitrogen until needed. Also known as apheresis. See also *stem cell transplantation.*

stem cell transplantation The use of stem cells as a treatment for cancer or other illness. The stem cells are removed (or obtained from a donor) first. Before the transplant is done, the patient receives high-dose chemotherapy and/or radiation therapy to destroy diseased cells. Then the stem cells are returned to the patient, where they can produce new blood and immune cells and replace the cells destroyed by the treatment. The stem cell preparation is infused into a vein and, once in the bloodstream, the stem cells act like homing pigeons by heading straight for the bone marrow space.

stenosis A narrowing. For example, aortic stenosis is a narrowing of the aortic valve in the heart.

stenosis, pulmonary See *pulmonary stenosis.*

stent A tiny tube that is commonly used to maintain the normal flow of blood in an artery that is in danger of being blocked by arteriosclerosis. Stents are often inserted in diseased coronary arteries to help keep them open after balloon angioplasty. The stent allows normal flow of blood and oxygen to the heart. Stents placed in narrowed carotid arteries appear to be useful for treating patients who are at elevated risk for stroke.

stereotactic Referring to precise positioning in three-dimensional space. For example, biopsies, surgery, or radiation therapy can be done stereotactically.

stereotactic needle biopsy See *biopsy, stereotactic needle.*

stereotactic radiation therapy See *radiation therapy, stereotactic.*

stereotactic radiotherapy See *radiation therapy, stereotactic.*

stereotactic surgery Surgery in which a system of three-dimensional coordinates is used to locate the site to be operated on.

stereotaxis Use of a computer and scanning devices to create three-dimensional pictures. Stereotaxis can be used to direct a biopsy, external radiation, or the insertion of radiation implants.

sternal rib See *rib, true.*

sternum　The long flat bone in the upper middle of the front of the chest. The sternum articulates (comes together) with the cartilages of the first seven ribs and with the clavicle (collarbone) on either side. The sternum consists of three parts: the manubrium (the upper segment of the sternum, a flattened, roughly triangular bone), the corpus (body) of the sternum, and the xiphoid process (the little tail of the sternum than points down). These sections of the sternum arise as separate bones, and they may fuse partially or completely with one another. Also known as breastbone.

steroid　One of a large group of chemical substances classified by a certain chemical structure. Steroids include drugs used to relieve swelling and inflammation, such as prednisone and cortisone; vitamin D; and some sex hormones, such as testosterone and estradiol.

steroid abuse　Use of substances containing steroids to increase muscle mass. Steroids can have many side effects when misused, including psychiatric problems, liver tumors, reduction in the size of male genitals, sterility, and heart damage.

stethoscope　An instrument that is used to transmit low-volume sounds such as a heartbeat (or intestinal, venous, or fetal sounds) to the ear of the listener. A stethoscope may consist of two ear pieces connected by means of flexible tubing to a diaphragm that is placed against the skin of the patient. The stethoscope has become one of the symbols of the medical profession. The origins of the stethoscope can be traced back to the French physician Laënnec, who in 1819 invented a crude model that consisted of a wooden box that served to help physicians hear the sounds within the chest cavity. It has undergone many modifications since then.

stiff baby syndrome　See *hyperexplexia.*

stillbirth　The birth of a dead baby, the delivery of a fetus that has died before birth for which there is no possibility of resuscitation. The distinction between a stillbirth and a miscarriage is arbitrary. The dividing line is variously set at 20 to 24 weeks of gestation. Before that time it is a miscarriage, and after that time it is a stillbirth.

Still's disease　See *arthritis, systemic-onset juvenile rheumatoid.*

sting, Africanized bee　See *bee sting, Africanized.*

sting, bee　See *bee sting.*

sting, insect　See *insect sting.*

stoma　An opening into the body from the outside that is created by a surgeon.

stomach　The digestive organ that is located in the upper abdomen, under the ribs. The upper part of the stomach connects to the esophagus, and the lower part leads into the small intestine. When food enters the stomach, muscles in the stomach wall create a rippling motion (peristalsis) that mixes and mashes the food. At the same time, juices made by glands in the lining of the stomach help digest the food. After about 3 hours, the food becomes a liquid and moves into the small intestine, where digestion continues.

stomach cancer　See *cancer, gastric.*

stomach emptying study　See *gastric emptying study.*

stomach flu　See *flu, stomach.*

stomach paralysis　See *gastroparesis.*

stomatitis, Vincent　See *acute membraneous gingivitis.*

stone, cystine kidney　See *cystine kidney stones.*

stone, kidney　See *kidney stone.*

stone, renal　See *kidney stone.*

stone, tonsil　See *tonsillolith.*

stool　The solid matter that is discharged in a bowel movement.

stool test　See *fecal occult blood test.*

storm supplies kit　See *disaster supplies.*

strabismus　A condition in which the visual axes of the eyes are not parallel and the eyes appear to be looking in different directions. In divergent strabismus, or exotropia, the visual axes diverge. In convergent strabismus or esotropia, the visual axes converge. The danger with strabismus is that the brain cones may come to rely more on one eye than the other, and the part of the brain circuitry that is connected to the less-favored eye may fail to develop properly, leading to amblyopia (blindness) in that eye. The classic treatment for mild to moderate strabismus is to cover the stronger eye with a patch, forcing the weaker eye to do enough work to catch up. Atropine eyedrops can also be effective in correcting moderate lazy eye. Severe strabismus may require surgery. Also known as lazy eye.

strain　**1** An injury to a ligament, tendon, or muscle that results from overuse or trauma.　**2** A hereditary tendency that originates from a common ancestor.　**3** To exert maximum effort.　**4** To filter.

strawberry hemangioma or strawberry mark　See *hemangioma, capillary.*

strep See *streptococcus.*

strep throat An infection caused by group A streptococcus bacteria that can lead to serious complications if not adequately treated. Treatment usually involves use of antibiotics. See *streptococcus.*

streptococcus A group of bacteria that cause a multitude of diseases. Under a microscope, streptococcus bacteria look like a twisted bunch of round berries. Illnesses caused by streptococcus include strep throat, strep pneumonia, scarlet fever, rheumatic fever (and rheumatic heart valve damage), glomerulonephritis, the skin disorder erysipelas, and PANDAS. Familiarly known as strep.

Streptococcus faecalis An old name for Enterococcus faecalis.

streptococcus, group A See *Streptococcus pyogenes.*

streptococcus, group B A major cause of infections, including those involving pregnant women and newborn infants. Group B strep can infect the mother's uterus, placenta, and urinary tract; in fact, it is present in the vagina of 10 to 25 percent of all pregnant women. Group B strep can be transferred between heterosexual couples via oral sex. Infections in the infant can be localized, or it may involve the entire body. In babies, strep infections are divided into early-onset and late-onset disease. Early-onset disease presents within the first 6 days of life, with breathing difficulty, shock, pneumonia, and occasionally infection of the spinal fluid and brain (meningitis). Late-onset disease presents between the seventh day and the third month of age, with a bloodstream infection (bacteremia) or meningitis. The bacteria can also infect an area of bone; a joint, such as the knee or hip; or the skin. Group B strep infection in a newborn is a serious and potentially life-threatening event, particularly because fever and warning signs are often minimal or absent and because the newborn's immune system is not mature. Early signs of infection can be as subtle as poor feeding, lethargy, and poor temperature control. Women with vaginal group B strep can transmit it to the infant before birth, after the membranes are ruptured, or during the delivery. In such cases, the infant has a 0.5 to 1 percent chance of contracting the early-onset type of infection. The risk rises with premature infants, infants born more than 18 hours after the amniotic membranes have ruptured, and infants whose mothers had fever, evidence of infection of the uterus lining, or infection of the urinary tract during labor and delivery. Because many infants today are discharged less than 24 hours after birth, there is growing pressure to culture all women during pregnancy for group B strep. Antibiotic treatment can be considered for culture-positive women before delivery. A positive culture alerts the infant's physician to watch for early signs of problems. Group B strep infection of the newborn is treated aggressively with antibi-

otics, usually in a neonatal intensive care unit, but the disease still carries a significant mortality rate. Prevention and early detection are critically important.

Streptococcus haemolyticus See *Streptococcus pyogenes.*

Streptococcus pneumoniae The most common cause of bacterial pneumonia and middle ear infection (otitis media) and the third most frequent cause of bacterial meningitis. Also known as pneumococcus.

Streptococcus pyogenes The bacterial cause of strep throat (streptococcal pharyngitis), impetigo, rheumatic fever, scarlet fever, glomerulonephritis, invasive fasciitis, strep skin infections, and rheumatic fever. Also known as Streptococcus haemolyticus and group A streptococcus. See also *PANDAS; rheumatic fever; strep throat; streptococcus; Sydenham chorea.*

stricture 1 An abnormal narrowing of a body passage, especially a tube or a canal. A stricture may be due, for example, to scar tissue or a tumor. 2 The process of narrowing a body passage.

stricture of the esophagus, acute See *esophageal stricture, acute.*

stricture of the esophagus, chronic See *esophageal stricture, chronic.*

stroke The sudden death of brain cells due to lack of oxygen, caused by blockage of blood flow or rupture of an artery to the brain. Sudden loss of speech, weakness, or paralysis of one side of the body can be symptoms. A suspected cerebrovascular accident can be confirmed by scanning the brain with special X-ray tests, such as CAT scans. Prevention involves minimizing risk factors, such as controlling high blood pressure and diabetes. Abbreviated CVA. Also known as cerebrovascular accident.

stroke prevention Methods of preventing the occurrence of a cerebrovascular accident. If a person has a transient ischemic attack (TIA), a neurological event with the symptoms of a stroke, the symptoms go away within a short period of time. TIAs are often caused by narrowing or ulceration of the carotid arteries, however, and if that is not treated, there is a high risk of major stroke in the future. A person who suspects that he or she has had a TIA should seek medical attention right away. An operation called a carotid endarterectomy can clean out the carotid artery and restore normal blood flow through the artery, markedly reducing the incidence of a subsequent stroke. In other cases, when a person has a narrowed carotid artery but no symptoms, the risk of stroke can be reduced with medications such as aspirin and ticlopidine (brand name: Ticlid). These medications act by partially blocking the blood-clotting function of the platelets in the patient's blood. Controlling other factors that contribute to strokes, such as high blood pressure and diabetes, is also important for stroke prevention.

stroke volume The amount of blood pumped by the left ventricle of the heart in one contraction. The stroke volume is not all the blood contained in the left ventricle; normally, only about two-thirds of the blood in the ventricle is expelled with each beat. Together with the heart rate, the stroke volume determines the output of blood by the heart per minute (cardiac output).

study 1 A procedure or an examination. 2 A research project.

Sturge-Weber syndrome A congenital, but not inherited, disorder that affects the skin, the neurological system, and sometimes the eyes and internal organs. The main sign of Sturge-Weber syndrome is a port-wine stain birthmark. Neurological symptoms of Sturge-Weber syndrome may include seizures and developmental delay. See also *port-wine stain.*

stuttering A speech disorder characterized by repetition of the sound of a word. Stuttering can usually be eliminated or significantly modified with speech therapy. See also *cluttering; communication disorder; speech disorder.*

subacute Rather recent onset or somewhat rapid change. In contrast, acute indicates very sudden onset or rapid change and chronic indicates indefinite duration or virtually no change.

subacute sclerosing panencephalitis A chronic brain disease of children and adolescents that occurs months to often years after an attack of measles and causes convulsions, motor abnormalities, mental retardation, and usually death. Abbreviated SSPE.

subarachnoid Literally, beneath the arachnoid, the middle of three membranes that cover the central nervous system. In practice, subarachnoid usually refers to the space between the arachnoid and the pia mater, the innermost membrane surrounding the central nervous system. It normally contains cerebrospinal fluid. See also *cerebrospinal fluid.*

subarachnoid hemorrhage A bleeding into the subarachnoid, the space between the arachnoid and the pia mater, the innermost membrane surrounding the central nervous system. Subarachnoid hemorrhage typically occurs when an artery breaks open in the brain, such as from a ruptured aneurysm. This can require emergency neurosurgical procedures.

subaortic stenosis Narrowing of the left ventricle of the heart, just below the aortic valve, through which blood must pass on its way up into the aorta. The narrowing cuts the flow of blood. Subaortic stenosis may be present at birth (congenital) or acquired as part of a specific form of heart disease known as idiopathic hypertrophic subaortic stenosis (IHSS). Treatment options include use of drugs and surgery. See also *idiopathic hypertrophic subaortic stenosis.*

subclinical disease An illness that is staying below the surface of clinical detection. A subclinical disease has no recognizable clinical findings. It is distinct from a clinical disease, which has signs and symptoms that can be recognized. Many diseases, including diabetes, hypothyroidism, and rheumatoid arthritis, are frequently subclinical before they surface as clinical diseases.

subcu See *subcutaneous.*

subcutaneous Under the skin. For example, a subcutaneous injection is an injection in which a needle is inserted just under the skin. Also known as subcu. Abbreviated subq.

subcutaneous hematoma See *hematoma, subcutaneous.*

subcutaneous injection An injection in which a needle is inserted just under the skin. A drug can then be delivered into the tissues below the skin. After the injection, the drug moves into small blood vessels and the bloodstream. Subcutaneous injection is used with many protein and polypeptide drugs, such as insulin, that, if given by mouth, would be broken down and digested in the intestinal tract.

subdural hematoma See *hematoma, subdural.*

subglottis The lower part of the larynx, the area from just below the vocal cords down to the top of the trachea.

sublingual Underneath the tongue. For example, a sublingual medication is a type of lozenge that is dissolved under the tongue.

sublingual gland A salivary gland that is located under the floor of the mouth, close to the midline. The sublingual gland is the smallest of the three major salivary glands (the parotid, submandibular, and sublingual glands).

subluxation Partial dislocation of a joint. A complete dislocation is a luxation.

submandibular gland A salivary gland that is located deep under the mandible (jawbone). The submandibular gland is the second largest of the three major salivary glands (the parotid, submandibular, and sublingual glands). Also known as submaxillary gland.

submaxillary gland See *submandibular gland.*

subq See *subcutaneous.*

subscapular Under the scapula. For example, the subscapularis muscle originates beneath the scapula.

subscapularis muscle A muscle that moves the arm by turning it inward (internal rotation). The tendon of the subscapularis muscle is one of four tendons that stabilize the shoulder joint and constitute the rotator cuff. Each of these four tendons hooks up to a muscle that moves the shoulder in a specific direction. See also *scapula.*

subtotal hysterectomy See *hysterectomy, partial.*

subungual onychomycosis, proximal white See *onychomycosis, proximal white subungual.*

succenturiate Substituting for or accessory to an organ. For example, a succenturiate spleen is an accessory spleen, one that is in addition to the primary spleen.

succenturiate placenta See *placenta, accessory.*

suction-assisted lipectomy See *liposuction.*

sudden infant death syndrome The sudden and unexpected death of a baby with no known illness, typically affecting sleeping infants between the ages of 2 weeks and 6 months. Abbreviated SIDS. Infants with a brother or sister who died of SIDS; babies whose mothers used heroin, methadone, or cocaine during pregnancy; infants born weighing less than 2,000 grams (4.4 pounds); children with an abnormal breathing pattern that includes long periods without taking a breath (apnea); and babies who sleep on their stomachs are at elevated risk for SIDS. Because babies who sleep on their stomachs are at least three times more likely to die of SIDS than babies who sleep on their backs, children's health authorities recommend always placing infants on their backs to sleep.

sudoriferous gland A small, tubular structure situated within and under the skin that discharges sweat through a tiny opening in the surface of the skin. Also known as sweat gland. See also *perspiration.*

sulcus A groove, furrow, or trench. The plural is sulci. In medicine, there are many sulci; an example is the superior pulmonary sulcus.

sulfa drug See *sulfonamide.*

sulfonamide One of the sulfa-related group of antibiotics, which are used to treat bacterial infection and some fungal infections. The sulfonamide family includes sulfadiazine, sulfamethizole (brand names: Thiosulfil, Forte), sulfamethoxazole (brand name: Gantanal), sulfasalazine (brand name: Azulfidine), sulfisoxazole (brand name: Gantrisin), and various high-strength combinations of sulfonamides. Sulfa drugs kill bacteria and fungi by interfering with cell metabolism. They were the wonder drugs before penicillin and are still used today. Because sulfa drugs concentrate in the urine before being excreted, treatment of urinary tract infections is one of their most common uses. Sulfa drugs can have a number of potentially dangerous interactions with prescription and over-the-counter drugs (including PABA sunscreens), and they are not appropriate for patients with some health conditions. Before people take sulfonamides, they should be sure their physicians know about any other medications they are taking and their full health history. Sulfa drug allergy is one of the more common allergies to medications.

summer cold See *hay fever.*

sun protection factor A measurement of a sunscreen's potency, expressed on a scale from two upward. Abbreviated SPF. Sunscreens with an SPF of 15 or higher provide the best protection from the sun's harmful rays. See also *ultraviolet radiation.*

sunscreen A substance that blocks the effect of the sun's harmful rays. Using lotions that contain sunscreen can reduce the risk of skin cancer, including melanoma. See also *ultraviolet radiation.*

superaspirin See *cox-2 inhibitor.*

superficial On the surface or shallow, as opposed to deep. For example, the skin is superficial to the muscles, and the cornea is on the superficial surface of the eye. See also Appendix B, "Anatomic Orientation Terms."

superficial spreading melanoma See *melanoma, superficial spreading.*

superior Above, as opposed to inferior. For example, the heart is superior to the stomach, and the superior surface of the tongue rests against the palate. See also Appendix B, "Anatomic Orientation Terms."

superior vena cava syndrome A condition in which the large vein that carries blood down to the heart (superior vena cava) is compressed. This compression may be caused by disease of any of the structures or lymph nodes surrounding this vein. Superior vena cava syndrome is characterized by swelling of the face, neck, and/or arms, with visible widening (dilation) of the veins of the neck.

Patients often have a persistent cough and shortness of breath. Other symptoms may include hoarseness, swelling around the eyes, fatigue, chest pain, headaches, and dizziness. Causes of superior vena cava syndrome include cancer and several benign conditions. Common forms of cancer that can cause superior vena cava syndrome are lung cancer, cancer of the lymph nodes (lymphoma), and cancer that has spread (metastasized) to the chest, most commonly breast and testicular cancer. Noncancerous causes include infections, such as tuberculosis, fungus infections, and syphilis; benign tumors, such as teratomas, thymomas, and dermoid cysts; aortic aneurysm; pericarditis; sarcoidosis; irradiation treatment to the chest; air in the chest (pneumothorax); and complications of central line catheters and congenital heart surgery. Diagnosis is made via observation of typical findings and is supported by identifying a cause for superior vena cava syndrome, a procedure that typically requires X-ray imaging or computerized axial tomography (CAT) or magnetic resonance imaging (MRI) scanning. Treatment is directed toward the underlying cause and therefore might include radiation, use of antibiotics, chemotherapy, use of clot-busting (thrombolytic) drugs, use of blood thinners (anticoagulants), balloon angioplasty, and even surgery. The outlook for patients with superior vena cava syndrome depends on the underlying cause. See also *vena cava, superior.*

supernumerary   Beyond the normal number, extra. For example, a supernumerary chromosome is an extra one beyond the usual number of 46, and a supernumerary digit is an extra finger or toe.

supernumerary digit   See *digit, supernumerary.*

supernumerary nipple   See *nipple, supernumerary.*

supernumerary placenta   See *placenta, accessory.*

supertaster   A person who has an unusually large density of taste buds, each surrounded by pain fibers. As a result, the person has an exquisite ability to taste accurately.

supination   Rotation of the arm or leg outward. In the case of supination of the arm, the palm of the hand faces forward.

supine   With the back or dorsal surface downward; lying face up, as opposed to prone. See also Appendix B, "Anatomic Orientation Terms."

supportive care   Treatment given to prevent, control, or relieve complications and side effects and to improve the patient's comfort and quality of life.

suppressant, cough   See *cough suppressant.*

suppressor T cell   See *T-suppressor cell.*

suppurative arthritis   See *arthritis, septic.*

supraglottis   The upper part of the larynx, including the epiglottis; the area above the vocal cords.

suprarenal gland   See *adrenal gland.*

supraspinatus muscle   The muscle that elevates the arm and moves it away from the body. The tendon of the supraspinatus muscle is one of four tendons that stabilize the shoulder joint and constitute the rotator cuff.

suprasternal notch   The V-shaped notch at the top of the breastbone (sternum).

surfactant   **1** A surface-active agent.   **2** A chemical that is secreted by the cells of the alveoli (the tiny air sacs in the lungs) and serves to reduce the surface tension of pulmonary fluids. Surfactant contributes to the elasticity of lung tissue.

surgeon   A physician who treats disease, injury, or deformity via operative or manual methods. A medical doctor who specializes in the removal of organs, masses, and tumors and in doing other procedures with a scalpel. The definition of *surgeon* has begun to blur in recent years as surgeons have begun to minimize the cutting, employing new technologies that are minimally invasive (such as using scopes and lasers). In England, a surgeon was once a practitioner without an MD degree but with the license of the Royal College of Surgeons.

surgery   The branch of medicine that employs operations in the treatment of disease or injury. Surgery can involve cutting, abrading, suturing, or otherwise physically changing body tissues and organs.

surgery, cataract   See *cataract surgery.*

surgery, fetal   The surgical treatment of a fetus before birth. Fetal surgery is usually done when the fetus is not expected to survive to delivery or to live long after birth unless fetal surgery is performed. Also known as prenatal or antenatal surgery.

surgery, retrograde intrarenal   See *retrograde intrarenal surgery.*

surgery, stereotactic   See *stereotactic surgery.*

surgery, Yag laser   See *Yag laser surgery.*

surgical menopause   See *menopause, induced.*

susceptibility gene, breast cancer   See *breast cancer susceptibility gene.*

suture **1** A type of bone joint in which two bones are held tightly together by fibrous tissue, as in the skull. **2** Thread-like material used to sew tissue. **3** To stitch a wound closed.

swallowing syncope The temporary loss of consciousness upon swallowing. See also *syncope, situational; vasovagal reaction.*

Swan-Ganz catheter See *catheter, Swan-Ganz.*

sweat See *perspiration.*

sweat chloride test See *sweat test.*

sweat gland See *sudoriferous glands.*

sweat gland tumor See *syringoma.*

sweat test A simple test that is used to evaluate a patient who is suspected of having cystic fibrosis (CF). The goal of the test is to painlessly stimulate the patient's skin to produce a certain amount of sweat, which may then be absorbed by a special filter paper and analyzed for chloride content. In a technique called iontophoresis, a minute, painless electric current is applied to the forearm or back, allowing penetration of a medication that maximizes sweat stimulation. Normal sweat chloride values are 10 to 35 milliEquivalents/liter; patients with CF usually have a value greater than 60 milliEquivalents/liter. Intermediate values (between 35 and 60 milliEquivalents/liter) may be seen in some CF patients and in some normal children. In those cases, the sweat test should be repeated. In a severely malnourished patient with CF, the sweat chloride may be normal; when the malnutrition is corrected, however, the test becomes positive. A few rare conditions that produce a false positive test include diseases of adrenal, thyroid, or pituitary glands; rare lipid storage diseases; and infection of the pancreas. Generally, children with these conditions are easily differentiated from patients with CF by their clinical condition, and molecular tests for CF can be done to clarify the situation. Also known as sweat chloride test. See also *cystic fibrosis.*

sweating The act of secreting fluid from the skin by the sudoriferous (sweat) glands. See also *perspiration; sudoriferous gland.*

sweating, gustatory Sweating on the forehead, face, scalp, and neck that occurs soon after ingesting food. Some gustatory sweating is normal after eating hot, spicy foods. Otherwise, gustatory sweating is most commonly a result of damage to a nerve that goes to the parotid gland, the large salivary gland in the cheek. In this condition, called Frey syndrome, the sweating is usually on one side of the head. Gustatory sweating is also a rare complication of diabetes mellitus. In that case, sweating may occur on both sides of the head, with mild or substantial severity. Gustatory sweating can be difficult to treat. It may be treated with oxybutynin chloride, propantheline bromide, and clonidine (brand name: Catapres). Recently, some success has been reported in the use of topical applications of glycopyrrolate, which is applied to the skin of the forehead and face, sparing the eyes and mouth. See also *Frey syndrome; diabetes mellitus.*

sweats, night See *night sweats.*

swimmer's ear See *ear infection, external.*

swimming pool granuloma See *granuloma, fish bowl.*

Sydenham's chorea A disorder that emerges after a bout of rheumatic fever and is most frequently seen in children. The choreaform movements associated with the disease are twisting. Sydenham's chorea can be treated with medication. See also *PANDAS; rheumatic fever.*

sylvatic plague See *plague, sylvatic.*

Sylvius, aqueduct of See *aqueduct of Sylvius.*

symmetric lipomatosis, multiple See *cephalothoracic lipodystrophy.*

sympathetic nervous system A part of the nervous system that serves to accelerate the heart rate, constrict blood vessels, and raise blood pressure. The sympathetic nervous system and the parasympathetic nervous system constitute the autonomic nervous system.

sympathetic ophthalmia Inflammation of the uveal tract of the uninjured eye (sympathizing eye) some weeks after a wound involving the uveal tract of the other eye (exciting eye). Also known as transferred ophthalmia.

symphysiotomy A surgical procedure that is used to effect an immediate dramatic increase in the size of the pelvic outlet to permit delivery of a baby. The cartilage of the area where the pubic bones come together (symphysis pubis) is surgically divided. This can be a lifesaver for the baby and requires months of healing for the mother.

symphysis pubis The area in the front of the pelvis where the pubic bones meet.

symptom Any subjective evidence of disease. In contrast, a sign is objective. Blood coming out a nostril is a sign; it is apparent to the patient, physician, and others. Anxiety, low back pain, and fatigue are all symptoms; only the patient can perceive them.

synapse A specialized junction at which a neural cell (neuron) communicates with a target cell. At a synapse, a neuron releases a chemical transmitter that diffuses across a small gap and activates special sites called receptors on the target cell. The target cell may be another neuron or a specialized region of a muscle or secretory cell. Neurons can also communicate through direct electrical connections (electrical synapses).

synchronic study A study that is done at a single point in time rather than over the course of a period of time (longitudinally).

syncope Partial or complete loss of consciousness, with interruption of awareness of self and surroundings and spontaneous recovery. Syncope accounts for 1 in every 30 visits to an emergency room. Syncope is due to a temporary reduction in blood flow and therefore a shortage of oxygen to the brain. This leads to lightheadedness or a "blackout" episode (loss of consciousness). Temporary impairment of the blood supply to the brain can be caused by heart conditions and by conditions that do not directly involve the heart. Heart conditions that can cause syncope include abnormal heart rhythms (heart beating too fast or too slow), abnormalities of the heart valves (aortic stenosis or pulmonic valve stenosis), high blood pressure in the arteries supplying the lungs (pulmonary artery hypertension), tears in the aorta (aortic dissection), and widespread disease of the heart muscle (cardiomyopathy). However, syncope is most commonly caused by conditions that do not directly involve the heart. These conditions include postural (orthostatic) hypotension, a drop in blood pressure due to changing body position to a more vertical position after lying or sitting; dehydration, which can cause a decrease in blood volume; blood pressure medications that lead to overly low blood pressure; diseases of the nerves to the legs in older people, especially those with diabetes or Parkinson's disease, in which poor tone of the nerves of the legs draws blood into the legs from the brain; high altitude; brain stroke or transient ischemic attack; and migraine attack. Another common form of noncardiac syncope is known as situational syncope because the fainting occurs after certain situations. Triggers for situational syncope include having blood drawn, urinating (micturition syncope), defecating (defecation syncope), swallowing (swallowing syncope), and coughing (cough syncope). In some individuals, one or more of these situations can trigger a reflex of the involuntary nervous system called the vasovagal reaction, which slows the heart, dilates blood vessels in the legs, and causes the person to feel nausea, sweating, or weakness just before fainting. A physician can detect many causes of syncope by taking a careful history. To diagnose the cause of syncope, the blood pressure and pulse are tested in lying, sitting, and standing positions. Blood pressures are measured in each arm, and the heart and nervous system are examined and tested. An EKG and other tests may be done including echocardiograms, rhythm monitoring tests (heart event recorders), and electrophysiologic testing for abnormalities of the heart's electrical system. When heart conditions are not suspected, tilt-table testing can be used. No treatment is needed for many noncardiac causes of syncope, as the person regains consciousness by simply sitting or lying down. The person is thereafter advised to avoid trigger situations. Older people should have their medications reviewed and be cautioned to slow the process of changing positions. Also known as fainting. See also *syncope, situational; tilt-table test; vasovagal reaction.*

syncope, coughing The temporary loss of consciousness upon coughing. See also *syncope; syncope, situational; vasovagal reaction.*

syncope, defecation The temporary loss of consciousness upon defecating (having a bowel movement). See also *syncope; syncope, situational; vasovagal reaction.*

syncope, micturition The temporary loss of consciousness upon urinating (micturation). See also *syncope; syncope, situational; vasovagal reaction.*

syncope, situational The temporary loss of consciousness in a particular kind of situation. The situations that trigger this reaction are diverse and include having blood drawn, straining while urinating or defecating, and coughing. The reaction can be caused also by emotional stress, fear, or pain. When experiencing the trigger condition, the person often becomes pale and feels nauseated, sweaty, and weak just before losing consciousness. Situational syncope is caused by a reflex of the involuntary nervous system called the vasovagal reaction. The vasovagal reaction leads the heart to slow down (bradycardia) while at the same time leading the nerves that serve the blood vessels in the legs to permit those vessels to dilate (widen). The result is that the heart puts out less blood, blood pressure drops, and circulating blood tends to go into the legs rather than to the head. The brain is deprived of oxygen, and the fainting episode occurs. Also known as vasovagal syncope, vasodepressor syncope, and Gower syndrome. See also *syncope; vasovagal reaction.*

syncope, swallowing The temporary loss of consciousness upon swallowing. See also *syncope; syncope, situational; vasovagal reaction.*

syncope, vasodepressor See *syncope, situational.*

syncope, vasovagal See *vasovagal syncope.*

syndactyly A condition in which fingers or toes are joined together. Syndactyly can involve the bones (bony syndactyly) or just the skin (cutaneous syndactyly, or webbing).

syndactyly, bony A condition in which the bones of fingers or toes are joined together.

syndactyly, complete A condition in which fingers or toes are completely joined together, with the connection extending from the base to the tip of the involved digits.

syndactyly, cutaneous A condition in which fingers or toes are joined together and the joining involves only the skin, not the bones.

syndactyly, partial A condition in which fingers or toes are partially joined together. Syndactyly can involve the bones or just the skin. With partial syndactyly, the connection extends from the base only partway up the involved digits.

syndactyly, Poland See *Poland syndrome.*

syndrome A combination of symptoms and signs that together represent a disease process.

syndromic Part of a syndrome. For instance, low-set ears are syndromic of Down syndrome.

synesthesia A condition in which the normal separation between the senses appears to have broken down. In synesthesia, sight may mingle with sound, taste with touch, and so on. People with synesthesia are six times more likely to be female than male. Most find their unusual sensory abilities enjoyable. People with synesthesia often report that one or more of their family members also had synesthesia, so it may in some cases be an inherited condition. Synesthesia can be induced by certain hallucinogenic drugs and can also occur in some types of seizure disorders.

synovia See *synovial fluid.*

synovial cyst, popliteal See *Baker cyst.*

synovial fluid The slippery fluid that lubricates joints. Also known as synovia.

synovial lining The lining of the joints, normally only one or two cell layers thick, that is responsible for the production of the joint fluid. Also known as synovium.

synovial osteochondromatosis A disorder of a joint that features a change of the normal synovial lining's cellular structure to form bone-cartilage tissue. Synovial osteochondromatosis is uncommon. It typically presents in young to middle-aged adults. Synovial osteochondromatosis leads to pain in the affected joint as well as limitation of the range of motion and often locking. The cause of synovial osteochondromatosis is unknown. Synovial osteochondromatosis generally affects only a single joint.

The most common joints involved are the knee, hip, or elbow. Synovial osteochondromatosis can be diagnosed with an imaging test of the joint, such as an X-ray, a computerized axial tomography (CAT) scan, or a magnetic resonance imaging (MRI) scan. Treatment of synovial osteochondromatosis typically involves surgical removal of the synovial lining.

synovial sarcoma See *sarcoma, synovial.*

synoviosarcoma See *sarcoma, synovial.*

synovitis Inflammation of the synovial membrane, the lining of the joints.

syphilis A sexually transmitted disease that is caused by Treponema pallidum, a microscopic organism called a spirochete. This worm-like, spiral-shaped organism infects people by burrowing into the moist mucous membranes of the mouth or genitals. From there, the spirochete produces a nonpainful ulcer known as a chancre. There are three stages of syphilis. The first (primary) stage is formation of the chancre, and it can last from 1 to 5 weeks. At this stage, syphilis is highly contagious. The disease can be transmitted via any contact with one of the ulcers, which are teeming with spirochetes. If the ulcer is outside the vagina or on the scrotum, the use of condoms may not prevent transmission. Likewise, if the ulcer is in the mouth, merely kissing the infected individual can spread syphilis. Even without treatment, the early infection resolves on its own in most women. However, 25 percent proceed to the secondary stage of syphilis, which lasts from 4 to 6 weeks. This phase can include hair loss; a sore throat; white patches in the nose, mouth, and vagina; fever; headaches; and a skin rash. There can be lesions on the genitals that look like genital warts but are caused by spirochetes rather than the wart virus. These wart-like lesions, as well as the skin rash, are highly contagious. The rash can occur on the palms of the hands, and the infection can be transmitted via casual contact. The third (tertiary) stage of the disease involves the brain and heart, and at this point the disease is usually no longer contagious. At this point, however, the infection can cause extensive damage to the internal organs and the brain; it can even lead to death. Diagnosis is made via blood test, either the rapid plasma reagin (RPR) or Venereal Disease Research Laboratory (VDRL) test. Treatment involves use of antibiotics. While syphilis is relatively easily treated with antibiotics in its earlier stages, late stage syphilis can leave permanent brain and nervous system damage despite an extended antibiotic course. See also *chancre; spirochete; syphilis, congenital; syphilis test, RPR; VDRL test.*

syphilis, congenital   Infection of a fetus or newborn with syphilis. Syphilis in a fetus can cause deformity, particularly of the long bones, or death. Syphilis infection acquired at birth is also dangerous. See also *TORCH screen.*

syphilis test, RPR   Rapid plasma reagin syphillis test, a blood test for syphilis that looks for an antibody that is present in the bloodstream when a patient has syphilis. A negative (nonreactive) RPR test is compatible with a person not having syphilis, but in the early stages of the disease, the RPR often gives false negative results. Conversely, a false positive RPR can be encountered in a patient with infectious mononucleosis, lupus, antiphospholipid syndrome, hepatitis A, leprosy, malaria, or, occasionally, pregnancy. See also *syphilis; VDRL test.*

syphilis test, VDRL   See *VDRL test.*

syringe   A medical device that is used to inject fluid into, or withdraw fluid from, the body. A medical syringe consists of a needle attached to a hollow cylinder that is fitted with a sliding plunger. The downward movement of the plunger injects fluid; upward movement withdraws fluid. Medical syringes were once made of metal or glass, and required cleaning and sterilization before they could be used again. Now most syringes used in medicine are plastic and disposable.

syringoma   A benign (noncancerous) skin tumor that derives from eccrine cells, specialized cells related to sweat glands. The skin lesions of syringoma usually appear during puberty or adult life, and they consist of small bumps 1 to 3 mm in diameter that form under the surface of the skin. The most frequent site is the eyelids and around the eyes, but other areas of the body can also be affected. There may be only one or a few lesions in a localized area, or numerous lesions may cover a wide area. Syringomas more frequently affect women than men, and they have a hereditary basis in some cases. They are also associated with Down syndrome, Marfan syndrome, and Ehlers-Danlos syndrome. Treatment of syringomas can be difficult, depending on their number and location. One method that seems to be effective and creates minimal scarring is the use of a hair-removal electric needle; another promising technique uses a CO_2 laser.

systemic lupus erythematosus   See *lupus erythematosus, systemic.*

systemic therapy   Treatment that reaches cells throughout the body by traveling through the bloodstream.

systemic-onset juvenile chronic arthritis   See *arthritis, systemic-onset juvenile chronic.*

systemic-onset juvenile rheumatoid arthritis   See *arthritis, systemic-onset juvenile rheumatoid.*

systolic   Referring to the time at which ventricular contraction occurs, which is called systole. Systolic pressure is the maximum arterial pressure during contraction of the left ventricle of the heart. In a blood pressure reading, the systolic pressure is typically the first number recorded. For example, in a blood pressure of 120/80 ("120 over 80"), the systolic pressure is 120 (that is, 120 mm Hg [millimeters of mercury]). A systolic murmur is a heart murmur heard during systole. See also *diastolic.*

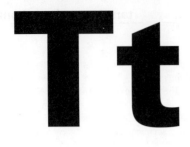

T Thymine, one member of the adenine-thymine (A-T) base pair in DNA.

t In genetics, translocation.

T cell A type of white blood cell that is made in the bone marrow and migrates to the thymus gland, where it matures, differentiates into various types of T cells, and becomes active in the immune system. T cells that are potentially activated against the body's own tissues are normally killed or changed (down-regulated) during this maturation process. There are several types of mature T cells. Most of the T cells in the body belong to one of two subsets known as T-4 cells and T-8 cells. T-8 cells are cytotoxic T lymphocytes that can produce cytokines, such as the interleukins, which in turn further stimulate the immune response. T-cell activation is measured to assess the health of patients with HIV. Also known as T lymphocyte. See also *natural killer cell; T-4 cell; T lymphocyte, cytotoxic; T-suppressor cell.*

T cell, CD4+ See *T-4 cell.*

T cell, CD8+ See *T lymphocyte, cytotoxic.*

T cell, peripheral A T cell that is found in the peripheral blood rather than in the lymphatic system.

T lymphocyte, cytotoxic A cell that expresses the CD8 transmembrane glycoprotein and is antigen specific. Abbreviated CTL. CTLs are able to search out and kill specific types of infected cells. When they find cells carrying the viral peptide they are looking for, they induce those cells to secrete proteins that attract nearby macrophages (specialized white blood cells). These macrophages then surround and destroy the infected cells. CTLs are particularly important in the immune response to viruses and cancer. Also known as TC cell. See also *CD8; T cell; T-suppressor cell.*

T1–T12 Symbols that represent the 12 thoracic vertebrae.

T-4 cell A T cell that expresses the CD4 transmembrane glycoprotein (CD4+ T cell). T-4 cells are active in the body's immune response, helping to turn on this system when it is challenged by an infection or by foreign matter in the body. HIV attacks T-4 cells, knocking out the body's ability to defend itself against infections. T-helper cells fall into two main classes: those that activate other T cells to achieve cellular inflammatory responses; and those that drive B cells to produce antibodies in the humoral immune response. These two classes of response are generally incompatible with one another and require coordination by substances called cytokines to promote one response while dampening the other. Also known as T-helper cell and TH cell. See also *CD4; T cell.*

T-4 count A test that counts the number of T-4 cells in the blood, for example, to assess the immune status of a patient with HIV. It is important to note that there are T-4 cells in the lymphatic system, and they may be more severely affected there than those in the bloodstream. Of the various ways to read a T-4 count test, the best indicator of health may be the absolute T-4 count, the actual number of T-cells per unit volume of blood. Also known as T-helper count. See also *helper/suppressor ratio; T cell.*

T-8 cell See *T-suppressor cell.*

T-helper cell See *T-4 cell.*

T-suppressor cell A T cell that expresses the CD8 transmembrane glycoprotein (CD8+ T cells). T-suppressor cells close down the immune response after invading organisms are destroyed. T-suppressor cells are sensitive to high concentrations of circulating lymphokine hormones, and they release their own lymphokines after an immune response has achieved its goal. This signals all other immune system participants to cease their attack. Some memory B-cells remain after this signal to ward off a repeat attack by the invading organism. Also known as T-8 cell. See also *CD8; T cell; T lymphocyte, cytotoxic.*

T-suppressor count A test that counts the number of T-suppressor (T-8) cells in the bloodstream. It appears that some T-8 cells secrete a substance that can kill HIV, so a high count is believed to be a good indicator for people with HIV (AIDS). See also *helper/suppressor ratio; T-suppressor cell.*

tabes dorsalis See *neurosyphilis, tabes.*

tablespoon An old-fashioned but convenient household measure of capacity that is equal to about 15 cc of liquid.

TACE Transarterial chemoembolization, a procedure in which the blood supply to a tumor is blocked (embolized) and chemotherapy is administered directly into the tumor. For example, TACE has been used to treat some liver cancers.

tache noire French for "black spot," to describe a small ulcer covered with a black crust at the site of a tick bite. A tache noire is characteristic of several tick-borne rickettsial diseases. See also *rickettsial diseases.*

tachy- Prefix meaning swift or rapid, as in tachycardia (rapid heart rate). From the Greek word *tachys,* meaning "swift."

tachycardia A rapid heart rate, usually defined as greater than 100 beats per minute.

tachypnea Abnormally fast breathing.

tactile Having to do with touch. For example, tactile signs of disease are signs that are perceptible by touch, such as roughness of the skin.

taenia 1 In medicine, a genus of large tapeworms, some of which are parasitic in humans. 2 In anatomy, a band or a structural line; specifically, several bands and lines of nervous matter in the brain. Also spelled tenia.

Taenia saginata See *beef tapeworm.*

Taenia solium A tapeworm that can parasitize people and can be contracted from undercooked or infested pork. Also known as the armed tapeworm, the pork tapeworm, and the measly tapeworm.

tag, ear See *ear tag.*

tag, preauricular See *ear tag.*

tag, skin See *skin tag.*

tail 1 A slender appendage, such as the tail of the pancreas. 2 The appendage that protrudes from the backside of an animal. A person can appear to have a tail due to the presence of extra segments of the coccyx.

taint To poison, infect, or spoil.

talipes See *clubfoot.*

talipes equinovarus The most common (classic) form of clubfoot. With this talipes equinovarus, the foot is turned in sharply, and the person seems to be walking on the ankle. See *clubfoot.*

talus The ankle bone, or the ankle itself. The ankle joint is formed by the talus and the bottom of the tibia and fibula, which rest upon it.

tamoxifen An antiestrogen that competes with estrogen for binding sites in target tissues such as breast tissue and blocks the effects of estrogen there. Tamoxifen was approved by the US Food and Drug Administration (FDA) to treat breast cancer, help prevent it in women at high risk, and treat women who have had surgery and radiation therapy for ductal carcinoma in situ, to lower the risk of invasive breast cancer arising from the intraductal carcinoma.

tampon A pack or pad that is used to stop or collect the flow of blood or other fluids. A tampon may be made of cotton, sponge, or another material. Tampons serve in surgery to control bleeding and are used to stop severe nosebleeds. Vaginal tampons collect the flow of menstrual blood.

tamponade, balloon See *balloon tamponade.*

tamponade, cardiac A life-threatening situation in which there is such a large amount of fluid (usually blood) inside the pericardial sac around the heart that it interferes with the performance of the heart. If cardiac tamponade is left untreated, the result is dangerously low blood pressure, shock, and death. The excess fluid in the pericardial sac acts to compress and constrict the heart. Cardiac tamponade can be due to excessive pericardial fluid, a wound to the heart, or rupture of the heart. Also known as pericardial tamponade.

tamponade, chronic A long-standing situation in which an excess of fluid inside the pericardial sac combines with thickening of the pericardial sac to progressively compress the heart and impair its performance.

tap, joint See *arthrocentesis.*

tap, spinal See *lumbar puncture.*

tapeworm A worm that is flattened like a tape measure and functions as an intestinal parasite, unable to live freely on its own but able to live within an animal's gut.

tapeworm, beef See *beef tapeworm.*

tapeworm, pork See *Taenia solium.*

TAR syndrome Thrombocytopenia–absent radius syndrome, in which the platelets needed for blood to clot normally are too few in number and the radius (the smaller of the two bones of the forearm) is absent, resulting in phocomelia (a "flipper" limb). The fibula (the smaller bone in the lower leg) is also often absent. The risk of bleeding due to having too few platelets is high in early infancy. About 40 percent of patients with TAR syndrome die within the newborn period due to hemorrhage. In the survivors, the platelet problem lessens with age. TAR syndrome is inherited in an autosomal recessive manner. The gene for it has not been identified. Also known as tetraphocomelia–thrombocytopenia syndrome.

tarsal cyst See *cyst, Meibomian.*

tarsal gland See *gland, Meibomian.*

tarsal tunnel syndrome A syndrome that is due to compression of the nerve in the ankle and foot, usually from the trauma of repetitive work involving the ankle. Abbreviated TTS. Obesity, pregnancy, hypothyroidism, arthritis, and diabetes predispose a person to TTS. Symptoms include numbness and tingling of the foot and toes, a "pins and needles" feeling at night, and feelings of weakness in the ankle and of poor coordination. The diagnosis of TTS can be suspected by history, made via examination (by finding Tinel's sign), and confirmed with a nerve conduction test. Early TTS is usually treated with modification of activities, use of a removable ankle brace, and use of anti-inflammatory medicines. Caught early, TTS is reversible. If numbness and pain continue in the foot and toes, a cortisone injection into the tarsal tunnel can help. In advanced TTS, particularly with profound weakness and muscle atrophy (wasting), surgery is done to avoid permanent nerve damage. The surgical procedure, called a tarsal tunnel release, relieves the pressure exerted on the nerve within the tarsal tunnel. TTS is analogous to carpal tunnel syndrome. See also *carpal tunnel syndrome; Tinel's sign.*

tarsus, bony See *bony tarsus.*

tartar The hardened product of minerals from saliva and foods that accumulates in plaque around the teeth. Dental plaque and tartar cause periodontal disease, including inflammation of the bone surrounding the teeth. Tartar can become as hard as rock, becoming removable only by a dentist or dental hygienist with special tools.

Tassinari syndrome A form of epilepsy that is associated with language difficulties. Tassinari syndrome surfaces around the age of 4, with receptive or expressive dysphasia and slowed learning. The patient may have absence, myoclonic, or focal seizures. The cause of Tassinari syndrome is unknown. Treatment involves use of seizure medications. The condition usually improves by adulthood. Also called continuous spike waves of slow sleep (CSWS). See also *dysphagia; epilepsy; seizure disorder.*

taste A perception that results from stimulation of a gustatory nerve. Taste belongs to the chemical sensing system. Tasting begins when molecules stimulate special cells in the mouth or throat. These special cells transmit messages through nerves to the brain, where specific tastes are identified. Gustatory, or taste, cells react to food and beverages. These surface cells in the mouth send taste information to their nerve fibers. The taste cells are clustered in the taste buds of the mouth and throat. Many of the small bumps that can be seen on the tongue contain taste buds. Smell contributes to the sense of taste, as does another chemosensory mechanism, called the common chemical sense. In this system, thousands of nerve endings—especially on the moist surfaces of the eyes, nose, mouth, and throat—give rise to sensations such as the sting of ammonia, the coolness of menthol, and the irritation of chili peppers. People can commonly identify four

basic taste sensations: sweet, sour, bitter, and salty. In the mouth, these tastes, along with texture, temperature, and the sensations from the common chemical sense, combine with odors to produce the perception of flavor. Flavor lets a person know whether he or she is eating a pear or an apple. Flavors are recognized mainly through the sense of smell. If a person holds his or her nose while eating chocolate, for example, the person will have trouble identifying the chocolate flavor—even though he or she can distinguish the food's sweetness or bitterness. That is because the familiar flavor of chocolate is sensed largely by odor.

taste bud One of the tiny, barrel-shaped endings of the gustatory nerve located around the base of the papillae (small bumps) on the tongue.

tattoo The permanent insertion of ink below the skin, using a sharp instrument. Humans have done tattooing for cosmetic and ritual purposes since at least the Neolithic era. Today the practice is made relatively safe by the use of nonreactive pigments; sterile, disposable needles; and sterile work conditions. Without these refinements, inks may cause inflammation, and infection is an ever-present danger. Persons who are prone to keloids should be aware that tattoos can trigger these heaped-up disfiguring scars. Ink lines may also spread or change color over the years, a fact of special concern for those interested in so-called "permanent cosmetics" (tattooed lip color, eyebrows, eyeliner, and the like). Tattooed skin requires some special care. Fresh tattoos should be kept clean, dry, and covered for the first day, and antibiotic ointment should be used for several days to promote healing and prevent infection. After it has healed, tattooed skin should be protected from UV rays with sunscreen to prevent fading and skin damage.

tattoo removal Removal of a tattoo, as with the use of lasers to destroy the ink itself. Multiple treatments may be necessary, depending on the size of the piece and the inks used. Some tattoos cannot be completely removed with lasers, and lasers may scar some types of skin.

Tay-Sachs disease A genetic metabolic disorder caused by deficiency of the enzyme hexosaminidase A (hex-A) that results in failure to process GM2 ganglioside, a lipid (fat) that then accumulates in the brain and other tissues. Abbreviated TSD. The classic form of TSD begins in infancy. The child usually develops normally for the first few months, but head control is lost by 6 to 8 months of age; the infant cannot roll over or sit up, spasticity and rigidity develop, and excessive drooling and convulsions become evident. Blindness and head enlargement occur by the second year. The disease worsens as the central nervous system progressively deteriorates. After age 2, constant nursing care is needed. Death generally occurs by age 5, due usually to cachexia (wasting away) or aspiration pneumonia. There are several forms of TSD. With juvenile TSD and adult TSD, the person has somewhat more hex-A and hence a later onset of clinical disease than with infantile TSD. All forms of TSD are inherited in an autosomal recessive manner and are due to mutation of the gene for the alpha subunit of hex-A that is on chromosome 15q23–15q24. The frequency of TSD is relatively high in Ashkenazi Jews (particularly those whose ancestors came from Lithuania and Poland). Knowledge of the biochemical basis of TSD now permits screening for carrier status and prenatal diagnosis. Also known as amaurotic familial idiocy, type 1 GM2-gangliosidosis, B variant GM2-gangliosidosis, hexosaminidase A deficiency, and hex-A deficiency. See also *Sandhoff disease.*

TB Tuberculosis.

TC-99 tetrofosmin scintimammography See *scintimammography.*

Td Adult diphtheria and tetanus toxoids. See *Td vaccine.*

Td vaccine A vaccine that is given to children over the age of 6 and to adults as a booster for immunity against diphtheria and tetanus.

teaspoon An old-fashioned but convenient household measure that is equal to about 5 cc of liquid.

technology, recombinant DNA See *recombinant DNA technology.*

teeth Plural of tooth.

telangiectasia, hereditary hemorrhagic See *hereditary hemorrhagic telangiectasia.*

telomerase The enzyme that is concerned with the formation, maintenance, and renovation of telomeres, the ends of chromosomes.

telomere The end of a chromosome. The ends of chromosomes are specialized structures that are involved in the replication and stability of DNA molecules. A telomere is a length of DNA that is made up of a repeating sequence of six nucleotide bases (TTAGGG). Small numbers of these terminal TTAGGG sequences are lost from the tips of the chromosomes, but the addition of TTAGGG repeats by the enzyme telomerase compensates for this loss.

temperature The specific degree of hotness or coldness of the body. The normal body temperature is generally considered to be 37° C (98.6° F). However, the normal body temperature may range between 36.1 to 37.2° C (97° and 99° F) during the day. The body temperature at the beginning of the day, when a person first arises, is called the basal temperature. If the body

temperature reaches 39.4 ° C (103° F) in a child or 40 to 40.5° C (104° to 105° F) in an adult, a physician should be consulted. See also *thermometer.*

temple The area just behind and to the side of the forehead and the eye, above the side of the zygomatic arch (checkbone) and in front of the ear.

temporal **1** Pertaining to the temple region of the head. For example, the temporal lobe of the brain is so named because of its anatomic location beneath the temple. **2** Pertaining to time, limited in time, temporary, or transient.

temporal arteritis See *arteritis, cranial.*

temporal bone A large irregular bone that is situated at the base and side of the skull. The temporal bone is connected with the mandible (the jawbone) via the temporomandibular joint.

temporal lobe The lobe of the cerebral hemisphere on the side of the brain just forward of the occipital lobe. The temporal lobe is located beneath the temple region of the head. The temporal lobe contains the auditory cortex, which is responsible for hearing. It is also the site of the seizure activity that is characteristic of temporal lobe epilepsy. See also *epilepsy, temporal lobe.*

temporary loss of consciousness See *syncope.*

temporary teeth See *primary teeth.*

temporomandibular joint The joint that hinges the lower jaw (mandible) to the temporal bone of the skull. Abbreviated TMJ. The TMJ is one of the most frequently used joints in the entire body, moving whenever a person eats, drinks, or talks. See *temperomandibular joint syndrome.*

temporomandibular joint syndrome A disorder of the temporomandibular joint (TMJ) that causes pain, usually in front of the ear(s), sometimes in the form of a headache. Pain in the TMJ can be due to trauma, such as a blow to the face; inflammatory or degenerative arthritis; or poor dental work or structural defects that push the mandible back toward the ears whenever the patient chews or swallows. Grinding or clenching the teeth due to stress is a frequent cause. Sometimes muscles around the TMJ that are used for chewing can go into spasm, causing head and neck pain, as well as difficulty opening the mouth normally. Treatment depends on the cause and severity of the problem and can range from use of a mouth guard or medication to prevent nighttime tooth grinding to surgery. See *temporomandibular joint.*

tendinitis See *tendonitis.*

tendon The soft tissue by which muscle attaches to bone. Tendons are somewhat flexible, but tough. When a tendon becomes inflamed, the condition is referred to as tendonitis.

tendon, Achilles See *Achilles tendon.*

tendonitis Inflammation of a tendon (the tissue by which muscle attaches to bone). Tendonitis most commonly occurs as a result of injury, as to the tendons around the shoulder or elbow. It can also occur as a result of an underlying inflammatory rheumatic disease, such as reactive arthritis or gout. Sometimes spelled tendinitis.

tenesmus Straining to defecate or urinate. Tenesmus refers especially to ineffectual and painful straining for an extended time. Straining to defecate is called rectal tenesmus; straining to urinate is called vesical tenesmus.

tenia See *taenia.*

tennis elbow See *elbow, tennis.*

tension **1** The pressure within a vessel, such as blood pressure (the pressure within the blood vessels). **2** Stress, especially stress that is translated into clenched muscles and bottled-up emotions. This type of tension is blamed for tension headaches.

tension, arterial See *arterial tension.*

tension headache See *headache, tension.*

tension, intraocular See *intraocular pressure.*

teratogen An agent that can disturb the development of an embryo or a fetus. A teratogen is capable either of terminating a pregnancy prematurely or, if the pregnancy persists, of damaging the fetus. The major classes of teratogens include radiation, maternal infections, maternal metabolic diseases, chemicals, and drugs. See also *teratogenic drug.*

teratogenic drug A drug that is capable of acting as a teratogen and interrupting a pregnancy or impairing the child. Drugs that are known teratogens include, but are not limited to, ACE inhibitors such as benazepril (brand name: Lotensin), captopril (brand name: Capoten), enalapril (brand name: Vasotec), fosinopril sodium (brand name: Monopril), lisinopril (brand names: Zestril, Prinivil), lisinopril and hydrochlorothiazide (brand names: Zestoretic, Prinzide), quinapril (brand name: Accupril), and ramipril (brand name: Altace); the acne medication isotretinoin (brand names: Accutane, Retin-A); alcohol, whether ingested chronically or in binges; androgens (male hormones); the antibiotics tetracycline (brand name: Achromycin), doxycycline (brand name: Vibramycin), and streptomycin; blood-thinners, such as

warfarin (brand name: Coumadin); seizure medications, including phenytoin (brand name: Dilantin), valproic acid (brand names: Depakene, Depakote, Valprotate), trimethadione (brand name: Tridione), paramethadione (brand name: Paradione), and carbamazepine (brand name: Tegretol); the antidepressant/antimanic drug lithium (brand names: Eskalith, Lithotab); antimetabolite/anticancer drugs methotrexate (brand name: Rheumatrex) and aminopterin; the antirheumatic agent and chelator penicillamine (brand names: Ciprimene, Depen); antithyroid drugs, such as thiouracil/propylthiouracil and carbimazole/methimazole; cocaine; the hormone DES (diethylstilbestrol); and thalidomide (brand name: Thalomid). Alcohol and illegal or unnecessary drugs should never be used by women who are pregnant or who plan to get pregnant. However, sometimes a medication that is necessary for health is also a teratogen: thyroid medication, blood thinners, and lithium are a few examples. Female patients who must take such medications should work carefully with their physicians to determine whether an alternative treatment is possible before and during pregnancy. In some cases the danger of birth defects is limited to a certain part of the pregnancy, and medication can be started again after that period has passed. Other medications can be safely restarted upon the baby's birth. Some medications also pass through breast milk, however, and if they cannot be avoided, the mother may need to choose formula feeding instead.

teratoma, ovarian See *ovarian teratoma.*

teres minor muscle A muscle that assists the lifting of the arm during outward turning (external rotation). The tendon of the teres minor muscle is one of four tendons that stabilize the shoulder joint and constitute the rotator cuff.

terminal ileitis See *Crohn's disease.*

test **1** An assay or examination. **2** A significant chemical reaction. **3** A reagent for a specific test. For specific tests, please see their alphabetical listings.

testes Plural of testis.

testicle See *testis.*

testicular cancer See cancer, *testicular.*

testicular self-examination A procedure for detecting the early signs of testicular cancer. Monthly, men should check the testes visually for new swelling or other changes on the skin of the scrotum, roll each testicle between thumb and fingers to detect internal growths, and check the cord (epididymis) on the top and back of each testicle for growths. A warm bath or shower relaxes the scrotum, making examination easier. Early detection of testicular cancer greatly improves the likelihood of successful treatment. See also *cancer, testicular.*

testis The male sex gland, located behind the penis in a pouch of skin called the scrotum. The testes produce and store sperm and are also the body's main source of male hormones, such as testosterone. These hormones control the development of the reproductive organs and other male characteristics, such as body and facial hair, low voice, and wide shoulders. Also known as testicle.

testosterone The principal androgenic hormone produced by the testes. Testosterone is made by the testes in response to luteinizing hormone from the pituitary gland. Androgens promote the development of adult male sex characteristics, such as deep voice; they strengthen muscle and bone mass; and they stimulate spermatogenesis, the production of sperm. High levels of testosterone appear to promote good health in men, lowering the risk of high blood pressure and heart attack, for example. High testosterone levels may also correlate with risky behavior, however, including increased aggressiveness and smoking, which may cancel out these health benefits. Testosterone may be given to treat medical conditions, including female (but not male) breast cancer. See also *androgen; testosterone replacement therapy.*

testosterone replacement therapy The practice of using testosterone to treat conditions in which the testes produce a deficient amount due to absence, injury, or disease. Testosterone is available in oral, IV, and patch forms. As with estrogen replacement therapy for women, dosing must be carefully calibrated to gain the greatest benefits and to minimize unwanted side effects. See also *testosterone.*

tetanus An often fatal infectious disease that is caused by the bacterium Clostridium tetani, which usually enters the body through a puncture, a cut, or an open wound. Tetanus leads to profound painful spasms of muscles, including "locking" of the jaw so that the mouth cannot open, and death. The C. tetani bacteria releases a toxin that affects the motor nerves, which stimulate the muscles. Prevention involves immediately cleaning and covering any open wound and getting a tetanus vaccination. The DPT, DTaP, DT, and Td vaccines all protect against tetanus. Regular boosters are necessary to ensure immunity. Unvaccinated people who get puncture wounds or cuts should get tetanus immunoglobulin and a series of tetanus shots immediately; those who have been immunized but are unsure of the date of their last tetanus shot should get boosters. Tetanus and diphtheria toxoids (Td) are recommended at age 11–12 years if at least 5 years have elapsed since the last dose of tetanus and diphtheria toxoid-containing vaccine. Subsequent routine Td boosters are recommended every 10 years. Also known as lockjaw.

tetany A condition that is due usually to low blood calcium (hypocalcemia) and is characterized by spasms of the hands and feet, cramps, spasm of the voice box (larynx), and overactive neurological reflexes. Tetany is generally considered to result from very low calcium levels in the blood. However, tetany can also result from reduction in the ionized fraction of plasma calcium without marked hypocalcemia, as is the case in severe alkalosis (when the blood is highly alkaline).

tetralogy of Fallot A combination of four heart defects that are present at birth and account for about 10 percent of all congenital heart disease:

- **Ventricular septal defect (VSD)** A hole between the two bottom chambers, the ventricles, of the heart that permits oxygen-poor blood from the right ventricle to mix with oxygen-rich blood from the left ventricle.

- **Pulmonary stenosis** Narrowing of the outlet to the pulmonary artery area with an abnormal pulmonary valve impeding blood flow from the right ventricle to the lungs.

- **Right ventricular hypertrophy (RVH)** Thickening and enlargement of the muscle of the right ventricle.

- **Overriding aorta** A case in which the aorta overrides or straddles the wall (the septum) between the ventricles, permitting oxygen-poor blood to flow through the VSD into the aorta.

Open-heart surgery is done on patients with tetralogy of Fallot in infancy or early childhood. Untreated tetralogy of Fallot is usually fatal before age 20. With open-heart surgery, the patient has an excellent chance of survival

tetraphocomelia–thrombocytopenia syndrome See *TAR syndrome.*

tetraploid Having four full sets of chromosomes: 4 copies of each autosomal chromosome plus 4 sex chromosomes. In humans, tetraploid is equal to 92 chromosomes.

thalamotomy A procedure that is performed via stereotaxic surgery and is designed to destroy part of the thalamus in order to relieve intractable pain, seizures, or involuntary movements, as in Parkinson's disease.

thalamus A large ovoid mass within the midbrain (the interbrain, connected to the cerebral hemisphere) that forms part of the walls of the third ventricle in the brain. The thalamus contains a number of distinct groups of cells or nuclei that function as relay centers for sensory and other impulses between the body and the brain and between the cerebellum, the basal ganglia, and the cerebral cortex. Destruction of part of the thalamus is called thalamotomy.

thalassemia A group of genetic disorders that involve underproduction of hemoglobin, the indispensable molecule in red blood cells that transports oxygen and carbon dioxide. All forms of hemoglobin are made up of two molecules: heme and globin. The globin part of hemoglobin is made up of four polypeptide chains. In normal adult hemoglobin (Hb A), the predominant type of hemoglobin after the first year of life, two of the globin chains are identical to each other and are called the alpha chains. The other two chains, which are also identical to each other but are different from the alpha chains, are called the beta chains. In fetal hemoglobin (Hb F), the predominant hemoglobin during fetal development, there are two alpha chains and two different chains called gamma chains. In thalassemia, there is a mutation (change) in one or both of the alpha or beta globin chains. Depending on which globin chain is affected, the mutation leads to underproduction or absence of that globin chain, a deficiency of hemoglobin, and anemia. The carriers of heterozygous forms of alpha and beta thalassemia have red cell anomalies that range from very mild to severe.

thalassemia, alpha A form of thalassemia that involves the alpha chain. If a fetus inherits two genes for alpha thalassemia, one from each parent, the disorder is lethal before birth: No alpha chains can be made, and without alpha chains, there can be no fetal hemoglobin. If the fetus inherits only one alpha thalassemia gene, it will survive and have no or few symptoms as a child, as there is another gene that is still able to make alpha chains.

thalassemia, beta See *thalassemia major.*

thalassemia major The most serious form of beta thalassemia, in which there is a mutation in both of the beta globin chains. This leads to underproduction or absence of beta chains, underproduction of hemoglobin, and profound anemia. Children with thalassemia major seem entirely normal at birth because at birth they still have predominantly fetal hemoglobin, which does not contain beta chains. The anemia emerges in the first few months of life and becomes progressively more severe, leading to pallor, fatigue, failure to thrive, bouts of fever due to infections, and diarrhea. The gene for thalassemia major is relatively frequent in people of Mediterranean origin. Children with thalassemia major inherit one thalassemia gene from each parent. Treatment based on blood transfusions is helpful but not curative. Gene therapy will, it is hoped, be applicable to this disease. Also known as beta thalassemia, Cooley anemia, and Mediterranean anemia.

thalassemia minor Also called thalassemia trait, the carrier state for thalassemia major. People who are carriers have just one beta thalassemia gene and are essentially normal, although they can transmit the gene to their offspring.

thalidomide A drug (brand name: Thalomid) that was used in the 1950s and early 1960s to treat morning sickness in pregnancy. The use of thalidomide had tragic results: When taken during pregnancy, it can cause a syndrome of congenital malformations in the developing fetus. Thalidomide was then not approved for marketing in the US and it was taken off the market in other countries. However, in 1998 it was approved by the US Food and Drug Administration (FDA) for the treatment of a skin condition that is due to leprosy (erythema nodosum leprosum). Thalidomide appears to modify the reaction of the immune system to the leprosy bacterium and thereby suppresses the skin reaction. It also appears to have other beneficial uses in the treatment of several different types of cancer, HIV-related ulcers, and some autoimmune diseases, including Behcet's disease and skin manifestations of dermatomyositis. One common side effect is peripheral neuritis (inflammation of the nerves). Thalidomide is a potent teratogen and should never be taken by women who are or could become pregnant. See also *thalidomide baby; thalidomide syndrome.*

thalidomide baby An infant who is affected by prenatal exposure to the drug thalidomide. In 1998, thalidomide again became available (to treat leprosy), and there is concern that babies may be born with the thalidomide syndrome as they were in the 1950s and early 1960s.

thalidomide syndrome A congenital malformation syndrome that is caused by maternal exposure to thalidomide. Although thalidomide syndrome is epitomized by the flipper-like limbs (phocomelia), thalidomide causes a wide range of birth defects, including absence of ears with deafness; defects of the muscles of the eye and of the face; absence or hypoplasia (underdevelopment) of the arms, especially affecting the radius and the thumb; thumbs with three joints; defects of the femur and of the tibia; and malformations of the heart, bowel, uterus, and gallbladder. The pattern of malformations depends on the time of intake of the drug. Thalidomide usually causes no malformations if taken before the 34th day or after the 50th day after the last menstruation. During the sensitive period, taking thalidomide causes the following sequence of malformations:

- 35th–37th day: absent ears and deafness
- 39th–41st day: absent arms
- 43rd–44th day: phocomelia with three fingers
- 46th–48th day: thumbs with three joints

If thalidomide is taken throughout the sensitive period, the baby may have severe defects of ears, arms, legs, and internal organs, and the baby may die. About 40 percent of thalidomide babies died before their first birthday.

Many thalidomide babies have lived into adulthood. They are now reaching middle age, and in some cases are facing new health problems from their exposure to the drug before their birth.

thelarche The time that breast development starts in girls.

therapeutic Relating to therapeutics, the branch of medicine that is concerned specifically with the treatment of disease. The therapeutic dose of a drug is the amount needed to treat a disease.

therapeutic abortion An abortion that is brought about intentionally. Also known as induced abortion.

therapeutic cloning Cloning designed as therapy for a disease. In therapeutic cloning, the nucleus of a cell, typically a skin cell, is inserted into a fertilized egg whose nucleus has been removed. The nucleated egg begins to divide repeatedly to form a blastocyst. Scientists then extract stem cells from the blastocyst and use them to grow cells that are a perfect genetic match for the patient. The cells created via therapeutic cloning can then be transplanted into the patient to treat a disease from which the patient suffers. In contrast to the goal of therapeutic cloning, the goal of reproductive cloning is to create a new individual, an idea that has stirred great controversy and met with almost uniform disapproval.

therapy The treatment of disease. Therapy is synonymous with treatment.

thermometer In medicine, a device used to measure the temperature of the human body. There are many types of medical thermometers, including oral thermometers (placed under the tongue), rectal thermometers (placed within the rectum), multipurpose thermometers (placed under the tongue, in the rectum, or under the armpit), eardrum thermometers (placed inside the ear), and basal thermometers (highly sensitive thermometers placed under the tongue or in the rectum to measure slight temperature changes indicating that ovulation has taken place in a woman). See also *fever; temperature.*

thiamine Vitamin B1, which acts as a coenzyme in the metabolism of the body. In its active form, thiamine participates in a range of biochemical reactions, including certain reactions that are important to carbohydrate metabolism. Deficiency of thiamine leads to the disease beriberi. See also Appendix C, "Vitamins."

thigh The thick, muscular portion of the leg that extends from the hip to the knee. The thigh has only one bone, the femur, which is the largest bone in the human body.

thighbone See *femur.*

third and fourth pharyngeal pouch syndrome See *DiGeorge syndrome.*

third stage of labor See *placental stage of labor.*

third ventricle One cavity in a system of four communicating cavities within the brain that are continuous with the central canal that contains the spinal cord. The third ventricle is a median (midline) cavity in the brain and is bounded by the thalamus and hypothalamus on either side. It communicates anteriorly (in front) with the lateral ventricles, and posteriorly (in back) with the aqueduct of the midbrain, also known as the aqueduct of Sylvius. All the ventricles are filled with cerebrospinal fluid, which is formed by choroid plexuses, structures that are located in the walls and roofs of the ventricles.

thoracentesis Removal of fluid from the space between the lungs and the chest wall (the pleural cavity) for diagnostic or therapeutic purposes using a needle inserted between the ribs.

thoracic Pertaining to the chest. For example, the thoracic aorta is the part of the aorta that lies within the chest.

thoracic aneurysm See *aneurysm, thoracic.*

thoracic aorta The part of the aorta that lies within the chest. The thoracic aorta starts after the arch of the aorta and runs down to the diaphragm, the great muscle that separates the chest from the abdomen. The thoracic aorta gives off numerous branches that supply oxygenated blood to the chest cage and the organs within the chest. Also known as aorta thoracica, aorta thoracalis, and pars thoracalis aortae. See also *aorta.*

thoracic duct A vascular structure that recirculates lymph from the lymphatic circulation into the bloodstream. The thoracic duct begins in the abdomen, tracks alongside the aorta and esophagus, and eventually joins with the left brachiocephalic vein.

thoracic outlet syndrome A condition that is due to compromise of blood vessels or nerve fibers between the armpit (axilla) and the base of the neck, usually because of compression of nerves or blood vessels between the neck and shoulders. Symptoms include pain, arm weakness, and numbness in the hands and fingers. Thoracic outlet syndrome can be caused by muscle development from some types of manual work or exercise, injury, or malformation. Treatment involves physical therapy and use of anti-inflammatory medication, and sometimes by surgery.

thoracic vertebrae The 12 vertebrae situated between the cervical (neck) vertebrae and the lumbar vertebrae. The thoracic vertebrae provide attachment for the ribs and make up part of the back of the thorax (chest). The thoracic vertebrae are represented by the symbols T1 through T12. See also *vertebra; vertebral column.*

thoracotomy An operation to open the chest, usually in order to gain access to the lungs or heart.

thorax The area of the body that is located between the abdomen and the neck. Within the thorax are the lungs, the heart, and the first section of the aorta. Also known as chest.

thrive, failure to See *failure to thrive.*

thrombectomy A procedure to remove a clot (thrombus) from an artery.

thrombi Plural of thrombus.

thrombin An enzyme that presides over the conversion of a substance called fibrinogen to fibrin, which promotes clotting.

thrombinogen See *prothrombin.*

thrombocyte See *platelet.*

thrombocythemia An abnormally high number of platelets in the blood. Also known as thrombocytosis.

thrombocytopenia–absent radius syndrome See *TAR syndrome.*

thrombocytosis See *thrombocythemia.*

thrombolytic agent See *clot-dissolving medication.*

thrombophilia The tendency to form thromboses (blood clots in arteries and veins).

thrombophlebitis Inflammation of a vein that occurs when a blood clot forms.

thrombosis, cavernous sinus See *cavernous sinus thrombosis.*

thrombosis, deep vein See *deep vein thrombosis.*

thrombotic disease due to protein C deficiency See *protein C deficiency.*

thrombotic thrombocytopenic purpura A life-threatening disease that involves embolism and thrombosis (plugging) of the small blood vessels in the brain. Abbreviated TTP. TTP is characterized by the presence of platelet microthrombi (tiny traveling clots composed of platelets, the clotting cells in the blood), thrombocytopenia (lack of platelets), hemolytic anemia (from the breakup of red blood cells), fever, kidney abnormalities, and nervous system abnormalities such as aphasia, blindness, and convulsions. TTP can be triggered by many drugs. Treatment may include plasma exchange with fresh or frozen plasma, dialysis, and corticosteroids.

thrombus A clot in a blood vessel or within the heart.

thrush A yeast infection of the mucous membranes within the throat and mouth. Thrush looks like a light or white coating on the affected tissue, and it may cause irritation. Thrush is seen most often in infants, young children, elderly people (especially those who wear dentures or take medications that lower output of saliva), and people with compromised immune systems. Diagnosis is made via observation, and it can be confirmed by culturing a saliva sample or cheek scraping. Treatment involves use of oral antifungal medications. See also *yeast; yeast infection.*

thymine One member of the base pair A-T (adenine-thymine) in DNA.

thymiosis See *yaws.*

thymus An organ that is located in the upper chest behind the breastbone and in front of the lower neck in which the immune cells called T lymphocytes mature and multiply in early life. The thymus begins to shrink after puberty.

thymus and parathyroids, hypoplasia of See *DiGeorge syndrome.*

thyroglobulin A protein that is found primarily in the thyroid gland. Some thyroglobulin can be found in the blood, and this amount may be measured after thyroid surgery to determine whether thyroid cancer has recurred. Thyroglobulin derived from pig thyroid glands is sometimes used to treat thyroid dysfunction. Abbreviated Tg.

thyroglossal cyst See *cyst, thyroglossal.*

thyroid binding globulin A blood protein that binds with the thyroid hormone thyroxine (T4).

thyroid gland See *gland, thyroid.*

thyroid hormone A chemical substance that is made by the thyroid gland and is essential for the function of every cell in the body. The thyroid gland uses iodine to make thyroid hormones, which help regulate growth and the rate of chemical reactions (metabolism) and are involved in the circadian rhythms that govern sleep, among other essential functions. The two most prominent thyroid hormones are thyroxine (T4) and triiodothyronine (T3). The thyroid gland also makes calcitonin, which is involved in calcium metabolization and bone strength, as well as other substances. Thyroid stimulating hormone (TSH), which is produced by the pituitary gland, acts to stimulate hormone production by the thyroid gland. The hypothalamus gland in the brain stimulates the pituitary gland to make TSH. See also *calcitonin; thyroxine; triiodothyronine.*

thyroid hormone organification defect IIb See *Pendred syndrome.*

thyroid scan An image taken of a patient's thyroid gland after the patient swallows radioactive iodine or technetium. The image shows the thyroid gland in action as it accumulates radioactive material. Thyroid scanning is used to determine how active thyroid tissue is in manufacturing thyroid hormone. This can help a physician determine whether inflammation of the thyroid gland (thyroiditis) is present. It can also show the presence and degree of overactivity of the gland (hyperthyroidism). Thyroid scanning is especially helpful in evaluating thyroid nodules, particularly after a fine-needle aspiration biopsy has failed to provide a diagnosis. A scan can reveal whether a thyroid nodule is functioning. A functioning nodule actively takes up iodine to produce thyroid hormone, and so it produces a localized "hot" area on the image. A nonfunctioning nodule does not take up iodine, and it produces a localized "cold" area. Most nodules, particularly if they are functioning, are not malignant.

thyroid stimulating hormone A hormone that is produced by the pituitary gland at the base of the brain in response to signals from the hypothalamus gland in the brain. Abbreviated TSH. TSH promotes the growth of the thyroid gland in the neck and stimulates it to produce more thyroid hormones. When the amount of thyroid hormones is excessive, the pituitary gland stops producing TSH, thus reducing thyroid hormone production. This mechanism maintains a relatively constant level of thyroid hormones circulating in the blood. Also known as thyrotropin.

thyroid stimulating immunoglobulin A form of immunoglobulin G (IgG) that can bind to thyroid stimulating hormone (TSH) receptors on the thyroid gland. Abbreviated TSI. TSIs mimic the action of TSH, causing excess secretion of thyroxine and triiodothyronine. The TSI level is abnormally high in persons with hyperthyroidism due to Graves disease.

thyroidectomy Surgery to remove part or all of the thyroid gland. Thyroidectomy might be done to remove a tumor or to treat hyperthyroidism or goiter (enlarged thyroid gland). Complications of the surgery can include vocal cord paralysis and accidental removal of the parathyroid glands, which are located behind the thyroid gland. Because the parathyroid glands regulate calcium metabolism, their removal can result in low calcium levels.

thyroiditis Inflammation of the thyroid gland. The inflamed thyroid gland can release an excess of thyroid hormones into the bloodstream, resulting in a temporary hyperthyroid state. When the thyroid gland is depleted of thyroid hormones, the patient commonly goes through a hypothyroid (low thyroid) phase. This phase can last for 3 to 6 months, until the thyroid gland fully recovers. Thyroiditis can be diagnosed with a thyroid scan or biopsy. For specific types of thyroiditis, please see their alphabetical listings.

thyrolingual cyst See *cyst, thyroglossal.*

thyrotropin See *thyroid stimulating hormone.*

thyroxine A hormone that is made by the thyroid gland and is one of the most important thyroid hormones. Four iodine molecules are attached to the molecular structure of thyroxine. Along with the more powerful thyroid hormone triiodothyronine (T4), thyroxine affects almost every process in the body, including body temperature, growth, and heart rate. Also known as T4.

TIA Transient ischemic attack.

tibia The larger of the two long bones in the lower leg. The tibia is familiarly known as the shinbone.

tibia vara A condition that is characterized by disturbance of normal growth in the inner part of the upper tibia. Tibia vara causes a bowlegged gait and can impair the knees significantly. It is most common in children of African descent. Treatment usually involves surgery, although a knee-ankle-foot orthosis brace may be used. Also known as Blount disease.

tibial bowing Improper growth of the tibia in the leg that causes bowlegs or other leg problems. The tibia may bow anteriorly (in the front) or posteriorly (in the back). See also *tibia vara.*

tic A repetitive movement that is difficult, if not impossible, to control. Tics can affect any group of muscles. The most common are facial tics, such as eye-blinking, nose-twitching, and grimacing. Tics that affect the muscles used to produce speech are known as vocal tics and can range from grunts or whistles to the repetition of complete words or phrases. Complex motor tics involve multiple sequenced movements and can include behaviors such as twirling in place, tapping a certain number of times, or stooping to touch the ground. Tics are believed to arise in differences in or damage to the basal ganglia, a structure deep within the brain that controls automatic movements and that also affects impulsivity. See also *coprolalia; echolalia; palilalia; tic disorder; Tourette's syndrome.*

tic disorder A disorder that is characterized by the presence of tics. If both motor and vocal tics are present for more than 6 months, the diagnosis of Tourette's syndrome may be made. Diagnosis is made via observation. Treatment is not usually recommended for minor tics that are not bothersome to the patient. When treatment is desired, medication choices include the blood pressure drugs guanfacine (brand name: Tenex) and catapres (brand name: Clonadine) and the atypical or older neuroleptics. See also *tic; Tourette's syndrome.*

tick bite A bite from a bloodsucking parasitic insect that punctures the skin with a sharp beak and burrows into the skin with its head. Tick bites can carry serious illness, including Rocky Mountain spotted fever, other forms of tick typhus, and Lyme disease. See also *tick-borne disease.*

tick-borne disease A disease that is carried by or caused by a tick. The tick-borne diseases in the US include babesiosis (a malaria-like infection), Colorado tick fever (generally in the western US), ehrlichiosis, Lyme disease, relapsing fever (also called tick fever, most common in the western US), Rocky Mountain spotted fever (throughout the US, but most prevalent in the west), tick paralysis, and tularemia (rabbit fever). Anyone working in the outdoors, especially in areas with tall grasses, shrubs, low-hanging branches, or leaf mold, is susceptible to being bitten by a tick. Ticks do not jump, crawl, or fall onto a person. They are picked up when clothing or hair brushes leaves or other objects that they are on. Ticks are generally found within 3 feet of the ground. After a tick is picked up, it crawls until it finds a likely site to feed. Ticks often find spots at the back of the knee, near the hairline, and behind the ears. The best way to prevent tick-borne diseases is to avoid being bitten by ticks.

t.i.d. A prescription abbreviation meaning three times a day. See also Appendix A, "Prescription Abbreviations."

tight foreskin See *phimosis.*

tilt-table test A test that involves placing a patient on a table with a foot-support, tilting the table upward, and measuring the blood pressure and pulse. Symptoms are recorded with the patient in diverse positions. The tilt-table test is designed to detect postural hypotension (orthostatic hypotension), a condition caused by changing body position from a prone, supine, or sitting position to a more vertical position. Poor tone of the nerves of the legs can cause a disproportionate distribution of blood to the legs, instead of to the brain, so the patient feels light-headed and may even faint. Tilt-table testing may be done when heart disease is not suspected of being responsible for an attack of syncope (fainting) or near syncope. Depending on the presence or absence of symptoms during the tilt-table test, persons with certain forms of temporary loss of consciousness may be admitted to the hospital for observation and further testing. See also *syncope; syncope, situational; vasovagal reaction.*

time, prothrombin See *prothrombin time.*

tinea barbae A ringworm infection of the bearded area of the face and neck, with swelling and marked crusting,

often with itching. In the days when men went to the barber daily for a shave, tinea barbae was called barber's itch. Effective antifungal treatments include terbinafine (brand name: Lamisil), itraconazole (brand name: Sporanox), and fluconazole (brand name: Diflucan).

tinea capitis Ringworm of the scalp. This disorder occurs most commonly in children, especially those in late childhood and adolescence. It appears as scalp scaling associated with bald spots. Effective antifungal tablets include terbinafine (brand name: Lamisil), itraconazole (brand name: Sporanox), and fluconazole (brand name: Diflucan).

tinea corporis Ringworm of the skin with characteristic spots that have an "active" outer border as they slowly grow and advance. Many antifungal creams can clear the condition in approximately two weeks.

tinea incognito Tinea corporis that has been modified by the application of high-potency topical steroids in a way that renders it no longer typical in appearance and makes it difficult to diagnose.

tinea unguium See *onychomycosis.*

Tinel's sign The sign that a nerve is irritated. Tinel's sign is positive when lightly banging (percussing) over the nerve elicits a sensation of tingling, or "pins and needles," in the distribution of the nerve. For example, in carpal tunnel syndrome, where the median nerve is compressed at the wrist, the test for Tinel's sign is often positive, eliciting tingling in the thumb, index, and middle fingers.

tinnitus Ringing in the ears. Tinnitus has many causes, including some medications (including aspirin and other anti-inflammatory drugs), diseases such as Ménière's disease, aging, and ear trauma.

tissue A group or layer of cells that perform specific functions. For example, muscle tissue is a layer of muscle cells.

titer The concentration of a substance in a fluid, such as the concentration of an antibody in blood. The titer reflects the amount of the substance in the fluid. Sometimes also spelled titre.

titre See *titer.*

TMA Trimethylaminuria. See *fish-odor syndrome.*

TMJ Temporomandibular joint.

TMJ syndrome Temporomandibular joint syndrome.

tobacco A South American herb (Nicotiana tabacum) whose leaves contain 2 to 8 percent nicotine and serve as the source of both smoking and smokeless tobacco and the basis of great health hazards.

toc-, toco- Prefix meaning childbirth, as in tocolysis (the slowing or halting of labor). Sometimes spelled tok- and toko-.

tocolysis The slowing or halting of labor during the birth process.

tocolytic Relating to the inhibition, delaying, or halting of labor. For example, a tocolytic drug is a medication that deters labor.

tocophobia Fear of childbirth.

tocus Labor, childbirth.

toddler's fracture See *fracture, toddler's.*

toe sign See *Babinski reflex.*

toenail A tough, protective plate that is produced by living skin cells in the toe. A toenail consists of several parts, including the nail plate (the visible part of the nail), the nail bed (the skin beneath the nail plate), the cuticle (the tissue that overlaps the plate and rims the base of the nail), the nail folds (the skin that enfolds the frame and supports the nail on three sides), the lunula (the whitish half-moon at the base of the nail), and the matrix (the hidden part of the nail unit under the cuticle). Toenails grow from the matrix. They are composed largely of keratin, a hardened protein that is also found in fingernails, skin, and hair. As new cells grow in the matrix, the older cells are pushed out and compacted, taking on the flattened, hardened form of the toenail. The average growth rate for toenails is 0.1 mm per day. The exact rate of nail growth depends on numerous factors, including the age and sex of the individual and the time of year. Toenails generally grow fastest in young people, in males, and in the summer. Toenails grow more slowly than fingernails. See also *nail; nail care.*

toenail, ingrown A common disorder, particularly on the big (great) toe, in which the corner of the nail curves down into the skin due to mistrimming of the nail or due to shoes being too tight. An ingrown toenail can be painful and lead to infection. Sometimes simply removing the corner of the nail from the skin is enough to cure this problem, although this might need to be done by a physician, podiatrist, or foot-care specialist. Any infection that is present requires treatment. In some cases the entire nail must be removed. If ingrown toenails are caused by congenital nail malformations, the nail bed can be treated to permanently prevent regrowth.

toes, six See *hexadactyly.*

tok-, toko- See *toc-, toco-.*

tongue A strong muscle that is anchored to the floor of the mouth. The tongue is covered by the lingual membrane, which has special areas to detect different types of tastes. The tongue muscles are attached to the lower jaw and to the hyoid bone, a small, U-shaped bone that lies deep in the muscles at the back of the tongue and above the larynx. On the top surface of the tongue are small nodules, called papillae, that give the tongue its rough texture. Between the papillae, at the sides and base of the tongue, are the taste buds, which are small bulb-like structures. The muscle fibers of the tongue are heavily supplied with nerves. Babies have more taste buds than adults, and they have them almost everywhere in the mouth, including the cheeks. The tongue aids in the formation of the sounds of speech and aids in swallowing.

tongue tie A minor congenital anomaly in which the flap of mucous membrane under the tongue (known as the frenulum) is unusually short and limits somewhat the mobility of the tongue. The name tongue tie reflects the folk belief that with this condition, a child cannot feed or speak properly because the tongue is "tied." This belief is unfounded. The medical term for this condition is ankyloglossia.

tonometry A standard eye test that is done to determine the fluid pressure inside the eye. Increased pressure is a possible sign of glaucoma, a common and potentially very serious problem if not detected and treated promptly. Adults over 40 should have tonometry every 3 to 5 years. The pressure inside the eye is measured from the outside. In most cases, the pressure can be measured without anything actually touching the eye. The patient looks at an instrument that blows a small puff of air into the eye and then uses a special kind of sensor (like a tiny radar detector) to detect the amount of indentation that the air puff causes on the surface of the eye. This indentation is normal and lasts only a fraction of a second. If patients need to have their eye pressure measured when this type of machine is not available (as in an emergency room), the pressure can be measured with an instrument that resembles a pen. One end of the instrument is placed on the surface of the eyeball. This feels like having a contact lens put in the eye. Tonometry does not cause significant pain and it is risk free. The risk is in not having tonometry and losing vision from undetected glaucoma.

tonsil A small mass of lymphoid tissue in the back of the throat (pharynx). There are usually two tonsils, one on either side of the posterior pharynx. Like other lymphatic tissue, the tonsils are part of the immune system and should not be removed without a sufficient reason.

tonsil stone See *tonsillolith.*

tonsillectomy The surgical removal of both tonsils.

tonsillitis Inflammation of one or both tonsils, typically as a result of infection by a virus or bacteria.

tonsillolith A tiny stone (calculus) in the tonsils. Such stones are found within little pockets (crypts) in the tonsils. These pockets typically form in chronic recurrent tonsillitis, and they harbor bacteria. Tonsilloliths are foul smelling because they tend to contain high quantities of sulfa. When crushed, they give off a characteristic rotten-egg smell and can cause bad breath. Tonsilloliths may also give a person the sense that something is caught in the back of the throat. Also known as tonsil stone.

tooth One of the structures within the mouth that allow for biting and chewing. Teeth have different shapes, depending on their purpose. The sharp canine and incisor teeth allow for biting, and the flattened, thick molars in the back of the mouth provide grinding surfaces for masticating food. All teeth have essentially the same structure: a hard crown above the gum line, which is attached to two or four roots by a portion called the neck. The roots are covered with a very thin layer of bone, and they keep the tooth embedded in the bones of the jaw. The exposed exterior of the tooth is covered with tough enamel. Under the enamel is a thick layer of dentin, and in the center is the pulp, which contains blood vessels and nerves.

tooth, cracked, syndrome See *cracked-tooth syndrome.*

tooth erosion The gradual loss of the normally hard surface of the tooth due to chemical, not bacterial, processes.

tooth pain, phantom See *phantom tooth pain.*

tooth root The lower two-thirds of a tooth. The roots are normally buried in bone, and they serve to anchor the tooth in position. The roots are covered with a thin layer of bone, and they are inserted into sockets in the bone of the jaw.

tooth root sensitivity Sensitivity of the tooth roots to cold, hot, and sour foods when they are no longer protected by healthy gum and bone. Chronic gum disease contributes to toothache due to root sensitivity. The bacterial toxins dissolve the bone around the roots and cause the gum and the bone to recede. Tooth root sensitivity may be so severe that the person avoids many foods. Treatment involves addressing the underlying gum disease and improving oral hygiene.

tooth, wisdom One of the large molars in the very back of the jaw. The human jaw has changed in size over the course of evolution, and wisdom teeth are no longer needed, but they continue to erupt in many individuals. If the jaw is too small to accommodate them, they may cause pain or crowd other teeth out of position. The wisdom teeth may need to be surgically removed.

toothache Pain in the tooth or gum. The most common cause of a toothache is a cavity or an injury to a tooth that exposes the pulp, which is heavily supplied by nerves.

tophaceous gout See *gout, tophaceous.*

tophi Plural of tophus.

tophus A nodular mass of uric acid crystals. Tophi are characteristically deposited in different soft-tissue areas of the body in chronic (tophaceous) gout. Even though tophi are most commonly found as hard nodules around the fingers, at the tips of the elbows, and around the big toe, they can appear anywhere in the body. They have been reported in unexpected areas such as in the ears, in the vocal cords, and around the spinal cord.

topical Pertaining to a particular surface area. For example, a topical agent is applied to a certain area of the skin and is intended to affect only the area to which it is applied. Whether its effects are indeed limited to that area depends on whether the agent stays where it is put or is absorbed into the bloodstream. Cortisone creams are topical medications.

TORCH screen A blood test that is designed to screen for a group of infectious agents known by the acronym TORCH, which stands for Toxoplasma gondii, other viruses (HIV, measles, and so on), rubella (German measles), cytomegalovirus, and herpes simplex. All these infectious agents are teratogens (agents that are capable of causing birth defects). The TORCH infectious agents affect 1 to 5 percent of all newborn babies and are among the leading causes of neonatal morbidity and mortality.

tornado supplies kit See *disaster supplies.*

torsion dystonia See *dystonia, torsion.*

torsion fracture See *fracture, torsion.*

torticollis The most common of the focal dystonias, a state of excessive or inadequate muscle tone in the muscles in the neck that control the position of the head. Torticollis can cause the head to twist and turn to one side. The head may also be pulled forward or backward. Torticollis can occur at any age, although most individuals first experience symptoms in middle age. It often begins slowly, and it usually reaches a plateau. About 10 to 20 percent of those with torticollis experience a spontaneous remission, but unfortunately the remission may not be long-lasting. Also known as spasmodic torticollis.

torticollis, congenital A deformity of the neck that is present at birth. Congenital torticollis is due to shortening of the neck muscles. Congenital torticollis tilts the head to the side on which the neck muscles are shortened, so that the chin points to the other side. The shortened neck muscles are principally supplied by the spinal accessory nerve. Also known as wryneck.

torticollis, spasmodic   See *torticollis.*

torus fracture   See *fracture, torus.*

total hysterectomy   See *hysterectomy, total.*

total parenteral nutrition   Intravenous feeding that provides patients with all the fluid and the essential nutrients they need when they are unable to feed themselves by mouth. Abbreviated TPN.

Tourette's syndrome   A genetic disorder that is characterized by the presence of chronic vocal and motor tics. The tics usually become evident between the ages of 6 and 18. The tics may be minor or debilitating. They may also vary in type and frequency over time. Strep infection can aggravate Tourette's syndrome. Emotional distress and stress also appear to influence the frequency of occurrence of tics. People with Tourette's syndrome tend to have an impulsive, quick, and frequently humorous disposition. Some experience episodes of rage that are difficult to control. Individuals with attention deficit hyperactivity disorder, obsessive-compulsive disorder, and autistic spectrum disorder are at increased risk of having Tourette's syndrome. Diagnosis of Tourette's syndrome is made via observation. Medications used to treat Tourette's syndrome include the blood pressure drugs guanfacine (brand name: Tenex) and catapres (brand name: Clonadine) and the atypical or older neuroleptics. Some patients have also found the nicotine patch to be useful as an adjunct to other medications. Therapy can help the patient develop social coping strategies and maintain a positive self-image. A gene for Tourette's syndrome has been mapped to chromosome 11 and is in band 11q23. Also known as Gilles de la Tourette's syndrome. See also *tic; tic disorder.*

toxemia   See *eclampsia.*

toxic multinodular goiter   See *goiter, toxic multinodular.*

toxic shock syndrome   A life-threatening syndrome that is characterized by the sudden onset of high fever, vomiting, diarrhea, and muscle aches, followed by low blood pressure (hypotension), which can lead to shock and death. There may be a rash resembling sunburn, with peeling of skin. Toxic shock syndrome occurs especially in menstruating women using tampons. It is caused by a toxin produced by Staphylococcus aureus bacteria growing under conditions in which there is little or no oxygen. Toxic shock syndrome is rare in women who do not use tampons and in men. See also *staphylococcus.*

toxin   A poison-produced by certain animals, plants, or bacteria.

toxo   See *toxoplasmosis.*

toxoplasmosis   An infection caused by a single-celled parasite called Toxoplasma gondii that can invade and damage tissues. Toxoplasmosis can be contracted by touching the hands to the mouth after gardening, cleaning a cat's litter box, or anything that has come into contact with cat feces. Toxoplasmosis can also be contracted by eating raw or partly cooked meat, especially pork or lamb, or touching the hands to the mouth after contact with raw or undercooked meat. The symptoms are similar to those of flu: fever, fatigue, headache, swollen lymph glands (lymphadenopathy), and muscle aches and pains (myalgia) that may last for a few days to several weeks. Persons with a weakened immune system are at risk for developing severe cases of toxoplasmosis. Toxoplasmosis is a well-known teratogen (an agent that can cause birth defects). If a pregnant woman is infected, the parasite can cross the placenta to the baby, with sometimes catastrophic consequences. Children born with toxoplasmosis (congenital toxoplasmosis) can have mental retardation, convulsions (epilepsy), spasticity, cerebral palsy, and partial or complete deafness and blindness. Also known as simply toxo.

TPN   Total parenteral nutrition.

trachea   A tube-like portion of the respiratory tract that connects the larynx with the bronchial parts of the lungs. Also known as windpipe.

tracheoesophageal puncture   A small opening that is made by a surgeon between the esophagus and the trachea. A valve is inserted to keep food out of the trachea but allow air into the esophagus to permit esophageal speech.

tracheostomy   Surgery to create an opening (stoma) into the windpipe. The opening itself may also be called a tracheostomy. A tracheostomy may be made as an emergency measure if the airway is blocked.

tracheostomy button   A small plastic tube that is placed in the opening (stoma) of a tracheostomy to keep it open.

tracheostomy tube   A small metal or plastic tube that keeps the stoma (opening) and the trachea in a tracheostomy open. Also known as a trach ("trake") tube.

trachoma   A chronic inflammatory disease of the eye and the leading cause of blindness. Trachoma is due to infection with the bacterium Chlamydia trachomatis. Transmission occurs mainly among children and from children to women caring for them. Key risk factors include inadequate supplies of water and low socioeconomic status. Trachoma affects approximately 500 million people worldwide, primarily in rural communities of the developing world and in the arid areas of tropical and subtropical zones. About 6 to 9 million people worldwide are currently blind due to trachoma and many more have suffered partial blindness due to trachoma. Australia is the only developed country where trachoma is still a significant health problem. The disease goes by a number of names, such as sandy blight.

traction   In medicine, a procedure for manually pulling a part of the body to a beneficial effect. See *traction, orthopedic.*

traction, orthopedic   The use of a system of weights and pulleys to gradually change the position of a bone. It may be used in cases of congenital defect or bone and joint injury to prevent scar tissue from building up in ways to limit movement and to prevent contractures in disorders such as cerebral palsy and arthritis.

trait   **1** In genetics, a genetically determined characteristic. **2** In medicine, a condition in the heterozygous state of a recessive disorder, as in sickle cell trait. **3** In psychology, a characteristic pattern of behavior.

tranquilizer   In pharmacology, a drug that calms and relieves anxiety. The first tranquilizer, chlordiazepoxide-hydrochloride (brand name: Librium), received FDA approval in 1960. Tranquilizers range in potency from mild to major, with increasing levels of drowsiness occurring as potency increases. They are prescribed for a wide variety of conditions but are used primarily to treat anxiety and insomnia. Most tranquilizers are potentially addictive, particularly those in the benzodiazepine family.

trans-   Prefix meaning across, over, or beyond, as in transplant operation (an operation in which an organ from one person is grafted into another person).

trans fat   See *trans fatty acid.*

trans fatty acid   An unhealthy substance that is made through the chemical process of hydrogenation of oils. Hydrogenation solidifies liquid oils and increases the shelf life and the flavor stability of oils and foods that contain them. Trans fatty acids are found in vegetable shortening and in some margarine, crackers, cookies, and snack foods. Trans fatty acids are also found in abundance in many deep-fried foods. Trans fatty acids wreak havoc with the body's ability to regulate cholesterol. In the realm of dietary dangers, trans fatty acids rank very high. It has been estimated that trans fatty acids are responsible for some 30,000 early deaths per year in the US. The toll of premature deaths worldwide is in the millions. Also known as trans fat.

transaminase, serum glutamic oxaloacetic   See *aspartate aminotransferase.*

transaminase, serum glutamic pyruvic   See *alanine aminotransferase.*

transcription   Making an RNA copy from a sequence of DNA (a gene). Transcription is the first step in gene expression.

transfer RNA   See *RNA, transfer.*

transferred ophthalmia   See *sympathetic ophthalmia.*

transfusion   The transfer of blood or blood products from one person (the donor) into the bloodstream of another person (the recipient). In most situations, transfusion is done as a lifesaving maneuver to replace blood cells or blood products lost through severe bleeding. Transfusion of one's own blood (autologous transfusion) is the safest method, but it requires advanced planning, and not all patients are eligible. Directed donor blood allows the patient to receive blood from known donors. Volunteer donor blood is usually most readily available and, when properly tested, has a low incidence of adverse events.

transfusion medicine   The practice of blood transfusion and blood conservation, complementary activities that ensure the best balance between safety and convenience during emergency care or surgery.

transient ischemic attack   An event that affects the central nervous system and has the signs and symptoms of a stroke but that goes away within a short period of time. Abbreviated TIA. A TIA is due to a temporary lack of adequate blood and oxygen (ischemia) to the brain. This is often caused by the narrowing (or, less often, ulceration) of the carotid arteries (the major arteries in the neck that supply blood to the brain). TIAs typically last 2 to 30 minutes and can produce problems with vision, dizziness, weakness, and trouble speaking. If a TIA is not treated, there is a high risk of a major stroke in the near future, usually within 90 days. A person who even remotely suspects a TIA should seek medical attention right away. Medication and/or a procedure to clean out the carotid artery and restore normal blood flow through the artery (carotid endarterectomy) can markedly reduce the risk of a subsequent stroke. Also known as mini-stroke.

transition, menopause   See *menopause transition.*

transitional cell carcinoma   See *carcinoma, transitional cell.*

translation   The process by which the genetic code carried by messenger RNA (mRNA) directs the production of proteins from amino acids.

translocation A structural chromosome rearrangement in which chromosome material is transferred from one chromosome to another. Translocation is the result of chromosome breakage.

transmission, perinatal See *vertical transmission.*

transmission, vertical See *vertical transmission.*

transplant The grafting of a tissue from one place to another, just as in botany when a bud from one plant might be grafted onto the stem of another. The transplanting of tissue can be from one part of a patient to another part (autologous transplantation), as in the case of a skin graft using the patient's own skin; or from one patient to another patient (allogenic transplantation), as in the case of transplanting a donor kidney into a recipient. See also *bone marrow transplant; heart transplant; kidney transplant; lung transplant.*

transsexual A person who desires or has achieved transsexualism.

transsexualism Consistently strong desire to change one's anatomical gender. Some transsexuals were misassigned gender at birth (for example, being anatomically male but raised as female), either on purpose or due to indistinct anatomy. Most, however, are perfectly normal physically. Transsexuals may dress and behave as individuals of the opposite sex, and they may choose to use hormones or surgery to develop desired secondary sex characteristics. Surgery to change the appearance of the external genitals is known as sex reassignment surgery. Surgery and hormonal treatments for gender reassignment are available for both male and female transsexuals. Transsexualism is distinct from transvestitism (cross-dressing), and it does not always indicate a change in the individual's sexual preference.

transudate A fluid that passes through a membrane, which filters out all the cells and much of the protein, yielding a watery solution. A transudate is a filtrate of blood. It is due to increased pressure in the veins and capillaries that forces fluid through the vessel walls or to a low level of protein in blood serum. Transudate accumulates in tissues outside the blood vessels and causes edema (swelling).

transurethral resection Surgery to remove tissue using a special instrument inserted through the urethra. The procedure may be performed, for example, to remove an enlarged prostate that is obstructing the flow of urine. Abbreviated TUR.

transvaginal ultrasound The creation of a picture called a sonogram by sending sound waves out through a probe inserted into the vagina. The waves bounce off the ovaries, and a computer uses the echoes to create the sonogram. Abbreviated TVS.

transverse A horizontal plane that passes through a standing body, parallel to the ground. See also Appendix B, "Anatomic Orientation Terms."

transverse fracture See *fracture, transverse.*

transvestite A person who dresses in the clothing of the opposite sex. Also known as a cross-dresser.

transvestitism Dressing in the clothing of the opposite sex. Transvestitism is distinct from both transexualism and homosexuality. Also known as cross-dressing.

trauma A physical or emotional injury.

trauma center A specialized hospital facility that is designed to provide diagnostic and therapeutic services for patients with injuries.

traumatic alopecia See *alopecia, traumatic.*

traumatology The branch of surgery that deals with injured patients, usually on an emergency basis. Patients who have suffered significant physical trauma, as from a car accident, may be cared for in a traumatology unit.

travelers' diarrhea Diarrhea that results from infections acquired while traveling to another country. Among the causes of travelers' diarrhea are enterotoxigenic Escherichia coli and a variety of viruses.

treadmill A machine with a moving strip on which one walks without moving forward. A treadmill was originally a wide wheel turned by the weight of people climbing on steps around its edge, used in the past to provide power for machines or as a punishment in prisons. The treadmill today serves as a device to maintain physical fitness. It is also an essential component of the exercise treadmill test, a stress test for heart disease.

treadmill, exercise See *exercise treadmill.*

tremor An abnormal, repetitive shaking movement of the body. Tremors have many causes and can be inherited, related to illnesses (such as thyroid disease), or caused by fever, hypothermia, drugs, or fear.

trench fever A disease borne by body lice that was first recognized in the trenches of World War I, when it is estimated to have affected more than 1 million people. Trench fever is still seen endemically in Mexico, Africa, Eastern Europe, and elsewhere. Urban trench fever occurs among homeless people and street alcoholics. Outbreaks have been documented, for example, in Seattle and Baltimore. The cause of trench fever is Bartonella quintana (also called Rochalimaea quintana), an unusual rickettsial organism that multiplies in the gut of the body louse. Transmission to people occurs when infected louse feces are rubbed into abraded (scuffed) skin or into the whites of the eyes. The disease is classically a 5-day fever, characterized by the sudden onset of high fever, severe headache, back pain and leg pain, and a fleeting rash. Recovery takes a month or more, and relapses are common. Also known as Wolhynia fever, shinbone fever, quintan fever, five-day fever, Meuse fever, His disease, His-Werner disease, and Werner-His disease. See also *Bartonella quintana; rickettsial disease.*

trench foot   A painful condition caused by exposure of the foot for several days. Trench foot was common during trench warfare in World War I and World War II, when soldiers stood for days and weeks in wet, muddy ditches without being able to change their footwear; today it is seen most frequently in urban homeless people. The feet become numb, turn red and then blue, develop blisters, and become infected. Gangrene may set in. Untreated trench foot can lead to the need for amputation due to gangrene; it can even lead to death.

trench mouth   See *acute membranous gingivitis.*

Treponema pallidum   The cause of syphilis, a worm-like, spiral-shaped bacterium called a spirochete that wiggles vigorously when viewed under a microscope.

triage   The process of sorting people based on their need for immediate medical treatment as compared to their chance of benefiting from such care. Triage is done in emergency rooms, disasters, and wars, when limited medical resources must be allocated to maximize the number of survivors. Triage in this sense originated in World War I. Wounded soldiers were classified into one of three groups: those who could be expected to live without medical care, those who would likely die even with care, and those who could survive if they received care.

TRICARE   See *CHAMPUS.*

triceps   The muscle that extends (straightens) the forearm. The triceps can be felt as the tense muscle in the back of the upper arm while one is doing push-ups. The triceps has three heads, or origins. Its full name is the triceps brachii.

Trichinella spiralis   The worm that causes trichinosis. Trichinella spiralis larvae can infest pigs and wild game. It hibernates in muscle tissue within a protective cyst. When a human or an animal eats meat that contains infective Trichinella cysts, the acid in the stomach dissolves the hard covering of the cyst and releases the worms. The worms pass into the small intestine and become mature within 1 or 2 days. After the adult worms mate, the females lay eggs. Eggs develop into immature worms,

travel through the arteries, and are transported to muscles. Within the muscles, each worm curls into a ball and encysts (becomes enclosed in a capsule). Infection occurs when these encysted worms are consumed in meat, continuing the cycle. Also known as pork tapeworm. See also *trichinosis.*

trichinellosis   See *trichinosis.*

trichinosis   A disease that is due to eating raw or undercooked pork or wild game that is infected with Trichinella spiralis larvae. Initial symptoms are abdominal discomfort, nausea, diarrhea, vomiting, fatigue, and fever. Next usually come headaches, fevers, chills, cough, eye swelling, aching joints, muscle pains, itchy skin, diarrhea, and constipation. With heavy infection, patients may experience difficulty coordinating movements and have heart and breathing problems. In severe cases, death can occur. The severity of symptoms depends on the number of infectious worms consumed in meat. To avoid trichinosis, meat should be cooked until the juices run clear or to an internal temperature of 77° Celsius (170° Fahrenheit); any piece of pork less than 15cm (6 inches) thick should be frozen for 20 days at -15° C (5° F) to kill any worms; and wild game meat should be cooked thoroughly (freezing wild game may not effectively kill all worms); all meat that is fed to pigs or other wild animals should be cooked first; meat grinders should be cleaned thoroughly; curing (salting), drying, smoking, and microwaving meat do not consistently kill infective worms. A person who thinks he or she has trichinosis should seek medical attention. Also known as trichinellosis.

trichobezoar   A wad of swallowed hair and food. Trichobezoars can sometimes cause blockage of the digestive system, especially at the exit of the stomach. See also *bezoar.*

tricuspid   Having three flaps or cusps. For example, the aortic valve and the tricuspid valve in the heart each have three cusps.

tricuspid valve   One of the four heart valves, the first one that blood encounters as it enters the heart. The tricuspid valve stands between the right atrium and the right ventricle, and it allows blood to flow only from the atrium into the ventricle.

tricyclic antidepressant   One of a family of medications that affect the neurotransmitters norepinephrine, serotonin, and acetylcholine. The tricyclic antidepressants are used to treat clinical depression, fibromyalgia, and other pain conditions.

trigeminal nerve   The chief nerve of sensation for the face, which is also the motor nerve that controls the muscles used for chewing. Problems with the sensory part of the trigeminal nerve result in pain or loss of sensation in the face. Problems with the motor root of the trigeminal nerve result in deviation of the jaw toward the affected side and trouble chewing. The trigeminal nerve is the fifth cranial nerve.

triglyceride The major form of fat, which consists of three molecules of fatty acid combined with one molecule of the alcohol glycerol. Triglycerides serve as the backbone of many types of lipids (fats). Triglycerides come from food and are also produced by the body. See also *triglyceride test*.

triglyceride test A simple blood test to measure the level of triglycerides in the blood. Triglyceride levels are influenced by recent fat and alcohol intake, so a person being tested should fast from food for at least 12 hours and abstain from alcohol for at least 24 hours before being tested. The normal level of triglyerides depends on the age and sex of the individual. Mild to moderate triglyceride increases occur in many conditions, including alcohol abuse, obstruction of the bile ducts, and diabetes. High levels of triglycerides (greater than 200 mg/dl) are associated with a heightened risk of heart disease. Markedly high triglyceride levels (greater than 500 mg/dl) can cause inflammation of the pancreas (pancreatitis). See also *triglycerides*.

triiodothyronine A hormone that is made by the thyroid gland. Triiodothyronine has three iodine molecules attached to its molecular structure. It is the most powerful thyroid hormone, and it affects almost every process in the body, including body temperature, growth, and heart rate. Also known as T3 and liothyronine.

trimester In obstetrics, one of the three divisions of three months each during pregnancy, in which different phases of fetal development take place. The first trimester is a time of basic cell differentiation. It is said to truly end at the mother's first perception of fetal movement, which usually occurs around the end of the third month. The second trimester is a period of rapid growth and maturation of body systems. A second-trimester fetus that is born prematurely may be viable, given the best hospital care possible. The third trimester marks the final stage of fetal growth, in which systems are completed, fat accumulates under the soon-to-be-born baby's skin, and the fetus at last moves into position for birth. This trimester ends with birth.

trimethylaminuria See *fish-odor syndrome*.

triple X See *XXX syndrome*.

triplo-X See *XXX syndrome*.

triploid Having three full sets of chromosomes: 3 copies of each autosomal chromosome plus 3 sex chromosomes. In humans, triploid is equal to 69 chromosomes.

trismus pseudocamptodactyly syndrome See *Hecht syndrome*.

trisomy 13 syndrome The presence of three copies of chromosome 13, rather than the normal two. Children with trisomy 13 syndrome are profoundly mentally retarded and have multiple malformations, commonly including scalp defects, hemangiomas (blood vessel malformations) of the face and nape of the neck, cleft lip and palate, malformations of the heart and abdominal organs, and flexed fingers with extra digits. The majority of trisomy 13 babies die soon after birth or in infancy. Also known as Patau syndrome.

trisomy 18 syndrome The presence of three copies of chromosome 18, rather than the normal two. Children with trisomy 18 syndrome have multiple malformations and mental retardation. They characteristically have low birth weight, small head (microcephaly), small jaw (micrognathia), malformations of the heart and kidneys, clenched fists with abnormal finger positioning, and malformed feet. The mental retardation is profound, and the IQ is too low to even measure. Nineteen out of 20 children with trisomy 18 syndrome die before their first birthday. Also called Edwards syndrome.

trisomy 21 syndrome See *Down syndrome*.

tRNA Transfer RNA.

trochanter One of the bony prominences toward the near end of the thighbone (the femur). There are two trochanters:

- **The greater trochanter** A powerful protrusion located at the proximal (near) and lateral (outside) part of the shaft of the femur. The greater trochanter is also called the major trochanter, the outer trochanter, and the lateral process of the femur.
- **The lesser trochanter** A pyramidal prominence that projects from the proximal (near) and medial (inside) part of the shaft of the femur. The lesser trochanter is also called the minor trochanter, the inner trochanter, and the medial process of the femur.

The trochanters are points at which hip and thigh muscles attach. The greater trochanter gives attachment to a number of muscles (including the gluteus medius and minimus, piriformis, obturator internus and externus, and gemelli muscles), and the lesser trochanter receives the insertion of several muscles (including the psoas major and iliacus muscles).

trochlear nerve   The nerve that controls the superior oblique muscle of the eye, one of the muscles that move the eye (extraocular muscles). Paralysis of the trochlear nerve results in rotation of the eyeball upward and outward (and, therefore, in double vision). The trochlear nerve is the fourth cranial nerve, and it is the only cranial nerve that arises from the back of the brain stem. It follows the longest course within the skull of any of the cranial nerves.

trophoblastic tumor, gestational   A tumor of women, in which cancer cells grow in the tissues that are formed following conception by the joining of sperm and egg. Gestational trophoblastic tumors start inside the uterus, the hollow, muscular, pear-shaped organ where a baby grows. This type of cancer occurs in women during the years when they are able to have children. There are two types of gestational trophoblastic tumors: hydatidiform mole and choriocarcinoma.

tropical typhus   See *typhus, scrub*.

true rib   See *rib, true*.

trunk bones   See *bones of the trunk*.

Trypanosoma cruzi   The microorganism that causes Chagas disease. See also *Chagas disease*.

trypanosomiasis, American   See *Chagas disease*.

TSH   Thyroid stimulating hormone.

TSI   Thyroid stimulating immunoglobulin.

Tsutsugamushi disease   See *typhus, scrub*.

TTP   Thrombotic thrombocytopenic purpura.

tubal pregnancy   See *pregnancy, tubal*.

tube   A long, hollow cylinder. There are many tube-like structures in the human body, such as the Eustachean tube in the ear. For specific types of tubes, see their alphabetical listing.

tuber   A lump or bump. For example, the backward protrusion of the heel is called the tuber calcanei or, alternatively, the tuberosity of the calcaneus. Small tubers are a characteristic finding in tuberculosis, and tubers in the brain are seen in tuberous sclerosis.

tubercle   A small tuber; a small lump or bump.

tuberculosis   A highly contagious infection that is caused by the bacterium Mycobacterium tuberculosis. Abbreviated TB. Tubercles (tiny lumps) are a characteristic finding in TB. Diagnosis is made via skin test, which if positive is followed by a chest X-ray to determine the status (active or dormant) of the infection. TB is more common in people with immune system problems, including AIDS, than in others. Treatment of active TB is mandatory by law in the US, and it should be available at no cost to the patient through the public health system. It involves a course of antibiotics and vitamins that lasts about 6 months. It is important to finish the entire treatment, both to prevent reoccurrence and to prevent the development of antibiotic-resistant tuberculosis. Quarantine is not needed for most patients with tuberculosis, but it is sometimes necessary. See also *tuberculosis, active; tuberculosis, antibiotic-resistant; tuberculosis, dormant; tuberculosis, miliary*.

tuberculosis, active   The presence of Mycobacterium tuberculosis infection with a positive chest X-ray. Treatment of active tuberculosis is mandatory by law in the US. See also *DOT; tuberculosis*.

tuberculosis, antibiotic-resistant   A variant of tuberculosis (TB) that is not affected by one or more of the antibiotics normally used to treat it. If the strain of TB is unaffected by more than one medication, it is called multi-drug-resistant (MDR) TB. A person with any form of drug-resistant TB needs care from a specialist who knows how to use stronger medications. These forms of TB are particularly contagious. Family members and other contacts of diagnosed patients may also need to take medications as a preventive measure.

tuberculosis, dormant   The presence of Mycobacterium tuberculosis infection without a positive chest X-ray. Treatment is not mandatory for dormant tuberculosis (TB), as with active TB, but it is a good idea because the bacterium could become active later. Treatment involves a course of antibiotics and vitamins.

tuberculosis, extrapulmonary   TB that occurs outside the lungs. For example, TB can be active in the lymph nodes or kidneys.

tuberculosis, MDR   Multi-drug-resistant tuberculosis. See *tuberculosis, antibiotic-resistant*.

tuberculosis, miliary   The presence of numerous sites of tuberculosis (TB) infection, each of which is minute. Miliary TB is caused by dissemination of infected material through the bloodstream.

tuberculosis, pulmonary   Tuberculosis (TB) in the lungs. Pulmonary TB is the most common form of active tuberculosis. It can be easily transmitted to others when someone who has it coughs.

tuberculosis vaccination   A vaccination for tuberculosis (TB). The vaccine, known as BCG (bacille Calmette

Guérin), is used in most developing countries to reduce the severe consequences of TB in infants and children. However, BCG vaccine has variable efficacy in preventing adult forms of TB and is, therefore, not routinely recommended for use in the U.S. and other developed countries. See also *BCG*.

tuberculous diskitis An infection of the spine that is seen most often in children. The main symptom is back pain. Untreated tuberculous diskitis can lead to inward or outward curvature of the spine. Imaging of the spine can find abscesses, some of which may have ossified (hardened). Also known as Pott's disease. Treatment involves antibiotics for extended periods.

tuberous sclerosis A genetic disorder that is characterized by abnormalities of the skin, brain, kidney, and heart. Skin abnormalities are present in all cases of tuberous sclerosis. They include tiny benign tumors (angiofibromas) on the face and depigmented areas anywhere on the body. The brain abnormalities of tuberous sclerosis are mainly benign cortical tumors (tubers) that cause seizures, developmental delay, and mental retardation. The kidneys in a person with tuberous sclerosis often contain multiple cysts and benign tumors (angiomyolipomas). The heart problems of tuberous sclerosis include arrhythmias and benign heart muscle tumors (rhabdomyomas). Diagnosis is made via clinical observation, for example, in a child with a seizure disorder who has white spots on the skin that are most easily seen under ultraviolet light. Tuberous sclerosis is inherited in an autosomal dominant manner and results from mutation of either one of two genes: the TSC1 gene on chromosome 9 or the TSC2 gene on chromosome 16. TSC1 and TSC2 encode products called hamartin and tuberin, respectively, which act as tumor suppressors. Two-thirds of cases of tuberous sclerosis are due to new mutations, and the other one-third are inherited from parents.

tubes See *fallopian tube.*

tubule A small tube.

tularemia A bacterial disease that is caused by infection with the bacterium Francisella tularensis, which lives in wild and domestic animals, most often rabbits, and can be transmitted to humans via contact with animal tissues, fleas, deerflies, or ticks. Hunters and other people who spend much time outdoors may be exposed by direct contact with an infected animal or carcass or by the bite of an infected flea or tick. Symptoms appear 2 to 10 days after exposure. Most often there is a red spot on the skin that enlarges and ulcerates, together with enlarged lymph nodes (swollen glands) in the armpit or groin. Ingestion of the organism may produce a throat infection, intestinal pain, diarrhea, and vomiting. Inhalation of the organism may produce a fever or a pneumonia-like illness.

Treatment involves use of antibiotics such as streptomycin, tetracycline, gentamycin, and tobramycin. Rubber or latex gloves should be worn when skinning or handling animals, especially rabbits. Wild rabbit and rodent meat should be cooked thoroughly before being eaten. One should try to avoid bites of deerflies and ticks and avoid drinking, bathing, swimming, and working in untreated water. A vaccine is recommended for people who are at highest risk such as hunters, trappers, and laboratory workers. Also known as rabbit fever and deerfly fever.

tumescent Swelling or slightly swollen. For example, tumescent liposuction involves pumping a solution beneath the skin, swelling it to facilitate suctioning out fat.

tumescent liposuction See *liposuction, tumescent.*

tumor An abnormal mass of tissue. Tumors can be benign or malignant (cancerous). There are dozens of different types of tumors. Their names usually reflect the kind of tissue they arise in and may also tell something about their shape or how they grow. For example, a medulloblastoma is a tumor that arises from embryonic cells (a blastoma) in the inner part of the brain (the medulla). Diagnosis depends on the type and location of the tumor. Tumor marker tests and imaging may be used; some tumors can be seen (for example, tumors on the exterior of the skin) or felt (palpated with the hands). Treatment is also specific to the location and type of the tumor. Benign tumors can sometimes simply be ignored, or they may be reduced in size (debulked) or removed entirely via surgery. For cancerous tumors, options include chemotherapy, radiation, and surgery. See also *blastoma; carcinoembryonic antigen test; desmoid tumor; ear tumor; epidermoid carcinoma; epithelial carcinoma; esophageal cancer; fibroid; syringoma; tumor marker.*

tumor debulking Surgically removing as much of a tumor as possible.

tumor marker A substance that can be detected in higher-than-normal amounts in the blood, urine, or body tissues of some patients with certain types of cancer. A tumor marker may be made by a tumor itself, or it may be made by the body as a response to the tumor. Tumor marker tests are not used alone to detect and diagnose cancer because most tumor markers can be elevated in patients who don't have a tumor, because no tumor marker is entirely specific to a particular type of cancer, and because not every cancer patient has an elevated tumor marker level, especially in the early stages of cancer, when tumor marker levels are usually still normal. Although tumor markers are typically imperfect as screening tests to detect occult (hidden) cancers, when a particular tumor has been found with a marker, the marker can be a means of monitoring the success or failure of treatment. The tumor marker level may also reflect the extent (stage) of the disease, indicate how quickly the cancer is likely to progress, and help determine the outlook. Examples of tumor markers include alpha-fetoprotein (AFP), carcinoembryonic antigen (CEA), human chorionic gonadotropin (HCG), lactate dehydrogenase (LDH), prostate specific antigen (PSA), and neuron-specific enolase (NSE).

tumor marker, CEA See *carcinoembryonic antigen test.*

tumor marker, NSE See *neuron-specific enolase.*

tumor registry Recorded information about the status of patients with tumors. Although a registry was originally the place (like Registry House in Edinburgh) where information was collected (in registers), the word *registry* has also come to mean the collection itself. A tumor registry is organized so that the data can be analyzed. For example, analysis of data in a tumor registry maintained at a hospital may show a rise in lung cancer among women.

tumor, sweat gland See *syringoma.*

tunica albuginea The whitish membrane within the penis that surrounds the spongy chambers (corpora cavernosa). The tunica albuginea helps to trap the blood in the corpora cavernosa, thereby sustaining erection of the penis.

tunnel Any passageway in the body that traverses solid tissue and is completely enclosed except for the ends, which are open and permit entrance to and exit from the tunnel. An example of a tunnel is the carpal tunnel.

TUR Transurethral resection.

turbinate A bone in the nose that is situated along the side wall of the nose and is covered by mucous membrane.

Turner syndrome The most common and important sex chromosome disorder in females, characterized by short stature, webbed neck, broad shield-like chest, wide-spaced nipples, increased carrying angle at the elbow (cubitus valgus), short fourth finger, and malformations of the heart and aorta. The intelligence of those with Turner syndrome is usually within the normal range (average IQ 90). Girls with Turner syndrome at the time of puberty do not experience the development of secondary sex characteristics such as breast enlargement. As women, they are infertile due to ovarian failure. The ovaries typically contain no follicles and look like streaks of fibrous tissue. The diagnosis of Turner syndrome is confirmed with chromosome analysis (karyotype). Turner syndrome is due to the presence of only one normal X chromosome and no other normal sex chromosome. A second sex chromosome may be present, but it is not structurally and functionally normal. However, the most frequent karyotype in Turner syndrome is 45, X, which is sometimes referred to as XO. The overwhelming majority of pregnancies with Turner syndrome conceptions result in miscarriages.

TVS Transvaginal ultrasound.

twin One of two children produced in the same pregnancy. Twins can develop from one ovum (egg) or from two ova (eggs). Twins who develop from a single ovum are called monozygotic or identical twins. They have identical genomes. Twins who develop from two ova that are fertilized at the same time are called dizygotic or fraternal twins. They are nonidentical and have different genomes.

tympanic membrane The eardrum, a thin membrane that serves as a partition between the external ear and the middle ear and transmits the motion of sound waves to the chain of bones in the middle ear.

tympanites See *tympany.*

tympano- Prefix indicating a relationship to the eardrum (tympanic membrane), as in tympanometry (a test that measures the function of the middle ear).

tympanometry A test that measures the function of the middle ear. Tympanometry works by varying the pressure within the ear canal and measuring the movement of the eardrum (tympanic membrane).

tympanoplasty A surgical operation to correct damage to the middle ear and restore the integrity of the eardrum.

tympanostomy tube See *ear tube.*

tympanum The cavity of the middle ear, which is separated from the outer ear by the eardrum.

tympany A hollow drum-like sound that is produced when a gas-containing cavity is tapped sharply. Tympany is heard if the chest contains free air (pneumothorax) or the abdomen is distended with gas. Also known as tympanites.

type I error See *alpha error.*

type II error See *beta error.*

type 1 GM2-gangliosidosis See *Tay-Sachs disease.*

typhoid See *typhoid fever.*

typhoid fever An acute illness characterized by fever caused by infection with the bacterium Salmonella typhi. Typhoid fever has an insidious onset, with fever, headache, constipation, malaise, chills, and muscle pain. Diarrhea is uncommon, and vomiting is not usually severe. Confusion, delirium, intestinal perforation, and death may occur in severe cases. The disease is transmitted through contaminated drinking water or food. Large epidemics are most often related to fecal contamination of water supplies or foods sold on the streets. A chronic carrier state—excretion of the organism for more than a year—occurs in approximately 5 percent of cases. Vaccination is recommended for people traveling to high-risk areas, such as the Indian subcontinent and developing countries in Asia, Africa, and Central and South America where there is prolonged exposure to potentially contaminated food and drink. Immunization is particularly recommended for anyone traveling to smaller cities, villages, and rural areas off the usual tourist itineraries. A person needs to complete the vaccination at least a week before travel so that the vaccine has time to take effect. Typhoid vaccines lose effectiveness after several years, and boosters are required. Typhoid vaccination is not 100 percent effective and is not a substitute for careful selection of food and drink.

typhoid Mary A chronic carrier of the agent of typhoid fever, or the chronic carrier of the agent of any other disease. Named for Mary Mallon, an Irish cook who was found to be a healthy typhoid carrier in the US early in the 20th century.

typhus, African tick One of the tick-borne rickettsial diseases of the eastern hemisphere, similar to Rocky Mountain spotted fever but less severe. Symptoms include fever, a small ulcer (tache noire) at the site of the tick bite, swollen glands near the site of the tick bite (satellite lymphadenopathy), and a red, raised (maculopapular) rash. Also known as fièvre boutonneuse. See also *rickettsial diseases*.

typhus, classic See *typhus, epidemic*.

typhus, endemic See *typhus, murine*.

typhus, epidemic A severe, acute disease with prolonged high fever up to 40° C (104° F), intractable headache, and a pink-to-red raised rash. The cause is a microorganism called Rickettsia prowazekii, which is found worldwide and is transmitted by lice. The lice become infected on typhus patients and transmit illness to other people. The mortality increases with age, and more than half of untreated persons age 50 or older die. Also known as European, classic, or louse-borne typhus and as jail fever. See also *rickettsial diseases*.

typhus, European See *typhus, epidemic*.

typhus, louse-borne See *typhus, epidemic*.

typhus, mite-borne See *typhus, scrub*.

typhus, murine An acute infectious disease characterized by fever, headache, and rash that are similar to, but milder than, those in epidemic typhus. Murine typhus is caused by the microorganism Rickettsia typhi (mooseri) and transmitted to humans by rat fleas (Xenopsylla cheopis). The animal reservoir includes rats, mice, and other rodents. Murine typhus occurs sporadically worldwide but is most prevalent in congested, rat-infested urban areas. Also known as endemic typhus, rat-flea typhus, and urban typhus of Malaya. See also *rickettsial diseases*.

typhus, Queensland tick One of the tick-borne rickettsial diseases of the eastern hemisphere, similar to Rocky Mountain spotted fever but less severe. Symptoms include fever, a small ulcer (eschar) at the site of the tick bite, swollen glands near the site of the tick bite (satellite lymphadenopathy), and a red, raised (maculopapular) rash. See also *rickettsial diseases*.

typhus, scrub A mite-borne infectious disease that is caused by the microorganism Rickettsia tsutsugamushi. Characteristic symptoms include fever, headache, a raised (macular) rash, swollen glands (lymphadenopathy), and a dark crusted ulcer, called an eschar or tache noire, at the site of the chigger (mite larva) bite. Scrub typhus occurs in the area bounded by Japan, India, and Australia. Also known as Tsutsugamushi disease, mite-borne typhus, and tropical typhus. See also *rickettsial diseases*.

typhus, tick See *Rocky Mountain spotted fever*.

typhus, tropical See *typhus, scrub*.

typhus, urban, of Malaysia See *typhus, murine*.

typist's cramp A dystonia that affects the muscles of the hand and sometimes the forearm and occurs only during handwriting. See also *dystonia, focal*.

tyrosinemia A genetic disorder that involves the metabolism of the amino acid tyrosine and is characterized by abnormally high levels of tyrosine in blood (hypertyrosinemia) and urine (tyrosinuria). There are several forms of tyrosinemia. Tyrosinemia type I is due to deficiency of fumarylacetoacetase, the last enzyme in the tyrosine catabolism pathway (the biochemical reactions that break down tyrosine). An acute form surfaces soon after birth, with the odor of cabbage and death from liver failure in infancy. A chronic form is characterized by chronic liver disease, rickets due to hypophosphatemia (low phosphate), and death in childhood. There is an association with liver cancer (hepatocellular carcinoma). Tyrosinemia type II is due to deficiency of the enzyme tyrosine transaminase and is characterized by the crystallization of tyrosine in painful thick areas on the palms and soles and in the cornea and often by mental retardation. Tyrosinemia types I and II are inherited in an autosomal recessive manner.

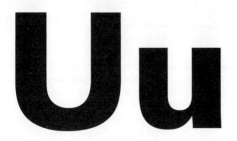

Uu

U   Uracil, one of the nucleotide bases in RNA.

UA   Urinalysis.

UAL   Ultrasonic-assisted liposuction. See *liposuction, ultrasonic-assisted*.

UBT   Urea breath test.

UDP-glucuronosyltransferase   A liver enzyme that is essential to the disposal of bilirubin, the chemical that results from the normal breakdown of hemoglobin from red blood cells. An abnormality of UDP-glucuronosyltransferase results in a condition called Gilbert syndrome. See also *Gilbert syndrome*.

ulcer   A lesion that is eroding away the skin or mucous membrane. Ulcers can have various causes, depending on their location. Ulcers on the skin are usually due to irritation, as in the case of bedsores, and may become inflamed and/or infected as they grow. Ulcers in the gastrointestinal tract were once attributed to stress, but most are now believed to be due to infection with the bacterium Helicobacter pylori. GI ulcers, however, are often made worse by stress, smoking, and other noninfectious factors.

ulcer, apthous   See *canker sore*.

ulcer bug   See *Helicobacter pylori*.

ulcer, duodenal   An ulcer in the lining of the duodenum, the first portion of the small intestine. See also *ulcer; ulcer, peptic*.

ulcer, esophageal   An ulcer in the lining of the esophagus that is corroded by the acidic digestive juices secreted by the stomach cells. See also *ulcer; ulcer, peptic*.

ulcer, gastric   An ulcer in the lining of the stomach that is corroded by the acidic digestive juices secreted by the stomach cells. See also *ulcer; ulcer, peptic*.

ulcer, peptic   An ulcer in the lining of the stomach, duodenum, or esophagus. Peptic ulcers affect millions of people in the US yearly. Ulcer formation is related to Helicobacter pylori bacteria in the stomach, use of anti-inflammatory medications, and cigarette smoking. Peptic

ulcer pain may not correlate with the presence or severity of ulceration. Complications of peptic ulcers include bleeding, perforation, and blockage of the stomach (gastric obstruction). Diagnosis is made via barium X-ray or endoscopy. Recent medical advances have increased the understanding of peptic ulcer formation, and improved and expanded treatment options are now available. Treatment involves use of antibiotics to eradicate H. pylori, elimination of risk factors, and prevention of complications.

ulcer, stasis   An ulcer that develops in an area in which the circulation is sluggish and the return of venous blood toward the heart is poor. A common location for stasis ulcers is on the ankles. Stasis refers to a stoppage or slowdown in the flow of blood (or other body fluid, such as lymph).

ulceration   The process or fact of being eroded away, as by an ulcer.

ulcerative colitis   See *colitis, ulcerative*.

ulcerative gingivitis   See *acute membranous gingivitis*.

ulcerative proctitis   Ulcerative colitis that is limited to the rectum. See also *colitis, ulcerative*.

ulcerative stomatitis   See *acute membranous gingivitis*.

ulna   The larger of the two long bones within the forearm. (The smaller one is the radius.) The ulna is on the same side of the arm as the little finger.

ulnar   Pertaining to the ulna, the larger bones in the forearm.

ulocarcinoma   Cancer of the gums. Ulocarcinoma is often associated with the use of smokeless (chewing) tobacco. Diagnosis is suspected by observation and confirmed with biopsy. Treatment may include radiation, chemotherapy, and surgery.

ultrasonic-assisted liposuction   See *liposuction, ultrasonic-assisted*.

ultrasound   High-frequency sound waves. Ultrasound waves can be bounced off tissues by using special devices. The echoes are then converted into a picture called a sonogram. Ultrasound imaging allows an inside view of soft tissues and body cavities without the use of invasive techniques. Ultrasound is often used to examine a fetus during pregnancy. There is no convincing evidence that any danger occurs from ultrasound during pregnancy.

ultrasound, Doppler   See *Doppler ultrasound*.

ultrasound, transvaginal   See *transvaginal ultrasound*.

ultraviolet A   See *ultraviolet radiation*.

ultraviolet B   See *ultraviolet radiation.*

ultraviolet C   See *ultraviolet radiation.*

ultraviolet radiation   Invisible rays that are part of the energy that comes from the sun. Abbreviated UV. UV radiation is made up of three types of rays: ultraviolet A (UVA), ultraviolet B (UVB), and ultraviolet C (UVC). UVC is the most dangerous type of UV light in its potential to harm life on earth, but it cannot penetrate the earth's protective ozone layer. UVA and UVB do penetrate the ozone layer and reach earth. UVA is weaker than UVB and less likely to cause sunburn, but it passes farther into the skin. Both UVA and UVB cause melanoma and other types of skin cancer; therefore, it is recommended that people use sunscreens that block both UVA and UVB radiation. The light from tanning lamps is like that from the sun and contains both UVA and UVB. Using tanning lights poses a major long-term risk of skin cancer. Electric arc lamps can also generate UV light to enable motion-picture projectors to show movies. Although UV light can damage health, it can also maintain or improve health. When UV light strikes human skin, it triggers the production of vitamin D, which promotes the growth of bones and teeth. See also *basal cell carcinoma; cancer, skin; squamous cell carcinoma; melanoma; sunscreen.*

umbilical cord   The cord that connects the developing fetus with the placenta while the fetus is in the uterus. The umbilical arteries and vein run within this cord. The umbilical cord is clamped and cut at birth, and its residual tip forms the bellybutton.

umbilical duct   See *yolk stalk.*

umbilicus   See *bellybutton.*

unconscious   **1** Interruption of awareness of oneself and one's surroundings; the lack of the ability to notice or respond to stimuli in the environment. A person may become unconscious due to oxygen deprivation, shock, injury, or use of central nervous system depressants such as alcohol and drugs.   **2** In psychology, the part of thought and emotion that happens outside everyday awareness.

unconsciousness, temporary   A partial or complete loss of consciousness; interruption of awareness of oneself and one's surroundings. When the loss of consciousness is temporary and recovery is spontaneous, it is referred to as syncope or, more commonly, fainting. Temporary unconsciousness may also occur with some types of seizures, from a head injury, or as part of a dissociative state. See also *dissociation; seizure; syncope.*

undulant fever   See *Brucellosis.*

unicornuate   Having one horn, or being horn shaped. For example, the uterus is normally unicornuate.

unilateral   Having, or relating to, one side. For example, a unilateral rash is one that is only on one side of the body.

uniparous   Having one offspring in a birth. See also *multiparous.*

unipolar depression   See *depression.*

United Network for Organ Sharing   A medical agency in the US that coordinates organ donations, including matching potential donors and recipients.

United States Public Health Service   The part of the Department of Health and Human Services (HHS) that is responsible for the public health of the US population. Abbreviated USPHS. USPHS administers a number of important health agencies, including the Food and Drug Administration (FDA), the Centers for Disease Control and Prevention (CDC), and the National Institutes of Health (NIH).

universal colitis   See *colitis, ulcerative.*

UNOS   United Network for Organ Sharing.

unresectable   Unable to be removed (resected) by surgery.

unsaturated fat   A fat that is liquid at room temperature and comes from a plant, such as olive, peanut, corn, cottonseed, sunflower, safflower, or soybean oil. Unsaturated fat tends to lower the level of cholesterol in the blood.

unsteadiness   Loss of one's equilibrium in respect to the environment, often with a feeling of almost falling and often as a result of bumping into something. There are many causes for unsteadiness, including problems in the cerebral or cerebellar portions of the brain, the spinal cord, vestibular system, or inner ear. See also *dizziness; lightheadedness; vertigo.*

upper GI series   A series of X-rays of the upper part of the gastrointestinal tract (the esophagus, stomach, and small intestine) that are taken after a patient drinks a barium solution. See also *barium solution; barium swallow.*

upper leg   See *leg, upper.*

urachus   A canal that connects the urinary bladder to the umbilicus (bellybutton) during fetal development. The urachus is normally obliterated, so it is usually a solid cord. Failure for the urachus to fill in leaves it open. The telltale sign of an open urachus is leakage of urine through the umbilicus. An open urachus is a malformation and needs to be surgically removed.

uracil   One of the nucleotide bases in RNA. Uracil takes the place in RNA that thymine occupies in DNA. Abbreviated U.

urate   A salt that is derived from uric acid. When the body cannot metabolize uric acid properly, urates can build up in body tissues or crystallize within joints. See also *gout; uric acid*.

urea   **1** A substance that contains nitrogen and is normally cleared from the blood by the kidney and excreted via the urine. Diseases that compromise the function of the kidney often lead to increased blood levels of urea, which can be measured by the blood urea nitrogen (BUN) test. See also *uremia*.   **2** A synthetic chemical that may be used to remove fluid from body tissues or the skin.

urea breath test   A procedure for diagnosing the presence or absence of the bacterium Helicobacter pylori, which causes ulcers. Abbreviated UBT. UBT may be used to demonstrate that H. pylori has been eliminated by treatment with antibiotics. UBT is based on the ability of H. pylori to break down urea, which is normally produced by the body in the presence of excess nitrogen and is then eliminated in the urine.

uremia   The presence of an excessive amount of urea in the blood. Uremia may be a sign of kidney disease or even kidney failure. See also *urea*.

ureter   One of the two tubes that carry urine from the kidneys to the bladder. Each ureter arises from a kidney, descends, and ends in the bladder.

urethra   The tube that leads from the bladder and transports and discharges urine outside the body. In males, the urethra travels through the penis and carries semen as well as urine. In females, the urethra is shorter than in the male, and it emerges above the vaginal opening.

urethral sphincter   A muscular mechanism that controls the retention and release of urine from the bladder. There are two urethral sphincters: the internal and external urinary sphincters. Part of the muscular bladder wall acts as the internal urethral sphincter and prevents urine from leaving the bladder to enter the urethra. This sphincter cannot be willfully controlled but is under involuntary control by the brain. A layer of muscle called the urogenital diaphragm supplies support for the contents of the pelvis and acts as the external urethral sphincter. It provides a second means of stopping the escape of urine from the body. This sphincter is under voluntary control.

urethritis   Inflammation of the urethra, the tube that leads from the bladder to the outside of the body. Urethritis can have a number of causes, including irritation and sexually transmitted diseases such as chlamydia.

Urethritis is closely associated with bacterial infection of the bladder (cystitis).

urethroscope   A device for examining the inside of the urethra.

URI   Upper respiratory infection. Infection of the air passages of the nose, the throat, and/or bronchial tubes.

uric acid   A substance that is produced when proteins are metabolized. In gout, elevated levels of uric acid are commonly found in the blood (hyperuricemia). However, only a small portion of people with hyperuricemia actually develop gout. See also *gout*.

uricaciduria   The presence of excess uric acid in the urine, which may be a sign of gout or kidney stones.

urinalysis   A test that is done in order to analyze urine. Because toxins and excess fluid are removed from the body in urine, analysis of urine can provide important health clues. Urinalysis can be used to detect certain diseases, such as diabetes, gout, and other metabolic disorders, as well as kidney disease. It can also be used to uncover evidence of drug abuse. Accurate urinalysis may require a "clean catch" of urine. Before a person gives a urine sample, he or she should drink plenty of fluids and wait until 1 or 2 seconds into the flow of urine before catching the urine in the receptacle. For some tests it is important to get the first urine of the day, which contains the highest concentration of toxins and other clues. For other tests, a 24-hour collection of urine may be needed.

urinary   Having to do with the function or anatomy of the kidneys, ureters, bladder, or urethra. For example, the urinary tract is the collection of organs of the body that produce, store, and discharge urine.

urinary bladder   See *bladder*.

urinary calculus   A stone in the urinary tract. A urinary calculus may be a kidney stone or it may be lower down in the ureter, bladder, or urethra.

urinary incontinence   The unintentional loss of urine due to loss of voluntary control over the urinary sphincters. One cause of urinary incontinence is overactive bladder, in which a sudden involuntary contraction of the muscular wall of the bladder results in urinary urgency, an immediate unstoppable need to urinate. See also *bedwetting; enuresis; urethral sphincter*.

urinary sphincter   See *urethral sphincter*.

urinary tract   The organs of the body that produce, store, and discharge urine. These organs include the kidneys, ureters, bladder, and urethra.

urinary tract infection   An infection of the kidney, ureter, bladder, or urethra. Abbreviated UTI. Not everyone with a UTI has symptoms, but common symptoms include a frequent urge to urinate and pain or burning when urinating. More females than males have UTIs. Underlying conditions that physically obstruct and impair the normal urinary flow, such as the formation of cysts within the urinary tract, can lead to complicated UTIs. Treatment usually involves increased fluid intake and use of antibiotics. In cases where physical obstruction is present, special medications or surgery may be necessary.

urine   Liquid waste. Urine is a clear, transparent fluid that normally has an amber color. The average amount of urine excreted in 24 hours is between 5 to 8 cups or 40 and 60 ounces. Chemically, urine is mainly a watery solution of salt and substances called urea and uric acid. Normally, it contains about 960 parts water to 40 parts solid matter. Abnormally, it may contain sugar (in diabetes), albumin (a protein, as in some forms of kidney disease), bile pigments (as in jaundice), or abnormal quantities of one or another of its normal components.

urine, blood in the   See *hematuria*.

urine pH   A measure of the acidity or alkalinity of urine. Checking urine pH is part of the routine urinalysis. Factors that affect urine pH include vomiting, diarrhea, lung disease, hormones, kidney function, and urinary tract infection.

urine test   See *urinalysis*.

urogenital   Relating to both the urinary system and the genital system (the interior and exterior genitalia).

urography   A method for examining the structure and functionality of the urinary system. A special dye is injected, and an X-ray machine records the dye's progress through the urinary tract. Urography is particularly useful for discovering cysts or other internal blockages.

urolithiasis   The process of forming stones in the kidney, bladder, and/or urethra. See also *kidney stone*.

urologist   A physician who specializes in diseases of the urinary organs in females and the urinary and sex organs in males.

urticaria   See *hive*.

USFDA   The United States Food and Drug Administration. See *Food and Drug Administration*.

Usher syndrome   The most common disease that diminishes both hearing and vision. Usher syndrome is a group of genetic disorders in which retinitis pigmentosa (an eye disease that causes vision to deteriorate over time) is combined with congenital deafness. The hearing loss in a patient with Usher syndrome occurs in both ears as a result of nerve deafness. Some patients also have balance problems because of lack of vestibular reflexes for balance. More than half of all deaf-blind people have Usher syndrome. The syndrome, named for the British ophthalmologist Charles Usher, is inherited in an autosomal recessive manner. There are three clinical types of Usher syndrome that illustrate the power of clinical observation and medical genetics to dissect one disease into many:

- **Usher syndrome type 1**   The combination of profound congenital deafness, loss of balance reflexes (vestibular areflexia), and retinitis pigmentosa that starts in adolescence and progressively impairs visual acuity. The vestibular areflexia is the defining feature of this type of Usher syndrome. Children walk later than usual and have difficulty with activities that require balance, such as riding a bicycle or playing sports. Mutations in at least six different places in the genome are known to cause Usher syndrome type 1. One of the genes is MYO7A.

- **Usher syndrome type 2**   The combination of congenital hearing loss that is not profound but predominantly affects the higher frequencies, variable vestibular impairment, and retinitis pigmentosa that develops in adolescence or early adulthood. Mutations in at least four different places in the genome are known to cause Usher syndrome type 2. One of the genes is USH2A, which encodes for a characteristic protein usherin.

- **Usher syndrome type 3**   The combination of normal hearing at birth, hearing loss that progresses over time, near-normal balance, and retinitis pigmentosa that develops in adolescence. At least three different types of mutations in a gene on chromosome 3q21–3q22, designated USH3A, can cause Usher syndrome type 3.

USPHS   United States Public Health Service.

ut dict   Abbreviation meaning "as directed." See also Appendix A, "Prescription Abbreviations."

uterine cancer   See *cancer, uterine*.

uterine fibroid   See *fibroid*.

uterine fornix   See *fornix uteri*.

uterine retroversion   See *uterus, tipped*.

uterine rupture   A tear in the uterus. A uterine rupture is a very serious situation. Causes include trauma, labor with an unusually big baby, multiple pregnancy (with twins, triplets, and so on), and vaginal delivery after a prior C-section (in which the old C-section scar ruptures). Uterine rupture can lead to hysterectomy, urologic injury, the need for blood transfusion, and even the death of the mother and baby.

uterine tube   See *fallopian tube.*

uterus   A hollow, pear-shaped organ that is located in a woman's lower abdomen, between the bladder and the rectum. The narrow lower portion of the uterus is the cervix (the neck of the uterus). The broader upper part is the corpus, which is made up of three layers of tissue. In women of childbearing age, the inner layer (endometrium) of the uterus goes through a series of monthly changes known as the menstrual cycle. Each month, endometrial tissue grows and thickens in preparation to receive a fertilized egg. Menstruation occurs when this tissue is not used, disintegrates, and passes out through the vagina. The middle layer (myometrium) of the uterus is muscular tissue that expands during pregnancy to hold the growing fetus and contracts during labor to deliver the child. The outer layer (parametrium) also expands during pregnancy and contracts thereafter.

uterus, prolapsed   A uterus that has moved from its normal position in the abdominal cavity into a different position, usually a lower position. Prolapsed uterus may occur because of underlying weak muscles or simply as a result of repeated term pregnancies. It can sometimes interfere with conception, cause difficulties during pregnancy, and contribute to pelvic pain. A prolapsed uterus can be treated by inserting a stabilizing device into the vagina called a pessary. Sometimes surgery is required.

uterus, tipped   A slight to dramatic placement of the uterus that orients it toward the back. A tipped uterus is common and usually causes no difficulty. In severe cases, it can affect choice of birth control method and cause pain in the pelvic area, especially during intercourse. Also known as uterine retroversion.

UTI   Urinary tract infection.

utility   In the analysis of health outcomes, a number between 0 and 1 that is assigned to a state of health or an outcome. Perfect health has a utility value of 1. Death has a utility value of 0.

UV   ultraviolet. See *ultraviolet radiation.*

UVA   ultraviolet A. See *ultraviolet radiation.*

UVB   ultraviolet B. See *ultraviolet radiation.*

UVC   ultraviolet C. See *ultraviolet radiation.*

uvea   An inner layer of the eye that includes the iris, the blood vessels that serve the eye (choroid), and the connective tissue between the iris and the choroid (the ciliary body).

uveitis   Inflammation of the uvea. Uveitis is a serious form of eye inflammation and requires aggressive treatment with medications to reduce the inflammation that can permanently impair vision. Uveitis can occur by itself or as a feature of an underlying disease, such as Behcet's disease, sarcoidosis, and others.

uvula   The anatomic structure that dangles downward at the back of the mouth and is attached to the rear of the soft palate.

uvulitis   Inflammation of the uvula. Uvulitis has many causes, including infection with a virus, fungus, or bacteria or the result of a side effect of a medication.

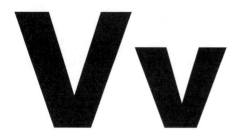

Vv

vaccination See *immunization.*

vaccination, children's See *children's immunizations.*

vaccine A microbial preparation of killed or modified microorganisms that can stimulate an immune response in the body to prevent future infection with similar microorganisms. Vaccines are usually delivered by intramuscular injection.

vagina The muscular canal that extends from the cervix to the outside of the body. It is usually 6 to 7 inches in length, and its walls are lined with mucous membrane. It includes two vaultlike structures: the anterior (front) vaginal fornix and the posterior (rear) vaginal fornix. The cervix protrudes slightly into the vagina, and through a tiny hole in the cervix (the os), sperm make their way toward the internal reproductive organs. The vagina also includes numerous tiny glands that make vaginal secretions.

vagina, septate A rare condition in which the vagina is divided, usually longitudinally, to create a double vagina. This situation can be easily missed by the patient and even by the physician on exam. If the patient becomes sexually active prior to diagnosis, one of the vaginas stretches and becomes dominant. The other vagina slips slightly upward and flush and can be difficult to enter.

vaginal birth after caesarean section See *caesarean section, vaginal birth after.*

vaginal fornix See *fornix uteri.*

vaginal hysterectomy See *hysterectomy, vaginal.*

vaginal introitus See *vaginal opening.*

vaginal opening The exterior opening to the vagina, the muscular canal that extends from the cervix to the outside of the female body. Also called vaginal introitus and vaginal vestibule.

vaginal vestibule See *vaginal opening.*

vaginitis Inflammation of the vagina. Vaginitis is a common condition and is often caused by a fungus. Symptoms include itching, burning, and discharge. Some factors predispose a woman to develop vaginitis. For example, women who have diabetes have vaginitis more often than other women. Treatment options include antifungal intravaginal creams and oral medications. See also *vaginitis, atrophic; yeast; yeast vaginitis.*

vaginitis, atrophic Thinning of the lining (endothelium) of the vagina due to decreased production of estrogen. Atrophic vaginitis may occur with menopause.

vaginitis, yeast See *yeast vaginitis.*

vaginosis, bacterial See *bacterial vaginosis.*

vagus nerve A remarkable nerve that supplies nerve fibers to the pharynx (throat), larynx (voice box), trachea (windpipe), lungs, heart, esophagus, and intestinal tract, as far as the transverse portion of the colon. The vagus nerve also brings sensory information back to the brain from the ear, tongue, pharynx, and larynx. The vagus nerve is the tenth cranial nerve. It originates in the medulla oblongata, a part of the brain stem, and wanders all the way down from the brain stem to the colon. Complete interruption of the vagus nerve causes a characteristic syndrome in which the soft palate droops on the side where damage occurred, and the gag reflex is also lost on that side. The voice is hoarse and nasal, and the vocal cord on the affected side is immobile. The result is difficulty swallowing (dysphagia) and speaking (dysphonia). The vagus nerve has several important branches, including the recurrent laryngeal nerve.

Valley fever Lung infection with the fungus Coccidioides immitis. The fungus is common in the sands of the deserts of the southwest, including the San Joaquin valley in California, after which it was named. Also called coccidiomycosis.

Valsalva maneuver A maneuver in which one tries with force to exhale with the windpipe closed, impeding the return of venous blood to the heart.

valve, heart See *heart valve.*

VAQTA A vaccine against hepatitis A. See also *hepatitis A; hepatitis A immunization.*

vara, tibia See *tibia vara.*

variant angina See *angina, Prinzmetal.*

varicella See *chickenpox.*

varicella vaccination See *chickenpox immunization.*

varicocele Elongation and enlargement of veins within the network of veins (pampiniform plexus) that leave the testis to form the testicular vein. A varicocele appears bluish through the scrotum, feels like a bag of worms, and can cause pain or discomfort.

varicose vein   A vein that has enlarged and twisted, often appearing as a bulging, blue blood vessel that is clearly visible through the skin. Varicose veins are most common in older adults, particularly women, and especially on the legs. Varicose veins can cause cramping pain and movement problems, or they may simply be a cosmetic concern. Treatment includes elevating the affected limb, wearing support hose to increase pressure on the vein, and in some cases surgery.

variola   See *smallpox.*

varix   An enlarged and convoluted vein, artery, or lymphatic vessel. Treatment of varices depends on where they are and whether they are causing problems. A varix in the esophagus can be caused by severe liver disease and can lead to bleeding. This form of varix can require tying up with a band to prevent dangerous bleeding.

vas deferens   The tube that connects the testes with the urethra. The vas deferens is a coiled duct that conveys sperm from the epididymis to the ejaculatory duct and the urethra.

vasa previa   A critically important condition in which blood vessels within the placenta or the umbilical cord are trapped between the fetus and the opening to the birth canal. Vasa previa carries a high risk that the fetus will die from blood loss due to a vessel tearing at the time the fetal membranes rupture or during labor and delivery. Another danger is lack of oxygen to the fetus. Vasa previa tends to occur with a low-lying or unusually formed placenta, an in vitro fertilization pregnancy, and multiple pregnancies (with twins, triplets, and so on). Vasa previa may not be suspected until the fetal vessel ruptures. Vasa previa can be documented as early as the 16th week of pregnancy via transvaginal ultrasound in combination with color Doppler imaging. When vasa previa is diagnosed, a C-section delivery is done to avoid an emergency.

vascular   Relating to blood vessels. For example, the vascular system in the body includes all of the veins and arteries. And, a vascular surgeon is an expert at evaluating and treating problems of the veins and arteries.

vascular bed   The vascular system, or a part thereof. For example, the pulmonary vascular bed describes the blood vessels of the lungs.

vascular endothelial growth factor   A gene that is responsible for the growth of blood vessels. Abbreviated VEG-F.

vascular headache   See headache, vascular.

vasculitis   A general term for a group of uncommon diseases that feature inflammation of the blood vessels.

Each of the vasculitis diseases is defined by characteristic distributions of blood vessel involvement, patterns of organ involvement, and laboratory test abnormalities. The actual causes of these vasculitis diseases are usually not known, but immune system abnormality is a common feature. Examples of vasculitis include Kawasaki disease, Behcet's disease, polyarteritis nodosa, Wegener's granulomatosis, Takayasu's arteritis, Churg-Strauss syndrome, giant cell arteritis (temporal arteritis), and Henoch-Schonlein purpura. Vasculitis can also accompany infections, such as hepatitis B; exposure to chemicals, such as amphetamines and cocaine; cancers, such as lymphomas and multiple myeloma; and rheumatic diseases, such as rheumatoid arthritis and systemic lupus erythematosus. Laboratory testing in a patient with active vasculitis generally indicates inflammation in the body, and depending on the degree of organ involvement, a variety of organ function tests can be abnormal. The ultimate diagnosis for vasculitis is typically established after a biopsy of involved tissue demonstrates the pattern of blood vessel inflammation. Treatment depends on the type and severity of the illness and the organs involved. Treatments are generally directed toward stopping the inflammation and suppressing the immune system. Typically, cortisone-related medications, such as prednisone, are used, as are other immune-suppression drugs, such as cyclophosphamide (brand name: Cytoxan). Also known as angiitis and vasculitides.

vasculitis, allergic   See *Churg-Strauss syndrome.*

vasoconstriction   Narrowing of the blood vessels that results from contraction of the muscular walls of the vessels. The opposite of vasoconstriction is vasodilation.

vasodepressor syncope   See *syncope, situational.*

vasodilation   Widening of blood vessels that results from relaxation of the muscular walls of the vessels. What widens in vasodilation is actually the diameter of the interior (lumen) of the vessel. The opposite of vasodilation is vasoconstriction.

vasodilator   An agent that acts as a blood vessel dilator, opening blood vessels by relaxing their muscular walls. For example, nitroglycerin is a vasodilator, as are the angiotensin converting enzyme (ACE) inhibitors.

vasomotor   Relating to the nerves and muscles that cause blood vessels to constrict or dilate.

vasomotor rhinitis   Inflammation of the nose (rhinitis) due to abnormal nerve control of the blood vessels in the nose. Vasomotor rhinitis is not allergic rhinitis. Decongestant medications are used to temporarily reduce swelling of sinus and nasal tissues leading to an improvement of breathing and a decrease in obstruction.

vasopressin   See *antidiuretic hormone.*

vasovagal attack   See *vasovagal reaction.*

vasovagal reaction   A reflex of the involuntary nervous system that causes the heart to slow down and, at the same time, affects the nerves to the blood vessels in the legs, permitting those vessels to dilate (widen). As a result, the heart puts out less blood, the blood pressure drops, and the blood that is circulating tends to go into the legs rather than to the head. The brain is deprived of oxygen, and a fainting episode (syncope) occurs. See also *syncope.*

vasovagal syncope   The temporary loss of consciousness in a particular kind of situation (situational syncope, or fainting) due to a vasovagal reaction. See also *syncope.*

VATER association   An association of birth defects that include vertebral anomalies, ventricular septal defects, and other heart defects; anal atresia (the lack of an anus at the end of the intestine); tracheoesophageal fistula (communication between the esophagus and trachea) with esophageal atresia (part of the esophagus not being hollow); radial dysplasia (abnormal formation of the thumb or the radius in the forearm); and kidney abnormalities. This remarkable pattern of malformations has occurred in many babies. The cause of the VATER association is unknown, although it is more common in the children of diabetic mothers than in others. Treatment involves surgery to correct the physical effects, as possible.

VBAC   Vaginal birth after caesarean section. See *caesarean section, vaginal birth after.*

VDRL test   Venereal Disease Research Laboratory test, a blood test for syphilis. A negative (nonreactive) VDRL test is compatible with a person not having syphilis. However, a person may have a negative VDRL and still have syphilis because in the early stages of the disease, the VDRL often gives false negative results. The VDRL test is sometimes positive in the absence of syphilis. For example, a false positive VDRL can be encountered in a patient with infectious mononucleosis, lupus, antiphospholipid antibody syndrome, hepatitis A, leprosy, malaria, and, occasionally, pregnancy. See also *syphilis.*

vector   In medicine, a carrier of disease or of medication. For example, in malaria a mosquito is the vector that carries and transfers the infectious agent. In molecular biology, a vector may be a virus or a plasmid that carries a piece of foreign DNA to a host cell.

VEG-F   Vascular endothelial growth factor.

vein   A blood vessel that carries blood that is low in oxygen content from the body back to the heart. The

deoxygenated form of hemoglobin (deoxyhemoglobin) in venous blood makes it appear dark. Veins are part of the afferent wing of the circulatory system, which returns blood to the heart. In contrast, an artery is a vessel that carries blood that is high in oxygen away from the heart to the body.

Velpeau hernia   See *hernia, Velpeau.*

velvet ant   A parasitic wasp that is common in most parts of the world, including the southern and southwestern US. Velvet ant stings can trigger allergic reactions that vary greatly in severity. Avoidance and prompt treatment are essential. In selected cases, allergy injection therapy is highly effective.

vena cava, inferior   A large vein that receives blood from the lower extremities, pelvis, and abdomen and then empties that blood into the right atrium of the heart.

vena cava, superior   The large vein that returns blood to the right atrium of the heart from the head, neck, and both upper limbs. The superior vena cava is located in the middle of the chest and is surrounded by rigid structures and lymph nodes. Structures bordering the superior vena cava include the trachea, aorta, thymus, right bronchus of the lung, and pulmonary artery. Compression of the superior vena cava by disease of any of the structures or lymph nodes surrounding it can cause superior vena cava syndrome. See also *superior vena cava syndrome.*

vena cava syndrome, superior   See *superior vena cava syndrome.*

venereal   Having to do with sexual contact. For example, a venereal disease is a sexually transmitted disease.

venereal disease   See *sexually transmitted disease.*

venereal warts   See *genital warts.*

venlafaxine   A unique antidepressant drug (brand name: Effexor) that is prescribed to treat depression. Venlafaxine is believed to affect the neurotransmitters serotonin, norepinephrine, and dopamine, but not monoamine oxidase (MAO). Venlafaxine is not usually indicated for use by people with kidney or liver disease, or by those with high blood pressure. Common side effects include sleepiness, insomnia, dry mouth, nervousness, nausea, and sexual dysfunction.

venous aneurysm   A localized widening and bulging of a vein. At the area of a venous aneurysm, the vein wall is weakened and may rupture.

venous catheterization   The insertion of a tiny tube (catheter) into a peripheral or central vein to deliver fluids or medication. Venous catheterization is the most frequently used method for administration of IV fluids. The most common complication of venous catheterization is infection at the site of the catheter (catheter sepsis).

vent To air one's feelings by putting problems into words.

ventilation 1 The exchange of air between the lungs and the atmosphere so that oxygen is exchanged for carbon dioxide in the alveoli (the tiny air sacs in the lungs). 2 When a person (or persons) airs out their feelings by putting their problems into words.

ventilator A machine that mechanically assists a patient in the exchange of oxygen and carbon dioxide, a process sometimes referred to as artificial respiration.

ventral Pertaining to the front or anterior of a structure. Something that is ventral is oriented toward the belly, toward the front of the body. For example, the bellybutton (umbilicus) is in the ventral midline. The opposite of ventral is dorsal. See also Appendix B, "Anatomic Orientation Terms."

ventricle A chamber of an organ. For example, the four connected cavities in the central portion of the brain are called ventricles.

ventricle, brain See *brain ventricle.*

ventricle, cerebral See *cerebral ventricle.*

ventricle, fourth See *fourth ventricle.*

ventricle, heart See *heart ventricle.*

ventricle, lateral See *lateral ventricle.*

ventricle, left The chamber of the heart that receives blood from the left atrium and pumps it out under high pressure to the body via the aorta. See also *heart ventricle.*

ventricle, right The chamber of the heart that receives blood from the right atrium and pumps it under low pressure into the lungs via the pulmonary artery. See also *heart ventricle.*

ventricle, third See *third ventricle.*

ventricular arrhythmia An abnormal, rapid heart rhythm (arrhythmia) that originates in the lower chambers of the heart (ventricles). Ventricular arrhythmias include ventricular tachycardia and ventricular fibrillation. Both are life-threatening arrhythmias that are commonly associated with heart attacks and scarring of the heart muscle from previous heart attacks.

ventricular fibrillation See *fibrillation, ventricular.*

ventricular septal defect A hole in the wall (septum) between the lower chambers of the heart (ventricles). Abbreviated VSD. VSDs are the most common birth defect that involves malformation of the heart. At least 1 baby in every 500 is born with a VSD. A VSD shunts blood from the left ventricle, where it is under relatively high pressure, into the right ventricle, which has to do extra work to handle the additional blood. The right ventricle may have trouble keeping up with the load, enlarge, and fail. The lungs also receive too much blood under too great pressure. The small arteries (arterioles) in the lungs thicken up in response, and permanent vascular damage can be done to the lungs. VSDs that are less than 0.5 square cm in area permit only minimal shunting of blood, so the pressure in the right ventricle remains normal and the heart and lungs function normally. Surgical repair is not recommended for small VSDs. No matter what size a VSD is, it carries an increased risk for infection of the heart walls and valves (endocarditis). To prevent endocarditis, anyone with a VSD should take antibiotics before dental and some other procedures. With a VSD greater than 1.0 square cm in area, there is a significant shunt into the right ventricle, excessive blood flow into the lungs, and elevated pressure in the arteries to the lungs (pulmonary hypertension). The child may have labored breathing and difficulty feeding, and he or she may grow poorly. Medically, a heart that has a large VSD should be kept strong, and vascular disease must not be allowed to develop in the lungs. Surgery should be done to close a large VSD. The prognosis for patients with VSD is generally excellent.

ventricular septum The wall between the two lower chambers (ventricles) of the heart.

ventricular tachycardia An abnormal heart rhythm that is rapid and regular and that originates from an area of the lower chamber (ventricle) of the heart. Ventricular tachycardias are life-threatening arrhythmias that are commonly associated with heart attacks and scarring of the heart muscle from previous heart attacks.

venule A little vein that goes from a capillary to a vein.

verbal child abuse See *child abuse, emotional.*

vernix A white, cheesy substance that covers and protects the skin of a fetus. Vernix is still all over the skin of a baby at birth. Vernix is composed of sebum (skin oil) and cells that have sloughed off the skin of the fetus. More formally known as vernix caseosa.

vernix caseosa See *vernix.*

verruca See *wart.*

verruga   See *wart*.

vertebra   One of 33 bony segments that form the human spinal column. Each vertebra has its own name and/or number. For example, the second cervical vertebra is known as the axis, or C2, vertebra. See also *vertebral column*.

vertebral artery   One of two key arteries located in the back of the neck that carry blood from the heart to the brain, spine, and neck muscles.

vertebral column   The 33 vertebrae that fit together to form a flexible, yet extraordinarily tough, column that serves to support the back through a full range of motion. The vertebral column also protects the spinal cord, which runs from the brain through the hollow space in the middle of the vertebral column. There are 7 cervical (C1–C7), 12 thoracic (T1–T12), 5 lumbar (L1–L5), 5 sacral (S1–S5), and 3 to 5 coccygeal vertebrae in the vertebral column, each separated by intervertebral disks. The first cervical vertebra, known as the atlas, supports the head. It pivots on the odontoid process of the second cervical vertebra, the axis. The cervical vertebrae end at their juncture with the thoracic vertebrae. The seventh cervical vertebra (the prominent vertebra, so named because of its long spiny projection) adjoins the first thoracic vertebrae. The thoracic vertebrae provide an attachment site for the true ribs and make up part of the back of the chest (thorax). This part of the spine is very flexible, to permit bending and twisting. The thoracic vertebrae join the lumbar vertebrae, which are particularly sturdy and large because they support the entire structure. The lumbar vertebrae are nonetheless quite flexible. At the top of the pelvis, the lumbar vertebrae join the sacral vertebrae. By adulthood, the five sacral vertebrae have usually fused to form a triangular bone called the sacrum. At the tip of the sacrum, the final part of the vertebral column projects slightly outward. This is the coccyx, better known as the tailbone. It is made up of three to five coccygeal vertebrae: small, rudimentary vertebrae that fuse together. Also known as the spinal column.

vertebral compression fracture   A fracture that collapses a spinal vertebra as a result of the compression of bone, leading to collapse of the vertebrae, similarly to the way a sponge collapses under the pressure of one's hand. Although they may occur without pain, such vertebral fractures often cause severe, band-like pain that radiates from the spine around both sides of the body. Over many years, spinal fractures decrease the height of the spine, and the person becomes shorter. Vertebral compression fractures are often linked to osteoporosis. Treatment usually involves use of pain medicine, rest, injury avoidance, and bracing, and in some cases surgery can be used. See also *vertebroplasty*.

vertebral rib   See *floating rib*.

vertebroplasty   A nonsurgical method for repairing osteoporosis back fractures, such as vertebral compression fractures. Vertebroplasty is performed by a radiologist, without surgery, and involves inserting a glue-like material (methylmethacrylate) into the center of the collapsed spinal vertebra to stabilize and strengthen the crushed bone. The methylmethacrylate is inserted through anesthetized skin with a needle and syringe, entering the midportion of the vertebra under the guidance of specialized X-ray equipment. Once inserted, the methylmethacrylate hardens to form a cast-like structure within the broken bone. Relief of pain comes quickly from this casting effect, and the newly hardened vertebra is then protected from further collapse. In addition to prompt pain relief, another advantage of vertebroplasty is improved mobility. Vertebrae that have collapsed to less than 30 percent of their normal height are poor candidates for this procedure. Also referred to as kyphoplasty.

vertex   The top of the head. For example, in a vertex presentation at birth, the top of the baby's head emerges first.

vertex birth   Birth in which the top of the baby's head emerges first. This is the most common presentation.

vertical   Upright, as opposed to horizontal. See also Appendix B, "Anatomic Orientation Terms."

vertical transmission   Passage of a disease-causing agent (pathogen) from mother to baby during the period immediately before and after birth. Transmission might occur across the placenta, in the breast milk, or through direct contact during or after birth. For example, HIV can be a vertically transmitted pathogen. Also known as perinatal transmission.

vertigo   A feeling that one is turning around or that things are turning about the person. Vertigo is usually due to a problem with the inner ear. See also *dizziness; lightheadedness; unsteadiness*.

vertigo, recurrent aural   See *Ménière's disease*.

vesical   See *bladder*.

vesicant   A substance that causes tissue blistering. Also known as vesicatory.

vesicate   To blister.

vesicatory   See *vesicant*.

vesicle   1 In dermatology, a tiny skin blister.   2 In anatomy, a small pouch.

vesicle, seminal See *seminal vesicle.*

vesicular Referring to the presence of one or more vesicles. For example, a vesicular rash features small blisters on the skin.

vesicular rickettsiosis See *rickettsialpox.*

vesiculitis Inflammation of a vesicle, particularly of the seminal vesicles behind the male bladder.

vesiculography The use of special X-ray equipment and a dye to examine the seminal vesicles and related structures. Vesiculography is most often used when prostate disease or cancer is suspected.

vessel A tube in the body that carries fluids. Examples of vessels are blood vessels and lymph vessels.

vessel, afferent See *afferent vessel.*

vessel, efferent See *efferent vessel.*

vestibular 1 Having to do with a structure that is a vestibule (entrance), such as the vestibule of the ear. 2 Having to do with the body's system for maintaining equilibrium.

vestibular apparatus The vestibule and three semicircular canals of the inner ear. Like an internal carpenter's level, these structures work with the brain to sense, maintain, and regain balance and a sense of where the body and its parts are positioned in space. See also *vestibular disease; vestibular system.*

vestibular disease A disorder of the vestibular apparatus, which is necessary for the sense of balance. A disease may cause vestibular problems by directly affecting the structure or integrity of the middle ear, by interrupting the feedback loop between these structures and the brain, or by affecting the parts of the brain that interpret data from the vestibular apparatus. Conditions known to impair vestibular function include acoustic neuroma, autism, Ménière's disease, multiple sclerosis, infection in the middle ear (otitis media), medications that are toxic to the ear (ototoxic), seizure disorders, syphilis, trauma, and vertigo. Diagnosis is made via neurological tests, in which the response to movement requests and questions about spatial positioning are observed. Diagnosis of vestibular disease may be confirmed by imaging inner ear structures or brain function. Treatment depends on the cause of the disease.

vestibular system A system that is composed of the vestibular apparatus, the vestibulocochlear nerve, and the parts of the brain that interpret and respond to information derived from those structures.

vestibule In medicine and dentistry, a space or cavity at the entrance to a canal, channel, tube, or vessel. For instance, the front of the mouth is a vestibule.

vestibule of the ear A cavity in the middle of the bony labyrinth in the inner ear.

vestibule, vaginal See *vaginal opening.*

vestibulocochlear nerve A nerve that is responsible for the sense of hearing and that is also pertinent to the senses of balance and body position. Problems with the vestibulocochlear nerve may result in deafness, tinnitus (ringing or noise in the ears), dizziness, vertigo, and vomiting. The vestibulocochlear nerve is the eighth cranial nerve.

vestigial Referring to a vestige (remnant) or a primitive structure and no longer believed to be important. For example, the appendix is considered a vestigial organ, and some infants are born with vestigial tails.

VHL syndrome von Hippel-Lindau syndrome.

viable Capable of life. For example, a viable premature baby is one who is able to survive outside the womb.

Vibrio A group of bacteria that includes Vibrio cholerae, the agent that causes cholera. Other species are common in salt and fresh water as well as soil. Vibrio move about particularly actively.

Vibrio cholerae One of the Vibrio bacteria, the agent that causes cholera. See also *cholera.*

vidian neuralgia See *cluster headache.*

Vincent gingivitis See *acute membraneous gingivitis.*

viral Of or pertaining to a virus. For example, if a person has a viral rash, the rash was caused by a virus.

viral hepatitis See *hepatitis, viral.*

viral infection An infection caused by the presence of a virus in the body. Depending on the virus and the person's state of health, various viruses can infect almost any type of body tissue, from the brain to the skin. Viral infections cannot be treated with antibiotics; in fact, in some cases the use of antibiotics makes a viral infection worse. The vast majority of human viral infections can be effectively fought by the body's own immune system, with a little help from proper diet, hydration, and rest. Treatment of other viral infections depends on the type and location of the virus and may include use of antiviral or other drugs.

viremia The presence of a virus in the blood. Viremia is analogous to bacteremia (the presence of bacteria in the blood) and parasitemia (the presence of a parasite in the blood). Viremia, bacteremia, and parasitemia are all forms of sepsis (bloodstream infection).

virion   A virus particle.

virology   The study of viruses.

virulence   The ability of an agent of infection to produce disease. The virulence of a microorganism is a measure of the severity of the disease it causes.

virulent   Extremely noxious, damaging, deleterious, and disease causing (pathogenic); marked by a rapid, severe, and malignant course; poisonous.

virus   A microorganism that is smaller than a bacterium that cannot grow or reproduce apart from a living cell. A virus invades living cells and uses their chemical machinery to keep itself alive and to replicate itself. It may reproduce with fidelity or with errors (mutations); this ability to mutate is responsible for the ability of some viruses to change slightly in each infected person, making treatment difficult. Viruses cause many common human infections and are also responsible for a number of rare diseases. Examples of viral illnesses range from the common cold, which is usually caused by one of the rhinoviruses, to AIDS, which is caused by HIV. Viruses may contain either DNA or RNA as their genetic material. Herpes simplex virus and the hepatitis B virus are DNA viruses. RNA viruses have an enzyme called reverse transcriptase that permits the usual sequence of DNA-to-RNA to be reversed so that the virus can make a DNA version of itself. RNA viruses include HIV and hepatitis C virus. Researchers have grouped viruses together into several major families, based on their shape, behavior, and other characteristics. These include the herpesviruses, adenoviruses, papovaviruses (papilloma viruses), hepadnaviruses, poxviruses, and parvoviruses, among the DNA viruses. On the RNA virus side, major families include the picornaviruses (including the rhinoviruses), calciviruses, paramyxoviruses, orthomyxoviruses, rhabdoviruses, filoviruses, bornaviruses, and retroviruses. There are dozens of smaller virus families within these major classifications. Many viruses are host specific, causing disease in humans or specific animals only.

virus, attenuated   A virus that has been weakened. A vaccine against a viral disease can be made from an attenuated, less virulent strain of the virus: a virus that is capable of stimulating an immune response and creating immunity but not of causing illness.

visceral leishmaniasis   See *leishmaniasis.*

visceral pericardium   The inner layer of the pericardium.

vision, central   See *central vision.*

vision, macular   See *central vision.*

vision, phantom   See *phantom vision.*

vision therapy   The use of special eye exercises to address eye defects, such as strabismus. Some vision therapists claim that eye exercises can help people with neurological or learning disabilities. Vision therapy is not proven for the latter use, although some patients do report improvement.

visual acuity   The clarity or clearness of vision, a measure of how well a person sees.

visual acuity test   See *eye chart test.*

visual field test   A test that measures the extent and distribution of the field of vision. A visual field test may be done via a number of methods, including termed confrontation, tangent screen exam, and automated perimetry. These tests may seem tedious but are not painful or uncomfortable. Many diseases can adversely affect the visual field, including glaucoma, strokes, high blood pressure (hypertension), diabetes, multiple sclerosis, and overactivity of the thyroid gland (hyperthyroidism). Medications, including the antimalarial drugs chloroquine (brand name: Atabrine) and hydroxychloroquine (brand name: Plaquenil), can also affect the visual field.

visual nerve   See *optic nerve.*

visual nerve pathways   See *optic nerve pathways.*

vital   Necessary to maintain life. For example, breathing is a vital function.

vitamin   An organic substance that naturally occurs in plants or animal tissue that is essential for normal metabolism of the body and to life. Vitamins play a part in dozens of crucial activities in the body: Some are antioxidants, preventing oxidation of cells and potentially preventing cancer; others permit or deny chemical reactions involved in sight, brain function, metabolism, nucleic acid synthesis, and the like. All vitamins are either available in food or can be made within the body. However, many people do not eat a diet that contains the minimum daily requirements of certain vitamins. Nutritionists suggest that the best way to ensure appropriate doses of vitamins is to eat a healthful diet, particularly one that is rich in green, leafy vegetables and carotene compounds. These foods offer many benefits that vitamin supplements cannot, including fiber, and probably include vitamin-like substances that have not yet been isolated. Lack of specific vitamins can lead to deficiency syndromes, such as rickets, beriberi, and anemia. Overconsumption of certain vitamins can also have consequences, ranging from minor to life threatening. Some vitamins are water soluble, and any excess is simply excreted in the urine. Others are fat-soluble and may build up in the body, potentially reaching dangerous concentrations. Vitamins may also interact with prescription and over-the-counter drugs, making them more or less potent. For these reasons, it is important to consult a physician before adding vitamin supplements to a daily regimen. See also Appendix C, "Vitamins."

vitamin P See *bioflavinoid.*

vitamin therapy The use of vitamins to prevent or cure disease. Many physicians now recognize the beneficial uses of antioxidant and other vitamins for a wide variety of conditions, often as complementary therapy to accompany medication or other treatments. One variant on this theme, megavitamin therapy, is still rather controversial. It is important to consult a physician before adding vitamin supplements to a health regimen. See also Appendix C, "Vitamins."

vitelline duct See *yolk stalk.*

vitiligo A condition in which the skin turns white due to the loss of pigment from the melanocytes, cells that produce the pigment melanin that gives the skin color. In vitiligo, the melanocytes are destroyed, leaving depigmented patches of skin. The hair that grows in areas affected by vitiligo may also turn white. The skin is not otherwise damaged. People with vitiligo must protect their skin from exposure to the sun. Affected areas of skin can become seriously sunburned while the surrounding skin tans. Also known as piebald skin and acquired leukoderma.

vitreous humor A clear, jelly-like substance that fills the middle of the eye.

vocal cord One of the two small bands of muscle that form a V-shape within the larynx. When a person breathes, the vocal cords relax, and air moves through the space between them without making a sound. When a person talks or sings, the vocal cords tighten up and move closer together. Air from the lungs is forced between them, making them vibrate to produce sound, much like the strings of a guitar. The tongue, lips, and teeth form that sound into words. See also *larynx.*

voice box See *larynx.*

void To urinate. The term void is also sometimes used to indicate the elimination of solid waste (defecation).

volar Pertaining to the palm or the sole. For example, the volar surface of the forearm is the portion of the forearm that is on the same side as the palm of the hand.

volume, stroke See *stroke volume.*

voluntary Done in accordance with the conscious will of the individual. The opposite of voluntary is involuntary. The terms voluntary and involuntary apply to the human nervous system and its control over muscles. The nervous system is divided into two parts: somatic and autonomic. The somatic nervous system operates the skeletal muscles, which are under voluntary control. The autonomic (automatic, or visceral) nervous system regulates individual organ function and is involuntary. For example, opening the mouth is voluntary, and blushing and the beating of the heart are involuntary. See also *autonomic nervous system.*

vomit 1 Matter from the stomach that is ejected in tandem with symptoms of nausea. When vomit is reddish or coffee-ground colored, it indicates serious internal bleeding. Also known as vomitus. 2 To expel vomit. Also known as peristalsis and emesis.

vomiting in pregnancy, excess See *hyperemesis gravidarum.*

vomiting of pregnancy, pernicious See *hyperemesis gravidarum.*

von Hippel-Lindau syndrome A genetic disease that is characterized by hemangioblastomas (benign blood vessel tumors) in the brain, spinal cord, and retina; kidney cysts, and kidney cancer (renal cell carcinoma); pheochromocytomas (benign tumors of adrenal-like tissue); and endolymphatic sac tumors (benign tumors of the labyrinth in the inner ear). Abbreviated VHL syndrome. The brain hemangioblastomas in VHL syndrome are usually in the cerebellum and can cause headache, vomiting, and gait disturbances or ataxia (wobbliness). The hemangioblastomas in the retina can cause vision loss and may be the initial sign of VHL syndrome. Renal cell carcinoma occurs in 40 percent of cases and is the leading cause of death. Pheochromocytomas can cause no symptoms or constant or intermittent high blood pressure. The endolymphatic sac tumors can diminish hearing, which is a key symptom of VHL syndrome. VHL syndrome is inherited in an autosomal dominant manner and is caused by a change that affects the VHL gene, a tumor-suppressor gene, on chromosome 3 (region 3p26–3p25). Molecular genetic testing for the VHL gene confirms the diagnosis of VHL syndrome. There is a 50 percent risk for each child of a person with VHL inheriting the VHL disease-causing mutation. Prenatal testing is available. Early recognition of VHL syndrome is important because it permits timely intervention and may be lifesaving. Treatment can involve neurosurgery.

von Recklinghausen disease   See *neurofibromatosis.*

Vrolik disease   See *osteogenesis imperfecta type II.*

VSD   Ventricular septal defect.

vulva   The female external genital organs, including the labia, clitoris, and entrance to the vagina.

vulvar pain, chronic   See *vulvodynia.*

vulvitis   Inflammation of the external genital organs of the female, often caused by the yeast Candida albicans. See also *yeast vulvitis.*

vulvodynia   Chronic pain in the area of the female vulva. The main symptom is pain, usually a burning irritation or rawness of the genitals. The pain may be constant or intermittent, localized or diffuse. It can last for months or longer, and it can vanish as suddenly as it started. The cause of vulvodynia is unknown. Many women with vulvodynia have a history of treatment for recurrent vaginal fungal infections. Treatments being tested include use of drugs, use of nerve blocks to numb the vulvar nerves, and biofeedback therapy to relax pelvic muscles. See also *vulvitis; yeast vulvitis.*

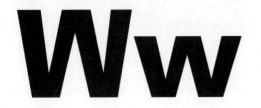

cause bleeding into the baby's brain (cerebral hemorrhage), underdevelopment (hypoplasia) of the baby's nose, and stippling of the ends (epiphyses) of the baby's long bones. See also *deep vein thrombosis*.

wart A local growth on the outer layer of the skin that is caused by a papillomavirus. Papillomavirus is transmitted by contact, either with a wart on someone else or a wart on oneself (autoinnoculation). Warts that occur on the hands or feet are called common warts. A wart on the sole of the foot is a plantar wart. Genital (venereal) warts are located on the genitals and are transmitted by sexual contact. Also known as verruca and verruga. See also *genital warts; human papilloma virus*.

wart, genital See *genital warts*.

wart, plantar A wart that grows on the sole of the foot. Plantar warts are different from most other warts. They tend to be flat and cause the buildup of a callus that has to be peeled away before the plantar wart itself can be seen. Plantar warts may attack blood vessels deep in the skin, and they can be quite painful. Plantar warts are caused by human papilloma virus (HPV) type 1, and they tend to affect teenagers. To avoid plantar warts, a child should be taught never to wear someone else's shoes. Plantar warts should be treated by a physician. Treatment may include freezing off the wart, excising it, or using an immersible ultrasound device to kill the wart. See also *human papilloma virus*.

wart, venereal See *genital warts*.

wasp sting A sting from a wasp, which can trigger allergic reactions that vary greatly in severity. Avoidance and prompt treatment are essential. In some cases, allergy injection therapy is highly effective.

water on the brain See *hydrocephalus*.

water-hammer pulse See *Corrigan pulse*.

wax dip See *paraffin dip*.

wax, ear See *earwax*.

WBC White blood cell.

WDWN Abbreviation for "well-developed, well-nourished," shorthand used by physicians when jotting down the results of a physical examination. For example, a WDWNWF would be a well-developed, well-nourished white female.

weaver's bottom Inflammation of the bursa that separates the gluteus maximus muscle of the buttocks from the underlying bony prominence of the bone that a person sits on (ischial tuberosity). Weaver's bottom is a form of bursitis that is usually caused by prolonged sitting on hard surfaces that press against the bones of the bottom or midbuttocks. Also known as ischial bursitis.

Waardenburg syndrome A genetic syndrome that features deafness, a white forelock (a frontal white blaze of hair), a difference of color between the iris of one eye and the other (heterochromia iridis), white eyelashes, and wide-set inner corners of the eyes. Abbreviated WS. The deafness of WS is typically present at birth and is bilateral, profound nerve deafness. The severity of WS varies, and about 40 percent of affected persons escape the deafness. The white forelock may be present at birth. The majority of individuals with WS have the white forelock or early graying of the scalp hair before age 30. WS is inherited in an autosomal dominant manner in which the heterozygous state (with one copy of the gene) is sufficient to cause the syndrome. The homozygous form of WS (with two copies of the gene) is a severe and fortunately rare disorder that features severe upper-limb defects and has been called Klein-Waardenburg syndrome. The gene for classic WS, symbolized WS1, is on chromosome 2 (in band q35) and is the PAX3 gene, which encodes a DNA-binding transcription factor that is expressed in the early embryo.

Waldenstrom macroglobulinemia A chronic low-grade type of lymphoma that is due to a malignant clone of plasma cells. These plasma cells multiply out of control, invade the bone marrow, lymph nodes, and spleen, and characteristically produce huge amounts of the antibody macroglobulin (IgM). The excess IgM causes the blood to thicken. Waldenstrom macroglobulinemia can occur in younger people but is usually seen in people over age 65. See also *lymphoma; plasma cell*.

warfarin An anticoagulant medication (brand names: Coumarin, Panwarfin, Sofarin) that is taken to treat blood clots or overly thickened blood. Some patients also take warfarin to reduce their risk of clots, stroke, or heart attack. Warfarin works by suppressing production of some clotting factors. Warfarin interacts with many other drugs, including some vitamins. These interactions can be dangerous and even life-threatening. A patient on warfarin should talk to a physician before taking any other prescription or over-the-counter drug. Warfarin taken by a woman during pregnancy can disturb the development of an embryo and a fetus and lead to birth defects. It can also

Wegener granulomatosis See *granulomatosis, Wegener.*

welt See *hives.*

Werner syndrome A premature aging disease that begins in adolescence or early adulthood and results in apparent old age by 30–40 years of age. Characteristic features include short stature, premature graying, early baldness, wizened face, beaked nose, cataracts, skin changes reminiscent of those in scleroderma, deposits of calcium beneath the skin, premature arteriosclerosis, and a tendency to diabetes and to tumors (especially osteosarcoma and meningioma). Werner syndrome is inherited in an autosomal recessive manner and is due to mutation in the RECQL2 gene, which encodes RecQ DNA helicase, an enzyme that catalyzes the unwinding of DNA.

Werner-His disease See *trench fever.*

West Nile virus A febrile disease that is transmitted from birds to mosquitoes and then to people. The virus is named after the area in which it was first found, in Uganda. West Nile virus occurs in parts of Africa and Asia and, infrequently, in Southern Europe, the Middle East, and the US. West Nile virus had never been seen in birds or people in the Western Hemisphere prior to an outbreak in summer 1999 in New York City. Since that time, it has spread across the US. Signs and symptoms include the sudden onset of drowsiness, headache and nausea due to encephalitis, pain in the abdomen, a rash, and swollen glands (lymphadenopathy). These features are usually but not always mild. Fatal cases tend to involve infants and small children under age 5, the aged, and people with impaired immune systems. Also known as West Nile encephalitis. See also *encephalitis.*

Western blot A technique in molecular biology that is used to separate and identify particular proteins.

WF Medical shorthand for white female.

wheezing A whistling noise in the chest during breathing. Wheezing occurs when the airways are narrowed or compressed.

whiplash injury A hyperextension and flexion injury to the neck, often a result of being struck from behind, as by a fast-moving vehicle in a car accident. The mechanics of whiplash injury are thought to be as follows: The victim may be first pushed or accelerated forward, pushing the body forward, but the head remains behind momentarily, rocking up and back, and some muscles and ligaments in and around the spine may be stretched or torn. These muscles, in a reflex action, contract to bring the head forward again, to prevent excessive injury. There may be overcompensation when the head is traveling in a forward direction as the vehicle decelerates. This may rock the head violently forward, stretching and tearing more muscles and ligaments.

Whipple disease A form of inability to absorb nutrients from the intestine that was described in 1907 by the pathologist, medical missionary, and Nobel laureate George H. Whipple, who first developed the disease. The symptoms are arthritis and then weight loss, cough, fever, diarrhea, hypotension (low blood pressure), abdominal swelling, increased skin pigmentation, and severe anemia. Whipple disease has been discovered to be due to a previously unknown type of bacteria, now named Tropheryma whippelii, which was reported in 2000 to have been grown in the laboratory, opening the way for the development of a simple blood test to diagnose the disease. Whipple disease is treated with antibiotics. Some patients relapse and need long-term, even life-long, treatment.

Whipple procedure A type of surgery that is used to treat pancreatic cancer and was devised by the US surgeon Allen Whipple. The head of the pancreas, the duodenum, a portion of the stomach, and other nearby tissues are removed.

whipworm A nematode (roundworm) that is also called Trichuris trichiura and is the third most common roundworm in humans. The whipworm is found worldwide, and whipworm infections are most frequent among children and in areas with tropical weather and poor sanitation practices. It is estimated that 800 million people are infected with whipworm worldwide. Infection with whipworm most often occurs without symptoms. Heavy infections, especially in small children, can cause gastrointestinal problems (such as abdominal pain, diarrhea, and rectal prolapse) and possibly growth retardation. Treatment involves use of the drug mebendazole or the drug albendazole.

white blood cell See *leukocyte.*

white blood cell count The number of white blood cells (WBCs) in the blood. The normal range for the WBC count varies among laboratories but is usually between 4,300 and 10,800 cells per cubic millimeter. It can be expressed in international units as $(4.3–10.8)\times10^9$ cells per liter. A low WBC count is called leukopenia. A high WBC count is termed leukocytosis. Also known as leukocyte count.

white coat hypertension A transient increase in blood pressure (hypertension) that is triggered by the sight of medical personnel in white coats (or other attire). Ideally, people so affected should do their best to relax when in the medical office.

white matter The part of the brain that contains myelinated nerve fibers. The white matter is white because it is the color of myelin, the insulation that covers nerve fibers.

white spots on the nails See *jogger's nails.*

white subungual onychomycosis, proximal See *onychomycosis, proximal white subungual.*

whitehead A familiar term for what is medically called a closed comedo. A comedo, the primary sign of acne, consists of a dilated (widened) hair follicle filled with keratin squamae (skin debris), bacteria, and sebum (oil). A whitehead is a comedo that has an obstructed opening to the skin. A closed comedo may rupture and cause a low-grade skin inflammatory reaction in the area.

WHO World Health Organization.

whooping cough See *pertussis.*

will, living See *living will.*

Willis, circle of See *circle of Willis.*

Wilms tumor A childhood form of kidney cancer. If the child has symptoms, the physician usually feels the child's abdomen to look for masses and runs blood and urine tests. A special X-ray to view the kidneys, called an intravenous pyelogram (IVP), may be done. Ultrasound and magnetic resonance imaging (MRI) may also be needed. If abnormal tissue is found, a biopsy is needed. In Wilms tumor, how the cancer cells look under a microscope (histology) is very important. The cancer cells can be of favorable histology or unfavorable histology (which includes focal and diffuse anaplasia). The child's chance of recovery and choice of treatment depend on the stage of the cancer (whether it is just in the kidney or has spread to other places in the body), how the cancer cells look under a microscope, tumor size, and the child's age and general health. Wilms tumor is curable in the majority of cases. Approximately 500 cases are diagnosed in the US annually. Today more than 90 percent of patients survive 4 years after diagnosis, which is an improvement over the 80 percent survival observed from 1975 to 1984.

Wilson disease An inherited disorder of copper metabolism that results in an abnormal accumulation of copper in the body. Although the accumulation of copper begins at birth, symptoms of the disorder do not appear until later in life, between the ages of 6 and 40. A diagnostic feature of the disease is a Kayser-Fleischer ring, a deep copper-colored ring around the edge of the cornea that represents copper deposits in the eye. The main clinical consequence of Wilson disease for about 40 percent of patients is liver disease. In other patients the first symptoms are nervous system or psychiatric symptoms or both and include tremor, rigidity, drooling, difficulty with speech, abrupt personality change, grossly inappropriate behavior and inexplicable deterioration of school or other work, neurosis, and psychosis. Without proper treatment, Wilson disease is always fatal, usually by age 30. If treatment is begun early enough, symptomatic recovery is usually complete, and a life of normal length and quality can be expected. However, if treatment is begun too late, recovery is only partial, and the disease is fatal. Wilson disease is inherited in an autosomal recessive manner and is due to mutation of the ATP7B gene on chromosome 13. The ATP7B gene encodes ATPase, a $Cu++$ transporting beta polypeptide that accounts for the basic problem in copper metabolism.

windpipe See *trachea.*

winter depression See *seasonal affective disorder.*

wisdom tooth See *tooth, wisdom.*

WM Medical shorthand for white male.

WNL Medical shorthand for within normal limits. For example, a laboratory test result may be WNL.

Wolff-Parkinson-White syndrome A condition that is caused by an abnormality in the electrical system of the heart, which normally tells the heart muscle when to contract. Abbreviated WPW syndrome. In WPW syndrome there is an extra electrical connection inside the heart that acts as a short circuit, causing the heart to beat too rapidly and sometimes in an irregular manner. WPW syndrome can be life threatening, although that is unusual. WPW syndrome can be treated via destruction of the short circuit, using a technique termed radiofrequency catheter ablation, in which wires are put in different places in the heart until the short circuit is found and can be destroyed with radio waves.

Wolhynia fever See *trench fever.*

womb See *uterus.*

word processor's cramp A dystonia that affects the muscles of the hand and sometimes the forearm and that occurs only during typing or use of a computer. Similar focal dystonias have also been called writer's cramp, pianist's cramp, musician's cramp, and golfer's cramp.

working memory See *memory, short-term.*

World Health Organization The subagency of the United Nations (UN) that is concerned with international health. Abbreviated WHO. Also known as Organisation Mondiale de la Santé (OMS).

wormwood The plant whose essence forms the basis of absinthe, a dangerous emerald-green liqueur. See also *absinthe.*

WPW syndrome Wolff-Parkinson-White syndrome.

wrist The part of the hand that is nearest the forearm and consists of the carpal bones and the associated soft tissues. The eight carpal bones are arranged in two rows. One row of carpal bones joins the long bones of the forearm (the radius, and, indirectly, the ulna). Another row of carpal bones meets the hand at the five metacarpal bones that make up the palm.

writer's cramp See *cramp, writer's.*

wryneck See *torticollis, congenital.*

WS Waardenburg syndrome.

Wt Abbreviation for weight. For example, "Wt 80 lbs" means "weight 80 pounds."

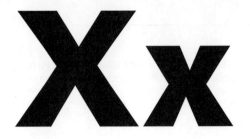

X In genetics and medicine, X chromosome.

X chromosome The sex chromosome that is found twice in normal females and singly, along with a Y chromosome, in normal males. The complete chromosome complement consists of 46 chromosomes, including the 2 sex chromosomes, and is thus conventionally written as 46,XX for chromosomally normal females and 46,XY for chromosomally normal males.

xanthelasma Tiny, slightly raised, yellowish plaques on the skin surface of the upper or lower eyelids. Xanthelasma is a harmless growth of tissue caused by tiny deposits of fat in the skin, and it is often associated with abnormal blood fat levels (hyperlipidemia). Xanthelasma is composed of lipid-laden foam cells called histiocytes. Treatment is directed toward any underlying lipid disorder when present. Dermatologists can remove the abnormal plaques. See also *xanthoma*.

xanthinuria A metabolic disorder that is caused by lack of an enzyme needed to process xanthine, an alkaloid found in caffeine; theobromine; theophylline; and related substances. Unchecked, xanthinuria can lead to kidney stone formation. Treatment involves avoiding foods and drinks that contain xanthine derivatives, such as coffee, tea, and cola. Xanthinuria is inherited in an autosomal recessive manner and is due to mutation of the gene on chromosome 2 that encodes the enzyme xanthine dehydrogenase.

xanthoma One of several conditions characterized by firm yellow, orange, or brown nodules deep in the skin (such as around the Achilles tendon, elbows, or knees) or mucous membranes. Although xanthomas themselves are harmless, they frequently indicate underlying disease, such as diabetes, lipid disorders (such as elevated blood cholesterol levels), or other conditions. They are composed of lipid-laden foam cells called histiocytes. Treatment is directed toward any underlying disorder when present. The nodules can be resected surgically for cosmetic purposes. Xanthoma is distinguished from xanthelasma by being a large nodule deep in the tissues as opposed to a plaque in the skin surface, but both can occur from lipid disorder. See also *xanthelasma*.

xanthoma, diabetic Xanthoma that is associated with poorly controlled diabetes mellitus. Treating the diabetes causes diabetic xanthomas to disappear.

xanthoma, disseminatum A type of xanthoma from chronically elevated blood fats (cholesterol and triglycerides) that is characterized by orange-to-brown nodules on the skin or mucous membranes.

xanthoma, eruptive Xanthoma that is linked to lipid disorders and is accompanied by a pink-to-red raised rash.

xanthoma, planar A type of xanthoma that is characterized by flat yellow-to-orange patches or pimples that cluster together on the skin.

xanthoma tendinosum Xanthoma that clusters around tendons and is associated with lipid disorders, including chronically elevated blood cholesterol levels.

xanthoma tuberosum Xanthoma that clusters near joints and is associated with lipid disorders, cirrhosis of the liver, and thyroid disorders.

xanthomatosis An accumulation of excess lipids in the body that is due to disturbance of lipid metabolism and marked by the formation of xanthomas. See also *xanthoma*.

xanthopsia A form of chromatopsia, a visual abnormality in which objects look as though they have been overpainted with an unnatural color. In xanthopsia, that color is yellow.

xanthosis Yellowing of the skin without yellowing of the eyes, as is seen in jaundice.

xenotransplantation Transplantation from one species to another (for example, from a baboon to a human).

xero- Prefix indicating dryness, as in xeroderma (dry skin).

xeroderma Abnormally dry skin. Xeroderma can be caused by a deficiency of vitamin A, systemic illness (such as hypothyroidism or Sjogren's syndrome), overexposure to sunlight, and medication. Xeroderma can usually be addressed with the use of over-the-counter topical preparations. If these products do not relieve the condition, the patient should see an aesthetician or a dermatologist for more specific remedies.

xeroderma pigmentosum A genetic disease that is characterized by such extraordinary sensitivity to sunlight that it results in the development of skin cancer at a very early age. Abbreviated XP. Children with XP can only play outdoors safely after nightfall. XP is due to defective repair of damage done to DNA by ultraviolet (UV) light. Whereas normal persons can repair UV-induced damage by inserting new bases into the DNA, XP patients cannot. A person with XP develops severe sunburn and eye irritation within minutes of exposure to sunlight. Other features of XP include very dry skin (xeroderma means extreme dryness of the skin), blisters on the skin, heavy freckling, and dark spots on the skin. XP is inherited in an autosomal recessive manner. Genes for XP reside in diverse locations, including chromosome regions 3p25, 9q22.3, 11p12–11p11, and 19q13.2–19q13.3. Avoiding UV light and using the highest level of sunscreen possible when exposure cannot be avoided helps prevent complications.

xerophagia   Having a tendency to eat a dry diet.

xerophthalmia   Dry eyes. Xerophthalmia can be associated with systemic diseases, such as Sjogren's syndrome, systemic lupus erythematosus, and rheumatoid arthritis; deficiency of vitamin A; and use of some medications. It results from inadequate function of the lacrimal glands, which produce tears. When xerophthalmia is due to vitamin A deficiency, the condition begins with night blindness and conjunctival xerosis (dryness of the eye membranes), progresses to corneal xerosis (dryness of the cornea), and in its late stages develops into keratomalacia (softening of the cornea). Treatment depends on the severity of the condition and ranges from artificial tears and ointments to plugging of the tear ducts. Also known as conjunctivitis arida.

xerosis   Abnormal dryness of the skin, mucous membranes, or conjunctiva (xerophthalmia). There are many causes of xerosis and treatment depends on the particular cause.

xerostomia   Dry mouth. Xerostomia can be associated with systemic diseases, such as Sjogren's syndrome, systemic lupus erythematosus, and rheumatoid arthritis; and it can be a side effect of medication and poor dental hygiene. Xerostomia results from inadequate function of the salivary glands, such as the parotid glands. Treatment involves adequate intake of water, use of artificial saliva, and good dental care. Untreated, severe dry mouth can lead to increased levels of tooth decay and thrush.

xiphoid process   The lower part of the breastbone. The xiphoid process has no particular function and ranges in size from miniscule to several inches in length.

X-linked   A gene on the X chromosome that travels with the X chromosome and therefore is part of the X chromosome. An X-linked disorder is associated with or caused by a gene on the X chromosome.

X-linked dominant   An X-linked trait that is expressed when one copy of the gene for that trait is present. In the case of an X-linked dominant disease, a single copy of the mutant gene on the X chromosome can cause the disease in a female. An example is a type of hereditary rickets called hypophosphatemic rickets. See also *autosomal dominant trait; X-linked recessive.*

X-linked recessive   An X-linked trait that expresses itself only when there is no different gene present at that spot (locus) on the X chromosome. For example, Duchenne muscular dystrophy (DMD) is an X-linked recessive disorder. A boy with DMD has the DMD gene on his sole X chromosome. Although it is much rarer, a girl can have the DMD gene on both her X chromosomes and have DMD. See also *autosomal recessive trait; X-linked dominant.*

X-ray   High-energy radiation with waves shorter than those of visible light. X-ray is used in low doses to make images that help to diagnose diseases and in high doses to treat cancer.

X-ray, AP   An X-ray picture in which the beams pass through the patient anteroposteriorly (from front to back).

X-ray, lateral   An X-ray picture that is taken from the side.

X-ray, PA   An X-ray picture in which the beams pass through the patient posteroanteriorly (from back to front).

X-ray therapy   The use of X-ray radiation to treat cancer. X-rays may be used inside or outside the body, depending on the type of tumor involved. See also *radiation therapy.*

XX   The sex chromosome complement of a normal human female. See also *X chromosome.*

XXX syndrome   A chromosome condition that is present in 1 in 1,000 females, due to the presence of three X chromosomes rather than the usual two. The condition is associated with increased height but no malformations. Intelligence ranges from above normal to mild retardation. The average IQ is 85 to 90. Learning problems may be helped with early special education. Also known as triple X and triplo-X.

XY   The most frequent sex chromosome complement in human males. See also *X chromosome; Y chromosome.*

xylitol   A sweetener that is found in plants and used as a substitute for sugar. Xylitol is called a nutritive sweetener because it provides calories, just like sugar. However, it is less likely than sugar to contribute to dental caries.

XYY syndrome   A chromosomal disorder that affects males only and is caused by the presence of an extra Y chromosome. Symptoms may include increased height, speech delays, learning disabilities, mild to moderate mental retardation, and behavioral disturbance. Also known as polysomy Y syndrome.

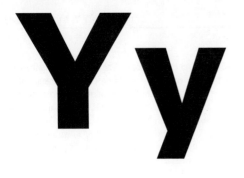

Y **1** In chemistry, the symbol for the element yttrium, an extremely rare metal that has been used in certain nuclear medicine scans. **2** In genetics, the Y chromosome.

Y chromosome The sex chromosome that is found, together with an X chromosome, in most normal males. The Y chromosome contains at least 20 genes, including the unique male-determining gene and the male fitness genes that are active only in the testis and are responsible for the formation of sperm. Other genes on the Y chromosome have counterparts on the X chromosome, are active in many body tissues, and play crucial "housekeeping" roles with the cell.

Y chromosome sex-determining region The region on the Y chromosome that decides the sex of the individual. Abbreviated SRY. SRY is necessary for male determination. It encodes the testis-determining factor. Mutations in SRY are responsible for XY females with gonadal dysgenesis who appear to be normal females at birth but at puberty do not develop secondary sexual characteristics (such as breasts), do not menstruate, and have scarred (fibrous) gonads without eggs. SRY is in chromosome band Yp11.3.

Y map The array of genes on the Y chromosome.

Yag laser surgery **1** The use of a laser to punch a hole in the iris, relieving increased pressure within the eye. Yag laser surgery is an office procedure that may be used for angle closure glaucoma and similar eye conditions. **2** Use of the Yag laser device to remove liver spots, café au lait spots, and some types of tattoos from the skin.

yard A measurement of length that is equal to 0.9 meters, 3 feet, or 36 inches.

yawn Involuntary opening of the mouth, accompanied by slowly breathing inward and then outward. Repeated yawning can be a sign of drowsiness, boredom, or depression. The yawn helps to open tiny air sacs (alveoli) in the lungs that can collapse during shallow breathing.

yaws A chronic infectious disease that occurs commonly in the warm, humid regions of the tropics. Yaws is characterized by bumps on the skin of the face, hands, feet, and genital area. Almost all cases of yaws are in children under 15 years of age. The organism that causes yaws is a spirochete, Treponema pertenue, which enters the skin at a scraped or cut spot. A painless bump (the mother yaw) arises and grows at this spot. Nearby lymph glands may become swollen. The mother yaw heals, leaving a light-colored scar. The mother yaw is followed by recurring (secondary) crops of bumps and more swollen glands. These bumps may be painless, or they may be filled with pus, burst, and ulcerate. In its late (tertiary) stage, yaws can destroy and deform areas of the skin, bones, and joints. The palms and soles tend to become thickened and painful ("dry crab yaws"). Diagnosis is confirmed via blood tests and via dark-field examination of the spirochete under a microscope. Treatment involves administration of a single shot of penicillin or another antibiotic, usually erythromycin or tetracycline. Also known as granuloma tropicum, polypapilloma tropicum, and thymiosis.

yd. Yard.

yeast A group of single-celled fungi that reproduce by budding. Most yeast is harmless, and yeast is commonly present without ill effect on normal human skin and mucous membranes, including the gastrointestinal (GI) tract. In the GI tract, the amount of yeast is usually controlled by helpful bacteria, although this balance can be upset by illness, immune-system problems, or antibiotic use. Some individuals also report that a diet high in sugars and starches can cause overproliferation, although this has not been medically proven. Extreme overproliferation of yeast can cause discomfort and disease. For example, the common yeast Candida albicans (once called Monilia) causes thrush and rashes, fingernail infections, vaginal infections, and a host of other problems in patients with immune deficiency. See also *Candida albicans; candidiasis; thrush; yeast infection; yeast rash.*

yeast diaper rash Infection in the diaper area of a baby that is caused by a yeast called Candida. Certain conditions, such as antibiotic use or excessive moisture, can upset the balance of microbes and allow an overgrowth of Candida. The infected skin is usually fiery red with areas that may have a raised red border.

yeast infection Overgrowth of yeast that affects the skin (yeast rash), mouth (thrush), digestive tract, esophagus, vagina (vaginitis), or other parts of the body. Yeast infections occur most frequently in moist areas of the body. Although Candida albicans and other Candida yeasts are the most frequent offenders, other yeast groups are known to cause illness, primarily in immunocompromised patients. These include Torulopsis, Cryptococcus, Mallasezia, and Trichosporon yeasts. Diagnosis is confirmed by culturing a stool or mucosa sample or a scraping from the affected area. Treatment involves use of topical or oral antifungal medications. Acidophilus, a helpful bacteria that normally helps to keep yeast in check, can also be used in supplement form or in yogurt with live cultures to treat yeast infection. See also *Candida albicans; candidiasis; thrush; yeast vaginitis; yeast rash.*

yeast rash A slightly raised pink-to-red rash that is caused by proliferation of yeast, usually in a moist area such as the groin. Yeast rash is most common in infants, but it can also occur on the skin of older children and adults. Treatment involves keeping the affected area clean and dry and applying topical antifungal medication. Also known as diaper dermatitis and nappy rash.

yeast vaginitis Infection of the vagina by Candida albicans, which characteristically causes itching, burning, soreness, pain during intercourse and urination, and vaginal discharge. Yeast vaginitis occurs when new yeast are introduced into the vagina or when the quantity of yeast in the vagina increases relative to the quantity of bacteria. Yeast vaginitis can be exacerbated by injury to the vagina, as from chemotherapy; immune deficiency, as from AIDS or cortisone-type medications; pregnancy or taking birth control pills; antibiotic use; or diabetes. Treatment involves use of topical or oral antifungal medications. During pregnancy, only the topical creams are used. Patients must take the full course of medication to prevent reinfection. The partners of sexually active women should also be treated. Some patients report that taking acidophilus supplements, eating yogurt with live acidophilus cultures, reducing the amount of sugar and starch in the diet, keeping the affected area clean, and wearing absorbent cotton underwear contribute to prevention of yeast vaginitis. See also *Candida albicans; yeast; yeast infection; yeast vulvitis.*

yeast vulvitis A yeast infection of the vulva. Yeast vulvitis commonly occurs with yeast vaginitis. Common symptoms include itching, burning, soreness, pain during intercourse and urination, and vaginal discharge. Treatment involves use of topical or oral antifungal medications. During pregnancy, only the topical creams are used. Patients must take the full course of medication to prevent reinfection. The partners of sexually active women should also be treated. Some patients report that taking acidophilus supplements, eating yogurt with live acidophilus cultures, reducing the amount of sugar and starch in the diet, keeping the affected area clean, and wearing absorbent cotton underwear contribute to prevention of yeast vulvitis. See also *Candida albicans; yeast; yeast infection; yeast vaginitis.*

yellow fever An acute, systemic illness that is caused by the Flavivirus taxon virus. In severe cases of yellow fever, infection causes a high fever, bleeding into the skin, and death of cells (necrosis) in the kidney and liver. The liver damage (hepatitis) causes yellowing of the skin from severe jaundice. Yellow fever once ravaged port cities in the US, but it is currently most common in tropical areas

of Africa and the Americas. The virus is transmitted by mosquitoes or, in a very few cases, monkey bites. Diagnosis is made via observation and, if necessary, culturing or examining blood samples. There is no cure for yellow fever, although antiviral medications may be tried. Yellow fever usually passes within a few weeks. Nonaspirin pain relievers, rest, and rehydration with fluids decrease discomfort. Yellow fever disease can be prevented with a vaccination. See also *yellow fever vaccination.*

yellow fever vaccination A live attenuated (weakened) viral vaccine for yellow fever. Yellow fever vaccination is recommended for people traveling to or living in the tropical areas in the Americas and Africa where yellow fever occurs. Because yellow fever vaccination is a live vaccine, it should not be given to infants or people with immune-system problems.

yellow jacket stings Stings from yellow jackets that can trigger allergic reactions of varying severity. Avoidance and prompt treatment (including diphenhydramine, brand name: Benadryl; and epinephrine, brand name: Epi-Pen) are essential. In selected cases, allergy injection therapy is highly effective for prevention.

Yersinia A family of bacteria that includes Yersinia pestis, which causes the bubonic, pneumonic, and septicemic plagues; Y. entercolitica, which causes intestinal infections, including mesenteric lymphadenitis, a condition that mimics appendicitis; and Y. pseudotuberculosis, which usually adversely affects only animals but can cause illness in immunocompromised patients. Both Y. entercolitica and Y. pseudotuberculosis have also been implicated in a viral form of arthritis. Infection with Yersinia bacteria can be treated with antibiotics. See also *plague.*

Y-linked A gene on the Y chromosome that is passed from father to son. See also *holandric inheritance.*

Y-linked inheritance See *holandric inheritance.*

yoga A relaxing form of exercise that was developed in India and involves assuming and holding postures that stretch the limbs and muscles, doing breathing exercises, and using meditation techniques to calm the mind. Yoga appears to have benefits for increasing physical flexibility and reducing internal feelings of stress. Yoga may be recommended as an alternative or complementary health-promoting practice.

yogurt Milk that is fermented with a culture of Lactobacillus (the milk bacillus) and often with acidophilus and other helpful bacteria. Some patients with yeast infections, particularly infections that are brought on by taking antibiotics, report that eating yogurt is helpful in alleviating symptoms. See also *probiotic.*

yolk bone See *zygoma*.

yolk sac The membrane outside the human embryo. The yolk sac is connected by a tube, the yolk stalk, through the umbilical opening to the embryo's midgut. The yolk sac serves as an early site for the formation of blood, and in time it is incorporated into the primitive gut of the embryo.

yolk stalk A narrow tube that is present in the early embryo that connects the midgut of the embryo to the yolk sac outside the embryo through the umbilical opening. Later in development, the yolk stalk is usually obliterated, but a remnant of it may persist, most commonly as a finger-like protrusion from the small intestine that is known as Meckel diverticulum. Also known as oomphalomesenteric duct, umbilical duct, and vitelline duct. See also *diverticulum, Meckel*.

youth The time between childhood and maturity.

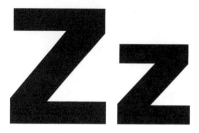

Z chromosome A sex chromosome in certain animals, such as chickens, turkeys, and moths. In humans, males are XY and females are XX, but in animals with a Z chromosome, males are ZZ and females are WZ.

zebra In medicine, an unlikely diagnostic possibility. It comes from an old saying in teaching medical students about how to think logically in regard to the differential diagnosis: "When you hear hoof beats, think of horses, not zebras." For example, when someone develops a mild transient cough, a virus infection is the most logical and likely cause, and tuberculosis is a zebra.

zinc A mineral that is essential to the body and is a constituent of many enzymes that permit chemical reactions to proceed at normal rates. Zinc is involved in the manufacture of protein (protein synthesis) and in cell division. Zinc is also a constituent of insulin, and it is involved with the sense of smell. Food sources of zinc include meat, particularly liver and seafood; eggs; nuts; and cereal grains. Recently, zinc has been touted as a treatment for the common cold. According to the National Academy of Sciences, the recommended dietary allowance of zinc is 12 mg per day for women and 10 mg per day for men.

zinc acetate A form of zinc that has been used as an emetic (something that causes vomiting).

zinc deficiency See *deficiency, zinc.*

zinc excess Too much zinc, which can cause gastrointestinal irritation, interfere with copper absorption to cause copper deficiency and, like too little zinc, cause immune deficiency. See also *zinc.*

zinc ointment A topical preparation that contains zinc and is applied to protect the skin from irritation or sunburn. Zinc ointment is also often the basis for commercial preparations for preventing diaper rash. It should not be used on skin that is already broken or irritated, however.

zinc oxide A form of zinc that has antispasmodic qualities.

zinc sulfate A form of zinc that can be administered in eyedrops. Zinc sulfate is used in some types of eye tests.

Zinsser disease See *Brill-Zinsser disease.*

zona pellucida The strong membrane that forms around an ovum as it develops in the ovary. The membrane remains in place during the egg's travel through the fallopian tube. To fertilize the egg, a sperm must penetrate the thinning zona pellucida. If fertilization takes place, the zona pellucida disappears, to permit implantation in the uterus.

zoonosis An infection that is known in nature to infect both humans and lower vertebrate animals.

zooparasite A living parasite, such as a worm or protozoa.

zoophilia A sexual disorder (paraphilia) that involves an abnormal desire to have sexual contact with animals. See also *paraphilia.*

zygoma The bone that forms the prominence of the cheek. Also known as zygomatic bone, zygomatic arch, malar bone, and yoke bone.

zygomatic arch See *zygoma.*

zygomatic bone See *zygoma.*

zygomycosis A dangerous infection that is caused by a water-borne fungus. Zygomycosis is seen most often in patients who are already ill with diseases that cause wasting, such as AIDS and poorly controlled diabetes. If unchecked, the fungal infection can spread to the lungs and other organs, the blood, the eyes, and the brain. Treatment involves controlling the underlying condition and attacking the infection with antifungal medications.

zygote The cell that is formed by the union of a male sex cell (sperm) and a female sex cell (an ovum). The zygote develops into the embryo, as instructed by the genetic material within the unified cell. The unification of a sperm and an ovum is called fertilization. See also *ovum; sperm.*

zygotic lethal gene See *gene, zygotic lethal.*

Appendix A

Prescription Abbreviations

Prescriptions are the traditional means by which a physician permits patients to obtain certain medications and/or supplies from pharmacies. The word *prescription* is derived from the Latin *prae*, meaning "before," and *scribere*, meaning "to write." This reflected the fact that a prescription had to be written before a drug could be prepared and administered to a patient. A number of abbreviations, many derived from Latin terms, are used on prescription forms and medication labels. These include the following:

ad lib   Use as much as one desires, or use at one's own discretion. From the Latin term *ad libitum*.

a.c.   Before meals. From the Latin term *ante cibum*.

b.i.d.   Twice a day. From the Latin term *bis in die*.

cap   Capsules.

da or daw   Dispense as written.

g, gm, or G   Gram.

gtt   Drops. From the Latin term *guttae*.

h   Hour.

mg   Milligram.

ml   Milliliter.

p.c   Take after meals. From the Latin term *post cibum*.

p.o   Take by mouth, orally. From the Latin term *per os*.

p.r.n   Take as necessary or when needed. From the Latin term *pro re nata*.

q.d   Take once per day. From the Latin term *quaque die*.

q.h   Take once every hour. From the Latin term *quaque* (every) and the abbreviation for hours.

q.i.d   Take four times per day. From the Latin term *quater in die*.

q.2h   Take once every 2 hours.

q.3h   Take once every 3 hours.

q.4h   Take once every 4 hours.

t.i.d   Take three times per day. From the Latin term *ter in die*.

ut dict   Take as directed. From the Latin term *ut dictum*.

Drug Caution Codes

Drug caution codes are abbreviations that are applied to medications to indicate caution. Drug caution codes provide valuable warnings to patients and their families. They include both universal codes that apply to all patients and specific caution codes that apply under certain circumstances. In the US, a system of stickers with pictographs may also be used to warn of specific side effects, such as drowsiness. Patients who see one of these codes on their prescriptions should talk to a pharmacist before using the medications.

Universal Caution Codes

D   Drowsiness

H   Habit forming

I   Interaction

X   S.O.S. (contains a substance, such as acetaminophen, that could cause problems; consult a pharmacist)

Specific Caution Codes

A   ASA (contains acetylsalicylic acid [aspirin])

C   Caution

G   Glaucoma

S   Diabetes

These code letters are cautions for patients with specific medical problems. A person with a medical problem, such as high blood pressure, might see the generic "C" code on a prescription bottle if the medication could raise his or her blood pressure.

Appendix B

Anatomic Orientation Terms

In anatomy, certain terms are used to denote orientation. For example, a structure may be horizontal, as opposed to vertical. Commonly used anatomic orientation terms include the following:

anterior The front, as opposed to posterior. For example, the breastbone is part of the anterior surface of the chest.

anteroposterior From front to back, as opposed to posteroanterior. Abbreviated AP. For example, when a chest X-ray is taken with the patient's back against the film plate and the X-ray machine in front of the patient, it is referred to as an AP view.

ascending Going upward. For example, the ascending aorta is the portion of the aorta that ascends, going upward as it leaves the heart to form the beginning of the arch of the aorta.

caudad Toward the feet (or tail, in embryology), as opposed to cranial.

cranial Toward the head, as opposed to caudad.

deep Away from the exterior surface or farther into the body, as opposed to superficial.

descending Going down. For example, the descending aorta is the portion of the aorta that descends, going downward from the top of the arch of the aorta.

distal Farther from the beginning, as opposed to proximal.

dorsal The back, as opposed to ventral.

external Situated on the outside.

horizontal Parallel to the floor; a plane that passes through the standing body parallel to the floor.

inferior Below, as opposed to superior.

internal Situated on the inside.

lateral Toward the left or right side of the body, as opposed to medial.

medial In the middle or inside, as opposed to lateral.

posterior The back or behind, as opposed to anterior.

posteroanterior From back to front, as opposed to anteroposterior. Abbreviated PA.

pronation Rotation of the forearm and hand so that the palm is down (or similar movement of the foot and leg, with the sole down), as opposed to supination.

prone With the front or ventral surface downward (lying face down), as opposed to supine.

proximal Toward the beginning, as opposed to distal.

sagittal A vertical plane that passes through the standing body from front to back. For example, the midsaggital, or median, plane splits the body into left and right halves.

superficial On the surface or shallow, as opposed to deep.

superior Above, as opposed to inferior.

supination Rotation of the forearm and hand so that the palm is upward (or similar movement of the foot and leg, with the sole upward), as opposed to pronation.

supine With the back or dorsal surface downward (lying face up), as opposed to prone.

transverse A horizontal plane that passes through the standing body parallel to the ground.

ventral Pertaining to the abdomen, as opposed to dorsal.

vertical Upright, as opposed to horizontal.

Appendix C

Vitamins

The term *vitamin* was coined in 1911 by the Warsaw-born biochemist Casimir Funk. Working at the Lister Institute in London, Funk isolated a substance that prevented nerve inflammation (neuritis) in chickens raised on a diet deficient in that substance. He named the substance "vitamine" because he believed it was necessary to life and it was a chemical amine. The *e* at the end was later removed when it was recognized that vitamins need not be amines. Vitamins soon became identified as they were noted to be associated with vitamin deficiency diseases. The letters (A, B, C, and so on) were assigned to the vitamins in the order of their discovery. The one exception was vitamin K, which was assigned its K (from Koagulation) by the Danish researcher Henrik Dam.

Vitamins are known to play a major role in both health maintenance and the treatment of certain diseases. The classic vitamins are divided into two categories, oil-soluble and water-soluble, based on how they are absorbed with the food we eat. The oil-soluble vitamins are vitamins A, D, E, and K and are absorbed with fats. There are nine water-soluble vitamins, thiamine (vitamin B1), riboflavin (vitamin B2), pyridoxine (vitamin B6), cyanocobalamin (vitamin B12), ascorbic acid (vitamin C), biotin, folic acid, niacin, and pantothenic acid. Other vitamins have more recently been described and are included below. Betacarotene is a plant pigment that is a precursor of vitamin A. Vitamins can be dangerous in overdose. The vitamins include:

ascorbic acid   Vitamin C.

beta carotene   Not actually a vitamin but a plant pigment that is a precursor of vitamin A. Betacarotene is an antioxidant that protects cells against oxidative damage that may predispose a person to cancer. Beta carotene is converted to the oil-soluble vitamin A, as needed. Food sources include vegetables such as carrots, sweet potatoes, and spinach and other leafy green vegetables; and fruits such as cantaloupes and apricots. Excessive carotene can temporarily yellow the skin, an innocuous condition called carotenemia that is commonly seen in infants who have been fed large amounts of mashed carrots.

bioflavinoid   Vitamin P.

biotin   Vitamin H.

calciferol   Vitamin D2.

cholecalciferol   Vitamin D3.

cobalamin   Vitamin B12.

folic acid   A member of the water-soluble, B vitamin family that is essential for cell growth and proliferation and for the proper utilization of vitamin B12 and vitamin C. Folic acid is an important factor in nucleic acid (RNA and DNA) synthesis. It is found in leafy green vegetables, liver and other organ meats, and whole grains. Deficiency of folic acid can lead to slow growth, diarrhea, oral inflammation, a decrease in all types of blood cells (pancytopenia), and megaloblastic anemia (anemia with abnormally large red blood cells). Inadequate folic acid during pregnancy raises the risk of neural tube defects in the fetus and of miscarriages. Also known as folate. Nonpregnant adults require 200 micrograms of folic acid per day. For pregnant women, typically 1 mg daily is recommend in the form of prenatal multi-vitamins.

niacin   Vitamin B3.

nicotinic acid   Vitamin B3.

pantothenic acid   Vitamin B5.

pyridoxine   Vitamin B6.

retinol   Vitamin A.

riboflavin   Vitamin B2.

thiamin   Vitamin B1.

vitamin A   An oil-soluble vitamin that is also known as retinol. Carotene compounds are gradually converted by the body to vitamin A. A form of vitamin A called retinal is responsible for transmitting light sensations in the retina of the eye. Vitamin A is found in egg yolk, butter, cream, leafy green vegetables, yellow fruits and vegetables, cod-liver oil, and similar fish-liver oils. Deficiency of vitamin A leads to night blindness and to diseases that affect the eyes and mucous membranes. Overdose of vitamin A can cause insomnia, joint pain, fatigue, irritability, headache, and other symptoms. The daily adult requirement is 900 micrograms.

vitamin A2   A form of vitamin A that is found only in the flesh of freshwater fish.

vitamin B1   Thiamin, a water-soluble vitamin, which acts as a coenzyme and is essential for a number of reactions in body metabolism. Vitamin B1 is found primarily in liver and yeast, and it is easily destroyed by cooking. Deficiency of vitamin B1 leads to beriberi, a disease of the heart and nervous system. The daily adult requirement is 1.2 milligrams.

vitamin B2   Riboflavin, a water-soluble vitamin, which is a component of two coenzymes in the oxidation-reduction processes that are important to body metabolism. Vitamin

B2 is found primarily in liver and yeast, and it is easily destroyed by cooking. Deficiency of vitamin B2 causes inflammation of the lining of the mouth and skin. The daily adult requirement is 1.5 milligrams.

vitamin B3 Niacin, a water-soluble vitamin, which is a component of coenzymes that are important in body metabolism. Vitamin B3 is found primarily in liver and yeast, and it is easily destroyed by cooking. Deficiency of vitamin B3 causes inflammation of the skin, vagina, rectum, and mouth, as well as mental slowing. Also known as nicotinic acid. The daily adult requirement is 16 milligrams.

vitamin B5 Pantothenic acid, a water-soluble, B vitamin that is widely distributed in nature. Pantothenic acid is virtually ubiquitous. It is present in foods as diverse as poultry, soybeans, yogurt, and sweet potatoes. No naturally occurring disease due to a deficiency of vitamin B5 has been identified, due to the ease of obtaining this vitamin. An experimental deficiency of pantothenic acid has, however, been created by administering an antagonist to pantothenic acid. This experiment produced disease, thereby demonstrating that pantothenic acid is essential to humans.

vitamin B6 Pyridoxine, a water-soluble vitamin, which is a cofactor for enzymes. Vitamin B6 is found primarily in liver and yeast, and it is easily destroyed by cooking. Deficiency of vitamin B6 leads to inflammation of the skin and mouth, nausea, vomiting, dizziness, weakness, and anemia. The daily adult requirement is 2 milligrams.

vitamin B12 Cobalamin, a water-soluble vitamin, which is an essential factor in nucleic acid synthesis. Vitamin B12 may affect vitamin C absorption. It is found primarily in liver and yeast, and it is easily destroyed by cooking. Deficiency of vitamin B12 leads to megaloblastic anemia, as can be seen in pernicious anemia. The daily adult requirement is 2 micrograms.

vitamin C Ascorbic acid, a water-soluble vitamin that is important in the synthesis of collagen, the framework protein for tissues of the body. Vitamin C is found in citrus fruits, tomatoes, berries, potatoes, and most vegetables. It may affect vitamin B12 absorption. Minor deficiency can cause gum bleeding, joint pain, nosebleeds, and easy bruising. Extreme deficiency can lead to scurvy, characterized by fragile capillaries, poor wound healing, and bone deformity in children. Overdose is not possible with this water-soluble vitamin, but overuse can cause diarrhea, painful urination, rash, and nausea. The daily adult requirement is 60 milligrams.

vitamin D An oil-soluble steroid vitamin that promotes absorption and metabolism of calcium and phosphorus and that is essential for tooth and bone growth. Under normal conditions of sunlight exposure, no dietary supplementation is necessary because sunlight promotes adequate vitamin D synthesis in the skin. Vitamin D is added to many common dairy products and breads, and it can also be found in saltwater fish and egg yolks. Deficiency can lead to osteomalcia (softening of bone) in adults and bone deformity (rickets) in children. The daily adult requirement is 10 micrograms.

vitamin D2 Calciferol, a synthetic form of vitamin D that is created by treating ergosterol (provitamin D2) with ultraviolet light waves. Vitamin D2 is important in normal bone metabolism. Vitamin D2 is largely supplied by the metabolism of vitamin D in the body.

vitamin D3 Cholecalciferol, a D vitamin that is needed for proper use of phosphorus, calcium, and vitamin A. It plays a steroid-like role in regulating cellular proliferation and differentiation. Vitamin D3 is important in normal bone metabolism. Also known as calcitrol. Vitamin D3 is largely supplied by the metabolism of vitamin D in the body.

vitamin E An oil-soluble vitamin that is vital for muscle, skin, blood vessel, and organ development and function. Dietary sources for vitamin E include nuts, nut and corn oils, wheat germ, liver, sweet potatoes, and green leafy vegetables. Deficiency if vitamin E can lead to anemia. The daily adult requirement is 10 milligrams.

vitamin H Biotin, which is actually considered part of the water-soluble, B vitamin family. It is a coenzyme essential for many enzyme functions. Normally produced by bacteria in the colon, biotin is also found in yeast, organ meats, legumes, egg yolks, whole grains, and nuts. The daily adult requirement is 60 micrograms.

vitamin K An oil-soluble vitamin essential to the normal clotting of blood. Vitamin K is normally made within the body by intestinal bacteria, but it is also found in many foods, including leafy green vegetables, yogurt, egg yolk, and fish-liver oils. Deficiency may occur following the administration of drugs that inhibit the growth of the vitamin-synthesizing bacteria or as a result of disorders affecting the production or flow of bile necessary for the intestinal absorption of vitamin K. In newborn babies, the absence of intestinal bacteria coupled with the absence of body stores of vitamin K may result in hemorrhagic disease of the newborn. This is a dangerous condition because there can be bleeding into critical organs such as the brain. This disorder can be prevented by the administration of vitamin K to the baby shortly after birth or to the mother during labor. Daily adult requirement is 65 micrograms.

vitamin P Bioflavinoids, a group of substances found with and essential to the use of vitamin C. They are essential for building collagen and capillary walls, among other functions.

What's on the CD-ROM?

This appendix provides you with information on the contents of the CD that accompanies this book. For the latest and greatest information, please refer to the ReadMe file located at the root of the CD. Here is what you will find:

- System Requirements
- Using the CD with Windows
- What's on the CD
- Troubleshooting

System Requirements

Make sure that your computer meets the minimum system requirements listed in this section. If your computer doesn't match up to most of these requirements, you may have a problem using the contents of the CD.

For Windows 9x, Windows 2000, Windows NT4 (with SP 4 or later), Windows Me, or Windows XP:

- PC with a Pentium processor running at 120 Mhz or faster
- At least 32 MB of total RAM installed on your computer; for best performance, we recommend at least 64 MB
- Ethernet network interface card (NIC) or modem with a speed of at least 28,800 bps
- A CD-ROM drive

Using the CD with Windows

To install the items from the CD to your hard drive, follow these steps:

1. Insert the CD into your computer's CD-ROM drive.
2. A window will appear with the following options: Install, Browse, Links and Exit.

   Install: Gives you the option to install the supplied software and/or the author-created samples on the CD-ROM.

   Explore: Allows you to view the contents of the CD-ROM in its directory structure.

   Links: Opens a hyperlinked page of web sites.

   Exit: Closes the autorun window.

If you do not have autorun enabled or if the autorun window does not appear, follow the steps below to access the CD.

1. Click Start ➪ Run.
2. In the dialog box that appears, type *d*:\setup.exe, where *d* is the letter of your CD-ROM drive. This will bring up the autorun window described above.
3. Choose the Install, Browse, Links, or Exit option from the menu. (See Step 2 in the preceding list for a description of these options.)

About the CD

The Webster's New World Medical Dictionary CD-ROM contains the complete text of the book in searchable electronic format. When you run the installation program, a program group will be created on your computer. You may then access the electronic dictionary from the Start menu.

Also on the CD is an appendix that lists, with brief descriptions, some of the more popular medications in use today; The CD also contains links to MedicineNet.com and other sites of interest.

Troubleshooting

If you have difficulty installing or using any of the materials on the companion CD, try the following solutions:

- **Turn off any anti-virus software that you may have running.** Installers sometimes mimic virus activity and can make your computer incorrectly believe that it is being infected by a virus. (Be sure to turn the anti-virus software back on later.)

- **Close all running programs.** The more programs you're running, the less memory is available to other programs. Installers also typically update files and programs; if you keep other programs running, installation may not work properly.

- **Reference the ReadMe:** Please refer to the ReadMe file located at the root of the CD-ROM for the latest product information at the time of publication.

If you still have trouble with the CD, please call the Customer Care phone number: (800) 762-2974. Outside the United States, call 1 (317) 572-3994. You can also contact Customer Service by e-mail at techsupdum@wiley.com. Wiley Publishing, Inc. will provide technical support only for installation and other general quality control items; for technical support on the applications themselves, consult the program's vendor or author.

Wiley Publishing, Inc.
End-User License Agreement

READ THIS. You should carefully read these terms and conditions before opening the software packet(s) included with this book "Book". This is a license agreement "Agreement" between you and Wiley Publishing, Inc."WPI". By opening the accompanying software packet(s), you acknowledge that you have read and accept the following terms and conditions. If you do not agree and do not want to be bound by such terms and conditions, promptly return the Book and the unopened software packet(s) to the place you obtained them for a full refund.

1. **License Grant.** WPI grants to you (either an individual or entity) a nonexclusive license to use one copy of the enclosed software program(s) (collectively, the "Software" solely for your own personal or business purposes on a single computer (whether a standard computer or a workstation component of a multi-user network). The Software is in use on a computer when it is loaded into temporary memory (RAM) or installed into permanent memory (hard disk, CD-ROM, or other storage device). WPI reserves all rights not expressly granted herein.

2. **Ownership.** WPI is the owner of all right, title, and interest, including copyright, in and to the compilation of the Software recorded on the disk(s) or CD-ROM "Software Media". Copyright to the individual programs recorded on the Software Media is owned by the author or other authorized copyright owner of each program. Ownership of the Software and all proprietary rights relating thereto remain with WPI and its licensers.

3. **Restrictions On Use and Transfer.**

   (a) You may only (i) make one copy of the Software for backup or archival purposes, or (ii) transfer the Software to a single hard disk, provided that you keep the original for backup or archival purposes. You may not (i) rent or lease the Software, (ii) copy or reproduce the Software through a LAN or other network system or through any computer subscriber system or bulletin-board system, or (iii) modify, adapt, or create derivative works based on the Software.

   (b) You may not reverse engineer, decompile, or disassemble the Software. You may transfer the Software and user documentation on a permanent basis, provided that the transferee agrees to accept the terms and conditions of this Agreement and you retain no copies. If the Software is an update or has been updated, any transfer must include the most recent update and all prior versions.

4. **Restrictions on Use of Individual Programs.** You must follow the individual requirements and restrictions detailed for each individual program in the About the CD-ROM appendix of this Book. These limitations are also contained in the individual license agreements recorded on the Software Media. These limitations may include a requirement that after using the program for a specified period of time, the user must pay a registration fee or discontinue use. By opening the Software packet(s), you will be agreeing to abide by the licenses and restrictions for these individual programs that are detailed in the About the CD-ROM appendix and on the Software Media. None of the material on this Software Media or listed in this Book may ever be redistributed, in original or modified form, for commercial purposes.

5. **Limited Warranty.**

   (a) WPI warrants that the Software and Software Media are free from defects in materials and workmanship under normal use for a period of sixty (60) days from the date of purchase of this Book. If WPI receives notification within the warranty period of defects in materials or workmanship, WPI will replace the defective Software Media.

   (b) WPI AND THE AUTHOR OF THE BOOK DISCLAIM ALL OTHER WARRANTIES, EXPRESS OR IMPLIED, INCLUDING WITHOUT LIMITATION IMPLIED WARRANTIES OF MERCHANTABILITY AND FITNESS FOR A PARTICULAR PURPOSE, WITH RESPECT TO THE SOFTWARE, THE PROGRAMS, THE SOURCE CODE CONTAINED THEREIN, AND/OR THE TECHNIQUES DESCRIBED IN THIS BOOK. WPI DOES NOT WARRANT THAT THE FUNCTIONS CONTAINED IN THE SOFTWARE WILL MEET YOUR REQUIREMENTS OR THAT THE OPERATION OF THE SOFTWARE WILL BE ERROR FREE.

   (c) This limited warranty gives you specific legal rights, and you may have other rights that vary from jurisdiction to jurisdiction.

6. Remedies.

(a) WPI's entire liability and your exclusive remedy for defects in materials and workmanship shall be limited to replacement of the Software Media, which may be returned to WPI with a copy of your receipt at the following address: Software Media Fulfillment Department, Attn.: *Webster's New World Medical Dictionary, Second Edition,* Wiley Publishing, Inc., 10475 Crosspoint Blvd., Indianapolis, IN 46256, or call 1-800-762-2974. Please allow four to six weeks for delivery. This Limited Warranty is void if failure of the Software Media has resulted from accident, abuse, or misapplication. Any replacement Software Media will be warranted for the remainder of the original warranty period or thirty (30) days, whichever is longer.

(b) In no event shall WPI or the author be liable for any damages whatsoever (including without limitation damages for loss of business profits, business interruption, loss of business information, or any other pecuniary loss) arising from the use of or inability to use the Book or the Software, even if WPI has been advised of the possibility of such damages.

(c) Because some jurisdictions do not allow the exclusion or limitation of liability for consequential or incidental damages, the above limitation or exclusion may not apply to you.

7. U.S. Government Restricted Rights.
Use, duplication, or disclosure of the Software for or on behalf of the United States of America, its agencies and/or instrumentalities "U.S. Government" is subject to restrictions as stated in paragraph (c)(1)(ii) of the Rights in Technical Data and Computer Software clause of DFARS 252.227-7013, or subparagraphs (c) (1) and (2) of the Commercial Computer Software - Restricted Rights clause at FAR 52.227-19, and in similar clauses in the NASA FAR supplement, as applicable.

8. General.
This Agreement constitutes the entire understanding of the parties and revokes and supersedes all prior agreements, oral or written, between them and may not be modified or amended except in a writing signed by both parties hereto that specifically refers to this Agreement. This Agreement shall take precedence over any other documents that may be in conflict herewith. If any one or more provisions contained in this Agreement are held by any court or tribunal to be invalid, illegal, or otherwise unenforceable, each and every other provision shall remain in full force and effect.